Case Studies in Geriatric Primary Care & Multimorbidity Management

KAREN L. DICK, PhD, GNP-BC, FAANP, FNAP

Associate Dean for Advanced Practice Programs
Graduate School of Nursing
University of Massachusetts Medical School
Worcester, Massachusetts;
Hebrew Senior Life
Boston, Massachusetts

TERRY MAHAN BUTTARO, PhD, AGPCNP-BC, FAANP, FNAP

College of Nursing and Health Sciences
University of Massachusetts Boston
Boston, Massachusetts;
Coastal Medical Associates
Salisbury, Massachusetts

ELSEVIER

3251 Riverport Lane
St. Louis, Missouri 63043

CASE STUDIES IN GERIATRIC PRIMARY CARE &
MULTIMORBIDITY MANAGEMENT

ISBN: 978-0-323-47998-1

Library of Congress Control Number: 2018961250

Executive Content Strategist: Lee Henderson
Senior Content Development Specialist: Heather Bays
Publishing Services Manager: Julie Eddy
Senior Project Manager: Tracey Schriefer
Design Direction: Maggie Reid

Printed in the United States of America

Last digit is the print number   9   8   7   6   5   4   3   2   1

  Working together
to grow libraries in
developing countries

www.elsevier.com • www.bookaid.org

ELSEVIER

This book is dedicated to our friend and colleague, Dr. Susan Russell Neary, whose legacy lives on through her colleagues and hundreds of former NP students who honor her memory through their commitment to care for the vulnerable and aged.

Carolyn Abbanat, MSN, APRN-BC
Nurse Practitioner
Boston Health Care for the Homeless
  Program
Boston, Massachusetts

Patricia Bailey, PhD, MSN, APRN, CNE
Assistant Professor
Graduate Online FNP Program
Chamberlain University
Downers Grove, Illinois

Jill Beavers-Kirby, DNP, MS, ACNP-BC, ANP-BC
Coordinator
Nursing Practitioner Programs;
Associate Professor
Mount Carmel College of Nursing
Columbus, Ohio

Jean Boucher, PhD, ANP-BC, AOCNP
Associate Professor & Director of DNP
  Program
Graduate School of Nursing
University of Massachusetts Medical School
Worcester, Massachusetts

Jemecia C. Braxton-Barrett, DNP, APRN, FNP-BC
Assistant Professor
College of Nursing
Walden University
Minneapolis, Minnesota

Dawn Carpenter, DNP, ACNP-BC, CCRN
Assistant Professor
Adult-Gerontology Acute Care Nurse
  Practitioner Track Coordinator
University of Massachusetts Medical School
Worcester, Massachusetts

Katharine Chapman, MSN, APRN, FNP-BC, CPNP-PC
Instructor
Frances Payne Bolton School of Nursing
Case Western Reserve University
Cleveland, Ohio

Marjorie Crabtree, DNP, ANP-BC, FNP-BC
Family Primary Care Provider
Harbor Community Health Center
Hyannis, Massachusetts;
Director of Education, NPACE (Nurse
  Practitioner Associates for Continuing
  Education)
Natick, Massachusetts

Cathleen Crowley-Koschnitzki, DNP, FNP-C, CNM, WHNP-BC, CNE
Associate Professor
FNP Track;
Sigma Theta Tau Phi Pi Chapter Counselor
Chamberlain College of Nursing
Downers Grove, Illinois

Evelyn G. Duffy, DNP, AGPCNP-BC, FAANP
Associate Professor;
Director of the Adult-Gerontology Nurse
  Practitioner Program;
Associate Director of the University Center
  on Aging and Health
Frances Payne Bolton School of Nursing
Case Western Reserve University
Cleveland, Ohio

Nicole Eckerson, RN, MS, FNP-C
Nurse Practitioner
Optum Health
Warwick, Rhode Island

Susan Feeney, DNP, FNP-BC, NP-C
Assistant Professor;
Family Nurse Practitioner Program
  Coordinator
Graduate School of Nursing
University of Massachusetts Medical School
Worcester, Massachusetts

Bethany Gentleman, MS, GNP-BC
Gerontological Nurse Practitioner
Private Practice
Hamilton, Massachusetts

Randy M. Gordon, DNP, FNP-BC
Assistant Professor
FNP Track
Chamberlain College of Nursing
Charlotte, North Carolina

Teresa L. Hagan, PhD, RN
Assistant Professor
School of Nursing
University of Pittsburgh
Pittsburgh, Pennsylvania

Lee Henderson, BA, MS (Ed.)
Executive Content Strategist
Elsevier Inc.
Philadelphia, Pennsylvania

Susan G. Henderson, BSN, RN, CLC, PCE
Perinatal Nurse II
AlphaCare
Philadelphia, Pennsylvania

Rebecca R. Hill, DNP, FNP-C, CN
Assistant Professor
MGH Institute of Health Professions;
Family Nurse Practitioner
Emergency Medicine
Massachusetts General Hospital
Boston, Massachusetts

Michaela Jones, DNP, MSN, AGPCNP-BC
Nurse Practitioner
Mount Sinai Hospital Selokoff Center for
  Occupational Medicine
World Trade Center Health Program
New York, New York

Terri LaCoursiere-Zucchero, PhD, RN, FNP-BC
Director of Nursing Education and Research
Boston Health Care for the Homeless
  Program
Boston, Massachusetts

JoAnn Lepke, APRN, MSN, MBA
Owner
DermaCare HI
Kapaa, Hawaii

Ruth Palan Lopez, PhD, GNP-BC, FGSA, FAA
Professor
MGH Institute of Health Professions
School of Nursing
Boston, Massachusetts

Brianna Morgan, MSN, AGPCNP-BC
Palliative Care Program Coordinator
Abramson Cancer Center
Pennsylvania Hospital
University of Pennsylvania Health System
Philadelphia, Pennsylvania

Nancy S. Morris, PhD, ANP-BC
Associate Professor
Graduate School of Nursing
University of Massachusetts Medical School
Worcester, Massachusetts

Tracy Murray, DNP, ACNP, FNP
Assistant Professor
MSN-FNP Program
College of Nursing
Chamberlain University
Downers Grove, Illinois

Susan Parker, DNP, APRN, GNP-BC, ACHPN
Coordinator DNP Program;
Lecturer
University of Massachusetts Lowell
Lowell, Massachusetts

Kenneth S. Peterson, PhD, FNP-BC
Assistant Professor
Graduate School of Nursing
University of Massachusetts Medical School;
Family Nurse Practitioner
Family Health Center of Worcester
Worcester, Massachusetts

Susan Sanner, PhD, APRN, FNP-BC
Associate Professor of Nursing
Family Nurse Practitioner Program
Chamberlain College of Nursing
Morrow, Georgia

Danielle Shih, MS, FNP-C, AE-C
Harvard Vanguard Medical
  Associates/Atrius Health
Family Medicine
Somerville, Massachusetts

Laura Struble, PhD, GNP-BC
Clinical Associate Professor
School of Nursing
University of Michigan
Ann Arbor, Michigan

Mary E. Sullivan, DNP, ANP-BC, ACNP-BC
Assistant Professor
Graduate School of Nursing
University of Massachusetts Medical School
Worcester, Massachusetts

Leslie-Faith Morritt Taub, PhD, ANP-C, GNP-BC, CDE, CBSM, CME (DOT), FAANP
Clinical Associate Professor;
Director Adult-Gerontology Primary Care
   NP Program
Rory Meyers College of Nursing
New York University
New York, New York

M. Elizabeth Teixeira, DrNP, APN, AGPCNP-BC, CDE
Assistant Professor
School of Nursing, Health, and Exercise
   Science
The College of New Jersey
Ewing Township, New Jersey

Laura J. Thiem, DNP, RN, FNP-BC, PMHCNS-BC, PMHNP-BC, CNE
Clinical Assistant Professor
University of Missouri-Kansas City
School of Nursing and Health Studies
Kansas City, Missouri

Patricia White, PhD, ANP-BC, FAANP
Associate Professor
DNP Program
Graduate School of Nursing
University of Massachusetts Medical School
Worcester, Massachusetts

Michelle Acorn, DNP, NP PHC/Adult, MN/ACNP, BScN/PHC, BA, CGP, CAP, GNC(C)
Nursing
University of Toronto
Toronto, Ontario, Canada

Margaret T. Andrews, DNP, RN, APRN, WHNP-BC, FNP-BC
Program Director
Nursing
South University
Richmond, Virginia

Jacqueline Aoughsten, DNP, RN, ACNP-BC
Assistant Professor
School of Nursing
University of Texas Medical Branch
Galveston, Texas

LaWanda Wallace Baskin, PhD, FNP-C
Assistant Professor
Graduate Nursing
Alcorn State University
Natchez, Mississippi

Sheryl Buckner, RN, PhD, ANEF
Assistant Professor
College of Nursing
University of Oklahoma
Oklahoma City, Oklahoma

Amy W. Bull, PhD, FNP-BC
Assistant Professor; Assistant Program Director, FNP specialty
Department of Advanced Nursing Practice
Georgetown University
Washington, District of Columbia

Cheryl Burkey-Wilson, DNP, ARNP, ANP-BC
Assistant Professor
Nursing
University of South Florida
Tampa, Florida

Kristen Childress, DNP, ARNP, FNP-BC, CWCN-AP, ARNP
Lecturer Part-Time
School of Nursing
Department of Psychosocial and Community Health Nursing
University of Washington
Seattle, Washington

Patti Christy, DNP, FNP-BC, APRN
Assistant Professor
Graduate Nursing
McNeese State University
Lake Charles, Louisiana

Diane Daddario, DNP, ANP-C, ACNS-BC, RN-BC, CMSRN
Adjunct Nursing Faculty
College of Nursing
Pennsylvania State University
University Park, Pennsylvania

Leonie DeClerk, DNP, APRN, FNP-BC
Clinical Assistant Professor
College of Nursing
University of Arkansas for Medical Sciences
Little Rock, Arkansas

Ruth E. Elsasser, ARNP-BC, DNP
Course Faculty
Family Nurse Practitioner Program/Graduate Studies
Frontier Nursing University
Hyden, Kentucky

Abimbola Farnide, PhD
Professor
College of Business
Columbia Southern University
Phoenix, Arizona

Linda Gambill, MSN/Ed, RN
Practical Nursing Program Director
Department of Health
Southwest Virginia Community College
Cedar Bluff, Virginia

Kristen Geyer, MSN, APRN, FNP-BC
Assistant Professor of Nursing
Yancey School of Nursing
Kentucky Christian University;
Family Nurse Practitioner
Spectrum Medical Care
Grayson, Kentucky

Ruth Gliss, MSN, RN, CNE
Professor of Nursing
Genesee Community College
Batavia, New York

Lorena C. Guerrero, PhD, ARNP, FNP-BC
Assistant Professor
School of Nursing
Pacific Lutheran University
Tacoma, Washington

Donna L. Hamby, DNP, RN, APRN, ACNP-BC
Clinical Assistant Professor
Director of the Doctor of Nursing Practice
   Program
College of Nursing and Health Innovation
Graduate Nursing Department
University of Texas Arlington
Arlington, Texas

Sonya R. Hardin, PhD, CCRN, ACNS-BC, NP-C FAAN
Professor;
Associate Dean Graduate Programs
College of Nursing
East Carolina University
Greenville, North Carolina

Tavane Harrison, RN, ARNP
Instructor of Nursing
Briar Cliff University
Sioux City, Iowa

Jenna Herman, DNP, APRN, FNP-BC
Family Nurse Practitioner Program
   Coordinator
Graduate Nursing
University of Mary
Bismarck, North Dakota

Judith M. Hochberger, PhD, RN
Assistant Professor
College of Nursing
Roseman University of Health Sciences
Henderson, Nevada

Heidi Holmoo, RN, BA, BScN, MScN, GNC(C), SANE-A
Professor of Nursing
Faculty of Health Sciences
Conestoga College
Kitchener, Ontario, Canada;
Nurse
Guelph General Hospital
Guelph, Ontario, Canada

Dawn Johnson, DNP, RN, Ed
Director of Nursing
Nursing Department
Great Lakes Institute of Technology
Erie, Pennsylvania

Georgina Julious Johnson, MSN, BSN, RN
Clinical Faculty
New Berry College
Lexington, South Carolina

Joanne M. Keefe, DNP, MPH, FNP-C
Instructor
Frontier Nursing University
Hyden, Kentucky

Andrea F. Knopp, PhD, MPH, FNP-BC
Associate Professor
School of Nursing
James Madison University
Harrisonburg, Virginia

Brenda Lee, ARNP-BC
Spine Surgery
Franciscan Spine Surgery Associates
Tacoma, Washington

Amber Littlefield, DNP, FNP-C, MEd
Family Nurse Practitioner
Frontier Nursing University
Hyden, Kentucky

Patti A. Parker, PhD, APRN, ACNS, ANP, GNP, BC
Assistant Clinical Professor
College of Nursing and Health Innovation
University of Texas at Arlington
Arlington, Texas

Faith Richardson, DNP RN MSN/FNP
Health & Wellness Advanced Practice Nurse
Kindle Health
Aldergrove, British Columbia, Canada

Dulce Santacroce, DNP, RN, CCM
Program Coordinator RN-BSN
Nursing
Touro University Nevada
Henderson, Nevada

Darla K. Shar, MSN, RN
Associate Director
Nursing
Hannah E. Mullins School of Practical
  Nursing
Salem, Ohio

Elizabeth Ubaldi, RN, BA, MN (CCNE)
Nursing Professor
Health Sciences
Sault College
Sault Ste. Marie, Ontario, Canada

Gretchen Elizabeth Wheelock, DNP, AANP-AGPCNP
Adult/Gero Primary Care Nurse Practitioner
Department of Nursing
Briar Cliff University
Sioux City, Iowa

Nancy Wiseman, MSN, RN
PN Instructor
Saline County Career Center
Marshall, Missouri

The graying of America is upon us: between now and 2050, the United States is projected to experience rapid growth in its older population. In 2050, the number of Americans aged 65 and older is projected to be 88.5 million, more than double its projected population of 40.2 million in 2010. We know the reality is that people are living longer due to declining mortality rates and are also living better lives despite multiple chronic health challenges. At the same time, a major shortage of health care clinicians who can competently care for our seniors exists, and we are glad that nurse practitioners and physician assistants are responsibly and successfully meeting this demand. However, faculty responsible for preparing future generations of health care providers may find that resources to help students develop the requisite skills and expertise to manage the challenging complexity of elder care are often inadequate. Our goal was to develop a text that could present evolving case studies of older patients with more than one presenting problem to better reflect the reality of primary care encounters today.

In the past, comorbidity was the term previously used to describe an additional health problem that develops in an individual with an *index* or *primary* health condition, but the concept of multimorbidity has emerged as a better description of the interacting nature of multiple chronic health care problems in an older adult. This book provides cases developed by practicing geriatric clinicians from across the United States (most based on actual encounters) that introduce patients of various ages, ethnicities, and genders, with various health and social problems, who move across the transitions of care with unfolding scenarios that will challenge the student to address a number of health conditions in collaboration with other interprofessional team members. Our hope is that faculty will be able to use this text and expand case discussions by sharing their own experiences and expertise in the classroom. Ultimately, our hope is that this text will contribute to student preparation and provide a strong foundation for their future practice caring for older adults.

Format

The text takes a unique three-part approach in preparing primary care students to think like expert geriatric clinicians. **Unit 1** provides a strong foundation in the *principles* of geriatric care with four introductory chapters: Physiology and Psychology of Aging, Untangling the Geriatric Assessment, Principles of Pharmacology in Geriatric Practice, and Palliative Care. **Unit 2** is a collection of 18 detailed, unfolding Exemplar Case Studies. These complex "worked" cases will demonstrate, with a unique and strong emphasis on "multimorbidity," how an expert advanced practitioner "thinks clinically" to provide care to older adults. The Exemplar Cases demonstrate expert advanced practice–level reasoning in the context of the multimorbidity, patient diversity, and succession of care settings that practitioners will encounter in clinical practice. Faculty can assign cases for review and discussion and add information as needed to challenge students in developing diagnostic reasoning; differential diagnoses; and selecting appropriate diagnostics, treatments, and patient/family education. To provide extensive *practice* in learning how to think like an expert, **Unit 3** features 22 exceptionally detailed and unfolding Practice Case Studies, featuring an emphasis on multimorbidity management in patients with diverse backgrounds and health care problems across varied health care settings. The practice cases provide students with opportunities to practice their developing skills as advanced practitioners and submit answers on

Evolve for grading and feedback. Space is provided for each answer in the printed book, so that students can jot down preliminary notes. Once the student is ready to submit answers to a given case, he or she can then submit them on Evolve. After clicking "Submit," the student's answers will automatically be emailed to the instructor by Evolve, and expert feedback for that case study will be "unlocked" for the student. As with the Exemplar Cases, faculty can expand the Practice Cases to facilitate additional discussion and engagement regarding patient care management. On the companion Evolve website, faculty will find an Instructor Guide to Practice Case Studies. This Instructor Guide provides more specific details on each Practice Case, including the age, gender, presenting problem or problems, co-morbidities, and practice settings. This additional information will allow faculty to assign cases to students based on specific characteristics, including disease state or age. In the Instructor Guide the cases are listed by actual patient problem (diagnosis or diagnoses) rather than the presenting complaint(s) that are provided for students. For example, Practice Case 5 is presented in the Instructor Guide as a case of a "68-year-old woman with chronic lymphocytic leukemia," but the student sees the case presented under the presenting complaints of fatigue and rhinitis. This differentiation is intended to allow faculty to assign cases with the knowledge of the actual diagnosis or diagnoses while requiring students to work through the cases to arrive at diagnoses and treatment plans.

CONTENTS

UNIT III   Practice Case Studies in Multimorbidity Management

Basic Case Studies   330

Advanced Case Studies 501

Principles of Geriatrics and Multimorbidity Management

CHAPTER 1

The Physiology and Psychology of Aging

Terry Mahan Buttaro

Populations around the world are aging. By 2050, there will be an estimated 83.7 million adults age 65 and older living in the United States.[1] This cohort will then represent 20.9% of the population in this country, and those older adults over age 85 who are often referred to as the "old-old" will then number 18 million.[1] Some of these older adults will live to be 100 years of age or even older,[2] which is the result of better care and understanding of diseases that can now be effectively controlled with behavioral changes (e.g., smoking cessation) and remarkable pharmacologic treatments. However, many of these elders will have multiple comorbidities that include, but are not limited to, Alzheimer's dementia, arthritis, cardiovascular disease, chronic obstructive lung disease, and hypertension.

The increasing number of aging adults in the United States and in other countries is a potentially consequential demographic change that could have widespread significance and affect economics, social structures, and health care throughout the world. Yet despite this knowledge, it is unclear what measures are being discussed and implemented in preparation for this seismic change. Even now there are not enough geriatricians in this country to care for our older patients. Currently there are about 7500 geriatricians in the United States, although the present projected need per 12 million older adults is 17,000 geriatricians.[2] The need for health care providers who (1) understand the pathophysiologic changes that accompany aging, (2) understand the distinction between normal changes of aging and disease, and (3) are skilled in the care of older adults with multiple comorbidities cannot be understated.

Aging is accompanied by both physiologic and psychological changes. Aging is not a disease process. It is normal, inevitable, and complex; it is not related to a single process, but a myriad of changes that can involve genetics, cellular changes, inflammation, simple wear and tear, and it is the subject of a host of other ongoing research initiatives.[3] Although aging is often thought to start in middle age, some changes do start as early as age 20.[4] As an example, atherosclerosis begins to develop at this time, lung tissue is already becoming less flexible, and the rib muscles are changing and becoming smaller. The result of these early pulmonary system changes is that ventilation is impacted.[4] Additional early aging changes occur in the gastrointestinal system because food absorption can be affected by a decrease in the number of digestive system enzymes.

For women, The Women's Health Initiative and other studies suggest that aging is possibly associated with menopause.[5] In addition to the cessation of menses, collagen production decreases, the layer of subcutaneous fat diminishes, and the dismay about sagging chins begins.

Men also notice physical changes. These occur at about the same time that women experience menopause. Prostate enlargement begins after age 40 and continues for the rest of their lives.[6]

However, these early physiologic changes are not dramatic and for most individuals, male or female, organ function is not significantly impacted until much later in life. Sometimes organ dysfunction is not apparent, even in older adults because they seem healthy, have no known comorbidities, and their laboratory values are normal. However, even seemingly healthy elders have physiologic aging changes that, when confronted with illness and/or dehydration, will become obvious (e.g., renal dysfunction). Still, it is important that all health care providers realize that people age differently depending on their lifestyle and health status, know that every patient is different, and that organ function is influenced not only by aging changes but also by disease processes.

Pathophysiology of Aging

There are many theories of aging and likely no single cause. Theories about aging are varied. The stochastic hypothesis suggests that aging changes occur haphazardly throughout the life span and it is the accumulation of these cellular injuries that affect function. Nonstochastic theorists argue that our cells are genetically preprogrammed for death and that aging changes are not random. It is likely that there is some truth to both these theories. Often people think that some of us live longer because we have "good genes," but we know too that people sense their bodies undergo changes in aging and will frequently state to their health care providers that "it is all a part of getting old."

Scientists continue to research the genetic components of longevity, as well as the aging process, and the results are controversial. There are some indications that genes (e.g., *APOE*), might play a role in longevity, but more studies are necessary to determine whether genetics plays a more important role than do patient lifestyle and environmental factors.[7,8] Researchers are also investigating epigenetics, the study of how lifestyle factors influence our genes and determine what role epigenetics plays in illness and/or in longevity. Understanding how chemicals, what we eat, how we exercise, and how other personal behaviors can possibly regulate gene function by modifying the biochemical processes in our bodies that turn genes both on and off will aid in health promotion and illness prevention for our patients and ourselves.

There are factors that are known to affect the aging process. At the cellular level, there is a decline in cell-mediated immunity. Additionally, apoptosis is considered to be a component of the decreased cellular function and atrophy that is associated with growing older.[3] Cellular death is actually a necessary element of cell turnover throughout our life span, and there are programmed pathways to promote cellular turnover and maintain body homeostasis.[9,10] Disruptions in programmed cellular function and homeostasis unfortunately do occur as years pass. Some causes of cellular dysfunction are possibly the result of inflammation, mitochondrial mutations or malfunctioning, and/or telomere shortening, which can result in genomic instability, oncogenesis, senescence, and apoptosis. However, there may be other aspects related to this dysregulation of cellular operation and it is suspected that human behaviors (e.g., obesity, diet, sedentary lifestyle) are contributing factors.[9,11] Whatever the mechanism is that influences the regulation of cellular dysfunction, the resultant outcome can include immunosenescence, sarcopenia, poor wound healing, a decreased ability to suppress cancer cells, and the development of neurodegenerative disease in aging.[9]

Other physiologic alterations that can affect tissue or cellular biology include the loss of homeostatic processes in the endocrine and immune systems. There can be a decrease in hormone production or secretion, as well as a diminished number of receptors in target organs. These changes can affect bone mass, lean muscle, immune function, and even impact our psychological well-being, resulting in fatigue or depression. Decreased B- and T-cell production affects an older adult's defense mechanisms. A decline in the number of B-cells will result in fewer antibodies, and fewer T-cells will disrupt the body's ability to effectively combat infectious processes or cancers.

There is also the concern about free radicals of oxygen and their impact on the aging process. Free radicals do not have a paired electron. These "free" molecules are thought to be the consequence of oxidative stress and result in cellular damage, as well as influencing aging processes throughout the body.[3]

It is the multiplicity of aging changes that occur in an older adult's body combined with multiple comorbidities that present a challenge for the health care provider. Human bodies do not age at the same pace; every person is different. Lifestyle and environment can also influence the aging process. Increasing the awareness of factors that impact health in older adults is important in preserving patient function and providing optimal care for everyone regardless of age.

Impact of Physiologic Processes on Aging Body Systems

SKIN

Skin is the primary barrier between our organs and the environment. The epidermis is comprised of five different layers, each with its own specific function. The two layers of the dermis lie below the epidermis, supporting the epidermis physically and by providing the epidermis with blood. Beneath the dermis is a subcutaneous layer of fat that provides the body with a layer of insulation and cushioning (Fig. 1.1). This fat layer diminishes as we get older and there is less protection from injury. Even a small bump can injure the aging skin, as well as the increasingly age-related vulnerability of the blood vessels in the dermis. The resultant damage: greater skin fragility,

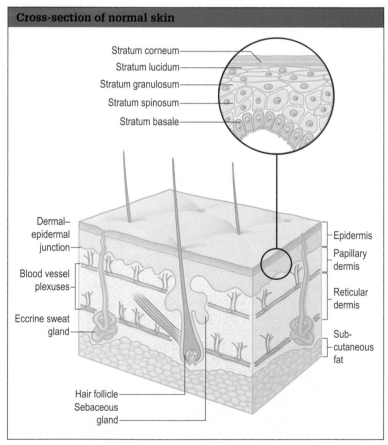

Fig. 1.1   Cross-section of normal skin. (From Guyuron, B., Eriksson, E., Persing, J.A., Chung, K. C., Disa, J. J., Gosain, A. K., ... Rubin, J. P. [2009]. *Plastic surgery: indications and practice* [1st ed.]. Philadelphia: Saunders.)

traumatic skin tears, bruises, senile purpura on the dorsum surface of hands and lower extremities, and delayed skin healing (Fig. 1.2).

Aging changes also cause the epidermis to begin to wrinkle and lose elasticity as we get older. This inelasticity is the result of intrinsic aging, but there are other skin changes (i.e., extrinsic aging or photoaging) that occur that are related to environmental insults, including pollutants and the sun. The daily insult of ultraviolet radiation is just one component of the external stressors that can affect skin and initiate cellular changes in the skin that damage the cell proteins and structure in the skin. Over a lifetime, the environmental damage combined with a series of intrinsic changes precipitated by reactive oxygen species result in epidermal thinning, dermal–epidermal separation, and a host of other skin changes. The effect is the obvious skin changes associated with aging: xerosis (skin dryness), laxity, itching, and the diminished ability of this remarkable organ to recover from injury. Lentigos (i.e., "liver spots"), skin cancers, barrier dysfunction, and decreased strength are the long-term sequelae of the skin changes (Fig. 1.3).[12]

In general, skin problems are as common in older adults as they are in the general population. Skin problems can be inherited or acquired (e.g., porphyrias). Some of the skin problems experienced in this age group are related to peripheral vascular disease, cancer, diabetes, or a systemic or

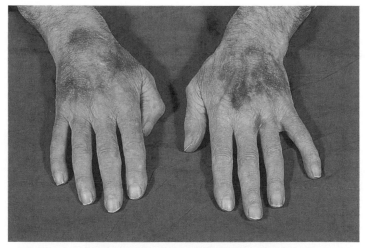

Fig. 1.2 Senile purpura. (From Forbes, C. D., & Jackson, W. F. [2003]. *Color atlas and text of clinical medicine* [3rd ed.]. London: Mosby.)

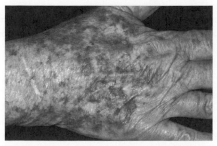

Fig. 1.3 Lentigo. (From Habif, T. P, Dinulos, J. G. H., Chapman, S., & Zug, K. A. [2018]. *Skin disease: diagnosis and treatment* [4th ed.]. St. Louis: Elsevier.)

metabolic disorder. Herpes zoster is especially prevalent in older adults, although herpes zoster also affects younger adults. Medication reactions, acne rosacea, atopic dermatitis, bullous pemphigoid, cellulitis, contact dermatitis, seborrheic dermatitis, herpes simplex, pediculosis, psoriasis, skin cancers, skin ulcers, infections (e.g., bacterial, fungal, tinea), and toxic epidermal necrolysis are among the many skin disorders that should be considered when a patient presentation indicates skin involvement.

NAILS

Nails are considered part of the integumentary system, as is the skin. Nails and skin are designed to help protect us and both change as we grow older. Nail disorders can be related to medications, an aging sign, or a sign of serious illness. Both fingernails and toenails should be examined routinely in men and in women (nail polish should be removed) and abnormalities appropriately identified and treated. Aging nails often are yellowed, thickened, and can have longitudinal ridges (Fig. 1.4). These are normal changes that occur with the passage of time and more easily identified than nail changes associated with some illnesses, although it is important to note that yellowed nails can also be associated with fungal infections, lymphoma, and other illnesses.[12] Brittle nails can be a sign of hypothyroidism. Any nail(s) that is/are misshapen or associated with clubbing (e.g., chronic obstructive pulmonary disease, malignancies and other illnesses), pitting (psoriasis), cuticle invasion (Lichen planus), spoonlike appearance (iron-deficiency anemia), splinter hemorrhages (bacterial endocarditis), longitudinal black or brown lines (melanoma or other cancer), and horizontal bands or ridges require further investigation and possible referral to dermatology for treatment.

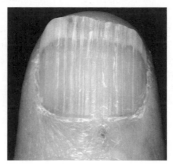

Fig. 1.4   Longitudinal ridging. (From Habif, T. P. [2016]. *Clinical dermatology* [6th ed.]. St. Louis: Elsevier.)

HEENT

We expect hair to turn gray or white as people age. For some, hair turns gray prematurely. Hair can also become thinner as people age and hair loss is not uncommon as people age, although hair loss can be congenital.

Hearing

Hearing and visual changes are especially important to identify in elders because vision and hearing loss can impact the quality of life and patient understanding of health care recommendations.[13] Throughout the world approximately 360 million people have some hearing loss.[14] In the United States, hearing loss is prevalent in older adults, yet many who could use hearing aids to improve their hearing do not.[13] For some people, it is access to an audiologist, for others the stigma or cost of hearing aids that prevents people with hearing problems from seeking care.

Conductive hearing loss can occur in aging, although usually this type of hearing loss in older adults is less common. Sensorineural hearing loss (i.e., presbycusis) is an expected aging change, although the cause is variable: genetic, illness, medications (e.g., furosemide), loud environmental noise, trauma, or just aging.[15] Sensorineural hearing loss or conductive hearing loss causes (e.g., cerumen impaction, cholesteatoma, infection [otitis media or externa], tympanic membrane rupture, trauma, tumors) or other causes of hearing loss as well should be excluded as a possible cause, no matter what the patient's age.

Health care providers caring for older patients should interview older adults who are hearing impaired in a quiet setting and write out the patient history and have the patient read it, if possible, to verify the patient's concerns. Reminding the patient to use their hearing aids or having an available hearing amplifying device can also be helpful when caring for hearing impaired patients.

Vision

Vision loss, although expected in older adults, sometimes is not as obvious to health care providers as hearing loss. We know that patients have cataracts corrected and health care providers in primary care probably do not check visual acuity or peripheral vision in older patients as often as we should. Yet many older adults experience vision loss for reasons other than lens opacities (i.e., cataracts). Peripheral vision is influenced by age, and any type of vision loss can increase the risk of falls and automobile accidents, as well as result in a decrease in an older adult's independence.

Presbyopia, a common age-dependent visual change, can occur as early as age 40. This results in difficulty focusing on anything up close. It is caused by a decrease in lens elasticity and the subsequent decrease in focus accommodation for near objects. Reading glasses or corrective surgery can improve vision.

Burning or stinginglike eye discomfort is a common complaint in primary care and is associated with dry eye. For some, visual acuity is significantly affected. The cause of dry eye can be a medication or disease (e.g., Sjögren's syndrome), but dry eye is a prevalent age-related problem caused by decreased tear production.

Serious eye disorders can affect visual acuity as people age and result in blindness. These include macular degeneration, retinal detachment, retinal artery occlusion, glaucoma, and chronic diseases (e.g., diabetes) that also affect a patient's vision.[16] In the retina, nerve cells and rods are decreased requiring more light to see. The macula atrophies and vision can be lost because of age-related macular degeneration (AMD). There are two types of macular degeneration, wet and dry. Wet AMD is considered more serious because it statistically causes more vision loss and frequently causes blindness. Dry AMD is more common, but the visual loss is slower (Fig. 1.5).

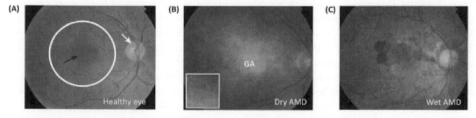

Fig. 1.5 (A–C) Clinical features of age-related macular degeneration (AMD). (From Carr, A. J. F., Smart, M. J. K., Ramsden, C. M., Powner, M. B., Cruz, L., & Coffey, P. J. [2013]. Development of human embryonic stem cell therapies for age-related macular degeneration. *Trends in Neurosciences, 36*[7], 385–395.)

Floaters occur because of posterior vitreous detachment. An increase in the number of floaters, or the development of a more cobweblike visual sensation, suggests a vitreous detachment. This type of retinal detachment is not associated with trauma; it is an actual retinal hole or tear. These can occur rapidly or over time. Other types of retinal tears can be caused by trauma or disease-related issues (e.g., diabetic retinopathy).

Increased ocular pressures decrease visual acuity caused by primary glaucoma (e.g., open angle, narrow angle, acute angle closure, chronic angle closure), secondary glaucoma (e.g., medication or trauma related), and congenital glaucoma. Whatever the cause, the risk of glaucoma increases with age and glaucoma can result in blindness.

Smell and Taste

Smell and taste changes are not limited to older adults, but often older patients present to primary care complaining that they cannot smell or taste their food. Smell is affected by smoking, rhinitis, sinusitis, nasal polyps, toxins, trauma, viral infections, medications, malignancy, neurologic diseases (e.g., Alzheimer's disease or Parkinson's disease), diabetes, and other illnesses, as well as a decrease in olfactory neurons associated with aging.[17,18] Determining the patient's concern—lack of smell (anosmia), decreased smell (hyposmia), or distorted smell (parosmia)—is important in trying to ascertain the cause of the patient's complaint. Often, the lost ability to smell can be related to a medication or an infection, but if these causes are excluded, further diagnostic testing will be necessary.

Olfactory loss is a common cause of taste disturbances, but in addition to affecting smell, medications can also cause dry mouth (xerostomia) or persistent taste dysfunction (dysgeusia). Dental caries, poorly fitting dentures, gingivitis, infections, and diseases also cause oral dryness or decrease taste.[19] Xerostomia can result in inflammation and mucous membrane ulceration, caries, and depending on the cause and severity of dry mouth, nutritional concerns.

Taste disturbances can be described as diminished (hypogeusia), not pleasant (aliageusia), or simply absent (ageusia). The differential diagnoses of taste disturbances are myriad and include, but are not limited to, medication side effects; irradiation of head and neck; malignancy; substance use; endocrine disturbances; and gastrointestinal, hepatic, metabolic, renal, and psychiatric disorders.[18] A decrease in taste buds is not uncommon in aging and is a consideration when an older patient complains of impaired taste, but the cause should not be presumed because it is essential to determine the cause.

Both smell and taste disorders can affect older adults in varied ways. There is the obvious concern about a serious disease or disorder causing the symptoms, but the lack of smell, even if innocuous, can affect patient safety (e.g., the ability to smell smoke). An alteration in taste will likely affect a patient's appetite possibly causing depression and/or nutritional deficiencies, weight loss, and increase the risk of frailty in the older patient.

Throat

Throat disturbances can be related to aging, as well as to medication side effects, brain diseases (e.g., dementia, Parkinson's disease), throat cancers, stroke, or past history of head or neck surgery. Swallowing difficulties increase with aging and can be related to poor dentition, periodontitis, missing teeth, dry mouth, or physiologic changes caused by diminished muscle mass and connective tissue plasticity.[20] The adverse outcomes associated with dysphagia are associated with dehydration, malnutrition, aspiration, pneumonia, and in some cases death.[20]

Vocal changes also occur, which can be the result of physiologic aging changes. As men age, the voice becomes higher pitched; in women, the aging process causes the voice to become lower in pitch.[21] In both sexes, the voice becomes weaker, more tremulous with aging, and there is less ability to project the voice or talk for long periods of time.[21] Other vocal changes (e.g., hoarseness) require further exploration to determine whether a pathologic process is the cause of the patient's symptoms.[21]

Respiratory

Respiratory issues in older adults are common, not only because of age-related changes, but also because over a lifetime the lungs are affected by infections of the respiratory system and environmental pollutants.[22] Cough and swallowing reflexes change as we age, resulting in aspiration. Not only are food and liquids aspirated, but gastric reflux can also be problematic, causing inflammation, as well as bronchiectasis and pneumonia.[22]

Age-related structural changes also occur. Muscle atrophy affects the diaphragm and respiratory musculature. Spinal deformity from osteoporosis or other disorders that cause kyphosis affect inspiration, as do obesity and restrictive lung disorders.[23] The result is chest wall rigidity, a decrease in the surface area of alveoli, loss of elastic recoil and surface area, and other changes.[22] A common complaint that results from these pulmonary changes is dyspnea, which is a significant symptom that reflects a new illness or disease progression in older adults.[24]

Dyspnea, which is described by some as shortness of breath or "I feel like I cannot get a good breath," is a significant symptom that reflects a new illness or disease progression in older adults and requires determination of the cause.[23] Shortness of breath has many causes and it is helpful to learn the following: Is this a new complaint? When do these symptoms occur? What is the patient doing at that time? Differentials that should be considered include anemia, asthma, anxiety, atrial fibrillation (or other arrhythmia), chronic obstructive pulmonary disease, heart failure, interstitial lung disease, restrictive lung disease, pneumothorax, pneumonia, and pulmonary emboli.

CARDIAC

Cardiac disease is a major cause of morbidity and mortality in the United States, as well as in other countries. Some changes in the cardiovascular system are related to hypertension, hyper-cholesterolemia, and hyperglycemia, as well as lifestyle choices (e.g., smoking). Physiologic changes include a decrease in "nitrous oxide mediated vasodilated responses"[25] throughout the vasculature in both men and women.[25] The cause is multifactorial, but it is likely the combination of oxidative stress (related to reactive oxygen species) and increased arginase (an enzyme), which limits nitrous oxide production. These processes combined with endothelial senescence, cause endothelial cell injury and dysfunction, as well as a decrease in vascular homeostasis.[25]

The result is arteriosclerosis, often referred to as the "hardening of the arteries." Arteriosclerosis consists of both atherosclerosis (i.e., plaque deposits within the arterial vasculature) and arterio-losclerosis (i.e., thickened and diseased arteriole intima within the small blood vessels). The complications of these pathologies consist of an increased risk of thrombotic blood vessel occlusions (e.g., stroke) and blood vessel wall weakness (e.g., abdominal aortic aneurysm).

Furthermore, as arteriosclerosis—a thickening and loss of elasticity throughout the arterial system—develops, the aorta and arteries become less pliable and more rigid. These "hardening of the arteries" changes increase left ventricular stiffness and afterload while decreasing left ventricular volume.[25] The result is cardiac hypertrophy, decreased blood flow throughout the vasculature, and an increase in oxygen requirements.[25] The ramifications of these changes are notable: patients with systolic hypertension will frequently have an associated decrease in diastolic blood pressure, as well as an increase in pulse pressure.[25]

Autonomic nervous system changes also associated with aging as older adults are not as responsive to beta adrenergic or parasympathetic stimulation.[25] This explains the cardiac decompensation that occurs when elders are stressed by illness or dehydration, as well as the increased episodes of orthostatic hypotension and syncope noted in older adults.[25]

The physiologic consequences of these changes, whether related to age or disease, are many. For older adults, these changes include a greater possibility of ischemia, atrial fibrillation, decreased vascular tone, systolic hypertension, valvular disease, heart failure, peripheral vascular disease, thrombosis, and renal dysfunction.[25]

GASTROINTESTINAL SYSTEM

The gastrointestinal system undergoes similar changes to those experienced in other organ systems. Poor dentition and periodontal disease can affect digestion if chewing is affected. Xerostomia can also decrease saliva production, although not every patient with dry mouth will experience hyposalivation, and for many patients the cause of hyposalivation is medication related.[26] Some patients do experience hyposalivation, and for them swallowing can be more challenging. Saliva plays an important role in deglutition (the act of swallowing) by moisturizing foods and enabling easier chewing and swallowing. Saliva also contains amylase, which is an enzyme that begins breaking down carbohydrate in foods as we chew.

Once food is chewed and swallowed, the food bolus enters the esophagus. Except in patients with oropharyngeal dysphagia these patients complain that they have difficulty swallowing and will cough or choke whenever they try to eat or drink. These episodes could be related to a neurologic problem, oropharyngeal motor and sensory aging changes that cause dysphagia, or even to an absent gag reflex.[27] Patients can complain of painful swallowing (odynophagia), which is often medication related, although acid reflux or varied infections also can also cause discomfort with swallowing.[28]

Slower movement through the gastrointestinal tract can be caused by an esophageal stricture, a motility disorder, or medications that affect the gastrointestinal system. The resultant decrease in esophageal motility and emptying can cause patients discomfort after meals.[28] Injury caused by alcohol, gastroesophageal reflux, aspirin, nonsteroidal antiinflammatory drugs (NSAIDs), or other medications can occur in the esophagus or stomach, resulting in esophagitis, gastritis, and in some cases bleeding.

Gastric atrophy is common in aging, causing a decrease in hydrochloric acid. Malabsorption is also possible, not only of food but of important proteins and nutrients. Changes in the gastric system can also be affected by previous surgery (e.g., gastric bypass) or by medications. Proton pump inhibitors and H_2 blockers, for example, can increase gastric pH and impede absorption of other medications.

Older adults are at risk for appendicitis, cholecystitis, cholelithiasis, diverticulitis, dyspepsia, peptic ulcer disease, gastroparesis, and gastric cancer, as well as other gastrointestinal disorders. However, elders sometimes are not aware of concerning symptoms or discount their symptoms as not important or serious. Older adults often consider dyspepsia or stomach discomfort unimportant, but the differential diagnoses of malignancy, volvulus, gallbladder or pancreatic disease, and other disorders should always be considered.[29]

Constipation is a common gastrointestinal complaint as people age. There are many causes of constipation (e.g., diet, lactose intolerance, malignancy, medications, electrolyte and endocrine disorders), but there is no clear pathophysiologic reason why older adults have constipation.[27] Anorectal dysfunction is possibly a factor in constipation (and in fecal incontinence), but it is not clear if this is an aging change.[27] Inadequate exercise, water intake, and fiber intake are associated with constipation, but medical disorders and malignancy as a cause should be discussed with the patient and family and not ignored. Treatment for constipation is also indicated to prevent abdominal discomfort, urinary tract infections, and fecal impaction.

The liver changes associated with aging are partly associated with a decrease in blood flow to the liver. Cross-linked undegradable protein aggregates known as lipofuscins are associated with reactive oxygen species that result in liver cell damage. Other pathophysiologic changes include inflammation, senescence, and organ dysfunction related to varied liver disorders (e.g., hepatitis, alcoholic and nonalcoholic fatty liver disease) and occur simultaneously.[30] It is primarily Phase 1 metabolism, the p450 system, which is affected, but ethnicity as well as age can affect medication clearance. All these factors can affect first-pass clearance and biotransformation. The result is that medication bioavailability can be increased, elevating the risk of medication toxicity in older adults.

Other organs in the gastrointestinal system include the gallbladder and pancreas. Older patients can certainly have gallbladder disease or pancreatitis, but the cause of these disorders is more likely to be associated with lifestyle choices or specific illnesses rather than aging changes.

RENAL

There are both structural and physiologic changes that influence renal function. Kidney injury can occur throughout life and for varied causes. Often the change is fleeting and possibly related to an illness and dehydration. When the illness and/or dehydration resolves, renal function returns to normal and often there is no significant impact on kidney function.

Aging changes (e.g., oxidative stress, inflammation) and disease (e.g., atherosclerosis, diabetes, hypertension, lupus erythematosus, other disorders) do affect renal function.[31] These changes can cause a decrease in the number of functioning nephrons over time. Structural changes (e.g., infarction, scarring or sclerosis) and medication-related nephrotoxicity are also possible causes of renal dysfunction.

Additionally, renal blood flow is an essential component of renal function. If blood flow is decreased for any reason, glomerular filtration is affected. Multiple factors regulate renal blood flow in an attempt to maintain a constant glomerular filtration rate (GFR).[32] These factors include autoregulation within the kidney itself, neural regulation of systemic arterial pressure by the sympathetic nervous system, and multiple hormonal and mediator regulators (renin angiotensin-aldosterone system, natriuretic peptides, bradykinin, etc.).

Renal blood flow does diminish in aging for a number of reasons. Diabetes and hypertension are definite kidney stressors and a definite cause of chronic kidney disease. However, degenerative changes, decreased perfusion, and other pathophysiologic aging changes also affect the number of functioning nephrons within the kidneys.[32] The result of these changes is that, by age 75, functioning nephrons can potentially be decreased by half and there can be some degree of chronic kidney disease.[32]

There are other causes of renal dysfunction. Hypertension, medications, infection (particularly sepsis), heart failure, and untreated urinary tract obstruction (from calculi, prostatic hypertrophy, or malignancy) can cause renal failure if untreated. These causes are frequently acute in nature, but older adults can have chronic changes and not be aware of renal changes unless they have significant chronic kidney disease.

The consequences of diminished kidney function can include decreased urinary output and the risk of fluid and electrolyte imbalances. Complications include normocytic anemia related to reduced erythropoietin production and possibly increased levels of hepcidin,[33] decreased sodium excretion, fluid retention, hypertension, congestive heart failure, hypocalcemia, hyperkalemia, and other electrolyte changes and hormonal imbalances.[34]

Other aging changes include an increase in glucosuria, even in patients who do not have diabetes. This is the result of decreased glucose reabsorption.[32] Higher doses of vitamin D are necessary because age-related renal dysfunction affects vitamin D availability, as well as causing secondary hyperparathyroidism and bone disease.[32]

Decreased renal function affects medication prescribing in older adults. For this reason it is essential that health care providers are aware of each patient's renal function.

GENITOURINARY

Bladder function issues are a common concern for patients as they age, and urinary incontinence is one of several geriatric syndromes that also includes delirium, dizziness, falls, frailty, and syncope. Types of urinary incontinence include urge incontinence, stress incontinence, functional incontinence, overflow incontinence, and mixed (a combination of stress and urge) incontinence. Delirium, depression, infection, and impacted stool are also associated with incontinence in older adults. From the patient's perspective, the bladder does not seem to hold as much urine without emptying, so older patients complain of frequent urination throughout the day and night. Urinary frequency and other symptoms, such as nocturia, urgency, incontinence, voiding symptoms, urinary dribbling, and the sensation that the bladder did not completely empty, are referred to as lower urinary tract symptoms (LUTS). Both men and women experience LUTS and many are concerned about the impact of incontinence in daily life. Shortening of the urethra as women age causes an inability of the urinary sphincter to contract efficiently and urinary incontinence can occur, but for both sexes the cause of urinary incontinence is really multifactorial.[35] Cognitive and functional impairment are certainly risk factors for incontinence, but medications (e.g., diuretics), overactive bladder, and a plethora of comorbidities are associated with urinary incontinence.[36] These include uninhibited detrusor contraction changes related to ischemic myopathy or neuropathy, cough-related incontinence, constipation, diabetes, hypercalcemia, neurologic conditions (e.g., stroke, neuromuscular disease), obstructive sleep apnea, and even anxiety and depression.[36]

As men age, they also experience LUTS that are similar to the symptoms that women experience (i.e., frequency, urgency, incontinence).[36] Additional concerns in older males can also include difficulty urinating, dribbling, painful urination, overactive bladder, and erectile dysfunction.[37] Erectile dysfunction has varied causes, but medications, diabetes, and cardiovascular disease are possible differentials that should be considered. Testosterone does decrease as men age, causing varied body changes that include a decrease in muscle and physical strength.[37] In some men, low testosterone levels can be related to erectile dysfunction, although cardiovascular disease is a more common cause of erectile dysfunction requiring careful investigation into the cause of the patient's concern. A decrease in testosterone can also be associated with a greater risk of cardiovascular disease.[37]

Sexual dysfunction also occurs in women as they age partly because of the decrease in hormonal changes at menopause, but arthritic pain, coronary artery disease, diabetes, hypertension, gynecologic conditions, and other comorbidities should be considered. Medications can also be contributing factors affecting sexual desire and lubrication. Unfortunately, older females are not often asked about their sexual health or offered treatment for easily remedied concerns such as vaginal dryness and pain during intercourse. Increased awareness of the importance of asking about discomfort during sex and lack of sexual desire are important considerations.

Prostatic hypertrophy symptoms become noticeable after age 50 for most men.[38] The urinary symptoms experienced by older men are possibly related to the way an increase in prostatic tissue changes the urethra and subsequently the urinary flow (e.g., prostatic tissue that grows inward will cause a man more symptoms that if the tissue grows outward).[38] Bladder outlet obstruction related to prostatic hypertrophy is always a concern and is associated with overflow incontinence, but some men will not sense the need to void.

Both men and women complain of nocturia. There are many reasons people wake up during the night to urinate. For some people, nocturia is caused by drinking coffee or alcohol late in the day or early evening, and for others it is simply drinking fluids later in the day. Medications and medical disorders (e.g., diabetes, urinary tract infection, overactive bladder, undiagnosed sleep apnea) can also cause nocturia, but the etiology can also just be an aging change. Frequently getting out of bed during the night to urinate can disrupt sleep, and there is always the potential risk of a fall in a frail elder or in an older adult with cognitive deficits. Asking about the presence of nocturia and determining the cause can improve sleep quality and perhaps decrease the risk of an untoward event.

Urinary tract infections (Table 1.1) are not uncommon in older adults and frequently are associated with urinary incontinence. Many older adults, especially women, chronically have bacteriuria in their urine, but they are asymptomatic. The causes of urinary tract infections in

TABLE 1.1 ■ **Criteria for Urinary Tract Infection**

Criteria	Comments
A. Without an indwelling catheter: Both criteria 1 and 2 present: 1. At least *one* of the following sign/symptom subcriteria (a–c) present: a. Acute dysuria or acute pain, swelling, or tenderness of the testes, epididymis, or prostate b. Fever or leukocytosis *and* At least *one* of the following localizing urinary tract subcriteria: i. Acute costovertebral angle pain or tenderness ii. Suprapubic pain iii. Gross hematuria iv. New or marked increase in incontinence v. New or marked increase in urgency vi. New or marked increase in frequency c. In the absence of fever or leukocytosis, then at least *two* or more of the following localizing urinary tract subcriteria: i. Suprapubic pain ii. Gross hematuria iii. New or marked increase in incontinence iv. New or marked increase in urgency v. New or marked increase in frequency	UTI should be diagnosed when there are localizing genitourinary signs and symptoms and a positive urine culture A diagnosis of urinary infection can be made without localizing symptoms if a blood culture isolate is the same as the organism isolated from the urine, and there is no alternate site of infection In the absence of a clear alternate source, fever or rigors with a positive urine culture in the noncatheterized resident or acute confusion in the catheterized resident will often be treated as UTI; however, evidence suggests most of these episodes are likely not from a urinary source Pyuria does not differentiate symptomatic UTI from asymptomatic bacteriuria Absence of pyuria in diagnostic tests excludes symptomatic UTI in residents of long-term care facilities
2. *One* of the following microbiologic subcriteria: a. $\geq 10^5$ cfu/mL of no more than two species of microorganisms in a voided urine b. $\geq 10^2$ cfu/mL of any number of organisms in a specimen collected by in-and-out catheter	Urine specimens for culture should be processed as soon as possible, preferably within 1–2 hours If urine specimens cannot be processed within 30 minutes of collection, they should be refrigerated Refrigerated specimens should be cultured within 24 hours
B. With an indwelling catheter: Both criteria 1 and 2 present: 1. At least *one* of the following sign/symptom subcriteria (a–d) present: a. Fever, rigors, or new-onset hypotension, with no alternate site of infection b. Either acute change in mental status or acute functional decline with no alternate diagnosis and leukocytosis c. New-onset suprapubic pain or costovertebral angle pain or tenderness d. Purulent discharge from around the catheter or acute pain, swelling, or tenderness of the testes, epididymis, or prostate	Recent catheter trauma, catheter obstruction, or new-onset hematuria are useful localizing signs consistent with UTI, but they are not necessary for diagnosis
2. Urinary catheter culture with $\geq 10^5$ cfu/mL of any organism(s)	Urinary catheter specimens for culture should be collected after replacement of the catheter (if current catheter has been in place >14 days).

cfu/mL, Colony-forming units per microliter; *UTI,* urinary tract infection.
Adapted from Stone, N. D., Ashraf, M. S., Calder, J., & Crnich, C. J. (2012). Surveillance definitions of infections in long-term care facilities: revisiting the McGeer criteria. *Infection Control & Hospital Epidemiology, 33*(10), 965–977.

women include changes in perineal flora that become more conducive to gram-negative bacilli.[39] However, immunosenescence, comorbidities, functional status, and other factors that influence the immune response (e.g., nutritional status, cancers) may play a role in any infection in an older adult.[39] Asymptomatic bacteriuria does not require pharmacologic treatment, but patients with symptomatic bacteriuria do require antibiotic therapy. Clinicians need to be aware that in older adults the clinical presentation of illness is not what is typically experienced in the care of younger adults. Elders may not recognize the classic symptoms associated with a urinary tract infection, and often older adults will not have the typical response associated with illness (i.e., a fever or leukocytosis). For that reason, it is important that health care providers consider an infectious etiology when an older adult has a change in cognitive or functional status, a change in oral intake, or a temperature increase of more than 2.4 degrees over baseline, as well as the classic symptoms commonly associated with a urinary tract infection (i.e., dysuria, frequency urgency, flank pain) (see Table 1.1).[39]

MUSCULOSKELETAL

Musculoskeletal disorders in aging are associated with changes that affect height, bones, muscles, and joints. All these disorders can affect function, mobility, and quality of life in older adults. In general, body weight increases but bone mass and lean muscle mass decrease in aging. Even older adults who have exercised their entire lives will experience some sarcopenia, which affects muscular function and strength, although continued exercise can help preserve muscle strength. Cartilage, ligament, and muscle changes throughout the musculoskeletal system result in stiffer joints and decreased range of motion. All these musculoskeletal alterations can compromise an adult's functional status and increase the risk of falls in elders.

Lyme Disease

Lyme disease is endemic in many areas throughout the United States. This bacterial infection is caused by *Borrelia*, which is a spirochete bacterium associated with a tick (*Ixodes scapularis*) bite. Often patients do not remember a tick bite and do not have the bull's eye rash associated with Lyme disease, but present to primary care complaining of muscle or joint pain often accompanied by fever. Sometimes only one joint is affected (e.g., a knee), but the concern could be pain is several joints; thus, Lyme disease should be a consideration in the differential diagnosis of muscle or joint pain.

Osteoarthritis

Osteoarthritis can cause pain, joint inflammation, and damage the synovial joints. Cartilage loss occurs in normal aging, but in osteoarthritis there is articular cartilage degeneration and degradation that occurs over time and is not repaired. Pain and immobility can occur. Weight-bearing joints are commonly affected, but osteoarthritis also develops in the cervical and lumbar vertebrae. As the disease process continues, patients develop painful bony protuberances known as Bouchard (proximal interphalangeal [PIP] joints) and Heberden (distal interphalangeal joints) nodes that affect function and motion. Patients' joints are affected differently, but trauma can play an initial role. In the weight-bearing joints, obesity as well as wear and tear can affect function (Fig. 1.6).[40]

Rheumatoid Arthritis

Rheumatoid arthritis (RA) is more common in younger adults but can develop in elders, especially in older men (age 60–80).[41] RA is not caused by aging, but is a systemic disease that often can have a genetic component. The disease starts slowly in some patients, but in older adults it can be abrupt. Patients note pain, edema, and morning stiffness in the PIP joint, metacarpophalangeal (MCP) joints, metatarsophalangeal (MTP) joints, and wrists. Fever and fatigue are common.[41]

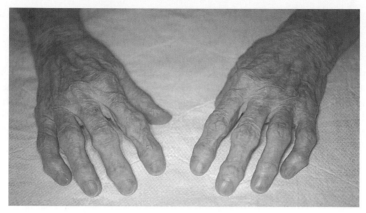

Fig. 1.6 Heberden nodes and Bouchard nodes in osteoarthritis. (From Swartz, M. H. [2010]. *Textbook of physical diagnosis: history and examination* [6th ed.]. Philadelphia: Saunders.)

Gouty Arthritis

Gouty arthritis (gout) does affect older adults, although it is associated with a metabolic disease and not really related to aging changes.[42] The pathophysiology of a gout attack is related to the deposition of urate crystals. These crystals are the result of increased levels of uric acid that occur with either decreased uric acid excretion or increased uric acid production. Obesity, alcohol, medications, genetic predisposition, and inflammation are possible precipitants. The gout attack itself is reflected in the presentation of pain (often in a MTP joint) usually, but not necessarily, in a single joint.[42] Diagnosis is based on identification of monosodium urate (MSU) crystals in synovial fluid, rather than serum uric acid levels, which can be normal at the time of the attack.[42] Pseudogout (acute calcium pyrophosphate [CPP] crystal arthritis) is related to calcium pyrophosphate dehydrate (CPPD) crystal deposition in synovial fluid. CPPD can also cause severe joint pain, often in a knee, but other joints also can be affected.[43]

Polymyalgia Rheumatica

Polymyalgia rheumatica (PMR) is an inflammatory disorder that most often affects people over 50 years of age.[44] The pathophysiology of PMR and its association with giant cell arteritis (GCA) is not clear. These disorders frequently exist together and affect older adults. Human leukocyte antigen (i.e., HLA-DR4 and associated allele polymorphisms) is identified in PMR.[44,45] There is possibly a genetic and immune relationship in PR, but the role of environment or infection is also questioned.

GCA is characterized as a vasculitis and affects large arteries (e.g., the aorta and temporal arteries), but cranial pain, headache, and visual disturbances are the symptoms that cause patients to seek care.[45] The inflammatory process associated with GCA results in granulomatous lesions on the walls of the affected arteries.[46] Some patients with GCA also will have symptoms primarily associated with PMR. These include an aching discomfort and a sensation of stiffness in a patient's neck, shoulders, and pelvis.[43-45] The onset of PMR can be acute or insidious and is sometimes associated with fever and lethargy.[43] Some patients are depressed and in others the diagnosis is complicated because the wrists, knees, and other joints are involved, blurring the diagnosis.[44]

Osteoporosis

Osteoporosis currently affects about 54 million people in the United States and costs about $19 million each year, primarily because of osteoporosis-related fractures and hospitalizations.[47] Defined as a T-score of −2.5, osteoporosis affects both men and women as they age causing a decrease in bone mass. The prevalence of osteoporosis has historically been greater in women as a result of lower bone mineral density and estrogen loss in menopause. Vertebral fractures occur equally in both sexes, but older men can have more serious sequelae.[48,49]

The pathophysiology of osteoporosis is related to decreased bone formation. Bone resorption, the elimination of decaying bone by osteoclasts, continues, but the decreased rate of bone formation cannot keep pace with the bone loss.[50] Because bone remodeling is altered, the bones become weaker and increasingly fragile.[51] For women, postmenopausal osteoporosis is prevalent, but there are other causes of osteoporosis that should be considered also. These causes are varied but contribute to the resultant bone loss and bone weakness. Genetics is one element, but several diseases (e.g., connective tissues disorders, gastrointestinal disorders, thyroid disease, hyperparathyroidism, chronic kidney disease) are also related to the development of osteoporosis.[52] Cigarette smoking, inadequate calcium consumption, vitamin D deficiency, excessive alcohol intake, and medications (especially corticosteroids and anticonvulsants) are among the other factors that cause bone loss.[50]

Common fracture sites include the distal radius, proximal femur, and vertebrae. In older adults new-onset acute back pain, especially in the mid to lower thoracic area, should raise concerns about a compression fracture.[53] Mild trauma in an elder either after a fall or lifting a heavy object can also result in an osteoporotic fracture, which can cause significant pain and need for hospitalization and pain management.[53] Some vertebral fractures do not cause pain but result in lost height and thoracic kyphosis.[54] These changes can decrease pulmonary function.[54] Hip fractures are usually considered the most serious of osteoporotic fractures because of the complications associated with hip fractures (e.g., blood loss, fat or pulmonary emboli, pain, and death).[54]

Neurologic Changes

Neurologic changes do occur in aging and can easily be missed during a health care visit with an older adult. Some changes are easily noticed and associated with aging, for example, visual and hearing changes. Psychomotor and motor-slowing changes might require more attentiveness by the health care provider, whereas a patient's muscle strength and speed can be more noticeable as a patient walks into the office or tries to get up from a chair.[55] The older adult's appearance, alertness, level of consciousness, and speech are important in any assessment because changes in any of these items can suggest alterations in the patient's neurologic state.[55]

As we age our brains become smaller. Porous changes in the blood-brain barrier can result in increased drug sensitivity (e.g., benzodiazepines, opioids) and other side effects. There can also be less coordination throughout the brain potentially causing cognitive dysfunction. Neurologic changes can be related to reduced cerebral perfusion, the result of age-related decline in cardiac output, and atherosclerotic and arteriosclerotic changes that occur in the brain and throughout the body.[56] In addition, there can be a decrease in the number of neurotransmitters and receptors, as well as decreased neuroreceptor receptiveness. Further cellular changes are caused by oxidative stress and inflammation within the cerebrovascular system. Other factors that can affect brain function include the age-related decrease in hormones, receptors, and neurotransmitters. Impaired glucose metabolism within the brain is a continuing concern because the brain requires a consistently stable level of glucose. If glucose levels within the brain are too high *or* too low, cognitive function and memory can be affected.

Aging changes can impart some degree of "benign senescent forgetfulness" in all of us.[57] We can forget words or someone's name, causing worry about developing dementia. Age does affect cognitive function in some ways. It can be more challenging to problem solve and learn new information, verbal fluency and spontaneous word finding is more challenging, and reaction time and information processing slows.

Yet the concerns we all have about dementia are well founded. Currently, approximately 5.4 million people in the United States have been diagnosed with Alzheimer's dementia, which is the sixth most common cause of death in the United States.[58] These numbers do not include the number of people with other common types of dementia (chronic traumatic encephalopathy, frontotemporal dementia, Parkinson's dementia, vascular dementia, etc.) or those people with undiagnosed cognitive dysfunction. The numbers also do not illustrate the cost of these disorders or the physical and psychological toll that families experience when caring for an older adult who is confused, does not recognize them, and may have distressing behavioral attributes associated with dementia. The pathophysiology of each of these brain diseases is different, and the cognitive deficits are similar in some ways and varied in others. For some people with Alzheimer's dementia, the disease is genetic and related to the $ApoE_4$ gene, which may be present in one-quarter of Americans. The pathology of Alzheimer's disease includes brain atrophy and neuritic plaques that include amyloid beta and neurofibrillary tangles with hyperphosphorylated tau proteins. Tangles result and spread throughout the brain causing dysfunction and dementia. Different cognitive domains (e.g., attention, language, orientation, and visuospatial function) can be affected in any of the dementias, but what is usually initially apparent in Alzheimer's dementia are the memory and thinking difficulties. There are different types of memory: declarative or explicit memory (e.g., conscious recollection), remote memory (e.g., what happened at grandma's house during the blizzard 10 years ago), semantic memory (e.g., colors), and procedural memory (e.g., how to drive a car). Alzheimer's dementia especially affects declarative memory (the ability to learn new information), but remembering in general is also an issue (e.g., where are the car keys).

Any concern about cognitive function in a patient requires careful screening and determining whether there are other causes of the patient's symptoms (e.g., depression, hypothyroidism, B_{12} deficiency, malignancy, medications, or normal pressure hydrocephalus). If these or other causes of cognitive dysfunction are not excluded, further diagnostics and mental status testing (e.g., Montreal Cognitive Assessment) are necessary. Early treatment of cognitive dysfunction is recommended.

Spinal Stenosis. This is an aging change causing a narrowing of the spinal canal and is usually associated with Paget's disease, osteophytes, and degenerative changes, as well as other disorders. Depending on the areas affected, patients can complain of back or leg pain, as well as weakness and possible paresthesias. Degenerative disk disease can also cause cervical discomfort or low back pain.

Motor Neuron Loss. This also occurs in aging.[59] The result is slower nerve conduction and a decrease in muscle strength and muscle mass throughout the body. In the spine, the age-related decrease in spinal motor neurons and myelin damage can also affect motor control.

Autonomic Nervous System. These changes are associated with blood pressure control and cerebral blood flow regulation. Ambulation and the ability of an older adult to adjust to both internal and external stimuli are also affected by changes in the autonomic nervous system.

The culmination of these and other neurologic changes can be problematic for elders. An older adult's awareness of the environment is diminished because of the multiple aging changes throughout their bodies, and they can subsequently be subjected to syncope, unexpected falls, and other traumatic injury.

Psychology of Aging

Psychological changes associated with aging are similar in some respects to physiologic aging changes, but every person is different. There are 95-year-old adults who live and continue to function happily and independently, whereas younger older adults can become very depressed or develop an early-onset severe dementia requiring constant care. For others, the very thought of aging is fraught with anxiety. How each of us approaches growing older is likely a combination of factors that include available support systems, finances, health, and our personalities. Some people are incredibly resilient in the face of overwhelming problems, whereas even minor worry in others can cause sleepless nights. Recognizing mental health issues in older adults is essential in primary care practice, yet it can be very challenging. Older adults can be vague about symptoms and often there are so many comorbid disorders and medications to review in a routine or follow-up care visit that there is little time to explore the common mental health issues that older adults and their families face.

Approximately one-fifth of adults older than age 60 have been previously diagnosed with a neurologic or mental disorder.[60] That diagnosis could be as simple as a headache or as serious as dementia or depression, which are both prevalent in older adults.[60] Many elders are anxious because they are worried about their health, finances, children, and the growing realization about death and dying. Another growing concern is the impact that substance use has on older patients.[60]

Despite the prevalence of mental health disorders in older adults and aging populations around the world, the availability of mental health services for this cohort is quite limited. There are not enough mental health professionals, and access to mental health services can depend on the patient's physical health, insurance, finances, an automobile or bus service, and willingness to talk to a health care provider about a mental health or cognitive concern. An additional issue in primary care is the health care provider's comfort, readiness, and time availability during an older patient's office visit to determine the presence of anxiety, depression, or cognitive dysfunction. Patients will complain about sleep problems, but they may not be aware of cognitive slowing or mood change. A patient who is reluctant to discuss their anxiety or depression, speaks a different language, does not hear well, or has a health literacy deficit also contributes to a provider's unawareness of the psychological issues confronting an elder. Asking the right questions (of the patient and with permission, of the family) and doing a thorough physical examination (perhaps in more than one office visit) can help elucidate concerning issues.[61]

ANXIETY

Anxiety in older adults is common and can be chronic or new. It is plausible that new-onset anxiety in an elder is related to a physiologic neurobiological disconnect between the amygdala and frontal areas of the brain.[62] However, it is more likely that it is the interplay of neurobiological influences, psychosocial issues, and possible comorbid illness(es) that result in an older adult's anxiety.[62] Whatever the cause of anxiety in elders, the result can be chronic and sometimes overwhelming distress, in addition to possible cognitive changes. There is also the association between anxiety and depression, not only in older adults but in other patient age groups as well. The cause is unclear, but afflicted patients can be more severely affected by the combination of symptoms associated with both of these disorders.

Anxiety is often unrecognized, but when it goes untreated it can be debilitating. Most elders with anxiety have generalized anxiety disorder, but there can be a relationship with other anxiety disorders (e.g., panic disorder, social phobia, obsessive-compulsive disorder, or previous history of trauma) that needs to be elucidated. Illness and medications are also associated with anxiety, and in some patients there can be a significant family history of anxiety and depression. Often patients will self-medicate with alcohol and or with drugs, possibly "borrowing" them from a neighbor or friend. Thus substance abuse in patients with anxiety is a concern. Older patients will not necessarily specifically complain of "anxiety," but can describe frequent worry, tired feeling, frequent tension, restlessness, irritability, and trouble sleeping. Reviewing the medications (including herbals and over-the-counter drugs) patients are taking and the amount of caffeine and alcohol ingested each day is necessary. Screening for anxiety with Generalized Anxiety Disorder-7 (GAD-7) is recommended and easily accessed (available at https://www.mdcalc.com/gad-7-general-anxiety-disorder-7) as is screening for an associated depression with the Geriatric Depression Scale (available at https://consultgeri.org/try-this/general-assessment/issue-4.pdf). However, a thorough physical examination and testing for a physical cause of the patient's anxiety (arrhythmias, hyperthyroidism, anemia, electrolyte imbalance, heart disease, etc.) should be conducted initially.

No one treatment is indicated for anxiety. Avoiding stimulants and caffeine can be helpful in some cases. Patients sometimes will ask for benzodiazepines. This category of medications works quickly and patients believe they help. Unfortunately, tolerance and dependence are possible and there are many adverse effects, especially for older adults, including falls, confusion, automobile accidents, and, if taken with alcohol or opioids, a greater risk of death. Effective and safer medication categories include antidepressants (e.g., serotonin reuptake inhibitors [SSRIs] and serotonin-norepinephrine reuptake inhibitors [SRNIs]). No one medication is considered the best because each person reacts differently to medications. However, a thorough medication review (including any over-the-counter and herbal medications the patient can be taking) to assess for potential drug–drug interactions is recommended for all patients. Older adults are especially susceptible to serotonergic effects of medications, so monitoring is necessary. Starting at the lowest dose possible with a slow titration if needed is recommended. Buspirone is another antianxiety medication that can be helpful for some patients. Encouraging healthy nutritional habits and daily exercise in capable older adults might also be beneficial, as well as meditation or yoga. If available, cognitive behavioral therapy or counseling is recommended.

DEPRESSION

Depression is associated with multiple causes in older adults. For some, it is possible that the depression has been long-standing (e.g., patients with a history of bipolar illness, major depression, persistent depressive disorder, or minor depression). For others, illness, financial concerns, grief, bereavement, and other losses are possible precipitants. Neurotransmitter changes in aging also can possibly cause depression.[63] The effects of comorbid disorders and psychosocial stressors are considered significant causes of depression in this age group with an estimated 20% of elders having "depressive symptoms."[61,63] In nursing homes, the incidence of depression is higher, approaching 50%.[63] The consequences of depression in older adults are significant: functional decline, cognitive dysfunction, and increased morbidity and mortality.[63] Because 25% of suicides occur in older adults and 75% of suicides in elders are patients with a history of depression, this is an important health care problem.

The presentation of depression in older adults can be unclear. Sometimes elders with depression will have somatic complaints about constipation or urinary issues rather than specific complaints of hopelessness or sadness.[63] Patient concerns that center around physical problems such as these need to be further evaluated to determine whether the patient does have an organic problem. Then, careful interviewing (including asking about a previous history of depression or bipolar illness) and screening for depression is important. Many primary care offices use the Patient Health Questionnaire (PHQ-9) to help identify patients who are depressed, but further screening with the Geriatric Depression Scale is indicated. Often, the health care provider specifically needs to ask the older patient if depression is a possible cause of his or her symptoms.[64] Of importance is determining whether the patient has a substance abuse problem as well as thoroughly reviewing all the patient's medications because many drug side effects can include depression. The diagnostic criteria (i.e., DSM-5) for depression should then be reviewed (http://images.pearsonclinical.com/images/assets/basc-3/basc3resources/DSM5_DiagnosticCriteria_MajorDepressiveDisorder.pdf).[65]

Concerns about the diagnosis, risk for suicidality or homicidality, and/or possible treatment should be discussed with a geriatric or mental health specialist.

MILD COGNITIVE IMPAIRMENT

Mild cognitive impairment (MCI), also known as prodromal dementia, is most commonly associated with memory loss (i.e., remembering names or appointments), but the ability to solve complex problems can also be compromised. The patient or one of the patient's family members notice that the patient has difficulty remembering and is concerned about the possibility that dementia is the cause.[66] Although initial testing should include a thorough physical examination, appropriate diagnostics, and screening for cognitive changes (e.g., the Montreal Cognitive Assessment) in the primary care office setting, neuropsychological testing is also recommended to determine possible deficits, associated domains, and the actual absence or presence of dementia. A medical cause cannot be deemed to be the cause of the patient's cognitive impairment for a diagnosis of MCI, so these need to be excluded before neuropsychological testing.

There are two categories of MCI. One category is associated with memory deficits and is known as amnestic MCI. Amnestic MCI is strongly associated with progression to Alzheimer's dementia. The second category of MCI, nonamnestic MCI, is associated with impairments in other cognitive functions (e.g., planning, judgment). There are four subsets of MCI, but none of them include a diagnosis of dementia. The four subsets of MCI include:

1. Single domain amnestic MCI: + memory loss, but no other deficits
2. Multiple domain amnestic MCI: + memory loss and other deficits
3. Single domain nonamnestic MCI: + impairment in a single, but not memory-related, cognitive domain
4. Multiple domain nonamnestic MCI: + impairment in multiple, but not memory-related, cognitive domain.[66]

Patients with MCI can have other symptoms that are often associated with dementia (e.g., depression, behavioral changes). A primary concern when a patient has MCI is the possible association and progression to Alzheimer's dementia or another form of dementia. Currently there is no specific treatment for MCI.

THE DEMENTIAS

Although memory loss is commonly associated with Alzheimer's dementia, other dementias and disorders also affect memory and function. Patients with dementia experience cognitive loss in at least one cognitive domain and often more than one. The cognitive losses progress over time, but patients with dementia frequently can also have behavioral changes. The differential diagnoses of dementias include Alzheimer's disease, frontotemporal dementia, vascular dementia, Parkinson's disease dementia, dementia with Lewy bodies, Huntington's disease, normal pressure hydrocephalus, and Creutzfeldt–Jakob disease. Alcohol, vitamins B_1 and B_{12} deficiency, pseudodementia, and other health problems also affect brain function causing confusion and dysfunction.

Each of these disorders, and other more uncommon dementias, has a different pathologic cause. Vascular dementia is associated with cardiovascular disease, and there are infarctions that occur throughout the brain. Patients with Lewy body dementia have "Lewy bodies" (e.g., α-synuclein inclusions) that cause anxiety, confusion, disorientation, memory loss, poor judgment, and the other symptoms associated with dementia.[67] Frontotemporal dementia is caused by neurodegeneration (cerebral tissue death) in the frontal temporal lobes.[67] There are three different clinical presentations associated with frontotemporal dementia, and each are different depending on the area affected.

The clinical presentation and pathophysiology can differ somewhat in all the dementias, but the result is intellectual dysfunction and behavioral changes. Dementia treatments are limited.

There are some treatment modalities (e.g., cholinesterase inhibitors or memantine, which is an NMDA receptor antagonist) for Alzheimer's disease, but their efficacy is limited, the disease progression is not arrested, some patients do not tolerate them well, and some patients see no change at all. Still, it is recommended to try cholinesterase inhibitors in patients with Alzheimer's dementia, as well as those with vascular dementia, Parkinson's disease dementia, and Lewy body dementia. Each patient's response to a medication should be monitored.

DELIRIUM

Delirium is often mistaken for dementia because the patient with delirium is confused and associated behavioral changes are common. Both delirium and dementia are characterized by cognitive impairment, but delirium is different. It is considered an acute, but reversible, confusional state frequently associated with alcohol, anesthesia, illness, medication, metabolic disorder, and a host of other causes. The onset of delirium is acute, but the episodes are transient and in some patients last weeks rather than just a few days. The delirious patient's mental status state fluctuates, and there are perceptual disturbances, as well as the decreased ability to focus. The pathophysiology of delirium is not clear. The cause may be related to a disruption of the neural network involving the upper brainstem's reticular activating system, neurotransmitter abnormalities (e.g., a decrease in acetylcholine or increase in dopamine), and proinflammatory factors.[68] Older adults are at risk for delirium, and in some cases delirium seems to be associated with an unmasking of a dementia.

Diagnosis and appropriate treatment of delirium are important. The diagnosis is primarily a clinical diagnosis, although there are screening tools that can help the health care provider identify delirium. The Confusion Assessment Method (CAM) Instrument is a valid and helpful tool (available at https://consultgeri.org/try-this/general-assessment/issue-13.pdf). Additionally, there are DSM-5 diagnostic criteria for delirium.

Delirium can present differently in patients because there are different types of confusional states. Patients can have a hyperactive delirium and be combative and/or agitated; a hypoactive delirium that is manifested by lethargy and confusion; or mixed delirium, which is a combination of both. Treatment of delirium is primarily supportive, but addressing the cause, instituting the specific therapies, and preventing injury are the goals of therapy.

SLEEP DISORDERS

Sleep disorders affect people of all ages and have varied causes. The complaint about sleep is a common one in primary care, but older adults, in general, do not sleep as well as younger adults. The reasons are myriad (nocturia, pain, sleep apnea), but there is also a physiologic cause in older adults. Nonrapid-eye-movement or slow-wave sleep decreases as we age and can even be nonexistent in older adults.[69] The result is more awakenings throughout the night.[69] Stress insomnia related to ongoing anxiety is another possible cause, as is caffeine, alcohol, sleep apnea, and poor sleep hygiene. A careful history should include exploration of psychophysiologic factors (i.e., the patient's expectation of sleep), sleep hygiene, psychiatric history (e.g., anxiety, depression), current medications, possible substance abuse, medications, and medical disorders (e.g., pain, dementia).[69]

Treatment should address those issues that can be corrected (e.g., restless leg syndrome, sleep apnea, pain) and behavioral changes that improve sleep (e.g., decreasing daily amount of caffeine, no evening alcohol, avoiding television or computer before bedtime). Cognitive behavioral therapy and stress relaxation techniques can be beneficial. In general, the medications for sleep are not recommended for older adults because of the cognitive and reaction time–related side effects. Doxepin, a tricyclic antidepressant, in doses less than 6 milligrams po at bedtime is a possible therapeutic, although the indication is to use doxepin only if the patient has depression-related insomnia. Low-dose mirtazapine in older adults with depression is an additional option.

References

1. Ortman, J. M., Velkoff, V. A., & Hogan, H. (2014). An aging nation: The older population in the United States. Retrieved from https://www.census.gov/prod/2014pubs/p25-1140.pdf.
2. Olivero, M. (2015). Doctor shortage: Who will take care of the elderly. Retrieved from http://health.usnews.com/health-news/patient-advice/articles/2015/04/21/doctor-shortage-who-will-take-care-of-the-elderly.
3. McCance, K. L., Grey, T. C., & Rodway, G. (2014). Altered cellular and tissue biology. In K. L. McCance, S. E. Huether, V. L. Brashers, & N. S. Rote (Eds.), *Pathophysiology: The biologic basis for disease in adults and children* (7th ed., pp. 49–97). St. Louis, MO: Elsevier.
4. National Institute on Aging. (2015). Health & Aging. Retrieved from https://www.nia.nih.gov/health/publication/aging-under-microscope/what-aging5.
5. Shuster, L. T., Rhodes, D. J., Gostout, B. S., Grossardt, B. R., & Rocca, W. A. (2010). Premature menopause or early menopause: Long-term health consequences. *Maturitas, 65*(2), 161.
6. Rodway, G., & McCance, K. L. (2014). Alterations of the aging reproductive system. In K. L. McCance, S. E. Huether, V. L. Brashers, & N. S. Rote (Eds.), *Pathophysiology: The biologic basis for disease in adults and children* (7th ed., pp. 800–914). St. Louis, MO: Elsevier.
7. Brooks-Wilson, A. R. (2013). Genetics of healthy aging and longevity. *Human Genetics, 132*(12), 1323–1338.
8. Fortney, K., Dobriban, E., Garagnani, P., Pirazzini, C., Monti, D., Mari, D., et al. (2015). Genome-wide scan informed by age-related disease identifies loci for exceptional human longevity. *PLoS Genetics, 11*(12), e1005728. http://doi.org/10.1371/journal.pgen.1005728.
9. Tower, J. (2015). Programmed cell death in aging. *Ageing Research Reviews, 23*(Pt A), 90–100.
10. McCann, S. A., & Huether, S. E. (2014). Structure, function, and disorders of the integument. In K. L. McCance, S. E. Huether, V. L. Brashers, & N. S. Rote (Eds.), *Pathophysiology: The biologic basis for disease in adults and children* (7th ed., pp. 1616–1664). St. Louis, MO: Elsevier.
11. Shammas, M. A. (2011). Telomeres, lifestyle, cancer, and aging. *Current Opinion in Clinical Nutrition and Metabolic Care, 14*(1), 28–34.
12. Yaar, M., & Gilchrest, B. A. (2012). Aging of skin. In L. A. Goldsmith, S. I. Katz, B. A. Gilchrest, A. S. n Paller, D. J. Leffell, & K. Wolff (Eds.), *Fitzpatrick's dermatology in general medicine* (8th ed.). New York, NY: McGraw-Hill. Retrieved from http://accessmedicine.mhmedical.com.ezproxy.simmons.edu:2048/content.aspx?bookid=392&sectionid=41138823.
13. Rooth, M. A. (2017). The prevalence and impact of vision and hearing loss in the elderly. *North Carolina Medical Journal, 78*(2), 118–120.
14. World Health Organization. (2017). Deafness and hearing loss. Retrieved from http://www.who.int/mediacentre/factsheets/fs300/en/.
15. Baldwin, K., Budzinski, C., & Shapiro, C. (2008). Acute sensorineural hearing loss: Furosemide ototoxicity revisited. *Hospital Pharmacy, 43*(12), 982–987, 1007.
16. Huether, S. E., Rodway, G., & DeFriez, C. (2014). Pain, temperature regulation, sleep and sensory function. In K. L. McCance, S. E. Huether, V. L. Brashers, & N. S. Rote (Eds.), *Pathophysiology: The biologic basis for disease in adults and children* (7th ed., pp. 484–526). St. Louis, MO: Elsevier.
17. Ropper, A. H., Samuels, M. A., & Klein, J. P. (2014). Disorders of smell and taste. In *Adams & Victor's principles of neurology* (10th ed.). New York, NY: McGraw-Hill. Retrieved from http://accessmedicine.mhmedical.com.ezproxy.simmons.edu:2048/content.aspx?bookid=690&sectionid=45424422.
18. Mahoney, M., Franklin, C. M., Reidy, P. A., Sheff, E. K., Kane, D. E., Ladd, E., et al. (2016). Smell and taste disturbances. In T. M. Buttaro, J. Trubulski, P. Polgar-Bailey, & J. Sandberg-Cook (Eds.), *Primary care: A collaborative practice* (5th ed., pp. 392–394). St. Louis, MO: Elsevier.
19. Calabrese, J. M., & Jones, J. A. (2016). Oral health. In J. B. Halter, J. G. Ouslander, S. Studenski, K. P. High, S. Asthana, M. A. Supiano, et al. (Eds.), *Hazzard's geriatric medicine and gerontology* (7th ed.). New York, NY: McGraw-Hill. Retrieved from http://accessmedicine.mhmedical.com.ezproxy.simmons.edu:2048/content.aspx?bookid=1923&sectionid=144520516.
20. Sura, L., Madhavan, A., Carnaby, G., & Crary, M. A. (2012). Dysphagia in the elderly: Management and nutritional considerations. *Clinical Interventions in Aging, 7*, 287–298.

21. American Academy of Otolaryngology – Head and Neck Surgery. (2017). The voice and aging. Retrieved from http://www.entnet.org/content/voice-and-aging.

22. Campbell, E. J. (2015). Aging of the respiratory system. In M. A. Grippi, J. A. Elias, J. A. Fishman, R. M. Kotloff, A. I. Pack, R. M. Senior, et al. (Eds.), *Fishman's pulmonary diseases and disorders* (5th ed.). New York, NY: McGraw-Hill. Retrieved from http://accessmedicine.mhmedical.com.ezproxy.simmons.edu:2048/content.aspx?bookid=1344&sectionid=72262213.

23. Amin, P., & Smith, A. M. (2014). Pulmonary disease. In R. J. Ham, P. D. Sloane, G. A. Warshaw, J. F. Potter, & E. Flaherty (Eds.), *Ham's primary care geriatrics* (6th ed., pp. 497–511). Philadelphia, PA: Elsevier.

24. Kernisan, L. (2014). Addressing dyspnea in older adults. In B. A. Williams, A. Chang, C. Ahalt, H. Chen, R. Conant, C. Landefeld, et al. (Eds.), *Current diagnosis & treatment: Geriatrics* (2nd ed.). New York, NY: McGraw-Hill. Retrieved from http://accessmedicine.mhmedical.com.ezproxy.simmons.edu:2048/content.aspx?bookid=953&sectionid=53375689.

25. Dai, X., Hummel, S. L., Salazar, J. B., Taffet, G. E., Zieman, S., & Schwartz, J. B. (2015). Cardiovascular physiology in the older adults. *Journal of Geriatric Cardiology*, *12*(3), 196–201.

26. Villa, A., Connell, C. L., & Abati, S. (2015). Diagnosis and management of xerostomia and hyposalivation. *Therapeutics and Clinical Risk Management*, *11*, 45–51.

27. Bitar, K., Greenwood-Van Meerveld, B., Saad, R., & Wiley, J. (2011). Aging and gastrointestinal neuromuscular function: Insights from within and outside the gut. *Neurogastroenterology and Motility: The Official Journal of the European Gastrointestinal Motility Society*, *23*(6), 490–501.

28. Hall, K. E. (2017). Aging of the gastrointestinal system. In J. B. Halter, J. G. Ouslander, S. Studenski, K. P. High, S. Asthana, M. A. Supiano, et al. (Eds.), *Hazzard's geriatric medicine and gerontology* (7th ed.). New York, NY: McGraw-Hill. Retrieved from http://accessmedicine.mhmedical.com.ezproxy.simmons.edu:2048/content.aspx?bookid=1923&sectionid=144526242.

29. McQuaid, K. R. (2017). Gastrointestinal disorders. In M. A. Papadakis, S. J. McPhee, & M. W. Rabow (Eds.), *Current medical diagnosis & treatment*. New York, NY: McGraw-Hill. Retrieved from http://accessmedicine.mhmedical.com.ezproxy.simmons.edu:2048/content.aspx?bookid=1843&sectionid=135709704.

30. Kim, H., Kisseleva, T., & Brenner, D. A. (2015). Aging and liver disease. *Current Opinion in Gastroenterology*, *31*(3), 184–191.

31. Bitzer, M. (2017). Renal disease. In J. B. Halter, J. G. Ouslander, S. Studenski, K. P. High, S. Asthana, M. A. Supiano, et al. (Eds.), *Hazzard's geriatric medicine and gerontology* (7th ed.). New York, NY: McGraw-Hill. Retrieved from http://accessmedicine.mhmedical.com.ezproxy.simmons.edu:2048/content.aspx?bookid=1923&sectionid=144525850.

32. Doig, A. K., & Huether, S. E. (2014). Structure and function of the renal and urologic systems. In K. L. McCance, S. E. Huether, V. L. Brashers, & N. S. Rote (Eds.), *Pathophysiology: The biologic basis for disease in adults and children* (7th ed., pp. 1319–1336). St. Louis, MO: Elsevier.

33. Poggiali, E., DeAmicis, M. M., & Motta, I. (2014). Anemia of chronic disease: A unique defect of iron recycling for many different chronic diseases. *European Journal of Internal Medicine*, *25*(1), 12–17.

34. Bonventre, J. V. (2014). Adaptation of the Kidney to Injury. In D. Kasper, A. Fauci, S. Hauser, D. Longo, J. Jameson, & J. Loscalzo (Eds.), *Harrison's principles of internal medicine* (19th ed.). New York, NY: McGraw-Hill. Retrieved from http://accessmedicine.mhmedical.com.ezproxy.simmons.edu:2048/content.aspx?bookid=1130&sectionid=79746357.

35. Jaipaul, N. (2017). Effects of aging on the urinary tract. Merck Manual. Retrieved from http://www.merckmanuals.com/home/kidney-and-urinary-tract-disorders/biology-of-the-kidneys-and-urinary-tract/effects-of-aging-on-the-urinary-tract.

36. DeBeau, C. E. (2014). Urinary incontinence. In R. J. Ham, P. D. Sloane, G. A. Warshaw, J. F. Potter, & E. Flaherty (Eds.), *Ham's primary care geriatrics* (6th ed., pp. 269–280). Philadelphia, PA: Elsevier.

37. Bhasin, S., & Basaria, S. (2014). Men's health. In D. Kasper, A. Fauci, S. Hauser, D. Longo, J. Jameson, & J. Loscalzo (Eds.), *Harrison's principles of internal medicine* (19th ed.). New York, NY: McGraw-Hill. Retrieved from http://accessmedicine.mhmedical.com.ezproxy.simmons.edu:2048/content.aspx?bookid=1130&sectionid=63651918.

38. Granville, L. J., & Suchak, N. (2014). Benign prostatic disease. In R. J. Ham, P. D. Sloane, G. A. Warshaw, J. F. Potter, & E. Flaherty (Eds.), *Ham's primary care geriatrics* (6th ed., pp. 542–553). Philadelphia, PA: Elsevier.

39. Bradley, S. F. (2014). Infectious diseases. In R. J. Ham, P. D. Sloane, G. A. Warshaw, J. F. Potter, & E. Flaherty (Eds.), *Ham's primary care geriatrics* (6th ed., pp. 512–534). Philadelphia, PA: Elsevier.

40. Pathology of the bones and joints. (2008). In W. L. Kemp, D. K. Burns, & T. G. Brown (Eds.), *Pathology: The big picture*. New York, NY: McGraw-Hill. Retrieved from http://accessmedicine.mhmedical .com.ezproxy.simmons.edu:2048/content.aspx?bookid=497&sectionid=11560302.

41. O'Dell, J. R., Imboden, J. B., & Miller, L. D. (2015). Rheumatoid arthritis. In J. B. Imboden, D. B. Hellmann, & J. H. Stone (Eds.), *CURRENT diagnosis & treatment: Rheumatology* (3rd ed.). New York, NY: McGraw-Hill. Retrieved from http://accessmedicine.mhmedical.com.ezproxy.simmons.edu:2048/ content.aspx?bookid=506&sectionid=42584899.

42. Schumacher, H., & Chen, L. X. (2014). Gout and other crystal-associated arthropathies. In D. Kasper, A. Fauci, S. Hauser, D. Longo, J. Jameson, & J. Loscalzo (Eds.), *Harrison's principles of internal medicine* (19th ed.). New York, NY: McGraw-Hill. Retrieved from http://accessmedicine.mhmedical.com. ezproxy.simmons.edu:2048/content.aspx?bookid=1130&sectionid=79751123.

43. Nakasato, Y., & Christensen, M. (2014). Arthritis and related disorders. In R. J. Ham, P. D. Sloane, G. A. Warshaw, J. F. Potter, & E. Flaherty (Eds.), *Ham's primary care geriatrics* (6th ed.). Philadelphia, PA: Elsevier.

44. Quismorio, F. P., & Johnson, D. K. (2016). Polymyalgia rheumatic and giant cell arteritis. In T. M. Buttaro, J. Trubulski, P. Polgar-Bailey, & J. Sandberg-Cook (Eds.), *Primary care: A collaborative practice* (5th ed., pp. 1159–1164). St. Louis, MO: Elsevier.

45. Helfgott, S. M., Todd, D. J., & Wei, K. (2016). Vasculitis. In T. M. Buttaro, J. Trybulski, P. Polgar-Bailey, & J. Sandberg-Cook (Eds.), *Primary care: A collaborative practice* (5th ed., pp. 1176–1180). St. Louis, MO: Elsevier.

46. Creager, M. A., & Loscalzo, J. (2014). Diseases of the aorta. In D. Kasper, A. Fauci, S. Hauser, D. Longo, J. Jameson, & J. Loscalzo (Eds.), *Harrison's principles of internal medicine* (19th ed.). New York, NY: McGraw-Hill. Retrieved from http://accessmedicine.mhmedical.com.ezproxy.simmons.edu:2048/content.asp x?bookid=1130&sectionid=79744168.

47. National Osteoporosis Foundation. (2017). What is osteoporosis and what causes it? Retrieved from https://www.nof.org/patients/what-is-osteoporosis/.

48. Lindsay, R., & Cosman, F. (2014). Osteoporosis. In. In D. Kasper, A. Fauci, S. Hauser, D. Longo, J. Jameson, & J. Loscalzo (Eds.), *Harrison's principles of internal medicine* (19th ed.). New York, NY: McGraw-Hill. Retrieved from http://accessmedicine.mhmedical.com.ezproxy.simmons.edu:2048/content.aspx?booki d=1130&sectionid=79744168.

49. Cawthon, P. M. (2011). Gender differences in osteoporosis and fractures. *Clinical Orthopaedics and Related Research, 469*(7), 1900–1905.

50. Malabanan, A. O. (2016). Metabolic bone disease: Osteoporosis and Paget disease of the bone. In T. M. Buttaro, J. Trubulski, P. Polgar-Bailey, & J. Sandberg-Cook (Eds.), *Primary care: A collaborative practice* (5th ed., pp. 960–970). St. Louis, MO: Elsevier.

51. Nelson, H. D. (2014). Osteoporosis. In R. J. Ham, P. D. Sloane, G. A. Warshaw, J. F. Potter, & E. Flaherty (Eds.), *Ham's primary care geriatrics* (6th ed., pp. 445–455). Philadelphia, PA: Elsevier.

52. Li, W. F., Hou, S. X., Li, M. M., Férec, C., & Chen, J. M. (2010). Genetics of osteoporosis: Accelerating pace in gene identification and validation. *Human Genetics, 127*(3), 249–285.

53. The regional musculoskeletal examination of the low back. (2012). In G. V. Lawry (Ed.), *Systematic musculoskeletal examinations*. New York, NY: McGraw-Hill. Retrieved from http://accessmedicine .mhmedical.com.ezproxy.simmons.edu:2048/content.aspx?bookid=384&sectionid=41842866.

54. Crowther-Radulewitz, C. L., & McCance, K. L. (2014). Alterations of musculoskeletal function. In K. L. McCance, S. E. Huether, V. L. Brashers, & N. S. Rote (Eds.), *Pathophysiology: The biologic basis for disease in adults and children* (7th ed., pp. 1540–1590). St. Louis, MO: Elsevier.

55. Galvin, J. E. Mental status and neurologic examination. In J. B. Halter, J. G. Ouslander, S. Studenski, K. P. High, S. Asthana, M. A. Supiano, et al. (Eds.), Hazzard's geriatric medicine and gerontology (7th ed.). New York, NY: McGraw-Hill. Retrieved from http://accessmedicine.mhmedical.com.ezproxy. simmons.edu:2048/content.aspx?bookid=1923&sectionid=144517915.

56. Puglielli, L., & Mattson, M. P. Cellular and neurochemical aspects of the aging brain. In J. B. Halter, J. G. Ouslander, S. Studenski, K. P. High, S. Asthana, M. A. Supiano, et al. (Eds.), *Hazzard's geriatric medicine and gerontology* (7th ed.). New York, NY: McGraw-Hill. Retrieved from http://accessmedicine. mhmedical.com.ezproxy.simmons.edu:2048/content.aspx?bookid=1923&sectionid=144523231.

57. Sloane, P. D., Warshaw, G. A., Potter, J. F., Flaherty, E., & Ham, R. J. (2014). Principles of primary care of older adults. In R. J. Ham, P. D. Sloane, G. A. Warshaw, J. F. Potter, & E. Flaherty (Eds.), *Ham's primary care geriatrics* (6th ed., pp. 3–17). Philadelphia, PA: Elsevier.
58. US against Alzheimer's. (2017). Retrieved from http://www.usagainstalzheimers.org/crisis.
59. Gonzalez-Freire, M., de Cabo, R., Studenski, S. A., & Ferrucci, L. (2014). The neuromuscular junction: Aging at the crossroad between nerves and muscle. *Frontiers in Aging Neuroscience, 6,* 208.
60. World Health Organization. (2016). Mental health and older adults. Retrieved from http://www.who.int/mediacentre/factsheets/fs381/en/.
61. Telerant, R., Eckstrom, E., Singer, C. M., & Luxenberg, J. (2014). Older patients. In M. D. Feldman, J. F. Christensen, & J. M. Satterfield (Eds.), *Behavioral medicine: A guide for clinical practice* (4th ed.). New York, NY: McGraw-Hill. Retrieved from http://accessmedicine.mhmedical.com.ezproxy.simmons.edu:2048/content.aspx?bookid=1116&sectionid=62687953.
62. Lenze, E. J., & Wetherell, J. L. (2011). A lifespan view of anxiety disorders. *Dialogues in Clinical Neuroscience, 13*(4), 381–399.
63. Diagnosis and management of depression. (2013). In R. L. Kane, J. G. Ouslander, I. B. Abrass, & B. Resnick (Eds.), *Essentials of clinical geriatrics* (7th ed.). New York, NY: McGraw-Hill. Retrieved from http://accessmedicine.mhmedical.com.ezproxy.simmons.edu:2048/content.aspx?bookid=678&sectionid=44833885.
64. Wagley, J. N. (2016). Mood disorders. In T. M. Buttaro, J. Trybulski, P. Polgar-Bailey, & J. Sandberg-Cook (Eds.), *Primary care: A collaborative practice* (5th ed., pp. 1654–1669). St. Louis, MO: Elsevier.
65. Diagnostic and Statistical Manual, 5th ed. (2017). Retrieved from http://images.pearsonclinical.com/images/assets/basc-3/basc3resources/DSM5_DiagnosticCriteria_MajorDepressiveDisorder.pdf.
66. Delirium and dementia. (2014). In S. C. Stern, A. S. Cifu, & D. Altkorn (Eds.), *Symptom to diagnosis: An evidence-based guide* (3rd ed.). New York, NY: McGraw-Hill. Retrieved from http://accessmedicine.mhmedical.com.ezproxy.simmons.edu:2048/content.aspx?bookid=1088&sectionid=61697830.
67. Boss, B. J., & Huether, S. E. (2014). Alterations in cognitive systems, cerebral hemodynamics and motor function. In K. L. McCance, S. E. Huether, V. L. Brashers, & N. S. Rote (Eds.), *Pathophysiology: The biologic basis for disease in adults and children* (7th ed., pp. 527–574). St. Louis, MO: Elsevier.
68. Delirium and dementia. (2013). In R. L. Kane, J. G. Ouslander, I. B. Abrass, & B. Resnick (Eds.), *Essentials of clinical geriatrics* (7th ed.). New York, NY: McGraw-Hill. http://accessmedicine.mhmedical.com.ezproxy.simmons.edu:2048/content.aspx?bookid=678&sectionid=44833884.
69. Czeisler, C. A., Scammell, T. E., & Saper, C. B. (2014). Sleep disorders. In D. Kasper, A. Fauci, S. Hauser, D. Longo, J. Jameson, & J. Loscalzo (Eds.), *Harrison's principles of internal medicine* (19th ed.). New York, NY: McGraw-Hill. Retrieved from http://accessmedicine.mhmedical.com.ezproxy.simmons.edu:2048/content.aspx?bookid=1130&sectionid=79725062.

CHAPTER 2

Untangling the Geriatric Assessment

Karen L. Dick

Mrs. Thompson is a 79-year-old woman who is new to a primary care practice. She comes to her visit today accompanied by her daughter with whom she is now living after the recent death of her husband. Mrs. Thompson had been very busy caring for him in the home since his cerebrovascular accident (CVA) a few years before. Mrs. Thompson has not seen a primary care provider in quite a while, and her daughter tells the provider of her concern for her mother's health, saying she had no idea about what she has had in terms of screening or evaluations. Her daughter reports that her mother has still been getting her medications renewed from her previous provider, but she does not have any of those records. She is worried her mother is neglecting herself and becoming more isolated. The provider begins to process how today's visit will be structured, as well as subsequent visits, with the goal of identifying the key areas and domains to focus on while establishing goals of care.

Introduction

The challenges of providing care for older adults within today's traditional model can be overwhelming for health care providers. Younger persons often have a *single* system problem or disease that can be easily managed with one intervention or, in some cases, a referral to a body system specialist. A 35-year-old with an acute ankle strain may be managed in primary care or may eventually need a referral to orthopedics. In comparison, older adults often present with a nonacute, ill-defined problem or problems involving *more than one* body system, which are likely the result of many interacting factors from multiple domains that are not always apparent. The traditional medical visit that uses a standard history and physical examination format is not thorough enough to gather enough information to help understand the connections between all the factors. An 80-year-old with heart failure, failing eyesight, depression, and frequent falls requires a more comprehensive and coordinated assessment to determine the interplay between the patient's medical problems, physical and emotional functioning, and social supports.

Caring for patients with these multiple coexisting chronic conditions, or what is referred to as multimorbidity, is very challenging. It is important for providers to use a person-centered approach that can take into account a number of key principles. These principles, as outlined by the American Geriatrics Society (AGS), include incorporating patient preference, interpreting the evidence, evaluating prognosis, considering clinical feasibility of treatment decisions, and choosing therapies that optimize benefit, minimize harm, and enhance the older person's quality of life.[1] The AGS details these principles in a free Multimorbidity Toolkit, which includes an algorithm called Approach to the Evaluation and Management of the Older Adult with Multimorbidity. This can be used as a guide for the management of older adults with multiple complex health problems (see https://geriatricscareonline.org/toc/multimorbidity-toolkit/TK011).

Comprehensive Geriatric Assessment

Promoting wellness, enhancing quality of life, and maximizing function require a methodology that assesses the older person's physical, nutritional, economic, cognitive, psychosocial, and environmental domains in addition to his or her medical conditions. The cornerstone of geriatric care has always been focused on maximizing the older adult's physical, cognitive, and social functioning, and to do that a more thorough and coordinated approach is required. Comprehensive geriatric assessment (CGA) is an evaluation of those areas that are key to detecting geriatric conditions and syndromes that are frequently unrecognized or not identified in this population. It addresses the need to understand the severity and impact of illness in an older person in a *broader* way. CGA has been described as not only a multidimensional diagnostic process that focuses on an individual's functional capacity but also as involving the development of an integrated plan for treatment and follow-up.[2] The underlying premise is that a systematic evaluation may identify treatable health problems, leading to better health outcomes.[3] To provide this kind of care, it is important to consider all the domains and areas that may affect an aged individual's health and well-being. To obtain a valid patient history, family, friends, or caregivers should be included as additional sources of information. Typically the assessment domains include:

Functional ability: Activities of daily living (ADLs) and instrumental ADLs (IADLs)

Physical health: Problems common in older adults and found during a history and physical (e.g., gait, continence, balance, visual/hearing deficits).

Cognition and mental health: Screening for cognitive impairment and depression

Medications: A review of the patient's current prescription and over-the-counter (OTC) medication use

Socioeconomic: The patient's social support network, living situation, home safety

Other: Advanced directives, driving

Although once primarily focused on tertiary or restorative strategies, geriatric assessment can also focus on primary and secondary prevention approaches. Geriatric assessment can be done routinely across all settings of care, including the primary care or specialty practice office; the emergency department (ED); a hospital, including in an acute geriatric evaluation unit; a nursing home; or at home. The scope of the assessment may vary depending on the plan of care, the setting, the patient's level of frailty, time constraints, and the availability of a multidisciplinary team.[4] Most models use a core team including a physician (usually a geriatrician), a nurse practitioner or physician's assistant, nurses, social worker, and other disciplines as needed. The team can be extended to include physical or occupational therapists, nutritionists, pharmacists, and psychologists or psychiatrists.[5] CGA has been shown to improve detection of geriatric problems, to reduce functional deterioration and mortality, to decrease nursing home admissions, and to increase patients' chances of living in their own homes at 6 to 12 months after the assessment[2,6-10] CGA performed in the home and in the acute care setting has been shown in meta-analysis and systematic reviews to be consistently beneficial for several health outcomes, including reduction of rehospitalizations and ED visits.[5]

There is no one standard model for CGA and no universal criteria that have been agreed on to identify which patients would be most likely to benefit. There is also considerable variation in approaches. Strategies include identifying patients based on age or a certain number of impairments or conditions, such as frailty, who could benefit from a more comprehensive evaluation. Targeted programs such as those done in the hospital before discharge may identify those patients who may be at risk for readmission and who may require more intense coordination of posthospital care. Because geriatric conditions are often associated with adverse surgical outcomes, assessment done before surgery may identify specific perioperative optimization strategies that can decrease the older patient's risk of postoperative complications. One example is the assessment of baseline cognition and function for all patients undergoing elective cardiac surgery to identify those patients with a preexisting cognitive impairment who are at risk of developing a postoperative delirium. Those patients can be flagged in the system and staff alerted to initiate specific protocols to maximize patient safety.

The annual wellness visit (AWV) for Medicare patients could be considered an abbreviated type of geriatric assessment because it directs primary care providers to screen for cognition, mood, and function along with preventative and health risk assessments. Details regarding the structure of the visit can be accessed through https://www.cms.gov/Outreach-and-Education/ Medicare-Learning-Network-MLN/MLNProducts/downloads/AWV_chart_ICN905706.pdf.

Programs may have specific domains that they emphasize in their evaluations of older patients, depending on the setting, and may use a variety of validated instruments. Again there is no one accepted, standard approach.

GERIATRIC SYNDROMES

Another important component of CGA is the screening and assessment for geriatric syndromes. Geriatric syndromes are multifactorial conditions that involve the interaction between age-related risk factors, chronic disease, and functional stressors.[11] It has been recognized over the last decade that geriatric syndromes contribute to poorer health outcomes for older adults.[12] It may be that a patient's deficits in individual systems viewed in isolation may not seem to amount to significant dysfunction or disability, but looked at collectively with a different lens, they may signal cause for great concern.[13] Consider the 80-year-old woman with diabetes who has impaired vision and peripheral neuropathy, obesity, a gait impairment from spinal stenosis, and an overactive bladder with urge incontinence who hurries to get to the bathroom in time to avoid being incontinent of urine. Each of her conditions by themselves may not signal great danger, but viewed together they clearly demonstrate her increased risk of falls. Geriatric syndromes include cognitive impairment, falls, frailty, and urinary incontinence. These syndromes are common, although often undiagnosed, and present a considerable threat to a patient's quality of life and functioning. Although geriatric syndromes are as prevalent as chronic diseases among older persons, they are not generally considered in a traditional medical evaluation.

ASSESSMENT DOMAINS

To complete a systematic assessment of an older adult that takes into account all the factors that could influence an individual's health and well-being, it is useful to refer to various mnemonics and tools that have been developed.

Mnemonics

AGING GAMES is an example of a mnemonic that stands for components of a geriatric evaluation that makes it easy to remember individual assessment domains.[14]

The actual assessment instruments that are used to measure these domains are not specified but can be individualized to the setting in which the assessment is performed:

AGING GAMES
A: Audiovisual
G: Gait and mobility
I: Insomnia
N: Nutrition
G: Gastrointestinal (GI)
G: Genitourinary (GU)
A: Assistance, ADLs/IADLs/advanced directives

M: Mood and memory

E: Environment + everyday activities

S: Sexuality

Another example is FEEBLE FALLERS ARE FRAIL developed by John Fleming and Kristy Scamehorn (available at https://www.pogoe.org/productid/18597). The FRAIL section can be performed by a social worker:

FEEBLE

F: Forgetful (memory testing, e.g. Mini-Cog, Mini-Mental State Examination [MMSE])

E: Eyes (vision testing)

E: Ears (hearing testing)

B: Brown bag of medications (pharmacy review)

L: Leaking (bowel/urinary incontinence)

E: Eat (nutritional assessment)

FALLERS

F: Fall (fall risk, gait, balance testing)

A: ADLs (functional assessment)

L: Lonely (depression screening)

L: Living (conditions at home, environment}

E: Expectations (goals/outcome anticipated from this assessment)

R: Rest (sleep disorders assessment)

S: Specialists (other physicians, providers, primary care physician [PCP])

ARE

A: Advanced directives, end-of-life planning

R: Ride (driving assessment)

E: ED visits (history of, emergency contacts, etc.)

FRAIL

F: Family (support, caregiver burden)

R: Religion (spiritual assessment)

A: Access (resources, transportation)

I: Income (financial issues)

L: Lifestyle (habits, alcohol, drug abuse, etc.)

A primary care practice might choose to use a standardized approach to assessing patients over a certain age by using a previsit questionnaire that can be completed in the waiting room on a tablet or online. Some practices may choose to mail the previsit questionnaire to new patients so that it can be completed before the first visit. Results can be incorporated directly into the electronic medical record (EMR). Staff can direct patients to complete self-report questionnaires, perform basic screening (cognitive and mood screens), and perform some standardized testing (vision, hearing, or gait/mobility). Deficits identified in key domains may trigger a more in-depth or comprehensive evaluation.

Patients can also be contacted ahead of the visit and asked to bring in all medicines including all prescribed medications, OTC preparations, vitamins, supplements, herbal, topicals, injectables, inhalants, and so forth. This is sometimes referred to as the brown bag review in which the patient is asked to put it all into a large brown bag to bring to the visit. Staff can sit down with the patient to generate a list of all medications including name of provider and date prescribed, as well as to inquire how and when the patient takes the medication. These types of reviews can be done for all new patients and at established intervals or if there is a change in the patient's condition. The Agency for Healthcare Research and Quality (AHRQ) has information related to doing the brown bag medication review in their Health Literacy Universal Precautions Toolkit (available at https://www.ahrq.gov/professionals/quality-patient-safety/quality-resources/tools/literacy-toolkit/healthlittoolkit2-tool8.html).

Commonly Used Screening Tools

As described previously, there are no standardized tools identified as the gold standard for use in a CGA. Choice of tool may depend on provider/practice preference, the setting, ease of use, and degree of patient burden. The screening tools described subsequently may be used as part of regular office visits, at a time of a patient's change in baseline, or as part of a more comprehensive assessment.

Hearing. Hearing impairments affect up to one-third of persons older than 65 and are associated with reduced cognitive and social function. These impairments may be often under-recognized and under-treated because patients may not self-report. If patients report yes to a question about having impaired hearing, they should be referred to an audiologist. Hearing deficits can be screened for by the whisper voice test, in which up to six random words are whispered at a set distance from one patient's ear while the other is covered. Patients are asked to repeat the words and fail the screening if they are unable to repeat half the words correctly.[15]

Vision. There are four eye conditions that have increasing prevalence with age: cataracts, macular degeneration, glaucoma, and diabetic retinopathy.[16] The majority of older adults have presbyopia and require corrective lenses. All of these conditions may lead to visual impairments that are associated with increased risk of falling, functional decline, and depression.[17] Screening in the office can be performed by asking: Do you have difficulty driving, watching TV, reading, or doing any of your daily activities because of your eyesight? The Snellen eye chart can also be used to screen for eye conditions. Patients fail the screening if they answer yes to the screening question or are unable to read the 20/40 line with glasses on and should be referred on for further evaluation by an ophthalmologist.

Physical Function. It is important for providers to assess physical function during every visit with an older patient whether it is at the initial assessment, an episodic visit, or part of a more comprehensive evaluation. A functional assessment assists the provider in focusing on the patient's baseline capabilities, facilitating early recognition of changes that may signify a need either for additional resources or for a medical workup.[18] Basic activities of daily living (BADLs) include six categories: bathing, toileting, transferring, dressing, continence, and feeding. These are all activities that patients need to perform on their own or would need assistance with to live in their own home. The Katz Independence in Activities of Daily Living Scale is the commonly used tool for assessing basic function in the home and clinical environments[19] (it is available at https://consultgeri.org/try-this/general-assessment/issue-2.pdf). Patients are scored as a yes/no for independence: a score of six indicates full function, four indicates moderate impairment, and a score of two or lower indicates significant impairment. An alternative tool is the Barthel Index, which measures 10 areas including walking and climbing stairs[20] (it is available at http://www.pmidcalc.org/?sid = 3403500&newtest = Y).

IADLs represent higher-level functions that lead to independence including shopping, meal preparation, laundry, housework, taking medications, handling finances, and travel including driving or using public transportation. The commonly used tool is the Lawton IADL Scale, which measures eight domains of function.[21] It is scored from 0 indicating low function, or dependent, to 8 indicating high function, or independent (it is available at https://consultgeri.org/try-this/general-assessment/issue-23.pdf).

Gait and Balance. Falls in older adults represent a major public health problem: more than one-third of those living in the community fall each year.[22] Falls are independently associated with functional decline. Patients who fall are at great risk for falling again.[23] Patients may not report a fall because they may not think it important or relevant to tell the provider unless specifically asked. Providers should ask their older patients the following three questions at regular intervals:

1. Have you fallen in the past month, months, or year?
2. Do you feel unsteady when standing or walking?
3. Do you worry about falling?

If the patient answers yes to any of these key screening questions, they are considered at increased risk of falling. Further assessment is recommended. Recognizing the patient's level of risk can lead to the identification of modifiable risk factors, as well as evidence-based interventions. The Centers for Disease Control and Prevention (CDC) has an initiative called the Stopping Elderly Accidents, Deaths and Injuries (STEADI), which uses evidenced-based clinical practice guidelines for the prevention of falls developed by both the AGS and the British Geriatrics Society. The CDC has developed a toolkit that has provider and patient materials (it is available from https://www.cdc.gov/steadi/). There are patient handouts including a patient guide to reducing the risk of falling, as well as a self-report fall risk assessment that patients could complete before a visit to their providers.

To assess a patient's risk of falls, tests of the patient's gait, balance, and functional reach can be easily done in any clinical setting. The toolkit contains instructions on various screening tools that can be used. A patient's gait can be observed while walking and performing maneuvers. The Timed Up and Go test (TUG) (Fig. 2.1) measures the patient's ability to stand from a seated position, walk 10 feet, turn, walk back, and sit down. Those who take longer than 12 seconds should receive further evaluation.[24] Another tool is the 30-second chair stand test, which tests leg strength and endurance and can be done in the office setting by asking a patient to cross their arms across their chest and stand repeatedly over 30 seconds without using the arms of the chair to stand.[25] The functional reach test is another screening test that is defined as the maximal distance an individual can reach forward beyond arm's length while maintaining a fixed base of support in the standing position without taking steps.[26] A patient at great risk of falling can be identified by the reach distance. Another test, the four-stage balance test (Fig. 2.2), has the patient stand in four different positions that get progressively harder to maintain. The stages include standing side by side, standing heel to toe, and standing on one foot. The patient is scored on the ability to hold the position for 10 seconds. If unable to hold a position, the patient is scored with a zero. Lower scores indicate balance issues and increased risk of falls.[27]

Cognition. As many as two-thirds of patients with dementia or probable dementia go undiagnosed by primary care providers.[28] Many patients are not diagnosed with a cognitive impairment until moderate to severe stages of disease. Early recognition would allow for treatment earlier in the

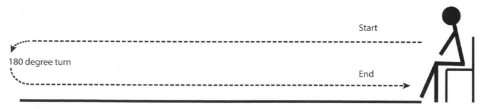

10 Feet

Fig. 2.1 Timed Up and Go test. (From Townsend, N. T., & Robinson, T. N. [2014]. Does walking speed predict postoperative morbidity? *Advances in Surgery*, 48[1], 53–64; data from Podsiadlo, D., & Richardson, S. [1991]. The timed "up & go": A test of basic functional mobility for frail elderly persons. *Journal of the American Geriatrics Society*, 39[2],142–148.)

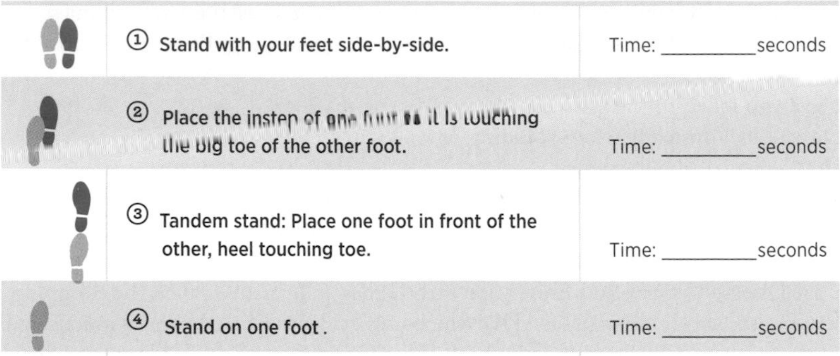

① Stand with your feet side-by-side.	Time: _____ seconds
② Place the instep of one foot so it is touching the big toe of the other foot.	Time: _____ seconds
③ Tandem stand: Place one foot in front of the other, heel touching toe.	Time: _____ seconds
④ Stand on one foot .	Time: _____ seconds

Fig. 2.2 Stage balance test. (From Centers for Disease Control and Prevention. The 4-stage balance test. [2017]. https://www.cdc.gov/steadi/pdf/4-Stage_Balance_Test-print.pdf.)

disease process and allow patients and families time to be educated and aware of future care-planning decisions. Evaluating cognitive function is a critical part of an assessment of an older adult and should be done on an ongoing basis to establish a baseline, as well as to identify changes. Incorporating cognitive testing into visits as a routine part of care may help ease the potential stress and anxiety that older adults may have about having their memory function tested. Even though the United States Preventative Services Task Force (USPSTF) has concluded that the evidence on screening for cognitive impairment in older adults is lacking and that the balance of benefits and harm cannot be determined, they have acknowledged the benefit of early detection of cognitive impairment.[28]

Primary care clinicians may not recognize cognitive impairment when using a routine history and physical examination[3,5] in as many as 76% of patients with dementia or probable dementia,[6-8] and most of these patients are not diagnosed until they are at moderate to severe stages of the disease.[9] Early identification of cognitive impairment would ideally allow patients and their families to receive care at an earlier stage in the disease process, which could lead to improved prognosis and decreased morbidity. Health, psychological, and social benefits from early recognition of dementia through education and improved decision making may make screening valuable, even if early treatment cannot alter the natural history of dementia by preventing or slowing the rate of cognitive decline.[10] The Medicare AWV, which is done in the primary care setting, provides an opportunity for primary care providers to complete cognitive screening using evidenced-based tools. In addition, any time an older adult has new memory concerns or other cognitive complaints, screening for cognitive impairment should be done. Family members or caregivers may also be the ones who first report personality changes, depression, deterioration of chronic disease without explanation, and falls or balance issues in their family member or client, and this should prompt an evaluation.

Regarding the Medicare AWV, the Alzheimer's Association convened an expert panel that made consensus recommendations for cognitive screening in the primary care setting as part of the provisions under the Affordable Care Act in 2011. They developed an algorithm that can be used during the AWV to evaluate cognition, and it is based on patient history and concerns of family or caregivers, as well as clinician observations. Several cognitive screening tools were chosen to be part of the algorithm based on the following criteria: administration time ≤5 minutes; validation in a primary care or community setting; psychometric equivalence or superiority to the MMSE; easy administration by nonphysician staff; and relatively free of educational, language, and/or cultural bias. The algorithm can be found on the Alzheimer's Association website and is available as part of their Cognitive Assessment Toolkit (see https://www.alz.org/documents_custom/

141209-CognitiveAssessmentToo-kit-final.pdf). The first step of the algorithm is a health risk assessment of the patient, clinical observations, patient self-reported concerns, and responses to queries. If signs and symptoms of possible cognitive impairment are present, then a brief structured patient assessment is done, as well as an assessment completed by family members or caregivers. If findings from the brief cognitive assessment trigger concerns, patients should be referred to a neurologist, neuropsychologist, or geriatrician where possible for a full dementia evaluation. Providers choose from the identified tools and may choose to repeat an assessment using one of the other tools to confirm alternative findings before referral or initiation of a full dementia workup. Patient assessment tools that are recommended by the algorithm include the Mini-Cog,[29] the Memory Impairment Screen (MIS),[30] and the General Practitioner Assessment of Cognition (GPCOG).[31] Informant tools include the Eight-Item Informant Interview to Differentiate Aging and Dementia, also known as the AD8 (Fig. 2.3),[32] as well as the Short Informant Questionnaire on Cognitive Decline in the Elderly (IQCODE).[33] All are validated tools with established scoring criteria. The Mini-Cog combines a three-word recall with clock drawing as the distractor. The MIS also combines word recall with distractor questions. The AD8 asks a series of eight questions and asks the informant to indicate if that there has been a change in a particular domain such as judgment, handling finances, or memory over the last several years. The IQCODE lists 26 everyday situations in which a person has to use their memory or intelligence. Examples of such situations include *knowing how to work familiar machines around the house* and *using his/her intelligence to understand what is going on and to reason things through.* Each situation is rated by the informant for the amount of change over the previous 10 years. There are other cognitive screening tools available including the Montreal Cognitive Assessment (MoCA)[34] and the St. Louis University Mental Status Examination (SLUMs).[35] Again, the choice of tool should be based on provider

If the patient has an accompanying reliable informant, they are asked the following questions. Otherwise, the AD8 is administered to the patient.

Has this patient displayed any of the following issues? Remember a "Yes" response indicates that you think there has been **a change in the last several years** caused by thinking and memory (cognitive) problems.

1) Problems with judgment (example, falls for scams, bad financial decisions, buys gifts inappropriate for recipients)?
2) Reduced interest in hobbies/activities?
3) Repeats questions, stories, or statements?
4) Trouble learning how to use a tool, appliance, or gadget (VCR, computer, microwave, remote control)?
5) Forgets correct month or year?
6) Difficulty handling complicated financial affairs (for example, balancing checkbook, income taxes, paying bills)?
7) Difficulty remembering appointments?
8) Consistent problems with thinking and/or memory?

Each affirmative response is one-point. A score of ≥ 2 is considered high-risk for cognitive impairment.

Fig. 2.3 AD8. (From Carpenter, C. R., DesPain, B., Keeling, T. N., Shah, M., & Rothenberger, M. (2011). The six-item screener and AD8 for the detection of cognitive impairment in geriatric emergency department patients. *Annals of Emergency Medicine*, 57(6), 653–661.)

preference and ease of administration because no one tool has been identified as superior to another.

Depression. Depression remains the largest category of psychiatric disorders in older adults and is associated with significant morbidity and mortality.[36] Depression is more common in people who also have other chronic illnesses such as heart disease or cancer or who have functional disabilities. Providers may mistake an older adult's symptoms of depression as a normal reaction to stressors such as death of a loved one, retirement, medical conditions, or loss of independence. Older adults themselves may share this belief and do not seek help. This may lead to under-recognition and under-treatment. An evaluation for depression should include a careful history with the chronology of the development of the patient's symptoms with the level of function. Information regarding the level of social contact, ADL patterns, sleep, and appetite should also be assessed. As with cognitive screening, providers should consistently screen for depression in an older adult on an ongoing established basis, as well as during times of a change in a patient's mood, cognition, or function. The most commonly used tools are the Patient Health Questionnaire (PHQ-9),[37] the Geriatric Depression Scale (GDS) Short Form,[38] and the Beck Depression Inventory (BDI).[39] Although there are many instruments available to measure depression, the Geriatric Depression Scale (GDS) (Fig. 2.4), first created by Sheikh and Yesavage in 1986, has been tested and used extensively with the older population. The Short Form is more easily used by physically ill and mildly to moderately demented patients who have short attention spans or

---

Ask the patient to choose the best answer for how he or she felt over the preceding week.

1. Are you basically satisfied with your life?	Yes/No
2. Have you dropped many of your activities and interests?	Yes/No
3. Do you feel that your life is empty?	Yes/No
4. Do you often get bored?	Yes/No
5. Are you in good spirits most of the time?	Yes/No
6. Are you afraid that something bad is going to happen to you?	Yes/No
7. Do you feel happy most of the time?	Yes/No
8. Do you feel helpless?	Yes/No
9. Do you prefer to stay at home rather than going out and doing new things?	Yes/No
10. Do you feel you have more problems with memory than most people?	Yes/No
11. Do you think it is wonderful to be alive now?	Yes/No
12. Do you feel pretty worthless the way you are now?	Yes/No
13. Do you feel full of energy?	Yes/No
14. Do you feel that your situation is hopeless?	Yes/No
15. Do you think most people are better off than you are?	Yes/No

Correct responses are the following:
Yes for questions 2, 3, 4, 6, 8, 9, 10, 12, 14, and 15.
No for questions 1, 5, 7, 11, and 13.
Give 1 point for each correct answer. A score greater than 5 suggests depression.

Fig. 2.4 Geriatric Depression Scale. (From Sheikh, J. I., & Yesavage, J. A. (1986). Geriatric depression scale (GDS). *Recent evidence and development of a shorter version.* In T. L. Brink (Ed.), *Clinical gerontology: A guide to assessment and intervention.* New York: The Haworth Press.)

who feel easily fatigued. It takes about 5 to 7 minutes to complete. Any positive score greater than 5 on the GDS Short Form should prompt an in-depth psychological assessment and evaluation for suicidality[40] (it is available at https://web.stanford.edu/~yesavage/GDS.html and has been translated into many languages).

Another tool, the Center for Epidemiologic Studies Depression Scale (CESD), was revised in 2004 to the CESD-R and has been used extensively in psychiatric testing and can be done via telephone and by self-administration.[41] It has also been used with older adults and the economically disadvantaged. It consists of 20 questions that cover nine symptoms of depression including areas such as sadness, guilt, sleep, appetite, and loss of interest. Patients are asked to identify the frequency of the symptom over the previous 2-week period. The range of possible scores is between 0 (for those who say "not at all or less than 1 day to all 20 questions") and 60 (for those who say "5–7 days" or "nearly every day for 2 weeks" for all 20 questions). The determination of a possible depressive symptom category ranging from major depression to no clinical significance is based on an algorithm.[41] The CESD-R is in the public domain and can be found at http://cesd-r.com/.

Nutrition. Older adults are at higher risk for nutritional deficits and malnutrition. Malnutrition affects older adults across all health care settings, affecting up to 60% of hospitalized older adults.[42] Approximately 40% to 50% of the population over 80 years of age suffers from sarcopenia, which is defined as loss of muscle mass and strength, making this condition a major geriatric clinical disorder and a key challenge to healthy aging. Older adults with sarcopenia are likely to have worse clinical outcomes and higher mortality compared with healthy individuals.[43] Aging, inadequate food intake, economic constraints, and acute and chronic medical conditions all contribute to malnutrition in the elderly.[42] Patients who are malnourished or who have lost weight are at an increased risk for hospitalization[44] and reduced function, including decreased mobility and a reduced capacity to perform ADLs, which affects independence and diminishes quality of life.[45] Therefore it is important to screen older adults for malnutrition to identify those who may be malnourished or at risk for malnutrition.

The Mini-Nutritional Assessment Short-Form (MNA-SF) is a screening tool that can be used with older adults and consists of six questions on food intake, weight loss, mobility, psychological stress or acute disease, presence of dementia or depression, and body mass index (BMI).[46] It can be completed by the provider and takes less than 5 minutes; no laboratory tests are required. Scores of 12 to 14 are considered normal nutritional status, 8 to 11 indicates at risk of malnutrition, and 0 to 7 indicates malnutrition. If patients are identified to be malnourished or at risk, a more comprehensive assessment and physical examination should be performed along with a 72-hour food intake log. The tool is available through the Hartford Institute for Geriatric Nursing at https://consultgeri.org/try-this/general-assessment/issue-9.pdf.

Driving. According to the National Highway Traffic Safety Administration (NHTSA), older Americans are overrepresented in traffic fatalities; they make up 9% of the population yet are involved in 13% of fatal crashes and 17% of pedestrian fatalities. The fatality rate for older drivers is 17 times higher than the rate for those 25 to 65 years of age.[47]

Drivers aged 85 years or older have among the highest per-mile crash rates and driving fatality rates.[47] Aging is associated with changes in perceptual, motor, and cognitive abilities that may affect an older adult's ability to drive safely. Cataracts and presbyopia can make it difficult to see the road; adjust to glare, low lighting, and darkness; and to judge distances. Deficits in limb strength, endurance, range of motion, and balance may impair motor function and reaction time. Cognitive impairments that may impair driving ability include memory loss (increased chances of getting lost), decreased insight (lack of awareness of impaired driving), or visuospatial problems (difficulty judging distance, turning, or staying in lanes). The ability to process several sources of information and to make a complex decision may also be impaired. In addition, older adults may be on medications that can affect safe driving by impairing level of alertness, attention, and reaction time.

Most older drivers have awareness of the deficits in their driving ability and make adaptive changes including driving only to familiar places during the day to avoid driving at night, or when traffic is less, or when bad weather is a concern. However, there are many instances when primary care providers find themselves in the position of having to deal with the issue of safe driving with their older patients. They may be asked by concerned family members or friends to address the subject, or it may be identified as a concern when there is a change in a patient's perceptual, cognitive, or motor abilities. Inquiring about an older patient's driving status is easily accomplished by incorporating it into the Medicare AWV.

Older adults can also be encouraged to review materials such as the Driving Safely While Aging Gracefully or the Drive Well Toolkit, which are both available from NHTSA. These and other printed materials could be made available in waiting rooms or mailed to patients before a visit.

The AGS publishes a detailed resource for primary care providers called *The Clinicians Guide to Assessing and Counseling Older Drivers*, which details an algorithm called Plan for Older Driver's Safety. It is available for free through the AGS website https://geriatricscareonline.org/ProductAbstract/clinicians-guide-to-assessing-and-counseling-older-drivers-3rd-edition/B022.

This resource provides guidance for identifying factors that put the older driver at risk and details use of the Clinical Assessment of Driving-Related Skills (CADReS) toolbox. CADReS is a toolbox of evidence-based practical, office-based functional assessment tools in the key areas of vision, cognition, and motor/sensory function related to driving. MAZE is a pen-and-paper test where subjects are asked to trace a path through a simple maze. It has been shown to be a proxy for the evaluation of visuospatial, planning, and judgment skills [48]

CADRes assesses the following areas:

General: Driving history, IADLs, medications, medication change

Vision assessment: Visual fields and acuity

Cognition assessment: MoCA, Trails Part B, clock drawing, MAZE

Motor sensory Assessment: Range of motion, proprioception, TUG, rapid pace walk

If patients are identified as being at risk, then patients should be referred to clinical specialists for specific targeted interventions such as physical therapy (PT), occupational therapy, ophthalmology, and so forth, or referred for a driving evaluation. Patient permission should be obtained before contacting caregivers, and this should be documented in the patient's health record. If the patient maintains decisional capacity and denies permission, their wishes must be respected. Primary care providers also need to have familiarity with their individual local and state regulations related to mandatory reporting of driving issues in their older patients.

COMBINATION TOOLS

The Rapid Geriatric Assessment tool (Fig. 2.5) screens for geriatric syndromes and it can be completed by patients and their caregivers in less than 4 minutes.[49] It screens for cognitive impairment, frailty, sarcopenia, and anorexia and it uses the following four instruments: the Simple "FRAIL" Questionnaire Screening Tool, the SARC-F Screen for sarcopenia, the Simplified Nutritional Assessment Questionnaire (SNAQ), and the Rapid Cognitive Screen (RCS). These tools were chosen because they can easily identify treatable conditions. They also have questions related to urinary incontinence, constipation, and advanced directives. The authors report that there are no copyrights on these screening tools and suggest that they be incorporated into EMRs without permission and at no cost (see http://aging.slu.edu/uploads/RGA_Algorithms_and_Pt_Info_Sheets_Updated_7_9_2016.pdf).

Saint Louis University
Rapid Geriatric Assessment

The Simple "FRAIL" Questionnaire Screening Tool
(3 or greater = frailty; 1 or 2 = prefrail)

<u>F</u>atigue: Are you fatigued?
<u>R</u>esistance: Cannot walk up one flight of stairs?
<u>A</u>erobic: Cannot walk one block?
<u>I</u>llnesses: Do you have more than 5 illnesses?
<u>L</u>oss of weight: Have you lost more than 5% of your weight
    in the last 6 mo?

From Morley JE, Vellas B, Abellan van Kan G, et al. J Am Med Dir Assoc 2013;14:392-397

Table I: SARC-F Screen for Sarcopenia

Component	Question	Scoring
Strength	How much difficulty do you have in lifting and carrying 10 pounds?	None = 0 Some = 1 A lot or unable = 2
Assistance in walking	How much difficulty do you have walking across a room?	None = 0 Some = 1 A lot, use aids, or unable = 2
Rise from a chair	How much difficulty do you have transferring from a chair or bed?	None = 0 Some = 1 A lot or unable without help = 2
Climb stairs	How much difficulty do you have climbing a flight of ten stairs?	None = 0 Some = 1 A lot or unable = 2
Falls	How many times have you fallen in the last year?	None = 0 1–3 falls = 1 4 or more falls = 2

From Malmstrom TK, Morley JE. J Frailty and Aging 2013;2:55-6.

SNAQ (Simplified Nutritional Assessment Questionnaire)

My appetite is
a. very poor
b. poor
c. average
d. good
e. very good

Food tastes
a. very bad
b. bad
c. average
d. good
e. very good

When I eat
a. I feel full after eating only a few mouthfuls
b. I feel full after eating about a third of a meal
c. I feel full after eating over half a meal
d. I feel full after eating most of the meal
e. I hardly ever feel full

Normally I eat
a. less than one meal a day
b. one meal a day
c. two meals a day
d. three meals a day
e. more than three meals a day

From Wilson et al. Am J Clin Nutr 2005;82:1074-81.

Rapid Cognitive Sreen (RCS)

1. **Please remember these five objects. I will ask you what they are later.** [Read each object to patient using approx. 1 second intervals.]
    Apple   Pen   Tie   House   Car
2. [Give patient pencil and the blank sheet with clock face.] **This is a clock face. Please put in the hour markers and the time at ten minutes to eleven o'clock.** [2 pts/hr markers ok; 2 pts/time correct]
3. **What were the five objects I asked you to remember?** [1 pt/ea]
4.   **I'm going to tell you a story. Please listen carefully because afterwards, I'm going to ask you about it.**

Jill was a very successful stockbroker. She made a lot of money on the stock market. She then met Jack, a devastatingly handsome man. She married him and had three children. They lived in Chicago. She then stopped work and stayed at home to bring up her children. When they were teenagers, she went back to work. She and Jack lived happily ever after.
What state did she live in? [1 pt]

Miscellaneous
Are you constipated? Y/N
Do you have worrisome incontinence? Y/N
Do you have an advanced directive? Y/N

From Malmstrom TK, Voss VB, Crus-Oliver DM et al. J Nutr Health Aging 2015;19:741-744.

Fig. 2.5 Rapid Geriatric Assessment tool. There is no copyright on these screening tools and they may be incorporated into the Electronic Health Record without permission and at no cost. (From Morley, J. B. (2017). *Rapid geriatric assessment. Clinics in Geriatric Medicine,* 33(3), 431–440.)

Its authors believe their tool can increase knowledge of geriatric syndromes and improve the quality of care given by primary care providers. They also suggest that it be incorporated into the Medicare AWV.[49]

Another tool is the G8 screening tool, which was developed specifically for older cancer patients in keeping with recommendations from the International Society of Geriatric Oncology that all cancer patients over the age of 70 be screened. The authors describe the utility of the tool as a way to screen older cancer patients to determine who could benefit from a more comprehensive geriatric assessment.[50] It consists of eight items, seven of which are from the MNA questionnaire, as well as age.

Summary

As critical as using validated assessment tools to establish a patient's baseline or to identify at-risk patients is, there are some practical challenges to performing them in a busy medical practice. Because of the multidimensional nature of older patients' problems and the presence of coexisting interacting medical conditions, a comprehensive evaluation can be time-consuming and costly. Primary care practices can make the process more efficient by incorporating screening tools that target the need for additional in-depth assessment, establishing processes for referral and consultation, and identifying time lines for reevaluation, especially during and after transitions of care.

Domain	Tools
Hearing/vision	Whisper test, Snellen
ADLs	Katz, Barthel
IADLs	Lawton
Gait/balance	TUG, functional reach, chair stand, four-stage balance test
Cognition	Patient: Mini-Cog, MIS,GPCOG, MoCA, SLUMs
	Informant: AD8, IQCODE
Depression	GDS, PHQ-9,CESD-R, BDI
Nutrition	MNA
Driving	CADReS

So let us go back to Mrs. Thompson to learn more about her health problems and to begin the process of outlining a plan of care. The provider learns that Mrs. Thompson has the following health problems: osteoporosis, chronic obstructive pulmonary disease (COPD), hypertension, and benign positional vertigo. She had a mechanical fall 3 years ago that resulted in a fractured right wrist with an open reduction internal fixation (ORIF) and a pelvic fracture, which required a 10-day stay in a subacute rehabilitation center. Using the first step of the AGS multimorbidity model, the provider asks the patient to describe her primary concern regarding her health. Mrs. Thompson reports she is very afraid of falling again and would like to go back to her home as soon as possible. She understands that her daughter is concerned for her, but thinks she is overreacting. Her other main complaint is that her daughter has taken her keys to her car away, and she is very unhappy stating: "I am a perfectly good driver I have been driving for 50 years." Her daughter has concerns regarding her mother's self-care abilities, and is worried that she is not eating or sleeping well and that she is very depressed.

The following is additional medical history including a review of systems (ROS) obtained during today's visit:

MEDICAL HISTORY

Medications: Albuterol (Proventil HFA) inhaler every 4 to 6 hours used as needed (prn), lisinopril (Zestril) 10 milligrams per mouth (po) daily, hydrochlorothiazide (HCTZ) 12.5 milligrams po daily, Caltrate + D3 two tablets daily, Ambien 10 milligrams po at bedtime (hs) prn.

Allergies: Seasonal.

Habits: Smoker 1 pack per day (PPD) × 35 years. Stopped for 2 years at age 75, began again before husband's death. Drinks two glasses a wine a night.

Past medical history: COPD, hypertension, osteoporosis, benign positional vertigo, pubic rami fracture.

Past surgical history: ORIF right wrist, total abdominal hysterectomy, benign breast cyst removal 15 years ago.

Family history: Father died at 84 from natural causes. Mother died age 78, cause unknown, was a heavy smoker. One brother, 76, has hypertension.

Personal and social history: Married 50 years, now widowed. Husband died 4 months ago. Three children, two live nearby, staying with one daughter. Worked as a medical records clerk in local doctor's office, retired at age 75, up until her husband's illness was still going into the office to help out. Still drives.

REVIEW OF SYSTEMS

General: Admits to being "very tired." Admits to diminished appetite: "I don't feel like eating, nothing interests me." Knows her clothes are getting very loose. Denies weakness.

Skin: Denies rashes or lesions.

Head, eyes, ears, nose, and throat (HEENT): Denies headache, dizziness, sore throat, has hearing aids but does not wear them, ran out of batteries, has trouble seeing both near and far vision, has no recall as to the date of her last eye examination.

Neck: Denies neck pain, lumps.

Respiratory: + shortness of breath with activity, has a productive morning cough, does hear herself wheezing at times. Denies recent respiratory infection, hemoptysis.

Cardiac: Denies chest pain, pressure, or palpitations.

Gastrointestinal: Denies difficulty swallowing, heartburn, nausea, vomiting, diarrhea.

Urinary: Admits to occasional urinary incontinence: "I have to run to the bathroom to avoid wetting myself." Denies urinary burning, flank pain.

Musculoskeletal: Does feel stiff "all over" in the morning, has to sit and drink two cups of tea and take a hot shower to get up and moving. Has a cane but does not use it. Denies back pain, leg pain. Does not take any medication for pain.

Peripheral vascular: Denies swollen legs, calf pain.

Neurologic: Poor sleep, takes Ambien but only gets about 4 to 5 hours of sleep, wakes up between 4 and 4:45 a.m. every morning. Taking the Ambien that was prescribed for her husband. Admits to not remembering things as well as she used to, has stopped reading the paper. Denies fainting, numbness, tingling.

Hematologic: Denies easy bruising, bleeding gums, history of anemia.

Endocrine: Denies temperature intolerance, sweating, thirst.

Psychiatric: + history of depression, used to take an antidepressant, cannot remember which one, feels very anxious and sad, knows she is smoking and drinking "too much."

PHYSICAL EXAMINATION

The physical examination reveals a quiet, slightly disheveled, frail-appearing woman with BMI of 20. According to the office protocol for patients over the age of 65, a Snellen, whisper test, Mini-Cog, and GDS were done by the medical assistant in the examination room before the provider came in for the visit. She was also asked about having an advanced directive. During the patient's history and physical, a TUG and a 30-second chair stand were done. She was also asked three questions related to falling, and although she had not had any falls in the previous year, she did admit she felt unsteady when walking and she worried about falling "all the time."

RESULTS

Snellen: 20/40 right eye, 20/50 left eye with glasses.

Whisper test: Unable to hear 6/6 whispered words on either ear.

Mini-Cog: Normal clock drawing, 2/3 items recalled.

GDS: Score of 9/15.

TUG: 30 seconds

Chair stand: The patient was unable to rise from a seated position to standing without using her arms to stand on five attempts and was scored as a 0.

The provider outlines for the patient and her daughter the medical problems areas that have been identified during today's visit:

Hypertension

COPD

Visual impairment

Hard of hearing

Low body weight

Dyspnea on exertion (DOE), cough

Fatigue

Gait disturbance/impaired balance

Depressed mood

    Impaired sleep pattern

    Increased alcohol intake

    Increased smoking

The provider explains to Mrs. Thompson and her daughter that additional evaluation is needed to complete the assessment. She and her daughter agree that she has a depressed mood that has likely had a major impact on her day-to-day functioning and contributed to her increased smoking, alcohol intake, and impaired sleep. The patient breaks down into tears and asks if there is anyone she could talk to about her grief. The provider discusses options for referral to a local geriatric social work practice. They discuss that a trial of an antidepressant may be beneficial and discussed further once blood work has been completed. The provider identifies that her gait disturbance/impaired balance needs a more thorough evaluation, and the plan is made to refer the patient to outpatient PT located near the daughter's home. In the meantime, the patient agrees to blood work (complete blood count [CBC], complete metabolic panel, thyroid panel, lipid panel, B_{12} level, vitamin D level), as well as a chest x-ray to evaluate the complaint of cough and weight loss. The patient signs a release form that will be sent to her previous provider to obtain her previous health records.

Once more data are collected and reviewed, the plan of care can be further developed. The provider will continue to be guided by the AGS multimorbidity algorithm to establish care that is based on best evidence, patient preference, and shared decision making. Interventions will focus on choosing therapies that will optimize benefit, minimize harm, and enhance Mrs. Thompson's quality of life.[1] The provider outlines the issues to be addressed on the next visit:

Advanced directives: The patient will be given a copy of the POLST form to review with her daughter and bring to the next visit.

Medication review: The patient is asked to bring all pill bottles, all OTC medications/vitamins/supplements and other preparations, including those of her husband, which she admits to still taking.

Nutritional status: The MNA form is given to the patient and her daughter because it will be reviewed with them at the next visit.

Driving: The patient is asked to refrain from driving until more information is available from the PT evaluation and until the patient has had her vision evaluated.

Health maintenance: A review of the patient's previous health record will help determine her immunization status, as well as the need for additional screening tests.

References

1. AGS. (2012). American Geriatrics Society Expert Panel on the care of older adults with Multimorbidity. Guiding principles for the care of older adults with multimorbidity: An approach for clinicians. *Journal of the American Geriatrics Society, 60*(10), E1–E25.
2. Ellis, G., Whitehead, M., O'Neil, D., Langhorne, P., & Robinson, D. (2011). Comprehensive geriatric assessment for older adults admitted to hospital. *Cochrane Database of Systematic Reviews,* (7), CD006211, doi:10.1002/14651858.CD006211.pub2.
3. Ward, K., & Reuben, D. (2017). Comprehensive geriatric assessment. In T. W. Post (Ed.), *UpToDate.* Waltham, MA: UpToDate.
4. Flaherty, E., & Resnick, B. (Eds.), (2014). *Geriatric nursing review syllabus* (4th ed.). New York: American Geriatrics Society.
5. Pilotto, A., Cella, A., Pilotti, A., Darajiati, J., Veronese, N., Musacchio, C., et al. (2017). Three decades of comprehensive geriatric assessment: Evidence coming from different healthcare settings and specific clinical conditions. *Journal of Post Acute and Long-Term Medicine, 18*(2), 192.e1–192.e11.

6. Kuo, H., Scandrett, K., Dave, J., & Mitchell, S. (2004). The influence of outpatient geriatric assessment on survival: A meta-analysis. *Archives of Gerontology and Geriatrics, 39*(3), 245–254.

7. Stuck, A., Egger, M., Hammer, A., Minder, C., & Beck, J. (2002). Home visits to prevent nursing home admission and functional decline in elderly people: Systematic review and meta-regression analysis. *Journal of the American Medical Association, 287*(8), 1022–1028.

8. Elkan, R., Kendrick, D., Dewey, M., Hewitt, H., Robinson, J., Blair, M., et al. (2001). Effectiveness of home based support for older people: Systematic review and meta-analysis. *BMJ: British Medical Journal, 323*, 1–9.

9. Huss, A., Stuck, A., Rubenstein, L., Egger, M., & Clough-Gorr, K. (2008). Multidimensional preventive home visits programs for community dwelling older adults: A systematic review and meta-analysis of randomized controlled trials. *Journal of Gerontology: Medical Sciences, 63A*, 298–307.

10. Bachmann, S., Finger, C., Huss, A., Egger, M., Stuck, A., & Clough-Gorr, K. (2010). Inpatient rehabilitation specifically designed for geriatric patients: Systematic review and meta-analysis of randomised controlled trials. *BMJ (Clinical Research Ed.), 340*, c1718.

11. Carlson, C., Merel, S., & Yukawa, M. (2015). Geriatric syndromes and geriatric assessment for the generalist. *Medical Clinics of North America, 99*, 263–279.

12. Morley, J. (2017). Rapid geriatric assessment: Secondary prevention to stop age-associated disability. *Clinics in Geriatric Medicine, 33*, 431–440.

13. Harlow, E., & Lyons, J. (2014). Assessment. In R. Ham, P. Sloane, G. Warshaw, J. Potter, & E. Flaherty (Eds.), *Ham's primary care geriatrics* (6th ed., pp. 31–43). Philadelphia, PA: Elsevier.

14. Birch, J. (2012). Functional assessment. Landon Center on Aging, Geriatric Education and Training. Retrieved from http://classes.kumc.edu/coa/Education/AMED900/FunctionalAssessment.htm.

15. Pirozzo, S., Papinczak, T., & Glasziou, P. (2003). Whispered voice test for screening for hearing impairment in adults and children: Systematic review. *British Medical Journal, 327*(7421), 967.

16. Kini, M., Leibowitz, H., Colton, T., Nickerson, M., Ganley, J., & Dawber, T. (1978). Prevalence of senile cataract, diabetic retinopathy, senile macular degeneration, and open-angle glaucoma in the Framingham eye study. *American Journal of Ophthalmology, 85*(1), 28–34.

17. Rosen, S., & Reuben, D. (2011). Geriatric assessment tools. *Mount Sinai Journal of Medicine: A Journal of Translational and Personalized Medicine, 78*, 489–497.

18. Gallo, J., & Bogner, H. (2006). The context of geriatric care. In J. Gallo, H. Bogner, T. Fulmer, & G. Paveza (Eds.), *Handbook of geriatric assessment* (4th ed., pp. 3–11). Sudbury, MA: Jones & Bartlett.

19. Katz, S., Ford, A., Moskowitz, R., Jackson, A., & Jaffe, M. (1963). Assessing self maintenance: Activities of daily living mobility and instrumental activities of daily living. *Journal of the American Geriatrics Society, 31*(12), 721–726.

20. Mahoney, F., & Barthel, D. (1965). Functional evaluation: The Barthel Index. *Maryland Medical Journal, 14*, 61–65.

21. Lawton, M., & Brody, E. (1969). Assessment of older people: Self-maintaining and instrumental activities of daily living. *The Gerontologist, 9*(3), 179–186.

22. Rubenstein, L., & Dillard, D. (2014). Falls. In R. Ham, P. Sloane, G. Warshaw, J. Potter, & E. Flaherty (Eds.), *Ham's primary care geriatrics* (6th ed., pp. 235–242). Philadelphia, PA: Elsevier.

23. Tinetti, M. E., & Kumar, C. (2010). The patient who falls: "It's always a trade-off. *JAMA: Journal of the American Medical Association, 303*(3), 258–266.

24. Mathias, S., Kayak, U., & Isaacs, B. (1986). Balance in elderly patients: The "get up and go" test. *Archives of Physical Medicine & Rehabilitation, 67*, 387–389.

25. Jones, C., Rikli, R., & Beam, W. (1999). 30-s chair-stand test as a measure of lower body strength in community-residing older adults. *Research Quarterly for Exercise and Sport, 70*, 113–119.

26. Duncan, P., Weiner, D., Chandler, J., & Studenski, S. (1990). Functional reach: A new clinical measure of balance. *Journals of Gerontology, 45*(6), M192–M197.

27. Rossiter-Fornoff, J., Walf, S., & Wolfson, L. (1995). A cross-sectional validation study of the FICSIT common data base static balance measures. *Journals of Gerontology, 50A*(6), M291–M297.

28. Moyer, V. (2014). Screening for cognitive impairment in older adults: U.S. Preventive Services Task Force recommendation statement. *Annals of Internal Medicine, 160*(11), 791–797.

29. Borson, S., Scanlan, J., Brush, M., Vitaliano, P., & Dokmak, A. (2000). The mini-cog: A cognitive "vital signs' measure for dementia screening in multi-lingual elderly. *International Journal of Geriatric Psychiatry, 15*(11), 1021–1027.

30. Buschke, H., Kuslansky, G., Katz, M., Stewart, W., Sliwinski, M., Echoldt, H., et al. (1999). Screening for dementia with the memory impairment screen. *Neurology*, *52*(2), 231–238.
31. Brodaty, H., Pond, D., Kemp, N., Luscombe, G., Harding, L., Berman, K., et al. (2002). The GPCOG: A new screening test for dementia designed for general practice. *Journal of the American Geriatrics Society*, *50*, 530–534.
32. Galvin, J. E., Roe, C. M., Powlishta, K. K., Coats, M. A., Muich, S. J., Grant, E., et al. (2005). The AD8: A brief informant interview to detect dementia. *Neurology*, *65*(4), 559–564.
33. Jorm, A. (1994). A short form of the Informant Questionnaire on Cognitive Decline in the Elderly (IQCODE): Development and cross- validation. *Psychological Medicine*, *24*, 145–153.
34. Nasreddine, Z., Phillps, N., Bedirian, V., Charbonneau, S., Whitehead, V., Colin, I., et al. (2005). The Montreal cognitive assessment MoCA: A brief screening tool for mild cognitive impairment. *Journal of the American Geriatrics Society*, *53*(4), 695–699.
35. Morley, J., & Tumosa, N. (2002). Saint Louis University Mental Status Examination (SLUMS). *Aging Successfully*, *12*(1), 4.
36. Fiske, A., Wetherell, J., & Gatz, M. (2010). Depression in older adults. *Annual Review of Clinical Psychology*, *5*, 363–369.
37. Spitzer, R., Kroenke, K., & Williams, J. (1999). Validation and utility of a self-report version of the prime-MD: The PHQ primary care study. Primary Care Evaluation of Mental Disorders. Patient Health Questionnaire. *JAMA: The Journal of the American Medical Association*, *282*(18), 1737–1744.
38. Sheikh, J., & Yesavage, J. (1986). Geriatric Depression Scale (GDS): Recent evidence and development of a shorter version. *Clinical Gerontology*, *5*, 165–173.
39. Beck, A. T., Ward, C. H., Mendelson, M., Mock, J., & Erbaugh, J. (1961). An inventory for measuring depression. *Archives of General Psychiatry*, *4*, 561–571.
40. Greenberg, S. (2012). The Geriatric Depression Scale (GDS). (2007). Try this: Best practices in nursing care to older adults. Retrieved from https://consultgeri.org/try-this/general-assessment/issue-4.pdf.
41. Eaton, W. W., Smith, C., Ybarra, M., Muntaner, C., & Tien, A. (2004). Center for Epidemiologic Studies Depression Scale: Review and Revision (CESD and CESD-R). In M. E. Maruish (Ed.), *The use of psychological testing for treatment planning and outcomes assessment: Instruments for adults* (pp. 363–377). Mahwah, NJ: Lawrence Erlbaum Associates Publishers.
42. Agarwal, E., Miller, M., Yaxley, A., & Isenring, E. (2013). Malnutrition in the elderly: A narrative review. *Maturitas*, *76*(4), 296–302.
43. Morley, J. (1997). Anorexia of aging: Physiologic and pathologic. *The American Journal of Clinical Nutrition*, *66*, 760–773.
44. Felder, S., Lechtenboehmer, C., Bally, M., Fehr, R., Deiss, M., Faessler, L., et al. (2015). Association of nutritional risk and adverse medical outcomes across different medical inpatient populations. *Nutrition*, *31*, 1385–1393.
45. Correia, M., & Waitzberg, D. (2003). The impact of malnutrition on morbidity, mortality, length of hospital stay and costs evaluated through a multivariate model analysis. *Clinical Nutrition*, *22*(3), 235–239.
46. Kaiser, M. J., Bauer, J. M., Uter, W., Donini, L. M., Stange, I., Volkert, D., et al. (2011). Prospective validation of the modified mini nutritional assessment short-forms in the community, nursing home, and rehabilitation setting. *Journal of the American Geriatrics Society*, *59*(11), 2124–2128.
47. National Highway Traffic Safety Administration. Issues Related to Younger and Older Drivers. http://www.nhtsa.gov/people/injury/olddrive/pub/Chapter1.html.
48. Staplin, L., Gish, K. W., Lococo, K. H., Joyce, J. J., & Sifrit, K. J. (2013). The Maze test: A significant predictor of older driver crash risk. *Accident Analysis & Prevention*, *50*, 483–489.
49. Morley, J. (2017). Rapid geriatric assessment. *Clinics in Geriatric Medicine*, *33*, 431–440.
50. Bellera, C., Rainfray, M., Mathoulin-Pelissier, S., Mertens, C., Delva, F., Fonck, M., et al. (2012). Screening older cancer patients: First evaluation of the G8 geriatric screening tool. *Annals of Oncology*, *23*(8), 2166–2172.

CHAPTER 3

Principles of Pharmacology in Geriatric Practice

Terry Mahan Buttaro ▪ Karen L. Dick

More than 10 years ago older adults living in the United States took 34% or more of the prescribed drugs in this country.[1] At that time this patient cohort also took 30% of the over-the-counter drugs.[1] Since that time the number of prescriptions in this country has increased substantially, and more than 40% of patients older than age 65 take five or more medications.[2] The reason for the increase in medication use is partly because many older adults are living longer and because of the number of comorbid disorders affecting many of our patients. These disorders include depression, heart disease, hypertension, hyperglycemia, and hyperlipidemia,[2] but many older adults have even more health problems (e.g., chronic obstructive lung disease, fatty liver disease, osteoarthritis, osteoporosis, urinary incontinence, history of chronic pain or malignancy). What the increase in comorbidities for this age group likely suggests is a still increasing number of prescriptions written not only by primary health care providers but also by a variety of other specialists (cardiology, endocrine, orthopedics, etc.). The increase in prescriptions also indicates a probable rise in rational polypharmacy, which is the use of more than one or two medications to treat a patient's medical condition. Rational polypharmacy is common in hypertension management when it is possible that three medication categories are necessary to help control the patient's blood pressure. Rational polypharmacy also is observed in patients with type 2 diabetes mellitus and in patients with severe mental health problems. There is a need for rational polypharmacy, but irrational polypharmacy occurs when health care providers forget to consider the pharmacodynamic and pharmacokinetic implications for patients taking multiple medications and neglect routine assessment for the continued need of so many medications. This is especially true in a population of patients with the probable likelihood of aging changes that affect the effectiveness of medication biotransformation and elimination, increasing the risk of an adverse drug reaction (ADR).

In the United States about 40% of adults have health issues,[3] 18% have a history of mental illness, and 9% have a substance abuse problem.[3] The top five health issues in older adults are: arthritic pain, heart disease, cancer, asthma, chronic obstructive lung disease, and Alzheimer's.[4] There are other concerns, however: one in five older adults has an alcohol or substance abuse problem, 36% to 40% are obese, elder falls result in 2.5 million emergency room visits yearly, and many older adults are depressed and have an income level below poverty level.[4]

Why is this information even important for us as health care providers? As the current care providers for many adults across the transitions of care (i.e., home to emergency room to hospital, to rehab to home), health care providers are caring for a population of adults facing aging and functional changes that affect their quality of life. Additionally, these patients are faced with experiencing a diminished quality of life, increased morbidity (both physical and psychological), and polypharmacy. The higher the number of medications an older adult takes, the more likely that person will have an ADR (e.g., hypoglycemia, falls) and require an emergency room visit and/or hospitalization; be faced with greater costs; and despite the good intentions of all health care providers, have a diminished quality of life.

Health care providers want to keep their patients comfortable and maintain their function. To do so, an understanding of geriatric aging changes that affect pharmacodynamics and pharmacokinetics is necessary. Not every patient is the same, and those changes associated with aging depend on many individual factors that include genetics, lifestyle and comorbidities. Additionally, there are many nonpharmacologic changes in aging that affect both medication prescribing and medication use in this population. Older adults often do not have the same illness presentations as do younger adults. Patients as they age may not develop a high fever even when they become significantly ill. Furthermore, an older adult patient can be vague about symptoms. Sometimes elders will complain of "some" abdominal discomfort, but they will be unclear in their description of the problem and will not really seem uncomfortable during the physical examination. For example, an older adult could have an abdominal infection, yet not have the same pain on examination that a younger person has with the same diagnosis.

Older adults may not take their prescribed medications on a regular basis either. Some of this might be forgetfulness or possibly concerns about cost. Health literacy and sensory changes (e.g., vision or hearing deficits) are problematic. Older adults may not hear the instructions for a medication well enough to understand them, or not have the capability to read the directions on the pharmacy label, open the pill container from the pharmacy, or discriminate one medication from another one. The issue of health literacy can be significant, even in older adults who would be considered well educated. Many factors affect health literacy. Understanding health care recommendations, navigating health care services, and making decisions about health care options can be complex and overwhelming. Cognitive decline can be a complicating factor and is certainly a possibility in aging adults. Memory and reasoning can both be affected by cognitive changes and, in the early stages of memory loss, may not be easily perceived during a health care encounter.

Additionally, health providers often speak a different language than the rest of the population. "Medicalese" is not easy to decipher for many patients, even for those who do not have cognitive changes. Patients and their families really need printed information to review after leaving the primary care office or clinic. To properly aid patient and family understanding of what is important, written instructions for older adults should be on one page, in bold print, and at the third- to sixth-grade level. For the patient simpler is better. Asking the patient and/or family to put the instructions on the refrigerator also can be a helpful reminder to take the medicine and call the health care provider if the medicine is causing an adverse effect.

Drug-Specific Factors in Geriatric Care

PHARMACODYNAMIC AND PHARMACOKINETIC CHANGES IN AGING

Pharmacodynamic Changes

Pharmacodynamic changes are not as significant as the pharmacokinetic changes that occur as we age. It is likely that there is a decrease in the number of receptors and receptor sensitivity throughout the body as we grow older. Diminished homeostatic mechanisms (e.g., changes in the hypothalamus and regulation of hormones, metabolism, fluid and electrolyte balance, energy, sleep) affect the relationship between the brain and the body and probably affect medication efficacy, as well as patient health and function.

There are also pharmacodynamic interactions that occur between medications. For example, there is the antagonistic interaction that occurs between aspirin and ibuprofen when taken together. The efficacy of aspirin will be decreased if taken with a nonsteroidal antiinflammatory drug (NSAID). This information is especially important to relate to patients who have an arterial stent designed to keep the artery open and are prescribed aspirin for its antiplatelet activity. In this situation, taking an NSAID could decrease the efficacy of the aspirin and cause occlusion of the stent, with ischemia as the end result.

Pharmacokinetic Aging Changes

Pharmacokinetic aging changes can have a more significant impact on an older adult than the pharmacodynamic aging changes. Absorption is not significantly affected by aging changes, although there are some considerations for health care providers caring for older adults.[5] A past medical history of a partial gastrectomy (not done as frequently as in the past) or bariatric or small bowel (especially the upper aspect of the small intestine) surgery is important to ascertain during history taking because depending on the operative procedure, medication absorption can be affected by a decrease in the surface area of the small bowel or the stomach, as well as a decrease in gastric hydrochloric acid related to stomach surgery.[6] Small bowel diseases can also affect the absorption of those medications and nutrients absorbed in the small bowel. Drug absorption can be somewhat affected by lifestyle because daily exercise will promote both drug absorption and distribution.

Medications also can affect absorption of other medications (e.g., antacids or iron supplements can interfere with the absorption of thyroid and other medications).[5] Proton pump inhibitors, H_2 blockers, and other drugs can lower gastric acid pH, and this change can decrease the absorption of some nutrients and drugs. The decrease in gastric acid and possible changes in the gastric environment affect drug bioavailability. As a result, some drug preparations are better absorbed than other drug preparations, which explains why calcium citrate is recommended for older adults, rather than calcium carbonate.

Drug Distribution. In older adults drug distribution is affected by (1) a smaller quantity of serum albumin and (2) body composition (i.e., a decrease in lean muscle mass and total body water, as well as an increase in body fat). Food availability is a concern for some of our older patients, but even obese older adults can be malnourished. A decrease in serum albumin is associated with undernourishment. A normal albumin level is usually 3.0 to 5.0 g/dL. If a patient is malnourished, has a low serum albumin, and is taking a medication that is highly albumin bound (e.g., warfarin), the unbound portion of the drug (in this example, warfarin) will be more available to disperse resulting in an increased amount of free warfarin and potential drug toxicity.

Body composition affects drug distribution in various ways. Obesity is increasing in patients across the lifespan, and as we age, most of us increase body fat and lose lean muscle mass. This happens even in healthy, athletic older adults, although to a lesser degree. From a pharmacologic viewpoint, it is the greater amount of body fat or a significant decrease in body weight or lean muscle mass that can affect drug distribution. Medications are either lipophilic or hydrophilic. Many drugs are lipophilic and are easily distributed to and stored in fat cells, but this can result in a diminished amount of the medication to be distributed throughout the body to their targeted receptors. For this reason, obese patients can, in some instances, require a higher dose of a medication because of the affinity a highly lipophilic drug has for the fat cells.[7] Furthermore, a lipophilic medication (e.g., diazepam) can accumulate in the central nervous system, which is significantly lipophilic, and in an older adult this can cause confusion, drowsiness, and even coma (especially if used in combination with a lipophilic opioid, such as fentanyl). This accumulation of a medication can be particularly problematic in older adults who also have associated chronic kidney disease (CKD) because elimination can be affected, further increasing the risk of an adverse reaction.

Hydrophilic drugs are similarly affected by aging changes. Distribution is reduced if a drug is hydrophilic because of less lean muscle mass and/or less body water. For example, if a frail older adult experienced depression while taking a lipophilic beta-blocker for angina, and is then prescribed atenolol, a hydrophilic, beta-1 selective, beta-blocker, he or she will likely require a larger dose of the medication.

Biotransformation. Liver changes in aging are interesting because not all medications are affected.[5] In general, liver function and drug metabolism are compromised as we age, although the extent can depend on an individual's overall health and comorbidities. Circulatory changes as we grow older can influence biotransformation. Diminished cardiac output, as well as the atherosclerotic and arteriosclerotic changes that occur over time, can decrease blood flow to the liver, affecting the first pass effect and drug metabolism. If there is a reduced first-pass effect, then there will be an increase in drug half-life and in drug bioavailability. The reduction in blood flow affects the Phase 1 and 2 metabolism, but it is the Phase 1 metabolism (the CYP450 system) that is primarily affected. Cirrhosis, hepatitis, hemochromatosis, and other liver diseases also can have a significant effect on the efficacy of the CYP450 enzymes.[8] The result of impaired biotransformation in the liver, for any reason, is a longer medication half-life and a greater risk of drug toxicity.[8] Additionally, infections, inflammation, heavy metal poisoning, porphyria, and some organ diseases (e.g., hypothyroidism, hyperthyroidism, lung cancer, pulmonary disease) are known to affect the drug metabolism of some specific medications.[7]

Elimination. This can be importantly affected by renal changes that occur over time; nephrons decrease and become less efficient, and the same circulatory changes that affect liver biotransformation and other organs affect renal perfusion and function. Tubular transport is also influenced by aging changes that can affect reabsorption and glucose and electrolyte balance.[9] Glucosuria can be increased and renal activation of vitamin D decreased, which in turn affects calcium absorption.[9] These are all aging changes that affect people as they get older. Hypertension, diabetes, and other disorders can also affect renal function, as can excess alcohol, smoking, medications (e.g., prolonged NSAID usage), contrast dye, and dehydration. All of these potential alterations in kidney function increase the risk of acute kidney injury in older adults. Acute tubular necrosis (i.e., prerenal injury) in older adults can occur because of dehydration, contrast dye, NSAIDs, and other medications.

Chronic Kidney Disease. This disease is common in older adults, and is sometimes related to aging. It is also related to comorbid diseases, especially cardiovascular disease, diabetes, and hypertension. Some individuals with CKD will have edema, but the diagnosis of CKD is not a clinical one; instead it is based on a decrease in glomerular filtration rate (GFR). Diagnosis of CKD is defined as (1) a GFR less than 60 mL/min/1.73 m² for 3 months or more with or without kidney damage or (2) structural or functional kidney damage that may or may not be associated with a decrease in GFR for longer than 3 months.[10]

Not every older adult has CKD. Most older adults do have a decline in creatinine clearance and are at risk for a resultant increase in drug half-life, even if the individual's serum creatinine is within the normal range.[5] For that reason, it is essential to consider kidney function in all older adults when prescribing medications. Many laboratories now include the GFR when a chemistry and renal profile is ordered (e.g., Chemistry 8), which is fortunate because GFR is a better estimate of renal function than creatinine clearance. The determination of an individual patient's actual creatinine clearance can be made with a 24-hour urine collection. However, it can be challenging for some older adults to collect an exact 24-hour urine and then deliver the urine collection to the laboratory.

When a GFR is not available, online calculators can be used by health care providers to get a better estimation of a patient's renal function, especially when the person is an older adult or has comorbidities associated with kidney dysfunction. There are disadvantages to some of the online calculators, and the calculators are less accurate than the 24-hour urine collection. Nevertheless, the calculators are readily available and helpful when a health care provider needs to consider an older adult's renal status to prescribe certain medications, and avoid serious renal dysfunction.

For instance:

A 74-year-old female with a history of asthma and osteoporosis presents to the office complaining of fever, chills, and cough for the past week. She has been using her inhaler but does not feel like it is helping. She feels she is getting worse, not better, but she has been keeping up with fluids.

The patient uses a Ventolin inhaler when necessary, which usually is in ragweed season and when she gets sick. Otherwise, she takes only vitamin D 2000 IU by mouth (po) each day and calcium citrate 250 milligrams, two pills po each day. She is allergic to penicillin (rash), sulfur (rash), and erythromycin (elevated liver transaminases).

Her blood pressure is 138/70, heart rate 102, respiratory rate 28, and temperature 100°F. There are no orthostatic changes. The physical examination suggests a right lower lobe pneumonia, and the health care provider orders a stat chest posteroanterior (PA) and lateral x-ray, complete blood count (CBC) and differential, and chemistry profile.

The chest x-ray results reveal a right lower lobe infiltrate. Her white blood cell count is elevated: 14,500/mm³ (normal 3200–9800/mm³). Her chemistry profile is normal with a blood urea nitrogen (BUN) of 18 milligrams/dL (normal 8–18 milligrams/dL) and serum creatinine of 1.1 milligrams/dL (normal 0.6–1.2 milligrams/dL).

The health care provider considers ordering levofloxacin, 750 milligrams po daily for 7 days knowing that the Infectious Disease Society of America suggests that dose for adults with comorbidity and a community-acquired pneumonia.[11] As the provider begins to write the prescription, he decides that based on the patient's age, he should calculate the patient's renal function. Using the online Chronic Kidney Disease Epidemiology Collaboration equation, the result of the patient's estimated creatinine clearance is

Female, age 74, serum creatinine 1.1., not African American
= creatinine clearance is 49 mL/min/1.73 mm²

The provider then researches the appropriate dose of levofloxacin and learns that for a creatinine clearance of 20 to 49 mL/min, the 750-milligrams dose of levofloxacin should be once every 48 hours, not every 24 hours. He further learns that with this patient's creatinine clearance, an alternate option is levofloxacin 500 milligrams po today, then 250 milligrams po daily for 7 days.

The health care provider discusses the risks and benefits of levofloxacin with the patient and decides to prescribe levofloxacin 500 milligrams po today, then 250 milligrams po daily for 6 days, knowing that this might be an easier regimen for the patient to remember and follow. He tells the patient he will call her in the morning, but he wants to see her in 48 to 72 hours to be certain she is improving.

The Chronic Kidney Disease Epidemiology Collaboration equation is available at https://qxmd.com/calculate/calculator_251/egfr-using-ckd-epi.

The National Kidney Foundation has recommended an online calculator available at https://www.kidney.org/professionals/kdoqi/gfr_calculator.

The Chronic Kidney Disease Epidemiology Collaboration equation is commonly used now. The National Kidney Foundation does not recommend using the Cockcroft–Gault calculator any longer. However, there is, as noted previously, an online calculator available on the National Kidney Foundation site. Their calculation requires a serum cystatin C concentration for their estimation of GFR because an elevated level is present earlier in kidney disorders and is considered to be a better measurement than serum creatinine. A benefit of cystatin C is that inflammatory conditions and patient diet and muscle mass do not affect cystatin C concentration.

It is important to remember that these calculators are only appropriate for calculating estimated GFR in adults with CKD. These calculators should not be used to estimate the GFR in children or in patients with acute kidney failure.

Additional Medication Dosing Considerations for Patients With Chronic Kidney Disease. Knowing a patient's GFR is important not only when prescribing antimicrobials (e.g., antifungals, fluoroquinolones, macrolides, tetracyclines, trimethoprim).[12] Many other medications (e.g., allopurinol, amantadine, metformin, rivaroxaban) can also be problematic and require dose reductions, especially if the patient's GFR is less than 30 mL/min.[13] In patients of all ages, even over-the-counter medications such as ranitidine (Zantac) and fexofenadine (Allegra) require renal dosing, although many health care providers may not be aware of this and the potential resultant adverse effects.[13]

Medication formulations (e.g., extended release) are also a concern when caring for older patients. Some drugs may not have been studied in older patients with renal dysfunction and unless there is clear information about the safety of an extended release formulation in a specific drug, these formulations should be avoided unless the patient's GFR is greater than 30 mL/min.

Neurodegenerative Aging Changes

Neurodegenerative changes in the brain alter the way medications work and they need to be taken into account when prescribing drugs for older adults. Changes in the blood-brain barrier, brain atrophy, inflammation, and pathology all affect cognitive function. These changes can make older adults more susceptible to medications and may account for an older adult's increased sensitivity to anesthesia, opioids, benzodiazepines, or hypnotics, although it is always important to remember that every individual is different. Additional potential pathologic brain changes include amyloid plaques, neuronal loss, vascular changes, cerebral amyloid angiopathy (i.e., amyloid plaques on arterial walls), lipofuscin deposits, and the many dementia-related diseases. The concern with neurodegenerative changes, whatever the cause, is that patients with these changes may be particularly susceptible to ADRs and yet not be able to recognize or verbalize them. When considered in combination with increased porosity of the blood-brain barrier and pharmacodynamic and pharmacokinetic aging changes, there needs to be increased attentiveness and concerns about possible ADRs, especially in patients with Alzheimer's and other dementias who are taking anticholinergic medications.[14] Anticholinergic medications block acetylcholine in the central and peripheral nervous systems as their primary function at the level of the muscarinic receptor. These drugs include medications used in the treatment of Parkinson's, as well as some antiemetics, antispasmodics, and bronchodilators, providing improved function and symptom relief. However, there are a number of other medications that have some degree of anticholinergic properties that are not desirable and put the older adult at risk for a number of unintended complications. These include impairment of working memory, attention and psychomotor speed, dry mouth, urinary retention, constipation, tachycardia, ataxia, and falls. There have been attempts to quantify the amount of exposure to help providers become more aware of the cumulative effect of multiple medications with anticholinergic properties, with medications commonly used to treat chronic medical conditions. There have been studies that have linked higher anticholinergic burden with cognitive impairment in older adults. A study by Gray and colleagues followed over 3000 patients 65 years and older over a 10-year period and tracked their cumulative anticholinergic use and found that 23.2% of patients developed incident dementia.[15] Another potential problem for patients with neurodegenerative diseases is QT prolongation.[14] Patients with Parkinson's are affected by drug interactions that occur with the combination of anti-parkinsonian and antihypertensive medications.[16] Hypotension is a definite risk, particularly with dopamine agonists, although loop and potassium-sparing diuretics for hypertension are considered safe.[16] Dopamine agonists should not be used for patients with orthostatic hypotension, dementia, or psychosis.[16]

Understanding the concept of anticholinergic burden from medications is key for providers when reviewing patients' medication regimes or considering adding new ones. Boustani and colleagues developed the Anticholinergic Cognitive Burden Scale (ACB), which includes 88 medications that have known anticholinergic activity. Medications are classified as having none or a possible score of one point, or definite anticholinergic activity scored as either two or three points. The authors of this scale tell us that each medication with a score of 2 or 3 may increase the risk of cognitive impairment by 46% over 6 years, and for each point increase in an ACB total score, a decline in Mini-Mental State Examination (MMSE) of 0.33 points over 2 years has been suggested.[17]

The following is an example of quantifying anticholinergic burden from multiple commonly used medications in one older adult:

HS is a 79-year-old female with overactive bladder (OAB), diabetes type 2, neuropathy, depression, hypertension, and benign positional vertigo. Medications include paroxetine 20 milligrams/day, acetaminophen PM 500 g at bedtime (hs), oxybutynin 5 milligrams ER per day, amitriptyline 50 milligrams hs, lisinopril 40 milligrams/day, and meclizine 50 milligrams/day as needed (prn). A quick check of the ACB scale tells us that paroxetine, acetaminophen PM, oxybutynin, amitriptyline, and meclizine each have a score of 3, which gives a total score of 15. As the authors of the ACB would suggest, this indicates that this patient has an elevated risk of developing cognitive impairment.

Goals of care for this patient would then include reviewing the need for these medications, considering stopping or switching to topical preparations or newer generation formulations, and counseling against the use of PM type products.

Caution and Caveats

The result of the aging changes that affect the volume of distribution in older adults (i.e., increased fat, decreased water and muscle mass), combined with liver and kidney changes that occur as we get older, is that the biologic half-life of medications can be prolonged in older adults. For these reasons, health care providers need to be more cautious when prescribing medications for patients over age 65. "Start low and go slow" has long been the mantra in geriatric care, and it is even more applicable today.

There is somewhat of a caveat to "Start low and go slow" slogan, however. We know that renal status is a serious concern in older adults and awareness of a patient's creatinine clearance is essential. However, when recommending antibiotic therapy for a patient of any age, it is also important to consider the "concentration-dependent killing" versus "time-dependent killing" efficacy of the chosen antibiotic.[18,19] Aminoglycosides are a concentration-dependent killing antimicrobial and can be effective even when a patient takes this category of antibiotics once a day. The reasoning is related to the medication's effectiveness in inhibiting bacterial growth. Concentration-dependent antibiotics suppress and eliminate bacteria because the high serum drug concentration helps effectively eradicate the organism causing the illness.[18,19] Cephalosporins, penicillins, and other β-lactams are time-dependent killing antimicrobials, and their antibacterial effectiveness requires more frequent dosing.[18,19]

Careful follow-up with patients requiring antibiotic therapy is also necessary. There are guidelines that suggest the correct amount of time that an antibiotic should be given for various infections, but each patient's response can be different. Many medications interact with antibiotics and can affect the intended response.[18]

Drug–Drug, Drug–Food, and Drug–Disease Interaction Concerns

Health care providers are usually aware of the potential for a drug–drug interaction. Still, we sometimes do not realize the extent of these interactions or consider the possibility that a patient's complaint is the result of an ADR or a drug–drug interaction. With now over 10,000 prescribable medications available to treat patient illnesses and disorders, plus the increasing number of herbal and over-the-counter drugs, the potential for serious side effects, especially in older adults with multiple comorbid diseases, has risen exponentially. Drug studies are rarely done on older adults with multiple comorbidities, so the effect of some medications on older adults, particularly those taking other medications, is not well known or easily recognized. Also, elders themselves do not realize that over-the-counter medications can have side effects that can compromise their ability to function optimally. For example, dizziness and drowsiness are common side effects of histamine H_1 antagonists, such as diphenhydramine (Benadryl), which are used to control allergy symptoms and for many older adults promote sleep. Yet histamine H_1 antagonists can be the cause of confusion, falls, and other accidents. Further drug–drug interactions that occur with histamine H_1 antagonists are caused by the interaction of histamine H_1 antagonists with acetylcholinesterase inhibitors, alcohol, opioids, and other medication categories.

It is primarily drug metabolism that is responsible for drug–drug, drug–herbal, or drug–food interactions. Hepatic aging changes do not affect all medications, although the decrease in blood flow associated with advanced age (e.g., arteriosclerosis and atherosclerosis) can increase drug bioavailability. It is the impact of the CYP450 system that is concerning because Phase 1 metabolism is affected by both age and ethnicity. For patients of all ages, inhibition of the CYP450 enzymes by a medication (e.g., diltiazem) will result in increased levels of other drugs metabolized by the CYP450 enzymes, whereas CYP450 induction (e.g., carbamazepine) by a medication will result in a decreased level of those drugs metabolized by the CYP450 enzymes. Hence, drug metabolism can be increased or decreased by the addition of a new drug, an herbal drug, or foods that affect the CYP450 system causing an increased or decreased amount of drug availability in the other medications a patient is taking.

Most health care providers are aware that warfarin toxicity is associated with several foods (e.g., vegetable greens rich in vitamin K decrease warfarin efficacy) that increase warfarin levels and possibly cause bleeding, but warfarin is also affected by botanicals and other drugs. Warfarin is metabolized by CYP 1A2, CYP 2D6, and CYP 3A4, which are all CYP450 enzymes. Amiodarone inhibits CYP3A4, CYP1A2, and CYP2c9 metabolism, increasing the plasma concentration of the two warfarin components (i.e., S-warfarin and R-warfarin) and causing an increase in the international normalized ratio (INR). Other medications that inhibit the CYP450 enzymes (e.g., fluconazole or fluoxetine) affected by warfarin will result in a similar increase in the INR.[20]

Grapefruit juice, a CYP3A4 CYP450 enzyme inhibitor, can interact with some cholesterol-lowering statin drugs, as well as other medications. However, not every drug in a specific medication category will result in an untoward reaction when eaten with grapefruit or grapefruit juice. There are drug–drug, drug–herbal, and drug–food interaction checkers that are easily accessed on the Internet, but local pharmacists can also be helpful in determining whether there are potential drug–drug or drug–food interactions for a patient or a health care provider.

Older patients, especially those with CKD, dementia, and/or a history of falls, are more likely to have a drug–disease interaction than other patients, so there needs to be increased understanding of the risks inherent in the care of these patients. NSAIDs and aspirin are readily available over the counter and are used regularly to relieve pain but are strongly associated with gastrointestinal bleeding in older adults. NSAIDs can also negatively affect patients with CKD by increasing fluid retention and potentially precipitating heart failure. Even in patients without CKD, NSAIDs are concerning because over time chronic NSAID use can affect renal function.

Patients with dementia can be harmed if prescribed anticholinergics, antiemetics, antipsychotics, or benzodiazepines or tricyclic medications. Some medications that are on the Beers List of Potentially Inappropriate Medications and the "STOPP/START Criteria for Potentially Inappropriate Prescribing in Older People: Version 2" are drugs that are known to affect disease states in older adults, and it is for this reason that these are recommended tools to review when prescribing medications for older patients.[21,22]

Patient-Specific Factors

POLYPHARMACY

Polypharmacy is not well defined, but it is estimated that almost one-half of older adults are taking at least one medication that is not effective or indicated medically.[23] In some instances, polypharmacy is related to inappropriate prescribing by a health care provider ordering a medication to treat a side effect of another medication. For many patients, polypharmacy is considered as rational. This concept is actually referred to as rational polypharmacy because patients will often need two or more medications to treat a comorbid disorder (e.g., chronic obstructive lung disease, diabetes, or hypertension). Some patients could have even more than these three disorders, possibly requiring up to 20 or more medications a day. Rational polypharmacy is based on the need to treat a medical disorder to a specific goal (e.g., hypertension, hypercholesterolemia, or hyperglycemia recommendations). Whether the polypharmacy is rational or not, there are definite risks to taking so many medications in a day. Patients are exposed to harm from a potential drug–drug, drug–food, or drug–disease reaction resulting in confusion, gastrointestinal bleeding, a fall, or worse, requiring emergency room visits and too often hospitalizations. The costs, economically to society and to the patient personally because of ADRs and their sequelae, are considerable.

FINANCIAL ISSUES IN GERIATRIC CARE

There is a cost to polypharmacy and the care of older adults that is unspoken and perhaps even unrealized. Medication expenses are not often explored with patients and families. The costs of health care and medications especially continue to rise. In 2015, $457 billion were spent on over-the-counter and prescription medications in the United States.[24] For many patients and families, the increasing cost of medications is a concern, and some of these medications, both prescribed and over the counter, are unnecessary. The government spends a notable amount of money (e.g., $18,424 per person in 2010) for each older adult's health care, but some older adults still cannot afford their medications, especially when in the "donut hole."[25]

The reality is that finances can be a significant issue for older adults. The projected average monthly social security benefit for someone retiring at full retirement age in 2017 is $2687.00 a month. For older adults, already retired, the average monthly social security benefit is only $1360.00 a month.[26] Medicare Part B can cost a patient $134.00 or more a month, plus required deductibles. Retirees also should purchase Medicare Part C and Part D, but those costs are variable depending on the chosen plan, plus each plan has associated deductibles and copays. These costs alone are estimated to be significant. When patients are unable to pay for their medications, some will take medications every other day or not take them at all. The result can be a greater risk of cardiac, diabetic, or other medical disorder complications.

Additionally, taking so many medications each day can be burdensome. The complexity alone for older adults with cognitive changes increases the risks of an ADR. However, avoiding polypharmacy is not simple when patients have varied health care problems and more than one health care provider (e.g., specialists). Still, as patients age they may need fewer meds to manage their blood pressure than they did in the past. Furthermore, as kidney function declines, many medication doses should be decreased, and some drugs eliminated, to decrease the risk of a fall or another type of adverse event. One recommendation for older adults is for their providers to try to decrease or discontinue one nonessential medication at each visit, and then discuss the plan for discontinuing or decreasing another medication at the next visit. Providers working with older adults need to be aware of the resources available for this process, which is referred to as *deprescribing*. This is the systematic process of stopping medications after weighing potential harm versus benefit within an individual's goals of care, taking into account quality of life and life expectancy, values, and preferences.[27] A number of tools have been developed to assist providers with deprescribing, and one example, the Good Palliative–Geriatric Practice algorithm by Garfinkle and Mangin, asks the following questions as a guide for decision making:

- Is there an evidence-based consensus for using the drug in its current dosing?:
- Do the known possible adverse reactions of the drug outweigh the possible benefit in old disabled patients?
- Any adverse symptoms or signs that may be related to the drug?
- Is there another drug that may be superior to the one in question?
- Can the dosing be reduced with no significant risk?[28]

Other resources can be found at http://deprescribing.org/.

Provider-Specific Concerns in Prescribing

ADVERSE DRUG EVENTS VERSUS ADVERSE DRUG REACTIONS

Adverse drug events (ADEs) need to be reported to the Food and Drug Administration (i.e., the FDA Adverse Event Reporting System). An ADE is a medical event not expected or related to a medication that causes a reaction that was unfavorable. The consequence of the ADE does not need to have a correlational relationship with the medication.

An ADR is different from an ADE. An ADR, although not intentional, can cause harm, even if the drug dosage was within normal limits. According to the Institute of Medicine report in 2000, more than 2 million ADRs occur each year.[29] Medical errors are responsible for almost 100,000 deaths each year, with approximately 7000 of these deaths related to an ADR.[29] Unfortunately, even now, it is suspected that these numbers do not reflect the magnitude of the problem because many ADRs are not reported.[29] What is especially compelling is the number of hospital deaths caused by an ADR. These are estimated to be 106,000 each year.[29] Unfortunately, we do not know the incidence and prevalence of ADRs that occur in primary care offices and ambulatory clinics throughout the country. The financial costs are staggering. The cause of so many ADRs is more drugs, more prescriptions, and more polypharmacy (rational or not), and as a result there are more drug–drug or drug–food interactions. Older adults are certainly more susceptible because of aging changes, but it is also true that some drug studies have limited numbers of participants, and not all include older adults in the studies, and comorbidities may or may not be factored into the study results. Also, health care providers are busy and may not (1) read the drug study results carefully, (2) review the pharmacodynamic or pharmacokinetic implications of medications they are prescribing, (3) consider older adults' liver/renal status/ethnic status (ethnicity can affect drug metabolism; some ethnic groups are more susceptible to some medication categories), or (4) remember to use electronic resources to check for potential drug–drug interactions.

Older adults also have significant risk factors that can predispose their susceptibility for an ADR. One risk factor, of course, is age. The others include a past history of an ADR, multiple comorbidities, multiple medications, a low body mass index (BMI), and lower creatinine clearance. Medication changes across the transitions of care; complexity of instructions; and patient, provider, or system errors also can contribute to an ADR.

Preventing ADRs in older adults is certainly feasible. Careful prescribing and deprescribing are helpful, when possible, but it is also important to recognize those subtle signs of a drug reaction in an older adult. Red flags for a possible ADR include bleeding, confusion, depression, falls, hallucinations, malnutrition, and renal failure. Yet often health care providers do not consider an ADR as the cause of these signs and symptoms; instead, they treat the patient by prescribing another medication, which can lead to a prescribing cascade. A patient who is told to take an NSAID for arthritis pain, has elevated blood pressure readings because of long-term use of NSAIDs, then has a calcium channel blocker prescribed for that elevation that then leads to ankle swelling, which leads to the decision to add a diuretic, which leads to the development of a gout attack is an example of a totally preventable cascade of events.

Drug Safety in Geriatric Care

Patient safety is one of the most distinctive features of quality care for all patients. All health care prescribers are responsible for the day-to-day stewardship of medication management in patient care. To best achieve that goal, each health care provider needs to incorporate a systematic routine with each patient encounter to avoid causing an adverse drug reaction. Although it may seem redundant, it is the health care provider (i.e., physician, physician assistant, or nurse practitioner) who is both obligated and accountable for each patient's safety. In geriatric care this responsibility can be more complicated because of the atypical presentations CYP450 older adults can have; the number of medications the older adult takes; the possible cognitive and sensory changes; and health literacy, adherence, mobility, and financial issues that accompany old age.

The recommended approach to safe prescribing includes each of the following:
- In older adults, a new symptom should be considered a potential drug–drug interaction until proven otherwise.[30]
- Medication reconciliation is required at every visit and needs to include the current dose of each medication. Encourage the "brown bag review" (i.e., patient brings *all* medications to the appointment):
  - All over-the-counter medications (e.g., vitamins, acetaminophen, NSAIDs, supplements) and herbals should be queried and documented.
  - Ask the patient/family member if any "borrowed" medications were obtained from friends or relatives for pain or other reasons.
  - If necessary, call the pharmacy to determine whether the patient has stopped refilling.
- Allergy review at each encounter with the documented specific adverse reaction (e.g., nausea versus angioedema versus previous ADR)
- Review patient comorbidities at each visit to be certain patient is stable:
  - Check routine renal status (every 3 months) and adjust patient medication doses appropriately. For example, if a patient with type 2 diabetes is taking metformin 1000 milligrams po twice a day, but the patient's estimated GFR has been slowing deteriorating over time and is now 40 mL/min/1.73 m^2, a dose reduction to metformin 1000 milligrams po once a day would be indicated. Then it would be necessary to carefully follow renal status every 3 months and discontinue the metformin if the estimated GFR falls below 30 mL/min/1.73 m^2.[31]
  - Check liver function periodically, especially in patients with fatty liver disease or cirrhosis.
- Check for drug–drug interactions (e.g., narcotic and benzodiazepine or histamine H_1 antagonist), drug–alcohol or food interactions (e.g., bleeding, dizziness, fainting, falls, depression), and drug–disease interactions (e.g., aspirin or NSAID use if peptic ulcer disease, NSAID use if hypertension, heart failure).
- Assess drug effectiveness.
- Avoid the prescribing cascade.

Recommended assessment at each visit:
- Complete review of symptoms
- Height and weight
- Blood pressure each arm; orthostatic blood pressures each visit
- Determine whether any there are any cognitive changes or depression
- Functional or sensory changes
- Determine health literacy

- Consider the following:
  - "The American Geriatrics Society 2015 Updated Beers List Criteria for Potentially Inappropriate Medications Use in Older Adults" is a well-respected resource available at http://onlinelibrary.wiley.com/doi/10.1111/jgs.13702/pdf.[21]
  - The "STOPP/START Criteria for Potentially Inappropriate Prescribing in Older People: Version 2" was released in 2015.[22]

Differential diagnosis:
- Is it a new problem or a side effect of a medication?
- Avoid attribution and cognitive errors:
  - There are many different types of errors in medicine, but cognitive errors and attribution errors are common:
    - Recommendations to avoid cognitive errors require the health care practitioner to review the patient's clinical presentation before deciding on a diagnosis or treatment:
      - What elements in the patient history and physical examination suggest or discount this diagnosis?
      - What are other possible causes of the patient's signs and symptoms?
      - What is the worst this could be?
      - Have I missed any "red flags" in this patient?
    - Attribution errors are associated with provider bias. The bias can be related to a patient's past medical history (e.g., the patient has a history or drug abuse) or to the provider's recent experiences caring for patients. One example of an attribution error in an older adult could be as simple as attributing the elder's abdominal pain to constipation and treating the constipation with a medication, when the patient's abdominal discomfort is caused by an abdominal blockage due to a tumor.

Treatment:
- Remember the "Goals of Geriatric Care":
  - Treat the patient's symptoms and disorders
  - Alleviate the patient's discomfort
  - Improve the patient's function and quality of life
- Is there a nonpharmacologic approach for treatment in this patient?
- Simplify prescriptions:
  - If starting a medication, try to stop a medication
  - One medication when possible (e.g., combination medications)
  - Once a day or twice daily medications:
    - Once a day is best, more than twice a day is challenging for most everyone to remember.
  - Avoid half pills
  - Write the reason for the medication on the patient's prescription and/or the patient instructions
  - Assess patient capabilities:
    - to pay for the prescription being written,
    - to open childproof medication bottles or blister packs,
    - to swallow a pill or capsule (some patients may need assessment to determine their ability to swallow some medications), and
    - to remember to take medications each day.
      - Does the patient need blister packs, an alarm, or other reminders for medication safety?
  - Explain (*and document the discussion of*) the medication risks, benefits, and importance of calling the health care provider if there are any adverse medication effects or patient concerns after starting the medication.

- Document the rationale for medication choices and the length of predicted treatment; this can be beneficial for colleagues who may be asked to cross-cover or comanage.
- Arrange a follow-up appointment to assess efficacy of the medication or any untoward effects
- Instructions need to be clear and organized, large print, one page, and at the third- to sixth-grade level.
  - Try to keep instructions to only three bullet points

Summary

The care of older adults is really best promoted and accomplished by the primary care providers who know their patients well and see them on a regular basis. This is a responsible undertaking, requiring patience, time, and attentiveness. Elder care cannot be rushed, and in some instances more than one visit may be necessary to accomplish the safe and responsible care that is needed. Encouraging appropriate immunizations, minimizing the number of medications an older adult takes each day, and promoting wellness will hopefully help decrease the hospitalizations and ADRs that compromise those goals. Our responsibility is to promote function and comfort, and we are accountable for the decisions we make, especially concerning the medications we prescribe. Pharmacologic therapy requires thoughtfulness, research, and due diligence. Due diligence in medicine demands that we do a comprehensive medication reconciliation with each patient, that we review allergies or untoward drug effects at each visit, that we determine whether a patient's symptoms are related to a medication (even if the patient has taken that medication for many years), that we consider the possibility of drug–drug interactions, and that we prescribe judiciously and carefully. Ours is a partnership with patients and sometimes with their family members to best provide care and comfort to an older generation.

References

1. American Public Health Association. (2005). Fact sheet: Prescription medication use by older adults. Retrieved from http://www.medscape.com/viewarticle/501879).
2. Kantor, E. D., Rehm, C. D., Haas, J. S., Chan, A. T., & Giovannucci, E. L. (2015). Trends in prescription drug use among adults in the United States from 1999-2012. *JAMA: The Journal of the American Medical Association, 314*(17), 1818–1830.
3. Dallas, M. E. (2016). More than half of Americans have a chronic problem: Study. *Psychology, Health & Medicine*. Retrieved from https://consumer.healthday.com/general-health-information-16/alcohol-abuse-news-12/more-than-half-of-americans-have-chronic-health-problem-study-716282.html. Oct. 25, 2016.
4. Vann, M. R. (2017). The 15 most common health concerns for older adults. Retrieved from http://www.everydayhealth.com/news/most-common-health-concerns-seniors/.
5. Katsung, B. G. (2015). Special aspects of geriatric pharmacology. In B. G. Katsung & A. J. Trevor (Eds.), *Basic & clinical pharmacology* (13th ed., pp. 1024–1032). New York: McGraw Hill.
6. Geraldo Mde, S., Fonseca, F. L., Gouveia, M. R., & Feder, D. (2014). The use of drugs in patients who have undergone bariatric surgery. *International Journal of General Medicine, 7*, 219–224.
7. Chen, J. (2017). Pharmacology in critical illness. In J. M. Oropello, S. M. Pastores, & V. Kvetan (Eds.), *Critical care*. New York: McGraw-Hill. Retrieved from http://accessmedicine.mhmedical.com.ezproxy.simmons.edu:2048/content.aspx?bookid=1944&sectionid=143516493.
8. Correia, M. A. (2015). Drug biotransformation. In B. G. Katsung & A. J. Trevor (Eds.), *Basic & clinical pharmacology* (13th ed., pp. 56–73). New York: McGraw Hill.
9. Doig, A. K., & Huether, S. E. (2014). Structure and function of the renal and urologic system. In K. L. McCance, S. E. Huether, V. L. Brashers, & N. S. Rote (Eds.), *Pathophysiology: The biologic basis for disease in adults and children* (7th ed., pp. 1319–1339). St. Louis, MO: Elsevier.
10. National Kidney Foundation. (2017). Clinical practice guidelines for chronic kidney disease: Evaluation, classification, and stratification. Retrieved from https://www.kidney.org/sites/default/files/docs/ckd_evaluation_classification_stratification.pdf.

11. Mandell, L. A., Wunderink, R. G., Anzueto, A., Bartlett, G., Campbell, D., Dean, N., et al. (2007). Infectious Diseases Society of America/American Thoracic Society consensus guidelines on the management of community acquired pneumonia in adults. *Clinical Infectious Diseases, 44*(2), S27–S72.

12. Vassalotti, J. A., Centor, R., Turner, B. J., Greer, R. C., Choi, M., & Sequist, T. D. (2016). Practical approach to detection and management of chronic kidney disease for the primary care clinician. *The American Journal of Medicine, 129*, 153–162.

13. Mallappallil, M., Friedman, E. A., Delano, B. G., McFarlane, S. I., & Salifu, M. O. (2014). Chronic kidney disease in the elderly: Evaluation and management. *Clinical Practice, 11*(5), 525–535.

14. Pasqualetti, G., Tognini, S., Calsolaro, V., Polini, A., & Monzani, F. (2015). Potential drug–drug interactions in Alzheimer patients with behavioral symptoms. *Clinical Interventions in Aging, 10*, 1457–1466.

15. Gray, S., Anderson, A., Dublin, S., Hanlon, J., Hubbard, R., Walker, R., et al. (2015). Cumulative use of strong anticholinergics and incident dementia. *JAMA Internal Medicine, 175*(3), 401–407.

16. Bitner, A., Zalewski, P., Klawe, J. J., & Newton, J. L. (2015). Drug interactions in Parkinson's disease: Safety of pharmacotherapy for arterial hypertension. *Drugs - Real World Outcomes, 2*(1), 1–12.

17. Boustani, M., Campbell, N., Munger, S., Maidment, I., & Fox, C. (2008). Impact of anticholinergics on the ageing brain: A review and practical application. *Ageing Health, 4*, 311–320.

18. Leekha, S., Terrell, C. L., & Edson, R. S. (2011). General principles of antimicrobial therapy. *Mayo Clinic Proceedings, 86*(2), 156–167.

19. Johansen, T. E. B., & Naber, K. G. (2014). Antibiotics and urinary tract infections. *Antibiotics*, Retrieved from C:/Users/tbuttaro/Downloads/Antibiotics%20and%20Urinary%20Tract%20Infections.pdf.

20. Busti, A. J., & Nuzum, D. S. (2015). The mechanism and drug interaction – Warfarin (Coumadin) and amiodarone (Cordarone). *Evidence-based Medicine Consult*. Retrieved from https://www.ebmconsult.com/articles/warfarin-coumadin-jantoven-amiodarone-cordarone-pacerone-interaction-dose-reduction.

21. The American Geriatrics Society 2015 Beers Criteria Update Expert Panel. American Geriatrics Society 2015 Updated Beers Criteria for Potentially Inappropriate Medication Use in Older Adults. Retrieved from http://onlinelibrary.wiley.com/doi/10.1111/jgs.13702/pdf.

22. O'Mahony, D., O'Sullivan, D., Byrne, S., O'Connor, M. N., Ryan, C., & Gallagher, P. (2017). STOPP/START criteria for potentially inappropriate prescribing in older people: Version 2. Retrieved from https://www.ncbi.nlm.nih.gov/pmc/articles/PMC4339726/.

23. Maher, R. L., Hanlon, J. T., & Hajjar, E. R. (2014). Clinical consequences of polypharmacy in elderly. *Expert Opinion on Drug Safety, 13*(1), 57–65.

24. Department of Health and Human Services (2016). *ASPE issue brief: Observations on trends in prescription drug spending*. Retrieved from https://aspe.hhs.gov/system/files/pdf/187586/Drugspending.pdf.

25. De Nardi, M., French, E., Jones, J. B., & McCauley, J.(2016). Medical spending of the U.S. elderly. National Bureau of Economic Research Working Paper No. 21270, 2015. Retrieved from https://journalsresource.org/studies/government/health-care/elderly-medical-spending-medicare.

26. Social Security Fact Sheet (2017). Retrieved from https://www.ssa.gov/news/press/factsheets/basicfact-alt.pdf.

27. Scott, I., Hilmer, S., Reeve, E., Potter, K., Le Couteur, D., Rigby, D., et al. (2015). Reducing inappropriate polupharmacy: The process of deprescribing. *JAMA Internal Medicine, 175*(5), 827–834.

28. Garfinkel, D., & Mangin, D. (2010). Feasibility study of a systematic approach for discontinuation of multiple medications in older adults. *Archives of Internal Medicine, 170*(18), 1648–1654.

29. U.S. Food and Drug Administration. (2016). Preventable adverse drug reactions: Focus on drug interactions. Retrieved from https://www.fda.gov/drugs/developmentapprovalprocess/developmentresources/druginteractionslabeling/ucm110632.htm.

30. Rochon, P. A., Gill, S. S., & Gurwitz, J. H. (2016). General principles of pharmacology and appropriate prescribing. In J. B. Halter, J. G. Ouslander, S. Studenski, K. P. High, S. Asthana, M. A. Supiano, et al. (Eds.), *Hazzard's geriatric medicine and gerontology* (7th ed.). New York: McGraw-Hill. Retrieved from http://accessmedicine.mhmedical.com.ezproxy.simmons.edu:2048/content.aspx?bookid=1923&sectionid=144519184.

31. Lipska, K. J., Bail, C. J., & Inzucchi, S. E. (2011). Use of metformin in the setting of mild-to-moderate renal insufficiency. *Diabetes Care, 34*, 1431–1437.

CHAPTER 4

Palliative Care

Susan Parker

Introduction

Palliative care is now part of mainstream health care, but there remains a good deal of misunderstanding as to what it really is. Many providers hesitate to make referrals to palliative experts for consultation believing that their patients will be reluctant or, worse yet, frightened. This is based on the belief that palliative care and hospice care are one and the same. By definition, palliative care is defined as follows:

- Palliative care is defined by the World Health Organization (WHO) as "early identification and impeccable assessment and treatment of pain and other problems, physical, psychosocial and spiritual."[1]
- Palliative care is not limited to symptom management. It must include the education and support to patients and families making decisions about goals of care and advanced directives.[2]

A brief history of palliative care and hospice will clarify the development of both and the current state of the specialty.

History of Palliative Care

The history of palliative care is intertwined with hospice in interesting and oftentimes confusing ways. Historically, health care providers have been reluctant to educate the patient about the limits of medical treatment. This, coupled with a lack of understanding on the part of the public regarding the limits to successful medical treatment, can lead to underutilization of palliative care services. These factors have slowed the development of palliative care. For example, consider an 82-year-old gentleman with extensive osteoarthritis and end-stage heart disease. He is readmitted to the hospital for the third time in 5 months for congestive heart failure (CHF). His echo shows an ejection fraction of 20%, and his activity level is severely impaired. His activity consists of mostly being in bed, or moving bed to chair, to the bathroom, and back to bed. He and his family inform the hospitalist that he wants everything done to take care of his problem of persistent shortness of breath. This includes a full code. With his poor ejection fraction and limited activity level, the likelihood that this man will resume a quality of life after cardiopulmonary resuscitation is unlikely. This patient's situation warrants a palliative consult as part of his initial workup to address his shortness of breath and his goals for quality of life.

The likelihood of a palliative care consult being ordered for this patient is dependent on several factors, most notably the training of the hospitalist and the availability of a viable palliative consult service in that hospital. Too often, even now in the 21st century, this patient's access to palliative care may be limited by:

- the hospitalist's belief that palliative care means hospice care and this patient is not ready to die,
- the nursing staff's concern that the family will be unduly upset if the palliative care consultant discusses death,

- the belief by the family that the patient will give up if the subject of death is brought up, and
- a concern that his Medicare will not cover the cost of this service.

Unfortunately, if no palliative consult occurs, the patient may miss out on receiving the one thing he really wants, relief of the shortness of breath. Because palliative care addresses the quality of life of the person and treatment of symptoms, the consultant need not discuss death at all. The focus of the consult may be solely on treatments to alleviate the shortness of breath.

Hospice began as a grassroots effort outside mainstream medical care. Members of the clergy, and then a few outspoken individuals who knew about the work of Dame Cicely Saunders (1963), pushed for the establishment of hospices in their area. Dame Saunders started the first modern hospice in Great Britain, called St. Christopher's, which has long been noted as the sentinel hospice of modern times. The term "hospice" comes from the medieval term for "way station for people on pilgrimages." There was a spiritual component to the care, and it is interesting to note that Dame Cicely Saunders, who started out as a nurse, furthered her education by becoming a social worker and then a physician as a way to "get people in medical care" to listen to her about the need for hospice care.

Physicians in the United States in the 1960s hesitated to prescribe narcotics to patients (even those with end-stage cancer) out of concern for them developing addiction or hastening death. Clergy and others were hearing about the distress of these patients and advocated for the start of hospices. Also in the 1960s, Dr. Elizabeth Kubler-Ross, a psychiatrist who worked with patients suffering from the effects of end-stage disease, noted that nurses and physicians did not communicate clearly and honestly with these patients. Studies done at this time showed that often these patients were put at the end of the hall in the hospital and nurses answered their call bells slowly. Dr. Kubler-Ross met resistance to treating people at end of life with dignity, respect, and open and honest communication. She developed the Five Stages of Grief Model describing these stages as denial, anger, bargaining, depression, and acceptance. She never intended that all people should go through all five stages in any rigid order.[3]

Another major player in the history of palliative care in the 1970s is Dr. Balfour Mount, a surgical oncologist at McGill University in Canada. The first to use the term "palliative care," Dr. Mount's inpatient palliative care unit provided compassionate communication and early treatment of symptoms, not just at the end of life, but early on when serious illness was diagnosed.[4]

In 1995 the Study to Understand Prognosis and Preferences for Outcomes and Risks of Treatment (SUPPORT), a randomized controlled trial with over 4000 patients funded by the Robert Woods Johnson Foundation for $29 million, demonstrated that:

- 46% of end-of-life patients had do not resuscitate (DNR) orders written only 2 days before death,
- less than 50% of the physicians caring for these patients knew about their patient's preferences for goals of care, and
- 50% of these patients had untreated moderate to severe pain.[5]

The alarming results of this study showed a lack of physician–patient communication regarding end-of-life wishes and degree of aggressiveness of medical treatment desired. Worse still, from a palliative care perspective, there was a lack of adequate pain control. It is also important to note that at this time in our history there were very few if any palliative care programs in acute care hospitals.

During the 1990s the speed at which palliative care moved forward into mainstream medical care was accelerated. In another landmark study, this time with the Institute of Medicine (IOM), Field and Cassel (1997) published the report *Approaching Death: Improving Care at the End of Life*.[6] Study findings demonstrated that physicians and caregivers failed to provide competent care to dying patients. As a result, the IOM called for steps to improve care for the dying: one, because Americans are living longer with more chronic illnesses than ever before in our history; and two, because this dying process takes place over weeks, months, or even years with chronic end-stage illness.

Other major developments in palliative care and hospice include the following:

1. **1978:** The start of the National Hospice and Palliative Care Organization (NHPCO) (see https://nhpco.org). This organization is now the "largest, nonprofit organization in the USA to represent the interests of hospice and palliative care programs, professionals, and patients and families."
2. **1986:** The start of the Hospice and Palliative Nurse's Association. This organization serves as a resource to promote the specialty of hospice and palliative nursing. It sets standards of practice and maintains programs for certification of nursing professionals (see https://www.hpna.org).
3. **1999:** The start of the Center to Advance Palliative Care (CAPC). This organization provides training, technical assistance, and support to palliative care providers. Its overall mission is to promote "palliative care to people with serious illness everywhere" (see https://www.capc.org/about/capc/).
4. **2004:** Release of *Clinical Practice Guidelines for Quality Palliative Care* (see https://www.hpna.org/multimedia/NCP_Clinical_Practice_Guidelines_3rd_Edition.pdf).
5. **2006:** The American Board of Medical Subspecialties recognized hospice and palliative medicine as a subspecialty, and fellowships in palliative care were started in the United States.
6. **2010:** Temel et al. demonstrated in a sentinel randomized control trial that palliative care can improve quality of life, improve mood, and prolong life in patients with nonsmall-cell lung cancer.[7]
7. **2010:** Affordable Care Act allows for a demonstration project by the Centers for Medicare and Medicaid Services (CMS) to provide palliative and hospice care for patients who are receiving aggressive medical treatment. This may result in the relaxing of hospice regulations in the future.

PALLIATIVE CARE MODEL

Palliative care as described by CAPC can be provided over time, and at any time in the course of a serious illness (Fig. 4.1). Read from left to right, the figure shows that the patient is diagnosed

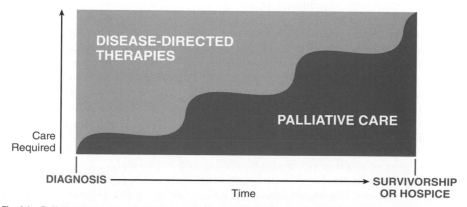

Fig. 4.1 Palliative care model. (From the National Consensus Project Clinical Practice. [2004]. *Guidelines for quality palliative care* [2nd ed.]. Richmond, VA: National Coalition for Hospice and Palliative Care.)

with a serious illness and, as needed, receives diagnostic services and treatment for life-prolonging therapy. Because many of the illnesses treated today are of a chronic nature, there may be relapses requiring more treatment, and perhaps hospital stays and inpatient therapy with transitions in care as the patient moves from acute care, to short-term rehabilitation, to home. These are the transitions in care and settings of care. Over time, the chronic illness becomes less responsive to life-prolonging therapy and worsening symptoms may require attention. As this occurs, palliative care is needed more than therapy for prolonging life (enlarging cross-section of palliative care and diminishing section of life-prolonging therapy). At the far end of the rectangle hospice is needed for end-of-life care. It is important to note that palliative care is provided as needed throughout the course of treatment to prolong life, as well as during the duration of hospice care.

This palliative care model guides the interdisciplinary team (IDT), setting the standard for practice for palliative care as it is provided in a variety of settings. For example, most tertiary acute care hospital with 300 beds or more have inpatient palliative care services. In these settings, a palliative care board certified physician is usually the medical director with a team of other physicians, nurse practitioners, physician assistants, social workers, and chaplains who make up the IDT. Most of these programs require that IDT members are board certified by their respective discipline. In the case of the nurse practitioner, for example, the certification requirements are 500 hours of supervised practice in palliative care, certification by a national board and state licensure, and successful scores on the palliative nurse practitioner examination.

Palliative care teams are also found in case management settings in the community, in hospices as a "prehospice service," long-term care facilities, assisted living facilities, rehabilitation hospitals, acute care hospitals, long-term care facilities, and, most recently, primary care. A recent article in the *Nurse Practitioner* described the increasing need for primary care nurse practitioners to integrate palliative care in their practices when hospice is not an option. Primary care practices are seeing increasing numbers of older patients who are living to advanced ages with chronic diseases for which there are often symptoms that require ongoing management. In addition, these patients need to be educated about the limits to medical care for their particular condition. This means that all healthcare providers need to have a comfort level and the skill set to manage the goals of care discussions (something for which many health provider programs have not prepared them).[8]

It is important to note that palliative care can be provided not only at any site of care, but it can and should be provided by clinicians at these sites whether or not they are "palliative care experts."

There are three levels of palliative care: primary, secondary, and tertiary.[9] Primary palliative care should be a part of what any clinician does in managing pain or other symptoms. In addition, primary care clinicians can and should facilitate goals of care and advanced planning conversations with additional training.[10] It also should be mentioned that clinicians in rehabilitation hospitals, long-term care facilities, and acute care hospitals can and should be integrating palliative care into their practice. Secondary palliative care is provided by consultants who are palliative clinicians, either board certified nurse practitioners, physician assistants, or physicians who can offer expert opinions for treating complex or difficult problems. Tertiary palliative care includes research and teaching in addition to expert level consultation.

The difference between hospice and palliative care is summarized in the Table 4.1. Additionally, hospice care in the United States is paid for by insurance companies, most notably Medicare, which has governed to a large extent what type of care will be provided.

The chart illustrates the shared elements between hospice and palliative care. Palliative care is threaded throughout hospice care because the goal of care is comfort. However, in palliative care the patient may still receive curative treatment, and there is no 6-month or less life expectancy requirement.

TABLE 4.1 ■ Differences Between Hospice and Palliative Care

Hospice	Palliative Care
• Comfort based rather than curative • Eligibility guidelines set by Medicare based on prognosis of 6 month or less • Eligible individuals sign onto hospice benefit • Covered under Medicare A benefit, Medicaid, and most private insurance • Intensive interdisciplinary support for patient and family	• Can receive/pursue curative, disease-modifying or life-prolonging treatment • Eligibility not based on life expectancy • Consultative in nature • Covered under Medicare B and most private insurance • Helps clarify goals of care together with family and medical team

COMMUNICATING WITH PATIENTS AND FAMILIES

Family can be defined in many ways. When providers consider communicating with a family member, the first step may be to recognize who can be spoken with about a patient's status. The cognitively intact patient easily identifies those who are family members. In the broader definition of family, these individuals may be blood relatives, legal relatives, or caring friends. The provider needs to have the patient tell them that it is permissible to share information with them. If the patient is no longer able to communicate clearly because of changes in cognitive status, perhaps because of a metabolic syndrome such as delirium or a more permanent condition such as dementia, then communication with family is usually with a designated individual. This person may have been designated by the patient before the illness ensued, such as the health care proxy in Massachusetts; a family member identified by the patient less formally, such as a caregiver who brings them to the hospital; or through a court-appointed guardian. Communication and confidentiality both must be ensured by the clinician.

There may be situations in which family members are estranged from a patient. Patients may identify a family member that they do not want to have involved in their care and clearly state this. In other situations, family members who have been out of contact with a patient may return. With a now shifting family dynamic, the family caregivers who have been present and the returned family negotiate roles and ways to communicate with each other and the patient.

Numerous studies have shown that communication between clinicians and patients and families about the seriousness of the illness, wishes for end-of-life care, and their hopes is seriously lacking. Some excellent strategies for clinicians to help them communicate in these situations were described by Peereboom and Coyle in their article on recommended communication approaches.[11] Using ask-tell-ask, the clinician first asks an open-ended question to find out certain information about the patient, such as how much they know about their condition, how they feel about their current situation, or what they are thinking. When the patient answers, the clinician knows how to answer, i.e., how much detail they really want to know, and can respond accordingly. The clinician's next comment is to provide the information. The third step in the ask-tell-ask cycle is to find out if the question was answered to the patient's satisfaction and what further direction the conversation can take.

Here is an example adapted from Peereboom and Coyle. The clinician in this situation is a nurse practitioner (PROVIDER):

PROVIDER: How are things going today?

PATIENT: Not great.

PROVIDER: You seem discouraged. Can you tell me what you are thinking?

PATIENT: I am really upset about what I was told about my illness.

PROVIDER: You do appear upset. What is your understanding of what you were told?

PATIENT: I was told by the oncologist that there is no more treatment for my cancer. That means it's all over.

PROVIDER: That sounds really hard to hear. Would you like to hear more about what **can** be done?

In this example, to the question "asked" the patient is at first reluctant to talk as can be seen by the very short response "Not great." The provider could respond in a number of different ways; i e , a simple, "I hope you are feeling better soon," could curtail the exploratory possibilities in this situation. By acknowledging and commenting the provider "tells" the patient how he appears or what message was received by the provider. This shows the patient the provider is paying attention through observation, as well as listening. Then by "asking" the next question in the logical flow of information the direction is set for discovering more about the patient and finding what the patient finds acceptable to talk about. This is the thread of ask-tell-ask. Through using this technique, the provider is guided as to how much depth to go into when delivering "bad news" and discussing difficult subjects.

Many authors have described the importance of body language as a nonverbal communication tool. As much as 90% of what we say is communicated through body language. Nonverbal communication becomes even more important when discussing sensitive issues and may be used by the clinician in assessing family dynamics for readiness or openness to hearing information about serious illness.

The ideal body positioning will include the clinician being situated at the same level as the patient. When the patient is lying in bed, the clinician should sit close to the patient, at the same level with eye contact, and in a relaxed body position (arms not crossed across the chest). In a family meeting, the clinician will position the chairs in a circle so that no one is at the head of the table (position of power). Clinicians should take into consideration that holding a laptop while entering information during the discussion can be seen by the patient or family as being an obstacle to open communication. The same can be said of holding a form while entering information during the conversation. Each clinician should evaluate the situation and facilitate communication through how they present themselves. When in doubt, the clinician should ask if it is alright to take notes during the conversation.

Clinicians are often distressed when having to communicate end-of-life information with patients and families. Described next is an example of how nurses in an oncology setting were given education in using the COMFORT model.[12]

A summary of this model and a description of the meaning of the acronym COMFORT is useful in this discussion about communication. First used to teach oncology nurses who experienced a high degree of distress in communicating end-of-life information, the COMFORT model focuses on the following:

Communication that provides education; is advocating; and provides caring, comfort, and a connection for the patient with the clinician, family, and others.

Orientation and opportunity describes how the clinician adjusts vocal tone, proximity for standing or sitting near the patient to the norm demonstrated by the patient and family.

Mindfulness is the conscious effort of the clinician to be attentive to the moment, actively engaged in the present, sensitive to context, nonjudgmental, and empathic.

Family refers to understanding a family climate. A family communication environment develops over time and is not created by the event of illness.

Openings will occur during transitions in care or when changes in the patient's status occur, and so forth, which may also have accompanying increased tension. This opening allows the nurse the opportunity to intervene to provide teaching and support.

Responding to patient and family needs.

Team structure and process of care assumes that nurses often serve as leaders during team meetings, and that role has tremendous influence on group communication.[13]

Consider this case example and the COMFORT Model:

Mr. Smith, a 71-year-old gentleman, was admitted to the hospital from a rehabilitation center where he had increasing respiratory distress. In the emergency department, he was found to be in respiratory failure with severe hypoxia. His past medical history includes chronic obstructive pulmonary disease (COPD), colon cancer, and advanced malnutrition. He has had multiple hospital admissions over the past 2 years, which were also for respiratory distress. He was admitted to the hospital and treated for acute on chronic respiratory failure complicated by pneumonia, an exacerbation of COPD, and new-onset rapid atrial fibrillation. Of note, he is under treatment for depression, he is a widower, and has a single-family home. It has been uncertain where he is going to live because of his declining condition. During your conversation with him he discloses that he and his daughter have a good relationship, but he does not want to be a burden.

Using the COMFORT Model, we can see that this is an *Opening* for mindful *Communication* that includes support, caring, education, and advocacy. In the present moment, during which the clinician takes the *Opportunity* to speak with the patient, the discussion is facilitated by the clinician being *Mindful* of the patient's presentation and sitting at eye level with the patient and speaking in a tone similar to that of the patient. The clinician will include the *Family* with the patient's permission, either during this discussion or perhaps by a telephone call during the meeting today or at another time to *Respond* to the needs and concerns of the entire caring support system. The communication is not complete until the clinician includes the *Team* through communication of the proceedings of this patient/family interchange.

Throughout this model of communication, it becomes readily apparent that assessing patterns of communication not only with the patient, but with the family, and the family's internal communication patterns can be pivotal in providing quality palliative care.

Assessing the family dynamic is a very important step in this communication process. Nurses, by the nature of the profession, are attuned to caring for patients and families and may be faced with a situation in which the patient and a family member or caregiver may be at a different stage of coping, or of a differing opinion as to how information should be shared. This can be very stressful for the clinician and very time-consuming. For example, the patient may want to know the details of their diagnosis, and the family member may want to "protect them" and asks the clinician to minimize the facts of the illness or to avoid the subject. In contrast, the family caregiver may be unaware of the seriousness of the illness and may not want to hear about the details or is alarmed that there is a need "now" for advanced directives. This mismatch of needs for support and education is very common in palliative care. The skilled clinician will be expected to facilitate communication. Using the steps previously described of ask-tell-ask and the therapeutic use of nonverbal communication can be very helpful.

Patient and family conflict is unfortunately very common in health care, and especially so in palliative care in which a patient's condition is expected to deteriorate, advanced care decisions need to be made, and caregiver burden may increase as the patient's need for care increases nearing end-of-life. Conflict within the family can have dire consequences for the patient. Communication among family members and communication between family members and the patient may be fractured so badly that important care decisions cannot be made. The division of labor as to who will do what for the patient who wants to live at home with family support may become difficult. Disagreement over who should be making decisions and what those decisions should be may occur because of old family tensions.

An example of an approach to addressing patient and family conflicts describes a process of assessment and clinical intervention (adapted from Lichtenthal and Kissane):

1. **Assessment of family for likelihood of conflict:** In this stage the clinician looks to see what the strengths of the family are and what the prior history of family communication styles have been. Families high in support, communication skill, and those who have conflict resolvers in the family are more capable of resolving conflicts. Families who do not have these tendencies will have more difficulty with conflict. In these cases, the additional skills

of the social worker on the team become invaluable in helping resolve conflicts and, if needed, facilitate a referral for family therapy.

2. **Clinical interventions:** This may need to be done on neutral ground when the clinician turns the focus of the intervention to

   a. the patient's needs primarily,

   b. the needs of the family members and patient, which are considered equally, and

   c. the need of the most at-risk person at that moment in time.

In each of these steps the communication involves active listening, self-disclosure of one's feelings without blaming another, explaining what the concern is, empathizing and demonstrating understanding of the other person's feelings, and then reframing the conflict as a problem that can be solved by the family if they work together with each other and the patient.[14]

Communication with the patient who is a child and the child's family has its special challenges. Pediatric palliative care is a field that has been slow in developing for reasons such as parents wishing to exhaust every possible treatment, clinicians being reluctant to "give up," and increased successes in life-prolonging treatment, and a misunderstanding of palliative care services as distinct from hospice care. Unfortunately, in many pediatric patients the end-of-life begins with birth because of a congenital defect or the disease presentation in early childhood. Even though life expectancy may have increased with the advent of 21st century medical care, the child lives with chronic illness during which he or she could benefit from palliative care. Studies have demonstrated that for pediatric palliative care to be successful, pediatric clinicians must develop a strong bond with the families and demonstrate their worth to the primary clinicians who are already providing care. The palliative service must provide innovative pain management techniques, continuity of care from hospital to home, a psychologist, end-of-life expertise, and bereavement support.[15]

Children under 7 to 8 years of age frequently view death as temporary, whereas adolescents have an understanding of death and are able to talk about their illness and its impact on them and their families. The IOM in 2003 described an urgent need for research on how to communicate with families who had a child with end-stage disease. Communication in many situations was seen as being uncaring, especially when parents were told there was nothing more to be done.[16]

Communication for Goals of Care and Advanced Care Planning

One role of the clinician in palliative care, particularly the nurse and the healthcare provider, is to develop the care plan for the patient with an end-of-life illness. According to the *Clinical Guidelines for Quality Palliative Care*, skilled communication is critical to develop a care plan that meets these criteria: "The care plan is based on the identified and expressed preferences, values, and needs, of the patient and family and is developed with professional guidance and support of the decision-making" (p. 14).[17]

Through working with the IDT, including the nurse, nurse practitioner or physician assistant, physician, social worker, and chaplain, this care plan is developed. Most patients will need to have a family meeting at some point. The patient may attend or not based on their preference or decision-making capacity. If the patient has decision-making capacity, it should be their decision to attend or not.

The setting, timing, atmosphere, and who is included in the family meeting are very important. In some circumstances, family members cannot be present physically, and can be conferenced in by speaker phone, teleconferencing, or videoconferencing. It is important that the patient's preference be honored in the selection of those family members to be present. Before the meeting it is important to state what the goals of the meeting are, and very often it is to discuss information about the patient's condition and choices for care.

An informational meeting at which the patient is going to be told their disease is progressing and cannot be treated further requires skill and planning. The clinician who actually delivers this information to the patient is often the physician, who may be the least prepared for this type of conversation. In actuality, there are many practices in which the nurse practitioner or physician assistant "tells the patient the bad news." Patients prefer to receive this information from the clinician most knowledgeable about their condition and treatment options, and in whom they have the most trust and an established rapport.

Robert Buckman set the stage a few years ago in helping us understand how to plan a way to deliver "bad news." Bad news is anything the patient thinks is a serious threat to their future. Dr. Buckman, an oncologist who has written several books on medical communication, trains clinicians in this skill because there was and still is a widespread lack of skill and experience in delivering bad news among clinicians. His emphasis is on strategy and not script, meaning there are no special words to be said. Trying to say words from a script not only sounds unreal; it is also rather insincere. However, a basic strategy that allows for modification according to the patient's needs and what comes up for discussion can be helpful. This strategy is made up of six steps that follow the acronym SPIKES:

1. **S: Setting the stage.** This means holding the patient/family meeting in an area that is private, with significant others present, and where the clinician is sitting down and makes a connection through eye contact and relaxed posturing. It is important at this step to let the patient know how much time the meeting will take so there is no last-minute rush and the conversation can be paced appropriately from the beginning.
2. **P: Perception of the patient.** The purpose of the first question asked by the clinician and directed to the patient/family is meant to assess their level of understanding of the patient's condition.
3. **I: Invitation.** The patient is asked what they would like to know about their test results, disease prognosis, treatment, and so forth. Not all patients want to know all the details. It is perfectly alright to address what they want to hear and not explain every aspect at this time. Some patients need time to assimilate information and may do so bit by bit over days or weeks.
4. **K: Knowledge.** The clinician is providing knowledge and information to the patient. It is important to use words that are not technical, such as "spread" instead of "metastasized". It is important to be sensitive. Tactlessness or being overly blunt will push the patient away and cause anger or hurt. It is best to give the information in small chunks, which allows the patient time to think and ask questions. Rather than say, "there is nothing more I can do for you," say, "I will continue to be involved in your care, and as you need it we will see that the treatment changes. You will not be alone in this."
5. **E: Emotions.** The clinician should respond to the patient's emotions first, then continue with teaching. By addressing the emotion, when you say something like, "you sound angry," the patient hears that you empathize.
6. **S: Strategy and Summary.** At this point near the end of the meeting it is important for the clinician to go back over what has been discussed so far. This lets everyone have an opportunity to review what was discussed and what may need further discussion now or at a later date. It is also the part of the meeting in which the clinician can discuss the patient's prognosis and treatment options.[18]

Depending on the patient and family situation, this type of meeting may be 30 minutes or so in length, and it is not recommended that the meeting continue past 60 minutes. This allows an opportunity for all participants to be heard in an environment of therapeutic communication without tiring people or rehashing information. Patients and family members often need an opportunity to absorb information after the meeting and have the opportunity for further discussion at another time.

Case Example

Setting the stage: You are the clinician and you have arranged a family meeting at your office having blocked out 30 minutes for this meeting in your private office in which there is comfortable seating for the four of you (note that this meeting is not held in an examination room). After welcoming the patient and his wife, you let them know you have a half-hour set aside for this discussion, and you let them know that if there are more questions you are available by telephone and you can have further discussion at the next office visit.

Perception of the patient. You say, "Mr. Smith, over the past few months you have needed to be admitted to the hospital three times. I saw in your hospital medical record that these admissions were caused by weakness and falls. Can you tell me what you think is the cause of these falls?" Mr. Smith responds, "Well I was putting a fan in the window this last time and tripped and fell." Mrs. Smith responds, "John, that is not entirely the way it happened. You haven't been eating well and you've been vomiting a lot." He nods sheepishly. "I guess that could have something to do with it."

Invitation: You ask, directing the question to both the patient and his wife, "Would you like to know more about the results of the tests at the hospital? I think the doctor in the hospital spoke with you." The patient answers, "I know I have cancer and I had an operation to remove some of it from my brain. I think that pretty well took care of things. I think it was just the hot weather that got me this time." His wife looks anxious then says, "I think we need to hear what the health care provider has to say." The patient answers looking a bit impatient, "All this talk is just a waste of time, but if you really want to OK."

Knowledge: You say, "I will tell you what I know as much as you want me to today and if you want to talk further you know we can do that at another time also. For now, let me tell you that the scan you had showed spread of the cancer to your liver. We know this can cause you to feel weaker, and it can upset your digestion." The patient looks very upset and says, "I wasn't expecting this. I had an operation and chemotherapy and they told me I was all done with it. I thought I was getting better." His wife is starting to cry. She says nothing.

Emotions: You say, "I can see this information is upsetting to you both." You hand his wife a tissue and move your chair a bit closer to his wife to touch her hand. She is receptive and appears to relax a bit. You say, "We can talk more about this now and what the next steps can be if you want. You will not be left alone with this, Dr. Jones and I will be caring for you as long as you want us to." The patient says, "I'm relieved that you just didn't say something like there is nothing more you can do for me. I want you and Dr. Jones to take care of me. What happens now? How much longer do I have to live? Is this thing going to kill me?" You know that there is no option for further chemotherapy, and clinical trial options are also not a possibility because of the patient's history of ischemic cardiomyopathy, atrial fibrillation, diabetes, and chronic kidney disease.

Summary and strategy: You say, "The cancer is very serious and we do not know for certain how much longer you have to live. What I can tell you is that there are some options open to you now. You can feel better, with little to no nausea and this may make you feel much better and perhaps stronger." The patient says, "That's kind of a relief." His wife says, "It is a relief to know we can do something. What else do you think we should do?" You say, "Let's talk more about what your wishes are and I have more information for you to think about."

As part of this type of conversation, patients often have further questions and are looking for suggestions as to what to read and what is available on the Internet and elsewhere. Recommended supplemental readings for these discussions include the following:

1. Many organizations purchase a pamphlet called *Five Wishes* and have it available for these discussions (available at https://agingwithdignity.org/docs/default-source/default-document-library/product-samples/fwsample.pdf?sfvrsn=2).
2. Many organizations also purchase the booklet *Hard Choices for Loving People* and use it as a handout with these discussions (available at https://www.amazon.com/Hard-Choices-Loving-People-Life-Threatening/dp/1928560067).

This conversation is a step in a series of multiple conversations that may occur over time in the care of this patient. Depending on how much time this has taken, and the amount of questions the patient and his wife have at this point, the meeting may now end. The next step should be another office visit to follow up or, if the discussion has turned in that direction, a consult for palliative care may be initiated.

Facilitating Palliative Care Communication in the Transitions of Care

In a perfect world, patients with a serious illness have spoken with their primary care providers and their wishes for care as the illness advances are known. Often this is not the case. Because of a lack of training received by the primary care clinician in advanced care planning, lack of time in patient interaction, or patient resistance, the patient remains a "full code" no matter what is occurring in his or her disease. All too often a chronic illness exacerbates or an unforeseen illness occurs and the patient is admitted to acute care. The acute care setting is a setting for palliative care to be introduced to patients and families. The palliative care team is available for advanced care planning discussions.

Palliative care clinicians tell us that too often the referrals they receive are too late in coming, especially in view of recent research that shows how patients with metastatic nonsmall-cell lung cancer feel better and live longer with palliative care. Transitions to the hospital from home could be reduced by providing palliative care to patients. Many of these patients want to be at home and simply need the education regarding what palliative care can offer them,[19] but clinicians need to be educated first. Researchers find that significant barriers exist to the timely referral to palliative care. Care and communication practices need to be streamlined, particularly in acute care, to improve patient care that is sensitive to their wishes. Timely referral to palliative care shows that both patient and family well-being are improved.[20] The time for a palliative care referral is any time the patient has a serious illness that has a detrimental impact as they see it on their quality of life.

Advance Care Plan

One of the major reasons primary care clinicians, hospitalists, oncologists, and other clinicians refer patients to palliative care is to help establish the goals of care. There may have been a preliminary discussion started by the referring clinician, or there may not have been. Using the communication tools just discussed, the palliative care clinician will proceed to help the patient and family develop the goals of care and the advance care plan (ACP). The ACP does not need to be completed by the palliative care clinician. Nurse practitioners and physician assistants in primary care are very well situated to help their patients and families with this because they may have come to know them well over time and trust is already established.

In the ideal situation, the ACP process is one in which the patient, family, and friends are guided through and educated about the risks and benefits of treatments. In this process they are given information, time to reflect on it, and time to ask questions. This is an organized approach to initiating conversations, considering the patient's values and current state of health. It should be noted that these conversations should be conducted when the patient is cognitively intact and capable of asking and answering questions. This means these conversations should occur well before a medical crisis.

There may be a lack of agreement about how much time the patient has left to live. If there is not some degree of urgency, clinicians are hesitant to bring up the subject of the ACP. Disagreement about this time left to live, otherwise known as accuracy of prognostication, is approached by some clinicians, and very commonly by palliative care clinicians, with tools that measure some aspect of physical ability. For example, the Palliative Performance Scale (PPS) measures the patient's ability to perform activities of daily living. Fully functional patients who are able to care for themselves and are mentally intact have a good prognosis. Patients who are totally bedbound, require assistance with all care, cannot eat, and are not alert have a very poor prognosis. Similarly, the Karnofsky Scale measures the patient's capabilities and is often used with the ECOG Performance Scale to clarify the prognosis of a patient who has cancer. Patients with cancer are given a prognosis based on their ability to perform activities in the ECOG Performance Status rating seen in the following table. Developed by the Eastern Cooperative Oncology Group (ECOG) in the 1980s, the purpose of this tool is to rate the patient's eligibility for hospice care. It can be considered a way to estimate life expectancy; the higher the score is, the shorter the life expectancy.

Grade	ECOG Performance Status[21]
0	Fully active, able to perform all predisease performance without restriction
1	Restricted in physically strenuous activity but ambulatory and able to perform work of a light or sedentary nature, e.g., light housework, office work
2	Ambulatory and capable of all self-care but unable to perform any work activities; up and about more than 50% of waking hours
3	Capable of only limited self-care; confined to bed or chair more than 50% of waking hours
4	Completely disabled; cannot perform any self-care; totally confined to bed or chair
5	Dead

Recent advances in clinical trials are providing more refined information to help in prognostication. Not surprisingly, studies look at genotypes and response to chemotherapy and other variables. In one study, findings suggested that advanced age is a major variable that worsens prognosis, at least in chronic lymphocytic leukemia.[22]

Another factor that makes it difficult to construct the ACP is the lack of readiness or sometimes denial on the part of the patient. Patients may be fearful that accepting less than all that is available for treatment may mean inferior care. This was seen recently in the political arena when reimbursing primary care clinicians through Medicare funding for working with patients on the ACP was seen as providing "death panels."[23] Inaccurate information stirred the public to be fearful of discussions regarding ACPs, saying that people would be dying sooner because of these discussions. Substantial data from studies have shown that people have improved quality of life when they are informed and provided education and support.

The purpose of the ACP is to provide guidance to clinicians, families, and friends regarding the wishes of the patient when he or she cannot voice their preferences for treatment. It also provides immunity to the clinician from litigation. By not treating the patient to the full extent of what is medically available for curative treatment when it is the patient's informed choice to withhold treatment, and it is in their best interest, the clinician has the confidence to withhold curative treatment. ACP discussions should be ongoing; as the patient's status changes, it is important to educate and support the patient. In this manner, the patient and family know things are on track, or if there is a significant change, they understand the implications.

There are two components of ACPs: first, the living will, which includes any plans related to treatment; and second, the information about who will take over making decisions when patients can no longer speak for themselves (surrogate decision makers or health care proxies). *Five Wishes* is a living will, and it partially fulfills the specifics required in the ACP in many health care settings. In Massachusetts, the Comfort Care Form served this purpose; however, this has been replaced by the Physician's Orders for Life Sustaining Treatment (POLST), which is now called the Medical Orders for Life Sustaining Treatment (MOLST). These forms are designed with check off boxes for questions regarding:

1. Cardiopulmonary resuscitation
2. Ventilation
3. Transfer to the hospital
4. Who is signing the form: patient, health care agent, guardian, parent/guardian
5. Signature of physician, nurse practitioner, or physician assistant

  6. Name of health care agent and name of primary care physician
  7. Intubation, ventilation, noninvasive ventilation
  8. Dialysis
  9. Artificial hydration
  10. Artificial nutrition

The intent of this form is to have the patient select treatment choices and their health agent, therefore covering all aspects of the ACP in one form that is transferrable from facility to home and during ambulance transport. This form must be signed by the clinician for it to be activated. Many of us in palliative care believe that this form is a starting point, not the end point in the advanced care planning process. Because patients may change their minds at any point in time, it is important to revisit the plans for further clarification as new developments occur in the patient's condition. Once again communication plays a major role in this care.

  More about the MOLST and POLST forms is listed here:

- They apply to inpatient and outpatient setting. They are DNRs for both the hospital and the community or out of the hospital.
- In the hospital, they may be referred to as DNRs, or Allow Natural Death (AND), or Comfort Care Only.
- In the community or out of the hospital, they may be known as a variation on the name: Medical/Provider/Physician Orders for Life Sustaining Treatment (MOLST/POLST).
- There are currently 15 states with fully implemented Orders for Life Sustaining Treatment documents and another 20 states that have a document in process (as of 2012). The POLST/MOLST forms have been available since 2009 in selected sites, and in 2014 they are widespread throughout Massachusetts.[24]

Patients living in Massachusetts can still select a health care proxy without the signature of an attorney or clinician. The health care proxy form can be made out in the patient's home and then signed by the proxy.

LEGAL ISSUES IN PALLIATIVE CARE

The delineation between what is an ethical issue and what is a legal issue is sometimes confusing. Legal issues are governed by laws, rules, and regulations. Ethical issues are standards that guide people in how they *should* act. The difference between the two can be staggering. In the example of a patient with end-stage COPD who has not made an ACP, the surrogate decision maker (his wife) believes he should have continued care requiring intubation and ventilator-assisted breathing when there is no hope of being weaned off the respirator. In this example of futile care, the wife has the legal authority to make the decision; however, many would argue that this is an ethically wrong decision.

  When considering legal issues in palliative care, the first concern is whether informed consent has been obtained, usually in the form of an ACP. If not, the second legal consideration is whether a decision-making capacity decision is needed, and if so, has it been done. Adults who are cognitively intact and of the legal age of 18 and older are considered to have the capacity to consent. If this is the situation, providing information in a way that ensures patients understand their medical status must be carefully done. Clinicians (including PROVIDERs) determine whether or not the patient has decision-making capacity. For patients to be deemed to have decision-making capacity they must:

  1. Be able to understand the information presented to them and state a treatment choice. For example, the patient states he does not want any further chemotherapy. He understands that he can voluntarily exit the clinical trial and he chooses to do so.
  2. Appreciate their situation and the consequence of their decision. To continue from the last patient scenario, the patient states he will continue to see his primary care provider

and continue treatment for his hypertension. He states that he knows the tumor may grow, and if it does, he may consider surgery if it is needed.

3. **Understand treatment options**. When asked, this patient says he knows he can continue chemotherapy, but he has decided instead to have medical treatment for his other conditions

4. **Voice their decision**. This patient says he wants to stop chemotherapy and he will risk having the tumor grow. He has decided to have different treatment now that will help him feel comfortable.

Another consideration for decision-making capacity is that it is not necessarily a global capacity. Patients may understand their medical condition but may be compromised in other areas of self-care. For example, perhaps they were taking care of themselves poorly at home and could not manage finances or the household. That does not matter; they only need to have an adequate understanding of their present medical condition.

This is different, however, in the situation of the patient who is in the advanced stages of dementia, amyotrophic lateral sclerosis, Parkinson's disease, multiple sclerosis, or in a coma. These patients will have significant brain damage and cannot make informed decisions. In other patients, communication may be difficult to impossible because of loss of motor control of the larynx or damage to Broca's area in the brain after an infarct. If there is no ACP for these patients, the family becomes the surrogate decision makers after the clinician has assessed that the patient does not have decision-making capacity. Each of these diseases may have a long disease trajectory of several years until end stage is finally reached, and then it may not be apparent to the family who may be accustomed to a slow decline.

Competency is a legal term about a patient's global capacity to make health care decisions. Competency is decided by a judge in a court of law, and it has strict legal ramifications. If a patient is deemed to be incompetent, then a surrogate is appointed. This is usually done in situations in which there is no ACP, no family, or the family is in conflict or otherwise incapable of making decisions for the patient. This situation is uncommon and usually avoided because court dates can be long in coming, the trial process is costly, and it takes time to locate a suitable guardian.

Advance care planning for children with end-stage/congenital disease or trauma requires special consideration not only for the child but the parents and siblings as well. The parents are the decision makers for very small children and infants. Older children and adolescents may very well understand their condition if it is explained in terms that are not technical. Advance care planning should take place with children and their families at a good time after the diagnosis, and not waiting until close to death. It should be integrated into the routine care of the child during office visits, if the child is hospitalized, or any time the parent asks a question about the disease. This openness and transparency to discussing the topic may take away the fear and uncertainty that may parents and children face.[25]

ETHICAL ISSUES IN PALLIATIVE CARE

Ethical issues in palliative care frequently involve situations in which patients are unable to state their choices in real time, and there may be no advance directive, or what is available for an advance directive seems counterproductive to the best interests of the patient. This is especially true in situations of futile care. For example, a 34-year-old patient who has schizoaffective disorder and tried unsuccessfully to commit suicide by jumping from a building. He sustained severe head injury, which the neurosurgeon explains to the family will never allow him to care for himself in any way. He is kept alive on a ventilator and attempts to wean him from the ventilator have been unsuccessful. The palliative care team arranges a family meeting at which the hospitalist explains that their son will need a feeding tube and a tracheostomy in the near future, but it is unlikely he will be successfully weaned off the respirator. There is no advance directive, and the family insists that the patient continue to be cared for in the hospital on the respirator because he is too young to die. Making plans with the family is at a stalemate. Situations such as these frequently require a consultation with the ethics committee, and then further action as warranted by the institution.

Moral dilemmas occur in situations such as this one and are often caused by needing to make a choice when the choices are equally undesirable. Clinicians may feel caught in a quandary. Guiding principles are available from the American Nurses' Association (ANA) Code of Ethics.[26] Clinicians feel there are 3 main types of moral dilemma. The first, *moral uncertainty*, can be illustrated in the example of a patient who refuses analgesics because of fear of addiction. Clinicians may feel that the severity of the disease and the degree of pain reported by the patient warrants an opioid, but in the end the patient has the right to decide whether or not to take the medication. This may become an uncomfortable situation for the clinician and may not feel morally right, especially in palliative care in which clinicians are educated extensively in ways to manage pain. The second, a *moral dilemma*, may be less common but can be very distressing for clinicians. This situation is one in which there may two or more decisions, all may be equally morally correct, but choosing one countermands the others. For example, a parent may be firm in not wanting a child to be allowed to die and wants surgery that has some, even if very little likelihood of saving the child's life. The child is old enough to tell the clinician that he does not want to hurt anymore and does not want any further painful treatment. The third type of moral problem is *moral distress*. In this situation, the clinician is bound by the protocol of the institution, but the action goes against the morals of the clinician. An example of this is nurses working in critical care who are caring for patients who are nonresponsive from an irreversible condition, and there is no plan to change the course of treatment. The nurses may feel this results in prolonged suffering for this type of patient situation. There have been studies to investigate whether moral distress is a reason for staff turnover in acute care, and it appears to be common enough that specialized programs are instituted to help nurses with moral distress.[27]

Caring for others is the moral principle on which ANA's Code of Ethics is largely founded. In this principle, autonomy of the patient is maintained when practice is based on compassion and respect of the worthiness, dignity, and worth of the patient as a person. Patients are given sufficient, accurate, and complete information so that they can make an informed decision. Paternalism is defined as making decisions for patients and is considered a violation of the patient's rights. This is true except in situations where:

1. the patient's capacity for making a decision is compromised; as discussed earlier, this is the situation in which the clinician determines the patient does not have decision-making capacity;
2. the patient is likely to be significantly harmed; and
3. the patient at another time will resume decision-making capacity.

Paternalism in palliative care may be very therapeutic and necessary. In the article "When Open-Ended Questions Don't Work: The Role of Palliative Paternalism in Difficult Medical Decisions," the authors provide a model of this style of communication (Fig. 4.2)

In the figure, reading from left to right, top to bottom, the patient is diagnosed with a life-limiting illness and is well enough to be self-directed with the information provided by the palliative care clinician. It is assumed that early in the disease process the patient has an adaptive coping style. This is not always true as the article describes, and it is important that the palliative care clinician assess the risk factors for maladaptive coping. Some of these risk factors are cognitive impairment, very young patient, serious mental illness, and so on. As the illness progresses, that patient is less self-directed because of weakness or other disease affect, and coping that was adaptive may now be maladaptive. When this occurs, it is important that the palliative clinician play a larger role in making decisions. Open-ended communication in this situation is not helpful

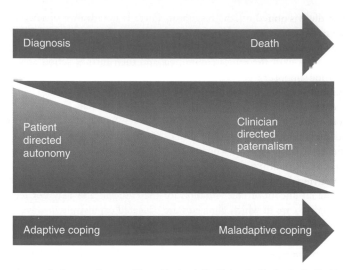

Fig. 4.2 Illness communication continuum. (From Roeland, E., Cain, J., Onderdonk, C., Kerr, K., Mitchell, W., & Thornberry, K. [2014]. When open-ended questions don't work: the role of palliative paternalism in difficult medical decisions. *Journal of Palliative Medicine,* 17[4], 415–420.)

to patients because they are not capable of making a choice that is helpful.[28] Roeland and colleagues based this on the assumptions that:

1. presenting treatment options that are unavailable or are not going to work causes more suffering,
2. life-limiting illnesses have a trajectory that will run out of treatment options,
3. the key to determining communication style is the assessment of the patient's coping skills, and
4. in maladaptive coping the palliative clinician should use focused, directive communication.

This model provides an ethical approach with a rational explanation as to why sometimes the best way to talk to the patient is to be very clear and direct but always compassionate. This seems counterintuitive, but in this example the technique is more clear:

Clinician: "Can you tell me what is going on with you?"

Patient: "I have no idea; I just want to get out of here."

Clinician: "I think it's time we talked about your cancer."

Patient: "I never even want to think about that!"

Clinician: "It is time we had a talk about your next steps in treatment."

Patient: "What good does talking do?"

Clinician: "You need to be cared for. Your treatment now should be to make you feel less uncomfortable."

Patient: "Yes, I would like to have less pain."

Clinician: "There is a medication I will prescribe for you called oxycodone. It will control the pain."

At each step the patient is not participating in the plan but is directed back to the topic by the clinician until a plan is arrived at.

In some situations, there is no agreement and the family (the patient is too physically incapacitated physically at this point) insists on futile care. Futile care can be defined as continuing treatment that has no possible chance of improving the patient's survival and may be causing suffering. This is usually the point at which the ethics and legal department of the institution intercede. In some situations, when there is no resolution, the organization (hospital usually) may not continue futile care. After a court hearing, a surrogate may be appointed or the family may be assisted in finding care elsewhere. This is a prolonged process, with many steps during which the clinicians continue to communicate with the family and offer support and education. The ethics committee also functions to provide support to the clinicians and brings objectivity with expertise to the situation.

Last, the principle of double effect is an important topic in this discussion of ethics. There may be treatment that has benefit but a side effect that is potentially harmful, as is the case with any medication or treatment in health care. The difference in palliative care, and more so in hospice care, is that the patient may die as a result. Family members must be educated about this possibility. The example of the clinician ordering morphine for respiratory distress in a patient with end-stage CHF should be explained to both the patient and family because not only may the respiratory distress be relieved, but the patient may lapse into a somnolent state and could die. This secondary effect is not considered a problem as long as the goal is to relieve suffering.

There are many examples of this in palliative care, and the take-home message is that if the intent of the order is for the relief of symptoms, and this is the goal of care agreed on by the patient, family as the surrogate, and the clinician, based on the medical situation of the patient, then no harm is done.

CULTURAL ASPECTS OF PALLIATIVE CARE

Culture plays a large part in how a person views the world and determines meaning and purpose in life. Culture also provides guidelines for living. Increasingly, clinicians and patients are from different cultural backgrounds. If the present trend continues, by 2060 56% of the population will be of an ethnic minority. This is a big increase from 2014 when 38% of our population claimed minority status.[29] This may mean a mismatch of cultural beliefs on many levels as the current trend of increasing cultural diversity continues. Take, for example, a clinical situation in which the clinician is from a minority group and is caring for a patient from another group. There is the potential for unclear communication and differing expectations. In a recent clinical situation, a patient, by assessment criteria, was found to be someone who would benefit from a palliative care consult. This patient was hospitalized with aspiration pneumonia related to the progression of his Alzheimer's disease. In addition to the dementia, he also had progressing cardiac disease with an ejection fraction of 20% and stage III kidney disease. The hospitalist (of Asian descent and known to be "unfriendly to the idea of hospice") was carefully approached for an order for a palliative care consult. The topic was presented as, "the patient's family is interested in advance care planning and has started a MOLST, but it should be revisited." Palliative care clinicians have experience in having this advance care conversation with the family because "they do it all the time." He was hesitant, but agreed after more discussion. Would a palliative care consult have been ordered automatically by another hospitalist more attuned to and culturally aligned with its benefits? It was interesting to note that this clinician was "known" to be resistant to advance care planning and hospice on general principles that may have been culturally based.

Clinicians, and especially the palliative care clinician, must be culturally competent. Providing care at end-stage disease involves making decisions on a deeply personal level that are founded to a great extent on cultural beliefs. Cultural competency is defined as the recognition of diversity, cultural awareness, and cultural sensitivity. The recognition that there is cultural diversity in every aspect of health care should be an everyday way of working with patients and colleagues. There will be individual differences in the patient's beliefs based on their experiences, education, and familiarity with the health care system as well. Many clinicians of minority groups develop an understanding of the potential benefits of palliative care after seeing the improved experiences of their patients. An example of this is a physician of Jewish Russian heritage who worked tirelessly on advanced care planning with his patients who were Russian immigrants. He explained that most of these patients were denied health care of any kind in Russia. They also had a deeply rooted distrust of authority figures and that included health care clinicians. When asked to consider the possibility of their illness having limited treatment possibilities and potentially poor outcomes from continued aggressive treatment, they refused. Any consideration of a decision other than for the "best care" (meaning care provided at a tertiary medical center) was unacceptable. Choosing other than the best care at a tertiary hospital and all it had to offer meant choosing less, which meant they were not deserving of the best care. This sometimes led to futile care. Our colleague was able to make some inroads with some of the patients because he understood their perception and expressed respect and understanding no matter what their choice of care was.

Cultural awareness on the part of the clinician requires a mindfulness and openness to different beliefs. For example, the patient may be culturally bound to operate within a family structure that governs decision making. In Asian families, the elder is respected, and a person nearing end-of-life may be viewed as a soon-to-be-honored ancestor. These families try to protect their loved one from the seriousness of his or her illness. Decision making may belong to the family, with the eldest male relative having the final say. The clinician, knowing this, would include the entire family in the advance care planning discussion and would not be surprised if the son voiced the decision for the patient, who did not attend the meeting.

Cultural sensitivity requires that the clinician assess the ways the patient communicates. For example, the patient of Asian heritage may be respectful of the authority the clinician has and may express this respect by saying "yes," without actually agreeing with the clinician. To get a truthful answer the clinician may need to be much more specific; instead of asking, "Do you want to hear more about your illness?" to ask "What do you want me to talk about today?" or "Who do you want me to talk to about your illness?" These questions require more of an answer on the patient's part and do not push into the taboo territory. Thoughtful use of translators is important. Children should not translate because it places them in a position of authority over their parents, and they may be asked to discuss information that the patient would not want them to know about. Communication style will vary among cultures; some patients will not appreciate a handshake, being looked at directly in the eyes, or being touched. As part of the clinical assessment, providers should pay attention to how the patient speaks to us and their family members and what words they use. For example, if the wife of a patient says, "I have been worried about his passing away," a good response would be to continue using the term "passing away" and to pick up on other acceptable words and use them as well. Providers should also consider the relative importance of telling the truth. In some cultures, telling the truth, such as saying that a patient has a very short time to live, is not done. It is believed to increase their suffering and instills a feeling of hopelessness. It may lead to a quandary of trying to decide when it is proper to push the discussion forward and when to hold back and continue taking our cue from the patient and family. Perhaps the best answer is to consider the concept of palliative paternalism in the cultural context. This would mean discovering who is the decision maker—patient, family, or a designated family member—and proceeding with the focused, compassionate conversation.

To summarize, some principles of culturally competent care include:

1. Clinicians should understand that our own culture sets certain expectations.
2. An assessment should be done of the culture(s) of the community in which care is provided.
3. Clinicians should be knowledgeable about the beliefs and values of patients.
4. Communication style should be adapted, if possible, to the culture of the patient.
5. Patients should be asked early in their care what their preferences are for end-of-life care.
6. If possible, a cultural facilitator should be found, such as someone of the same culture. Translators can be of invaluable service not only for translation of discussions but to enhance our understanding of the culture.

7. If possible, the office or hospital should be a culturally friendly environment. This may include wall hangings and pictures that depict scenes from patients' cultures.

Cambodian Culture Example. Health care is provided in the context of the community, which may have shifting cultural groups over time. As refugees are assimilated into a community, the health care system adapts to provide for these groups. One such group, the Cambodian community, provides us with an opportunity to examine the cultural impact on care. As background, consider that most adult Khmer (Cambodian) refugees are Buddhists. This religion is based on the belief that all people suffer and that birth, death, and other losses are inevitable. The cause of suffering is having the desire for things and life itself, and the way to end suffering is to give up desire. To do this, Buddhists must follow certain ways of believing and thinking about how to get to a desire-free state. Buddhism does give hope to its followers who believe that a better life is possible once the person detaches. According to an old Buddhist tradition, there are four basic human needs: a place to live, food, clothing, and medicine.[30]

The Cambodian refugee views health as a balance of yin and yang, the elements of "hot" and "cold," and the "winds." To be balanced the person must eat properly, take medicine, and practice certain procedures. These procedures, including coining, pinching, cupping, and so forth, are meant to restore balance. Coining is the practice of rubbing a coin across the skin of the chest, upper arms, neck, and back, which can cause ecchymosis. Clinicians may be surprised to see this and be concerned that the patient is being hurt by family members. Cupping is lighting cotton on fire in the base of a cup, which is placed on the skin to cause a vacuum. This can cause circular marks on the patient's back next to the spine where the cups are usually placed.[30]

Many Cambodian patients will also be taking Chinese medicines, which are trusted and readily available, as well as herbs and roots for medicinal purposes. If clinicians do not know about these alternative medicines they may prescribe medications that interact adversely. A Cambodian patient may not readily give information about these medications and treatments because of their reluctance to disclose personal and private information, which is a tendency that is also inherent in their culture.

Perhaps the bigger concern, particularly in palliative care, is what the Cambodian refugee has had to do to survive having lived through the Pol Pot regime in the Cambodian holocaust (1975–1979). During this time there was mass murder of millions, concentration camps, starvation, and torture. Cambodian refugees reprocess these experiences at end-of-life with suffering and survival guilt. Their suffering can be great and related to choices they had to make during the holocaust. Similar to other Asian cultures, the Cambodians tend to "protect" the elder who is at end-of-life from the knowledge of a poor prognosis, and in some cases the Cambodian refugee has an almost mystical faith in Western medicine so that giving up even futile care is difficult.[30] It is important to consider these aspects of the Cambodian culture because any one of them may influence the choices the patient makes in regard to end-of-life care.

In summary, cultural influences greatly influence whether or not palliative care is accepted and how it is provided. Clinicians must be aware of their own cultural beliefs and those of their patients and colleagues to practice effectively.

SPIRITUAL ASPECTS OF PALLIATIVE CARE

Spirituality in the US health care system is practically a nonentity. Clinicians are schooled in pathophysiology, anatomy, pharmacology, psychology, and many other "ologys," but there is literally no place in the curriculum for spirituality other than to say it should be recognized in our patients in some way, but that way is understudied. This cannot be the case when the topic turns to palliative care. Spiritual care must be considered, and not just by the chaplain and the social worker. All clinicians on the team need to be aware of the spiritual needs of the patient and family for quality care to be provided.

Spiritual care does not need to be religious care, although it may be. Spirituality, while hard to describe, may be easily identified when patients appear to be searching for meaning to their lives or a connectedness to something larger than life. Spirituality is greatly influenced by culture, as is religion. Religion, on the other hand, is much more easily seen because there are established rituals, sacred objects, and texts. Called a life review, commonly seen in patients nearing the end-of-life, patients look for a meaning to their life in answers to these questions: "Why is this happening to me now?" "Is God angry with me?" "Will I be remembered or missed after I die?" Suffering can be intense for patients during this process, particularly if they feel they have come up short. The average clinician has not been prepared to understand spiritual suffering, how to assess it, or how to provide care for it. In fact, many clinicians would argue that this is not a part of their role and may ignore the signs of suffering or totally defer this care to chaplains and social workers. Patients at the end-of-life, on the other hand, expect clinicians to provide spiritual care.[31] Studies have shown that patients may be ready for this care and these conversations, but clinicians are not. It becomes especially important to provide spiritual care for patients who are experiencing existential suffering.

Existential suffering is often described as a loss of meaning or purpose, loss of connectedness to others, thoughts about the dying process, struggles around the state of being, difficulty in finding a sense of self, or loss of hope. Cicely Saunders introduced the concept of total pain, which included physical, social, psychological, and spiritual suffering. Existential suffering, which is difficult to define because so many have a different view of it, is perhaps best said to be distress that incorporates some but not all three of the factors Saunders described as total pain. These types of suffering are connected. For example, a patient may experience severe cancer pain (physical pain) that he tries to endure in the context of his stoical family (social pain), which he fears he brought on himself by smoking all his life (psychological pain) and hopes that by managing his suffering he has control over his life (spiritual suffering). For many patients who have been motivated throughout their lives by the drive to achieve, being very ill and unable to achieve or having nothing to look forward to accomplishing leaves them feeling empty. Patients experiencing existential suffering may present clinically with depression, anxiety, and suicidal ideation and may say they want to die. Patients may begin to experience insomnia because they fear they will die in their sleep. From this it becomes apparent that being able to identify spiritual suffering is important to the overall care of the patient.[32]

Spiritual Assessment

Clinicians should assess the spiritual needs of patients routinely as part of advance care planning; however, clinicians as a rule do not conduct spiritual assessments. The reasons for this are unclear, and they may be rooted in the clinician's lack of education in how to do a spiritual assessment and their concern that this may be information that is too personal to delve into. As part of the advance care planning conversation, and over time as it is reviewed, the clinician establishes a trusting relationship with the patient and family. In these discussions, the clinician has the opportunity to find out what patients value and their beliefs, goals, and hopes. This is fundamental to a spiritual assessment. The HOPE spiritual assessment tool is useful in the clinical setting and is presented in Table 4.2. Some, if not all, of these questions should be asked as part of each advance care planning discussion.[33]

Spiritual Care

The role of the clinician in providing spiritual care will vary depending on the practice setting, but the overall elements are the same: an assessment followed by listening and discussion with teaching and support. Teaching in spiritual care takes the form of clarifying information about the illness and treatment, as well as providing information about referral sources. Clinicians are not expected to provide religious or spiritual education. In primary care, for example, the time available to spend with the patient may be limited and spiritual intervention may seem to be

TABLE 4.2 ■ HOPE Spiritual Assessment Tool

Mnemonic	Questions to Ask Patient
H	What is your source of hope, meaning, comfort? What sustains you, what keeps you going?
O	Do you consider yourself to be a part of organized religion? How is this important to you? Are you a member of a community that supports you? How does it help you?
P	Do you have personal spiritual beliefs? What are they? How has your illness affected them? What makes your life most worth living?
E	Are your beliefs in alignment with your illness and your thoughts about end-of-life? Based on your beliefs have you thought about what you would want for treatment at the end-of-life?

Adapted from Anandarajah, G., & Hight, E. (2001). Spirituality and medical practice: Using the HOPE questions as a practical tool for spiritual assessment. *American Family Physician, 63*(1), 87.

impossible. The intervention may be simply listening to patients in a way that makes it possible for them to feel safe enough to say things that concern them about the meaning of their life. For primary clinicians who have come to know their patients through repeated office visits, this could be a pattern of interaction with these patients over time. In a recent study of how experienced palliative care nurses provided spiritual care there were major themes, such as "being with," "listening to," and "engaging in." "Being with" referred to the clinician's openness and accepting of whatever the patient said without judgment; "listening to" and "engaged in" meant the clinician paid attention to what was being said and was engaged in the conversation without distraction.

INTIMACY AND SEXUALITY IN PALLIATIVE CARE

Sexuality and intimacy are important components of a palliative care assessment. There is research available to demonstrate that patients want to discuss these issues with clinicians. Unless the patients are asked, they may be hesitant to bring up the subject, perhaps not wanting to take up the clinician's time with what may seem to be an unimportant issue. So why is this not a part of the palliative care assessment on a routine basis? As with the spiritual assessment, clinicians are not routinely educated in sexual assessment in the setting of end-stage disease. It is often assumed that the patient is too sick to think of such things, but this is far from the truth. Many patients are sexually active up until the final weeks and days of their lives.

The first step may be for clinicians to view sexuality and intimacy on a broader scope and to just start talking to their patients about sexuality and intimacy. In a palliative care qualitative study, the researchers found that patients described what intimacy and sexuality meant to them:

> If my partner sees me as being sexual even though ... you think you're deformed, but you're not. I think it's their attitude that helps me with my attitude about myself. See, I don't think sexuality is anything to do with the act of sex. (p. 632)[34]
> You know what is important to me right now in my life?.... At home I should be there for the family and be as loving as I can and I know that my disease is progressing and I don't have very much longer to live ... I want to be as nice as I can as a mother, as a wife and daughter. (p. 633)[34]

As these comments illustrate, some patients feel that by continuing in roles that let them be close to family members they are maintaining intimacy. Other patients want to continue having sexual relations and feel very sad that they cannot, or if there is the possibility and the capacity they will certainly continue. The diagnosis of having an end-stage disease and being under care with chemotherapy is not necessarily an impediment. This was one of the themes in the study and illustrated in these comments:

What are you supposed to do when it says something is deadly when you get it [chemotherapy] on your hands, yet they're putting it inside your body—that's pretty scary. So you know it's floating around in your body so it can be passed on … but we went ahead anyway. We just went for it. (p. 632)[34]

We asked the doctor and we asked the nurse if it was ok because I was taking chemo. Never saw a doctor change to so many different colors of red in all your life. I think that we were the first person to ask that. (p. 633)[34]

Or by this example of this questions and others like it that never were asked or answered.

I am so shy to ask them and maybe the same with them. Maybe they are waiting for the patient to ask them.… Sometimes the patient is shy and somebody has to bring it to their attention. (p. 363)[34]

How intimacy was impacted by illness was examined in a quality improvement study conducted in two inpatient hospitals. The results in this population of patients (average age 58), 60% of whom were male, suggested that the patients were concerned with issues of intimacy and sexuality and wanted help with these issues. Recommendations for clinicians were to routinely conduct a sexual assessment and treat modifiable factors. Some of these modifiable factors that could improve sexuality are depression and fatigue, which are symptoms that palliative care clinicians treat patients for routinely. Education to patients and their partners about the barriers and safety precautions around sexual techniques was seen as being important, i.e., use of pillows to protect mastectomy sites and lubricants to protect vaginal walls thinned by loss of estrogen.[34]

Assessing sexuality can be a challenge, but there are tools to assist the clinician, two of which have been in use for years by oncology nurses. These are shown in Table 4.3. The first, is the

TABLE 4.3 ■ **Comparison of PLISSIT and BETTER Models**

PLISSIT Model	BETTER Model
P = Permission: The clinician is open and honest and initiates a discussion about sex; patients are reassured that their feelings are shared by other patients	**B** = Bring up the subject of sexuality: Let the patient know it is an acceptable topic for discussion and get baseline information
LI = Limited information: Patients are given limited information specific to their condition; i.e., what to do about low libido and body image issues	**E** = Explain that sexuality is a quality-of-life issue and is an important issue for clinicians to address
SS = Specific suggestions: Patients are given information about sexual positions for comfort, methods for expressing closeness and intimacy, and interventions to provide for vaginal lubrication and to diminish fatigue	**T** = Tell the patient there are many resources, and assist them in finding them
IT = Intensive therapy: Patients are referred for counseling by a trained specialist (sex therapy)	**T** = Time the discussion to be appropriate to the patient's needs; bring this up at a point early in the care and revisit the topic when wanted/needed
	R = Record the sexuality discussion in the health care record

Adapted from Kaplan, M., & Pacelli, R. (2011). The sexuality discussion: Tools for the oncology nurse. *Clinical Journal of Oncology Nursing, 15*(1), 15–17.

PLISSIT Model, which is a four-step process that asks the patient permission to broach the topic and then the clinician proceeds to educate the patient in ways to solve the immediate sexual problem with very specific recommendations. The intent of this is to focus the conversation, limit the possibility of overwhelming the patient, and allowing time to accomplish the assessment as a beginning step to be continued if needs change or if there are additional problems. The clinician is not expected to be a sex therapist, and any issue that is out of the ordinary or complex can be referred to a trained specialist. The BETTER Model describes a way for the clinician to bring up the subject and reassure the patient. Patients are also provided with resources and educated as to how possible side effects of the treatment could affect their sexuality. In both models, it is important to note that the clinician is the one to broach the topic, letting the patient know that it is important and permissible to discuss the topic of sex.[35]

In summary, clinicians need to step outside their comfort zone and conduct a sexual assessment for patients at end-of-life. The assumption that serious illness means no interest in sex and no capability to enjoy intimacy is untrue. Many patients are waiting for the clinician to begin the dialogue.

Social Aspects of Care: The Family Caregivers

Against the backdrop of serious illness, with the considerations of cultural and spiritual influences, and the management of symptoms, patients receiving palliative care will require increasing amounts of care over time as their condition deteriorates. Much of this care falls to the family caregiver, or network of family caregivers. Family caregivers may be spouses, adult children, siblings, partners, friends, or others. The definition of family is changing over time with the changes in life expectancy, divorce rates, legalization of same-sex marriages in some states, economic and workforce changes, and so forth. A family can be said to be a unit of people who may be related by blood, legal ties, bonds of friendship, or living arrangements. Family may be people who in some way know and care about each other. The definition has loosened since the 1950s when the nuclear family of husband, wife, and children lived under one roof with perhaps one or more grandparents.

Caregivers are, by and large, adult women in their 40s to 60s caring for an adult female relative. There is an increasing number of older caregivers in their 70s and older, and this may increase as older people continue to age and live into their 100s. Caregiver stress is often associated with the caregiver taking the responsibility of too many roles such as caring for children, working, and caregiving of the older person as well. The number of spouses caring for aging spouses with Alzheimer's disease or other diseases is increasing. This may result in the older caregiver neglecting his or her needs and developing an illness as well. The importance of family caregivers cannot be overemphasized. Their care is often the determining factor as to whether or not a patient can remain at home as the patient becomes increasingly debilitated. The family caregiver is unpaid and sometimes unappreciated.

Family caregivers often appreciate teaching and support provided by clinicians and especially appreciate those who visit the patient in the home where oftentimes the care is more personalized and extends for a prolonged period of time. Education, support, and encouragement are frequently required with periods of respite care (where someone else takes in or cares for the patient for a period of time, such as adult daycare, homemakers, and personal care attendants). Providing support to family caregivers can make the difference in helping ensure a successful at-home care program during palliative care. Table 4.4 summarizes the importance of caregivers and why it is necessary to support them in their role.

TABLE 4.4 ■ Characteristics of Caregivers

Caregiver Needs	Explanation
1. Family caregivers typically have unmet needs and problems	Caregivers: • Are prone to physical and psychological morbidity • Approximately 50% of caregivers are below population norms on physical health and rates of probable depression and anxiety • Are responsible for numerous tasks, such as symptom management • Are financially disadvantaged • Become socially isolated • Report unmet needs (typically aligned with lack of information about the caregiver role) • Have needs equal to and/or greater than the needs of patients
2. Confounding factors affect the caregiving role	Caregivers: • Have very limited firsthand exposure to death and dying • Are often excluded from information and care planning and consequently feel underprepared for their role
3. Caregivers have the potential for positive outcomes and gains	Caregivers: • Can contemporaneously improve the care of palliative care patients • Have the potential (with suitable support) to gain positive outcomes from the role • Are pivotal to achieving "successful" home care (where most people prefer to die) • Make a remarkable economic contribution to health care • May significantly enhance the well-being of patients when they are well supported

Adapted from Hudson, P. & Payne, S. (2011). Family caregivers and palliative care: current status and agenda for the future. *Journal of Palliative Medicine, 14*(7), 864–869.

Overview of Pain and Pain Assessment

Pain is the number one symptom of concern in palliative care, and is often classified by itself aside from dyspnea, fatigue, nausea, vomiting, and so on. Perhaps because it is so prevalent, and its treatment so complex, it receives this special designation. The treatment of pain, especially from the viewpoint of the palliative care clinician who is asked to consult for pain management, is multifocal. It involves not only the assessment of pain in the individual patient with recommendations for treatment but also support and education to the primary clinician who writes the orders or prescription. Many times this is because the primary clinician is unfamiliar with the dosing that may be required for adequate pain management.

BARRIERS AND FACILITATORS IN PAIN ASSESSMENT AND MANAGEMENT

There are several barriers to adequate pain management. In a recent systematic review, the findings suggested that the patient, caregivers (family, friends, and others), the prescribing clinician, and the health care system were significant barriers to effective pain assessment and treatment in patients with cancer. Unfortunately, despite the education that clinicians have concerning pain assessment, i.e., pain is what the patient says it is,[36] clinicians were still using "objective pain assessments" (the patient had to look like he was in pain). This led to mistrust on the part of the patient who did not feel believed. This in turn resulted in patients not reporting pain going

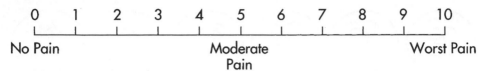

Fig. 4.3 Numeric pain scale.

forward and a likelihood of the patient suffering needlessly and an undermined patient–clinician relationship. This study demonstrated that pain scales and objective assessment of the patient, while necessary, were only a part of a pain assessment. Patients want and need to have their pain assessed holistically and individually. This holistic assessment takes into consideration the physical, emotional, cultural, and spiritual aspects of the perception of pain. Patients in this study were most concerned with how pain interfered with their daily life, and wanted this interference managed rather than the complete absence of pain per se. Communication between sites of care during transitions in care needed to be strengthened so that successful management of pain was continued at the new site of care or the challenges of pain management were reassessed. Overall, including the patient in choices of pain management, some of which were nonpharmacologic and fostering the patient's ability to self-manage pain, could lead to improved outcomes in pain management.[37]

Many patients and families are concerned that the patient will become addicted to narcotics and believe that postponing taking opioids until the patient is nearing death is the best choice. Others believe that administering opioids at end-of-life hastens death. Educating patients and families is part of the process to improving pain management while assessing their beliefs, and working within their belief system may provide the best answer. There are several ways to accomplish this, and two examples will be discussed here.

The first example incorporates some of the elements of cultural competence previously discussed. When viewed as part of pain assessment, how the patient and family view pain will determine how much they disclose in a pain assessment and how they express pain. Some cultural groups will be stoic, thinking pain is part of God's plan and that enduring it is a sign of strength, or that it is unacceptable to complain of pain. Stoic pain behavior, or not showing signs of pain such as grimacing, crying, or moaning, can lead to an inaccurate pain assessment and suffering. Some of these cultural groups report lower numbers on pain scales, but this does not mean that the tools are ineffective; rather, it means that pain assessment should be conducted within the entire context of the culture. Some cultures will equate the use of opioids with end-of-life and will reserve use until then, and other cultures perceive opioids as medication for euthanasia. Pain scales used effectively for minority groups include the numeric pain rating scale and the visual analog scale with faces (Figs. 4.3 and 4.4). Patients can mark on the tool where their pain is. Pain 5/10, for example, signifies moderate pain on the numeric pain scale.

In the visual analog scale, the downturn of the mouth and sad eyes signifies moderate pain. These scales must be used in tandem with a thorough pain assessment that incorporates these elements: when did the pain start, what does it feel like, where does it radiate, and what makes it better or worse.

A second way to assess and manage pain was described in a quality improvement study conducted to assess the personal pain goals of patients. Patients developed a personalized pain management plan in which they were asked to describe the pain level they would find to be acceptable. Their pain description was not linked to a pain scale but rather to their perception and description of pain. Next, they were educated as to the types of analgesics available for their pain with the possible side effects and ways to manage these. Patients became more active participants not only in their own pain assessment but in their treatment. The researchers noted that traditional pain scales "fixate on numbers" rather than personal goals for pain management. These patients

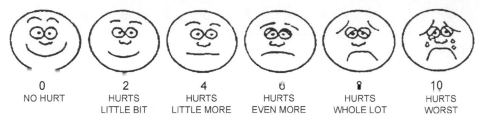

0	2	4	6	8	10
NO HURT	HURTS LITTLE BIT	HURTS LITTLE MORE	HURTS EVEN MORE	HURTS WHOLE LOT	HURTS WORST

Fig. 4.4 Wong-Baker FACES pain rating scale. (From Wong-Baker FACES Foundation [2016]. Wong-Baker FACES® Pain Rating Scale. Retrieved with permission from http://www.WongBakerFACES.org. Originally published in *Whaley & Wong's Nursing Care of Infants and Children.* © Elsevier.)

had improved satisfaction and reported that the clinicians listened to their concerns and focused on providing quality care rather than being focused on numbers.[38]

Assessing and educating the patient and family about how analgesics work, clarifying terms, and not using the word "narcotic" and instead using the term "opioid" is sometimes helpful. For the purposes of this discussion the following terms and definitions are helpful:

1. **Addiction:** Refers to a disease state that has genetic, environmental, and psychosocial factors. It is characterized by impaired control over a behavior or substance use, with compulsive use of a substance or behaviors despite possible harm. Note that behaviors are included in this definition because addiction to smoking, gambling, sex, shopping, use of street drugs, and so forth may have serious consequences to the quality of life and interfere with pain management.
2. **Physical dependence:** Refers to the body's adaptation to a drug or behavior that can be manifested by abrupt cessation or dose reduction.
3. **Tolerance:** Refers to the bodily adaptation with repeated exposure to the drug or the behavior over time. It is important to note that increased doses of opioids may be necessary because of disease progression and not just tolerance.
4. **Pseudo-addiction:** Refers to the patient asking for pain medication "on the hour" when the pain is not adequately managed. This is a problem of insufficient dosing in the first place.
5. **Diversion:** Refers to the use of legally prescribed medications by others for whom the drug was not intended.[39]

Addiction can be present in patients with end-stage disease and their pain requires careful assessment of the patient's background and habits. Patients may not be forthcoming in disclosing their use of addictive substances or behaviors, which may become apparent during an inpatient stay when the patient does not have access to the "drug of choice" and may present with withdrawal symptoms. In the outpatient setting, the patient may not respond to analgesics as expected and require larger doses at the outset of pain management, or may admit to addictive behaviors. In these circumstances, the clinician should obtain toxicology screening and adjust analgesia accordingly. These patients usually require a treatment contract that outlines the limits of treatment and the required activity of the patient and ongoing toxicology screening. The majority of patients at end-stage disease do not have an addiction and should be counseled that taking opioids does not make them an addict. Addictive behaviors are present well before the patient starts to take the medication, and if there is a problem, the patient will be assessed and treated in such a way that their pain is managed.

Key to managing pain is assessing the type of pain the patient is experiencing and the factors that influence pain perception. In Fig. 4.5 the factors influencing pain perception are summarized. Physical factors include changes in sensorium, damage to the nervous system, rest, fatigue, nutrition, hydration, and the disease itself. Psychological factors such as depression, mental illness, and grief may negatively impact that patient's ability to see the pain experience as being controllable. Social

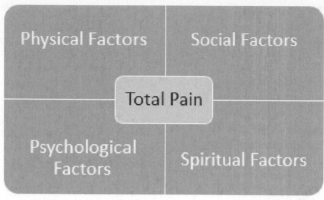

Fig. 4.5 Total pain perception.

factors such as isolation, family support, and a sense of connectedness greatly influence the patient's ability to see the effectiveness of treatment. Spiritual factors can give meaning to the pain experience or cause the patient to suffer greatly.

Pain assessment is unfortunately not well done in the United States, especially in children or in cognitively impaired patients who present special challenges. In a landmark study Ferrell and colleagues found that cognitively impaired elders were under-treated for pain.[40] This continues to be the case for reasons not entirely known, but efforts are being made to improve this. In one study, researchers found that pain management was improved when nurses asked these specific questions:

1. Do you have any pain right now?
2. Do you have pain every day?
3. Does pain keep you from sleeping at night?
4. Does pain keep you from participating in activities?
5. Do you tell the nurse about your pain?
6. Does the nursing staff ask you about your pain?
7. Would you prefer to take medication for your pain?[41]

This supports the notion that individual consideration of the patient, rather than just asking for a number on a rating scale, improves pain assessment.

TYPES OF PAIN

Pain types can be categorized as acute, chronic, malignant, nociceptive, neuropathic opioid-induced, and mixed. Additionally, visceral pain refers to pain originating from the hollow organs, which is diffuse and difficult to localize; somatic pain originating from muscle and bone; and referred pain. Acute pain occurs after an injury, infection, sudden increase in pressure in an enclosed space, or other factors. For acute pain the pain sensation is immediate, the cause is known, and the duration is less than 3 months. Chronic pain can be caused by multiple causes including chronic diseases such as diabetic neuropathy. The duration of chronic pain is 3 months or longer and often includes damage to the nervous tissue and remodeling of neurons. Malignant pain is associated with tumor growth and may increase in intensity rapidly as the tumor compresses or erodes adjacent organs, nerves, blood vessels, or other body structures. Nociceptive pain is defined as pain that is caused by stimulation of the peripheral nociceptors, which in turn transmit pain signals to the central nervous system (CNS). A burn is a good example; when the finger touches the hot stove, burned nociceptors are stimulated, pain receptors in the CNS activate the consciousness,

TABLE 4.5 ■ Pain Type, Characteristics, and Treatment

Nociceptive Pain Characteristics	Nociceptive Pain Treatment	Neuropathic Pain Characteristics	Neuropathic Pain Treatment
Cramping	ASA, NSAIDs	Flashing	Gabapentin
Crushing	NSAIDs	Lancinating	Pregabalin
Cutting	APAP/Codeine #3	Numb	Methadone
Gnawing	APAP/Hydrocodone	Radiating	Corticosteroids
Pounding	APAP/Oxycodone	Burning	Tricyclic antidepressants;
Pressing	Tramadol	Shooting	i.e., desipramine
Sharp	Morphine	Stabbing	
Squeezing	Oxycodone		
Tender			
Throbbing			

APAP, Acetaminophen or Tylenol; *ASA*, aspirin; *NSAIDS*, nonsteroidal antiinflammatory drugs.

and the motor response results in the finger being removed from the stove. In neuropathic pain, neurons are damaged over time; for example, with multiple sclerosis the myelin sheath is destroyed, resulting in increased transmission of pain signals. With shingles, the neurons are damaged by the varicella virus, again causing aberrant pain signals. Many other diseases cause neuronal damage and result in neuropathic pain, and it should be noted that pain assessment can be quite complex with the combination of acute and chronic pain and/or mixed pain syndromes of neuropathic and nociceptive pain requiring treatment at the same time. Opioid-induced pain may occur when patients develop hyperalgesia after receiving an opioid and pain increases rather than lessens. The reasons for this are under study, but it is thought that the opioid disrupts transmitters on the neuron surface and activate the *N*-methyl-D-aspartate (NMDA) receptor in a way that is similar to neuropathic pain. Last, there is breakthrough pain, which is described as the pain felt when long-acting analgesics on the whole are managing pain until pain transmission overrides the analgesia. This may or may not be related to episodic pain, which is caused by an activity that momentarily worsens the pain experience.

How patients describe their pain will help determine its type, location, and whether or not it is nociceptive or neuropathic in origin (Table 4.5). Nociceptive pain is well managed with nonsteroidal antiinflammatory drugs (NSAIDs) and opioids as a rule. Neuropathic pain is not as receptive to opioids (with the exception of methadone) as nociceptive pain and is best controlled with neuroleptics and anticonvulsants.

PAIN PERCEPTION AND METABOLISM OF ANALGESICS

Pain perception and successful pharmacologic treatment are connected. One theory of pain perception, the Gate Control Theory, explains that pain is recognized in the brain only after the gate in the spinal cord has been sufficiently stimulated by impulses conducted along neurons activated by neurotransmitters (serotonin, acetylcholine, GABA, dopamine, norepinephrine, epinephrine, and glutamate).[42] Pharmacologic treatment of moderate and severe pain is directed at the opioid receptors: kappa, delta, and mu and the NMDA receptor. Opioids, such as morphine, oxycodone, fentanyl, and levorphanol, activate the mu receptors making them effective in the treatment of nociceptive pain.[43] Methadone and ketamine activate the NMDA receptors, which make them more effective in the treatment of neuropathic pain.[44]

Pain management is also dependent on how quickly medications are metabolized in the patient's system. This is dependent on the patient's individual characteristics (kidney, liver, cardiac, and respiratory function), age-related factors (metabolism is different in pediatric and geriatric

TABLE 4.6 ■ Some Drugs That Inhibit or Induce Opioid Metabolism

CYP450 Inhibitors	CYP450 Inducers
• Amiodarone	• Rifampin
• Quinidine	• Dexamethasone
• Chlorpromazine	
• Duloxetine	
• Escitalopram	
• Bupropion	
• Moclobemide	
• Ranitidine	
• Celecoxib	

Adapted from Gudin, J. (2012). Opioid therapies and cytochrome P450 interactions. *Journal of Pain and Symptom Management, 44*(6S), S4–S14.

patients), and enzyme systems (cytochrome P450 3A4). This system may activate, inhibit, or intensify the action of certain drugs by regulating how quickly the drug is metabolized. Medications that are taken jointly with opioids may act as inhibitors or inducers and will affect metabolism of the opioid as well (Table 4.6). If at all possible, clinicians should use opioids that are not metabolized via the CYP450 system (morphine, hydromorphone, oxymorphone, and tapentadol) and, if this is not possible, a careful assessment of all the other medications being taken and renal and hepatic function should be done. Understanding that the CYP450 system will affect drug metabolism will guide the clinician in prescribing the safest, therapeutic dose.[42]

THE WORLD HEALTH ORGANIZATION CLASSIFICATION AND TREATMENT OF PAIN

WHO developed a three-step ladder for analgesia for cancer patients that is also used in palliative care for patients who have a variety of end-stage diseases (Fig. 4.6). At step 1, the patient experiences mild pain, which should be treated with NSAIDs, acetaminophen, and adjuvants if needed (there will more discussion about these later). At step 2, the patient experiences moderate pain, which should be treated with low-dose opioids combined with an NSAID or acetaminophen such as acetaminophen with codeine, acetaminophen with hydrocodone, acetaminophen with oxycodone, or tramadol. At step 3, the patient experiences severe pain, which is treated with opioids such as morphine, oxycodone, fentanyl, hydromorphone, and methadone. These and other medications in this class should be titrated to the effective dose, and clinicians should understand that there is no ceiling dose to these drugs. As the patient's disease progresses, the doses may need to be increased substantially for more adequate pain management.

Pharmacologic Treatment

Step 1   World Health Organization Pain Ladder Medications. At step 1 of the WHO pain ladder nonopioids, such as acetaminophen and products that include acetaminophen, can provide adequate pain relief. Assessing the total dosage of all products that a patient may be taking is wise to ensure that the total dosage of acetaminophen does not exceed 2000 milligrams/day in patients. Hepatic damage can occur over time with doses of 2000 milligrams/day with normal liver function, and in dosages more than 3000 milligrams/day acute hepatic damage can occur.

NSAIDs and step 1 analgesics are very effective for mild pain management and act as antiinflammatory, analgesic, and antipyretic agents. Examples of these include aspirin, ibuprofen (e.g., Motrin), and naproxen (e.g., Naprosyn). NSAIDS are particularly useful in relieving bone pain and dysmenorrhea. The mechanism of action includes the inhibition of prostaglandins by blocking

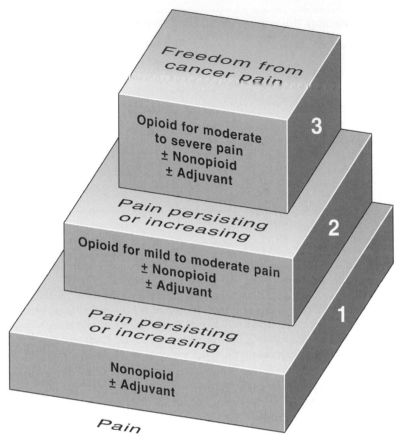

Fig. 4.6 World Health Organization pain ladder. (From the World Health Organization [1996]. *Cancer pain relief*. Geneva, Switzerland: World Health Organization.)

cyclooxygenase. Prostaglandins are rich in the periosteum of the bone and in the uterus, as well as other locations. A unique NSAID, choline magnesium trisalicylate, does not affect bleeding time, platelet aggregation, and platelet 5-HT release or plasma thromboxane levels when given in therapeutic dosages. However, gastrointestinal (GI) bleeds and renal dysfunction can still occur. Celecoxib (Celebrex) is a selective cyclooxygenase-2 inhibitor that was hypothesized to provide analgesia with reduced risk of GI bleeding. Despite short-term GI benefits (6 months), this benefit did not appear to continue with longer-term use. Additionally, there was no reduction in renal effects commonly seen in the older NSAIDs, and the analgesic effect was not superior to the older NSAIDS.[36]

Unfortunately, there are several side effects of NSAIDs, and there is a ceiling effect (increasing the dose will not improve analgesia but will substantially increase the risk of side effects). Side effects include:

1. gastric toxicity with bleeding,
2. inhibition of platelet aggregation (increases risk of bleeding), and
3. renal dysfunction.

NOTE: There is risk of an of adverse effect increasing with the concomitant administration of corticosteroids.

Step 2 World Health Organization Pain Ladder Medications. Most of the step 2 medications are composed of weak opioids combined with acetaminophen or NSAIDs. An exception to this is tramadol, which is available in an immediate release (IR) formula; an extended release (ER) formula (Ultram ER); and a combination drug, tramadol with acetaminophen (Ultracet). Tramadol is a class IV controlled substance with some of the same side effects and should not be used concomitantly with opioids. Serotonin syndrome can occur with the administration of this medication and the concomitant administration of any of the following medications: selective serotonin uptake inhibitors (SSRIs), serotonin and norepinephrine reuptake inhibitors (SNRIs), and tricyclic antidepressants (TCAs). Tramadol also should not be administered to patients with a history of seizure disorders. Seizures are likely to recur if tramadol is administered.[36]

Step 3 World Health Organization Pain Ladder Medications. Opioids are the mainstay of step 3 medications. The most commonly used opioids include:
1. Morphine (e.g., MS Contin, Oramorph, Kadian, Avinza)
2. Hydrocodone (e.g., Vicodin/Lortab)
3. Hydromorphone (e.g., Dilaudid)
4. Fentanyl (e.g., Duragesic)
5. Methadone (e.g., Dolophine)
6. Oxycodone (e.g., OxyContin, Roxicodone)
7. Oxymorphone (Opana)[36]

These medications block the release of neurotransmitters that are involved in the processing of pain. The side effects may be respiratory depression, sedation, constipation, nausea, sweating, pruritus, urinary retention, and/or hormonal changes.

Morphine is considered the gold standard against which other opioids are compared and dosed. In tables of equianalgesic dosing, the morphine equivalent daily dose (MEDD) is calculated when analgesia is being rotated (switching to another drug). These tables are a guide, and each patient should be considered individually. Patients will have their opioid rotated when the dose achieved consistently does not produce pain reduction or the side effects are making it impossible for the patient to maintain a quality of life. Side effects can include CNS toxicity, with myoclonus and hyperalgesia (increased pain sensation). Lesser side effects include constipation, nausea and vomiting, and sleepiness, which can be managed without changing the opioid.

Morphine is available as an elixir of concentrations up to 20 milligrams/mL, immediate release (IR) tablets, sustained release tablets, capsules containing sustained release beads, suppositories, and parenteral versions. Starting dose in the elderly opioid-naive patient is 5 milligrams by mouth (po). Respiratory suppression does not occur when doses are started low and titrated up slowly to the therapeutic level. There is no ceiling to morphine dosing, and patients are given doses to achieve the desired pain control. Oxycodone is a synthetic opioid and is superior to morphine for patients with renal disease because there are no active metabolites. Patients receive this orally or rectally because there are no parenteral forms of this drug available in the United States. Table 4.7 lists the major opioids used in palliative care with the equianalgesic dosing.

An example of drug rotation includes the following: Mr. Johnson has metastatic cancer with severe pain, which has been treated with ER morphine 100 milligrams po every 12 hours and with six doses of as needed (prn) morphine IR for the past 4 days. He has now developed nausea and vomiting, which is typical of malignant pain, and it is increasing and intensifying. The clinician's assessment findings are that Mr. Johnson has a creatinine of 2.0 with signs of delirium. Although the choice may be to treat the delirium and nausea and vomiting with another drug (polypharmacy is to be avoided if possible), the much better choice would be to rotate to another drug and route, particularly because the pain is rapidly escalating. The clinician decides to rotate the patient to hydromorphone. This is an excellent choice because much less of this drug will be needed (potentially

TABLE 4.7 ■ **Equianalgesic Dose Table**

Drug	PO Route	IV, SC	Comments
Morphine sulfate	30 milligrams	10 milligrams	—
Oxycodone	20–30 milligrams	—	—
Dilaudid (hydromorphone)	7.5 milligrams	1.5 milligrams	—
Dolophine (methadone)	7.5 milligrams	3.75 milligrams	Very long half-life
Duragesic (fentanyl) Exception because this is absorbed through the skin and many factors can interfere of foster absorption	25-μm patch = approximately 50 milligrams po morphine in 24 hours	—	25-μm patch = 1 milligrams/hr IV morphine

Adapted from Coyle, N., Layman-Goldstein, M., & Hunter-Johnson, L. (2015). Pain assessment and pharmacological/nonpharmacological interventions. In Matzo, M., & Sherman, D. W. (Eds.), *Palliative care nursing: Quality care at the end of life* (4th ed., pp. 432–485). New York: Springer.

reducing the delirium) and the subcutaneous route will bypass the gut, managing the nausea and vomiting. The conversion calculations are as follows:

Morphine ER po 100 milligrams every 12 h × 2 = 200 milligrams/24 hr

Morphine IR po 60 milligrams in 24 hours (10-milligrams tabs × 6 prn doses) = 60 milligrams/24 hr

Mr. Johnson has had 260 milligrams of morphine in 24 hours.

MEDD calculation: 30 milligrams po morphine = 1.5 milligrams hydromorphone subcutaneously (see Table 4.3).

Calculate from the 30/1.5 ratio, 20 milligrams morphine = 1 milligrams hydromorphone, so 260 milligrams (the 24-hour dose) divided by 20 = 13 milligrams of hydromorphone in 24 hours.

For the CADD pump: this is an hourly rate of 13 divided by 24 = 0.541 milligrams or an hourly rate of 0.5 milligrams.

Adjuvant Medications

There are several classes of medications that act as adjuvants in pain management. Synthetic glucocorticoids, particularly dexamethasone, which is stronger and longer acting than cortisone, is commonly used in treating pancreatic cancer, lymphedema, bone pain caused by tumor growth, bowel obstruction, and cord compression. Inflammation in the pancreas can cause pain because this organ is covered by a capsule that limits its space. When there is increased pressure of the pancreas pushing against the capsule there is pain. The same can be said of cord compression, tumor growth with bone pain, and bowel obstruction. Increased swelling in a confined space causes pain, which is relieved by the reduction of swelling caused by inflammation. Antidepressants, tricyclics such as amitriptyline, and SNRIs such as duloxetine are used in the treatment of neuropathic pain. Gabapentin and pregabalin alter the manner in which sodium and calcium cross the neuronal membrane, inhibiting the transmission of pain impulses. Both of these drugs are frequently used for neuropathic pain. Intravenous (IV) lidocaine is used for refractory neuropathic pain, whereas lidocaine patches are available for local pain, but it may take several weeks to work. If opioid resistance pain occurs, then ketamine is the drug of choice. It can be administered orally, subcutaneously, and topically as subanesthetic dosages (<1 milligrams/kg) for very effective treatment of refractory pain.[45] Cannabinoid extracts are under study for the relief of pain in cancer patients. Used for many years for relief of nausea and vomiting and as an appetite stimulant, research may suggest that cannabinoid extracts can reduce pain.

Considered adjuvants to pain management, surgical and radiologic therapies can reduce pain. Celiac plexus blocks can control pain in the abdominal cavity (particularly useful for pancreatic cancer) and blockade of the superior hypogastric sympathetic ganglion can reduce pain in the pelvic region. These are only two of the possible ganglion blocks that can be used to control advanced cancer pain.[39] Radiation therapy and cyber knife excision of tumors can be very useful in reducing tumor bulk, which in turn reduces pain.

Polypharmacy is a concern in palliative care and is defined as ordering the same class of drug, for the same reason, by the same route, with the same speed of action. An example of this would be morphine IR 15 milligrams po and oxycodone IR 30 milligrams po, whereas morphine SR 60 milligrams po and morphine IR 15 milligrams po is not polypharmacy. The latter is an example of a long-acting medication with prn dosing for breakthrough pain.

Other basic principles of analgesia in palliative care and end-of-life care include:

1. Anticipate pain, do not chase pain. Medications should be dosed so there is 24-hour coverage.
2. Opioids should be started at a low dose and titrated up to therapeutic effect.
3. SR medications should be instituted *after* 3 to 4 days of immediate-acting medication administration and a 24-hour dose is established.
4. Whenever possible the oral route is preferred.
5. There is no ceiling effect for opioids.
6. Fentanyl patches are started (rotated to) after immediate-acting opioids have been in place. It takes 12 hours for this medication to be effective and 24 to 48 hours for it to clear the patient's system. Clinicians should remember that the MEDD for fentanyl is 25 mcg, fentanyl to 50 milligrams of po morphine, or 1 milligrams of IV morphine per hour.
7. Increases in basal doses of SR opioids are calculated based on the prn doses needed in 24 hours and the current basal dose.
8. Patients who have substance abuse issues should be managed with adequate pain medication, including opioid for severe pain. Toxicology screening and treatment contracts are necessary for these patients.
9. Pain perception is multifactorial.
10. The key to adequate pharmacologic management is ongoing assessment of the pain control and the patient's goals for pain management.
11. Remember the axiom for titration of opioid doses in the elderly: start low and go slow.

Psychological Treatment

Because pain perception is multifaceted, it is not surprising that psychological treatment plays a major part in the management of pain. Consider this case example:

Joe is a retired carpenter who worked until 2 years ago with a group of close friends in the trades. They shared good times after work, which usually included a few beers every night on the way home from work. Joe lost his wife of 40 years around the time of his retirement. They did not have any children, and most of Joe's family has also died. Six months ago Joe was diagnosed with metastatic nonsmall-cell lung cancer. He has been at home, isolated from his former work friends who admit they are embarrassed to have not gone to see him, but he "just looks awful since he lost 40 pounds." Joe is being treated for severe right-sided chest pain. He admits to being depressed and has anxiety with panic attacks. He wants more medication or a least a higher dose so he does not have to feel anything. The IDT is concerned that he may be saving the tablets up to take all at the same time. Part of their intervention will be a referral for cognitive behavioral therapy (CBT).

Psychological distress is thought to increase with the increased intensity of cancer pain. Increased psychological distress increases pain perception. Both of these processes can result in a patient with considerable suffering. CBT that addresses catastrophizing, and which enables that patient to feel more in control, can improve pain management. Some of the components of CBT are distraction, humor, and changing the patient's internal dialogue of hopelessness to one of action and optimism. This gives patients increased control in their pain management. The overall goal of CBT is to assist patients to be more active and to improve their problem-solving ability regarding pain, rather than to feel powerless and hopeless. Patients are educated in the cause of pain, ways to manage it, and the action of medications and therapies.

An assessment is done to determine whether or not CBT could benefit the patient. During the clinical interview the clinician reviews the patient's current distress level, health history, social history, family history, and medications. A psychophysiologic evaluation may be done (although this is usually impractical in the setting of a patient suffering from severe pain). Brain activity such as event-related potentials (ERPs), positive electron imaging (PET scans), functional magnetic resonance imaging (fMRI), and electroencephalograms (EEGs) can be used to link physiologic activity to feelings and thinking. More commonly, patients are asked to keep a diary of their pain as it relates to activities and thoughts. The psychological assessment of the patient may be conducted by a clinician as part of a routine visit using common tools such as the Mini-Mental Status Examination (for short-term memory loss), the Montreal Cognitive Assessment tool (better sensitivity and sensitivity for memory loss), or the Patient Health Questionnaire (PHQ) for depression. With the assessment done, CBT can be initiated, along with medication, if indicated. If there are signs of suicidal ideation as in the example, the patient may need to be interviewed more thoroughly to determine suicide risk with an inpatient stay if indicated for safety until the imminent threat is resolved.[46]

Treatment with CBT is multidimensional. Patients are expected to improve their activity level and their engagement in pleasurable activities, reducing emotional distress and suffering. Patients are expected to actively participate in this therapy (note pain may be treated pharmacologically until the emotional distress is reduced and hopefully the pain is reduced as well). CBT is a very active process, and patients must be willing and able to participate in the treatment.

From the example, Joe will be interviewed by the clinician to determine the baseline pain presentation. The social worker will conduct the PHQ-9 to assess for depression and will begin educating the patient in therapies for depression if indicated. He is thoughtful about the threat of suicide and states he wants to stick around a while longer if he can feel better. Analgesics will be prescribed as needed, and he asks to be started on an antidepressant. He is in agreement with having CBT, for which he will have to keep a diary of what he is thinking when he feels pain. He understands there may be other activities that are required of him while he is receiving CBT and will try it to do what he can.

Summary

Palliative care is now part of mainstream health care. This has been a gradual process, with multiple factors influencing its incorporation. Communication skills need to be fine-tuned in palliative care because of the nature of decision making associated with advance care planning. Health care providers are capable of initiating advance care planning and should have the MOLST/POLST discussion with their patients and families, but few providers have been educated in this process as part of their academic programs. This can result in a delay in having these discussions, and in some cases they do not occur at all. Similarly, patients with end-stage disease should be offered discussion about their spiritual and sexual needs. Of the many symptoms that patients with end-stage experience, pain is at the top of the list. Pain assessment and management varies from individual to individual, with guidelines for management established by WHO. Depending on the type of pain, its severity, and preferences of the patient, the clinician should carefully assess the pain and treat when appropriate for the achievement of the patient's pain treatment goals.

References

1. World Health Organization. WHO definition of palliative care. Retrieved from http://www.who.int/cancer/palliative/definition/en/.
2. Center to Advance Palliative Care. (2016). Retrieved from http://capc.org/about/capc/.
3. Elizabeth Kubler-Ross 5 Stages of Grief. Retrieved from http://www.businessballs.com/elisabeth_kubler_ross_five_stages_of_grief.htm.
4. McGill/Palliative Care. Retrieved from https://www.mcgill.ca/palliativecare/portraits-0/balfour-mount.
5. Connors, A. F., Dawson, N. V., & Desbiens, N. A. (1995). A controlled trial to improve care for seriously ill hospitalized patients. The Study to Understand Prognoses and Preferences for Outcomes and Risks of Treatments (SUPPORT). *JAMA, 74*(20), 1591–1598.
6. Field, M. J., & Cassel, C. K. (Eds.). (1997). *Approaching death: Improving care at the end of life*. Washington, DC: National Academies Press.
7. Temel, J. S., Greer, J. A., Muzikansky, A., Gallagher, E. R., Admane, S., Jackson, V. A., et al. (2010). Early palliative care for patients with metastatic non-small-cell lung cancer. *The New England Journal of Medicine, 363*(8), 733–742.
8. Cleary, S. (2016). Integrating palliative care into primary care for patients with chronic, life-limiting conditions. *The Nurse Practitioner, 41*(3), 42–48.
9. Meire, D. (2011). Increased access to palliative care and hospice services: Opportunities to improve value in health care. *The Milbank Quarterly, 89*(3), 343–380.
10. Wheeler, M. S. (2016). Primary palliative care for every nurse practitioner. *The Journal for Nurse Practitioners: JNP, 12*(10), 647–653.
11. Peereboom, K., & Coyle, N. (2012). Facilitating goals-of-care discussions for patients with life-limiting disease-communication strategies for nurses. *Journal of Hospice and Palliative Nursing, 14*(4), 251–258.
12. End-of-Life Nursing Education Consortium (ELNEC) Communication Module. Retrieved from https://cjon.ons.org/sites/default/files/N075441051676053_first.pdf.
13. Goldsmith, J., Ferrell, B., Wittenberg-Lyles, E., & Ragan, S. L. (2013). Palliative care communication in oncology nursing. *Clinical Journal of Oncology Nursing, 17*(2), 163–167.
14. Lichtenthal, W. G., & Kissane, D. W. (2008). The management of family conflict in palliative care. *Progress in Palliative Care, 16*(1), 38–45.
15. Edlynn, E. S., Derrington, S., & Morgan, H. (2013). Developing a pediatric palliative care service in a large urban hospital: Challenges, lessons, and successes. *Journal of Palliative Medicine, 16*(4), 343–348.
16. Crozier, F., & Hancock, L. E. (2012). Pediatric palliative care: Beyond the end of life. *Pediatric Nursing, 38*(4), 198–227.
17. Clinical Practice Guidelines for Quality Palliative Care (3rd Ed.). National Consensus Project for Quality Care. Retrieved from https://www.hpna.org/multimedia/NCP_Clinical_Practice_Guidelines_3rd_Edition.pdf.
18. Baile, W. F., Buckman, R., Lenzi, R., Glober, G., Beale, E. A., & Kadelka, A. P. (2000). SPIKES—A six step protocol for delivering bad news: Application to the patient with cancer. *The Oncologist, 5*, 302–311.
19. Lowney, S. E. (2017). Care transitions at the end of life among Medicare beneficiaries. *Nursing, 47*(6), 36–43.
20. Broom, A., Kirby, E., Good, P., Wootton, J., & Adams, J. (2012). Specialists' experiences and perspectives on the timing of referral to palliative care: A qualitative study. *Journal of Palliative Medicine, 15*(11), 1248–1253.
21. ECOG Performance Status. Retrieved from http://ecog-acrin.org/resources/ecog-performance-status.
22. Nabhan, C., Mato, A., Flowers, C., Grinblatt, D. L., Lamanna, N., Weiss, M. A., et al. (2017). Characterizing and prognosticating chronic lymphocytic leukemia in the elderly: Prospective evaluation on 455 patients treated in the United States. *BMC Cancer, 17*(198), 1–11.
23. Doc Bill Medicare. Retrieved from https://www.usatoday.com/story/news/2017/02/09/kaiser-docs-bill-medicare-end—life-advice-death-panel-fears-reemerge/97715784/.
24. MOLST. Retrieved from http://molst-ma.org/about.
25. Advance Planning in Pediatric Hospice/Palliative Care Part One. Retrieved from https://www.nhpco.org/sites/default/files/public/ChiPPS/ChiPPS_ejournal_Issue-38.pdf.
26. ANA. Retrieved from http://nursingworld.org/DocumentVault/Ethics-1/Code-of-Ethics-for-Nurses.html.

27. Grace, P. J., Robinson, E. M., Jurchak, E., Zollfrank, A. A., & Lee, S. M. (2014). Clinical ethics residency for nurses: An education model to decrease moral distress and strengthen nurse retention in acute care. *The Journal of Nursing Administration, 44*(12), 640–646.

28. Roeland, E., Cain, J., Onderdonk, C., Kerr, K., Mitchell, W., & Thornberry, K. (2014). When open-ended questions don't work: The role of palliative paternalism in difficult medical decisions. *Journal of Palliative Medicine, 17*(4), 415–420.

29. New Census Bureau Report Analyzes U.S. Population Projections. Retrieved from https://www.census.gov/newsroom/press-releases/2015/cb15-tps16.html.

30. Keovilay, L., Rasbridge, L., & Kemp, C. (2000). Culture and the end of life. *Journal of Hospice and Palliative Nursing, 2*(4), 143–151.

31. Ronaldson, S., Hayes, L., Aggar, C., Green, J., & Carey, M. (2017). Palliative care nurses' spiritual caring interventions: A conceptual understanding. *International Journal of Palliative Nursing, 23*(3), 194–201.

32. Bates, A. T. (2016). Addressing existential suffering. *British Columbia Medical Journal, 58*(5), 268–273.

33. Chrash, M., Mulich, M., & Patton, C. M. (2011). The APN role in holistic assessment and integration of spiritual assessment for advance care planning. *Journal of the American Academy of Nurse Practitioners, 23*, 530–537.

34. Holder, R., Kelemen, A. M., & Pettit, C. (2016). Have a Seat at the Sex Café: Discussing and Managing Intimacy Concerns and Sexual Symptoms in Patients with Serious Illness. Retrieved from http://c.ymcdn.com/sites/www.hnmd.org/resource/resmilligramsr/2016_annual_conference/PallCare_HaveaSeatSexCafe_Ke.pdf.

35. Kaplan, M., & Pacelli, R. (2011). The sexuality discussion: Tools for the oncology nurse. *Clinical Journal of Oncology Nursing, 15*(1), 15–17.

36. Pasero, C., & McCaffery, M. (2011). *Pain assessment and pharmacological management.* St. Louis, MO: Mosby.

37. Luckett, T., Davidson, P. M., Green, A., Boyle, F., Stubbs, J., & Lovell, M. (2013). Assessment and management of adult cancer pain: A systematic review and synthesis of recent qualitative studies aimed at developing insights for managing barriers and optimizing facilitators within a comprehensive framework of patient care. *Journal of Pain and Symptom Management, 46*(2), 229–253.

38. Zylla, D., Larson, A., Chuy, G., Illig, L., Peck, A., Van Peursem, S., et al. (2017). Establishment of personalized pain goals in oncology patients to improve care and decrease costs. *Journal of Oncology Practice, 13*(3), e266–e272.

39. Coyle, N., Layman-Goldstein, M., & Hunter-Johnson, L. (2015). Pain assessment and pharmacological/noproviderharmacological interventions. In M. Matzo & D. W. Sherman (Eds.), *Palliative care nursing: Quality care at the end of life* (4th ed., pp. 432–485). New York: Springer.

40. Ferrrell, B. A., Ferrell, B. R., & Rivra, L. (1995). Pain in cognitively impaired nursing home residents. *Journal of Pain and Symptom Management, 10*(8), 591–598.

41. Monroe, T. M., Misra, S., Habermann, R. C., Dietrich, M. S., Bruehl, S. P., Cowan, R. L., et al. (2017). Specific physician orders improve pain detection and pain reports in nursing home residents: Preliminary data. *Pain Management Nursing, 16*(5), 770–780.

42. Gudin, J. (2012). Opioid therapies and cytochrome P450 interactions. *Journal of Pain and Symptom Management, 44*(6S), S4–S14.

43. Pasternak, G. W., & Pan, Y. (2015). Mu opioids and their receptors: Evolution of a concept. *Pharmacological Reviews, 65*(4), 1215–1357.

44. Jamero, D., Borghol, A., Vo, N., & Hawawini, F. (2016). The emerging role of NMDA antagonists in pain management. *U.S. Pharmacist, 36*(5), HS4–HS8. Retrieved from https://www.uspharmacist.com/article/the-emerging-role-of-nmda-antagonists-in-pain-management.

45. Fromer, E., & Ficek, B. (2012). Management of pain in the elderly at the end of life. *Drugs and Aging, 29*(60), 286–305.

46. Kerns, R. D., Marcus, K. S., & Otis, J. (2001). Cognitive-behavioral approaches to pain management for older adults. *Topics in Geriatric Rehabilitation, 16*(3), 24–33.

Exemplar Case Studies in Multimorbidity Management

Weakness

Kenneth S. Peterson

Case Study Scenario

It is 3:45 p.m. on a busy Wednesday afternoon in your family primary care clinic. You have been attending to urgent visits since 1 p.m. and have two more patients to see before 5 p.m. The triage nurse notifies you that she just added a walk-in patient to your schedule. She offers you a brief history that reveals the patient will be Maria Santiago, a 72-year-old Spanish-speaking female with complaints of weakness and blurred vision.

1. What is your plan?

There are three important matters to consider at the start of this encounter. The first responsibility is to think about the approach the health care provider should take to address the patient's presenting problem. Clinical reasoning, differential diagnosis, and symptom analysis are components of the scientific process that health care providers use to investigate patients' concerns.[1] The second matter is directly related to the first and involves consideration of language concordance with the patient. This is important because empirical evidence suggests a strong link between patient–provider communication, health care delivery processes, and patient outcomes.[2] A third matter to contemplate, albeit less of a priority but still worthy, is the notion of primary care practice-based management for patients with chronic illness. Primary care providers encounter numerous barriers to chronic care delivery such as limited orientation to illness monitoring, disease management, insufficient office systems, and limited time for dealing with complex encounters.[3] Efficient use of time becomes essential in producing high-quality health care outcomes for patients with chronic illness.[3]

Primary care providers use the diagnostic or clinical reasoning process to work through simple and complex diagnostic possibilities to reach treatment decisions and manage immediate, intermediate, and chronic care for patients.[1,4-6] Weakness and blurred vision in an older adult can signify a multitude of diagnostic possibilities. At this time, the health care provider should be thinking about engaging in a problem-solving process.

A hypothesis-oriented inquiry is a good beginning strategy. The provider starts with an inductive process to generate nonspecific and specific inferences.[1,4,6] These generalized inferences or hypotheses are used to direct the health care provider toward the advanced health assessment techniques that will best aid in determining the data to be gathered for continued interpretation and analysis.[1,5] This strategy will help focus on the patient's problems and gather the additional specific data needed to ensure accurate diagnosis. The provider should begin to think about looking for clues. Eliciting a history of present illness (HPI) is a good place to start. Obtaining this initial evidence through a series of open-ended questioning techniques will help consider the important contextual information such as the environmental, physiologic, and pathophysiologic mechanisms involved with the patient's presenting symptoms.[4]

In this encounter, the health care provider is challenged with evaluating a patient with symptoms that are potentially the result of both serious and complicated health care disorders. The acuity level of the patient will first need to be determined, and this will help guide the extent of the assessment and decisions for overall management. The provider usually will need a more complete symptom analysis, and the simplest method is determining the seven characteristics of the symptom (onset, location, duration, characteristics, aggravating/relieving factors, radiation, timing) as described during the taking of the HPI.[1,5]

History of Present Illness. Maria tells you that she experienced a new onset of right arm weakness (onset) and blurred vision at 7 a.m. earlier in the day (associated factors). She relates that she has weakness in that extremity, but is without pain (character). The weakness is significant enough that she lost strength in her handgrip and dropped her toothbrush (severity). With further questioning, she denies that the weakness occurred or is present in other extremities or areas of her body (location). She states that the weakness is still present (duration), but as the time has progressed, the right arm feels less weak than it did earlier in the day (pattern). She notes that what also made her come in so urgently today was the result of an additional problem that occurred while cooking her oatmeal. She comments that shortly after leaving the bathroom and while cooking at the stove, she experienced an episode of blurred vision. She describes the vision change as if she was seeing double. She felt as though she was going to lose her balance and fall so she moved to the sink for better support and to be away from the stove. While standing at the sink and attempting to regain her balance, she said she starting seeing doubles of the trees outside her apartment window. She immediately became nauseated but denies vomiting. She notes that the blurred vision lasted for about 2 hours and then resolved.

2.   What are the next steps in the diagnostic reasoning process?

Determining a list of differential diagnoses and prioritizing the probable diagnosis for Maria's symptoms requires eliciting more information about her past medical and surgical history, current medications, social history including daily habits and family history, and a pertinent review of systems. Differential diagnoses for Maria's upper extremity weakness and blurred vision include but are not limited to deconditioning, nutritional deficits, multiple sclerosis, alteration in her diabetes, thyroid abnormalities, anemia, dehydration, visual disturbances, cardiac rhythm disorders, central nervous system (CNS) infection, migraine, brain tumor, seizure, trauma/fall, subarachnoid hemorrhage, transient ischemic attack (TIA), stroke, and vertigo.

Past Medical History. Hypertension (HTN), diabetes mellitus type 2 (DM II), degenerative joint disease (DJD), chronic allergic rhinitis, peripheral neuropathy, gastroesophageal reflux disease (GERD), hypothyroidism, peripheral arterial disease (PAD), coronary artery disease (CAD) hyperlipidemia, allergy to penicillin (PCN).

Past Surgical History. Cholecystectomy at age 39, angioplasty with stent placement at age 66.

Medications Reconciled by the Triage Nurse
    Clopidogrel bisulfate 75 milligrams, 1 tablet by mouth (po) daily
    Gabapentin 100 milligrams, 1 capsule po at bedtime
    Isosorbide mononitrate ER 30 milligrams, 1 tablet po daily
    Levothyroxine sodium 75 micrograms, 1 tablet po daily
    Metformin 500 milligrams, 1 tablet po twice daily with food
    Simvastatin 20 milligrams, 1 tablet po at bedtime
    Valsartan 80 milligrams, 1 tablet po daily
    Nitrostat 0.4 milligrams sublingual tablet as needed (prn) for chest heaviness
    Cetirizine 10 milligrams, 1 tablet po daily prn

Social History and Habits. Born in Puerto Rico and moved to the continental United States at age 15; lives alone in a one-bedroom apartment in a two-building 36-unit housing complex for individuals 50 years and over; completed grade 9; divorced since she was 46 years old; 1 adult son and 1 adult daughter who live locally; a former tobacco smoker (3 pack-years) who quit at age 25, no concerns for current or past alcohol or other substance use.

Family History. Mother died age 82 of complications from dementia. Father died age 57 of myocardial infarction (MI). Sister alive age 68 with CAD, HTN, hypothyroidism, DM II. Children: 1 male age 50 with depression, HTN, DM II; 1 female age 52 with HTN, DM II, breast cancer stage II.

3.   What additional history would be helpful at this time?

Eliciting more detail about her right arm concern is important in determining the cause of Maria's right arm weakness. In diagnostic reasoning, the health care provider tries to consider the relationship of the patient's presentation concerns (i.e., the HPI symptoms) to other symptoms that the patient might also have. This helps test a hypothesis and determine the extent of the problem. The provider is then able to consider the relation of the probable physiologic or pathophysiologic mechanisms that may be contributing to a patient's specific symptom. This represents the further interpretation and refining of the evidence phase of the diagnostic reasoning process.[1,4,5]

Case Study, Continued

Maria tells you that earlier in the day she experienced weakness in her arm and then blurring of her vision. She notes that soon after waking up and tending to her usual morning routine, she noticed that her right arm (dominant) felt heavy when she was brushing her teeth. She said she dropped the toothbrush two times before finishing. With some gentle prodding from you, she further details the right arm as feeling weak but not painful. She says that she didn't think much of it and thought maybe the sensation was the result of lying on her right side most of the night.

Maria tells you that she called her daughter after lunch because the symptoms were still present. Her daughter states that she left work as soon as she could, picked up her mother, and drove her to the clinic. You sense some nervousness and anxiety developing on the part of the daughter during the discussion. Maria tells you she is worried because she still feels her vision is not normal. She says, "Ay Dios Mio!" (Oh My God!). Maria's daughter asks you, "What do you think is going on?"

4.   How do you respond?

Efficiency with time management is key, particularly when considering the seriousness of a patient's symptoms, but maintaining empathy as the provider works against the clock is essential. Addressing the family member's anxiety early in the encounter helps foster trust and enhance the patient–provider relationship (it will also save time in the end). Establishing and maintaining trust in the patient–provider relationship is essential. This is significantly important in managing patients who come from one of the many marginalized ethnic or racial groups in the United States. Patient outcomes related to states of anxiety, well-being, and recovery are influenced by trust.[7] When patients feel trust in their relationship with providers, they engage more often in preventive services, adhere better to medication and other treatment recommendations, and maintain long-term relationships.[7]

5.   What are the key differentials you would consider given the information you know about Maria's current and past history?

Maria presents with weakness of her right upper extremity and blurring of her vision. The best approach to identifying key differentials is to rely on the cognitive process of diagnostic reasoning. Novice providers are likely to rely more on an effortful, analytical method that incorporates deductive reasoning to determine the diagnosis. More experienced providers are likely to rely more on cognitive shortcuts and rapid pattern matching used in heuristics over a slower deductive analytical approach.[8] Whether one process is chosen over the other or both, it is helpful to begin to think about each symptom in isolation. The provider can organize thoughts into categories such as simple, common, less urgent etiologies or complex, serious, acute, or chronic etiologies. In this case Maria's right upper extremity weakness could be thought of as a symptom of overall age-related deconditioning or as a sequela of a space-occupying lesion in the cranium. The blurring of her vision could also be associated with age-related changes in her vision or as a manifestation of a neurologic degenerative disorder such as multiple sclerosis. These two symptoms are also possibly the dual manifestations of one neurologic process (e.g., a cerebral infarct).

The diagnostic reasoning involved in the evaluation of Maria's symptoms must include consideration of all aspects of her medical history and ongoing aspects of her medical management. When thinking about her symptoms in the context of both her present and past history, as well as her ongoing medical management, the health care provider begins to deliberate whether Maria's symptoms are related to an episodic illness or metabolic or neurologic concern.

6. So how best should a health care provider narrow the possible causes of Maria's problems?

The next important consideration for the health care provider is to think about the potential differential diagnoses for Maria's symptoms. This must also be done while contemplating whether her manifestations are related to episodic illness or a metabolic or neurologic concern. At this time, it is necessary to engage in further history taking, as well as a review of systems and functional health patterns. It may also be the time to consider the key aspects of physical examination in relationship to her symptoms and the three categories mentioned previously.

While considering the evolving list of potential differentials, think carefully about whether these symptoms are a manifestation of an episodic illness or metabolic or neurologic concern. Then think about which questions are the most important to ask. The review of systems approach should focus on questions about Maria's constitutional symptoms (e.g., a recent illness; symptoms of fever, chills, sweats, and weight loss).

Review of Systems
> **General**: Denies any constitutional symptoms such as fever, chills, and sweats; she has had no weight loss over the course of the past 6 months. Before this morning, she has not felt ill or been exposed to any others with known communicable illness.
>
> **Head, eyes, ears, nose, and throat (HEENT)/neck:** She denies any face, head, or scalp pain or tenderness. She notes that other than the blurring of her vision today she has had no changes to her acuity or lateral vision. She reports no speaking or swallowing concerns or hoarseness. She has not experienced neck problems or injury to her head or neck.
>
> **Cardiac:** She denies chest pain, shortness of breath, or palpitations. She does not describe lightheadedness or dizziness. She denies paroxysmal nocturnal dyspnea (PND).
>
> **Respiratory:** She denies cough, shortness of breath, dyspnea, or wheezing.
>
> **Musculoskeletal:** She continues with chronic tenderness of her knees bilaterally when ambulating stairs. She denies any new-onset pain, joint swelling, or stiffness.
>
> **Neurologic:** She denies any recent headaches, dizziness, or fainting sensations. She has not noticed any new sensations of pain in her feet other than the burning she often experiences from her peripheral neuropathy. She has not dropped items or felt that her upper extremities have been unusually weak. She denies any "pins and needles" feeling in her hands, arms, or legs.
>
> **Endocrine/metabolic:** She is very consistent at checking her blood glucose levels twice a day and reports her levels range from 150 to 200. These are consistent with blood glucose levels in the past. She states she is voiding regularly and feels hydrated. She has not had chills or felt unusually warm.

Hematologic: She denies fatigue out of the ordinary. She has not noticed any recent bruises on her skin or extremities. She has not noticed any blood in her stool.

Sleep/rest: She denies any changes in her sleep duration and pattern. She reports feeling rested as her usual.

Physical activity/activities of daily living (ADLs): She denies any concerns with self-care. She reports feeling well walking one flight of stairs in her building and during shopping activities with her daughter. She does not engage in daily physical activity other than getting around her building and shopping with her daughter.

Nutrition: She reports no changes to her usual diet or food access or preparation activities. She enjoys her fruits and vegetables and eats 2 to 3 servings per day.

Case Study, Continued

Maria's symptoms of arm weakness and subsequent blurred vision occurred over the course of the morning. She continues to notice weakness in her arm, but the visual disturbance is improving. She states that these symptoms were never present before this event. She has not experienced a recent illness from what she has told you.

7.   What are your working differential diagnoses at this time?

The provider determines that these are transient focal symptoms and suggestive of a neurologic condition, which raises concern for cerebrovascular diagnoses such as acute stroke, minor ischemic stroke, or TIA. The provider is aware that these symptoms are also commonly associated with other neurologic diagnoses such as seizure, migraine, and syncope. The etiology of the transient upper extremity weakness could also include peripheral nerve compression or nerve root compression.

8.   What physical examination should be performed for these particular neurologic considerations?

The physical examination for patients who present with cerebrovascular concerns should include vital sign measurement, a thorough cardiovascular examination, and a comprehensive neurologic examination. Cerebrovascular ischemia often produces elevations in blood pressure (BP).[9] The vital sign assessment and cardiovascular examination should include the patient's BP and assessment for carotid bruits and cardiac arrhythmias.

Maria presents with an acute neurologic problem. The approach to her physical assessment should be a focused neurologic examination. The American Academy of Neurology offers guidelines for a screening neurologic examination. They recommend that the examination for patients presenting with neurologic complaints should be adequate for detection of neurologic disease.[5] Elements of the neurologic examination should correspond to the patient's presenting symptoms of extremity weakness and blurring vision. In this case motor and sensory testing of the upper and lower extremities is essential. Cranial nerve testing should be comprehensive and include all dimensions of vision assessment (cranial nerves II–VI).

Maria's physical examination would include assessment of her mental status, cranial nerves, motor system, sensory system, and reflexes. Assessment of her mental status should include level of alertness, appropriateness of responses, and orientation to date and place.

Assessment of her cranial nerves should incorporate vision with emphasis on visual fields and a funduscopic examination. Pupillary light reflex, eye movements, and hearing should be included. Attention to facial strength with emphasis on smile and eye closure should also be included.

Assessment of her motor system should take into consideration strength determination with shoulder abduction, elbow extension, wrist extension, finger abduction, hip and knee flexion, and ankle dorsiflexion. Observation of gait should be included and focused on casual movement, heel walk, toe walk, and tandem walk.

Assessment of her sensory system should be included with attention to one specific area such as toes. The examination should involve light touch, pain/temperature, or proprioception.

Assessment of her reflexes should include the deep tendon reflexes of the biceps, patellar, and Achilles tendons. Plantar responses should also be included.

Physical Examination

Vital signs: Height 62 inches; weight 210 pounds; temperature 98.4°F; BP sitting left arm 150/90, right arm 152/90, standing left arm 148/90, right arm 146/90; respiratory rate 16, oxygen saturation 98%.

General: Well appearing female in no apparent distress sitting on edge of examination table with her daughter present.

Skin: Intact with no obvious pigment changes or cyanosis, warm and slightly reduced turgor over hand, numerous seborrheic keratosis lesions are present on her posterior thorax.

Head: Normocephalic with thinning hair distribution.

Eyes: Sclera clear, no conjunctival injection or drainage.

Ears: Tympanic membranes visualized with mild graying, no effusions.

Nose: Nares patent, moist mucosa, mild erythema of turbinates bilaterally.

Throat: Mild erythema of posterior pharynx, uvula midline, no tonsillar hypertrophy or exudate.

Neck: No lymphadenopathy, thyroid not appreciated, full range of motion.

Heart: Regular rate and rhythm, normal S1, S2, no murmurs, no bruits or thrills over the precordium, no carotid bruits or thrills.

Lungs: Respirations smooth without effort, slightly diminished breath sounds at bases, no adventitious sounds.

Breasts: Symmetric, no palpable lesions.

Abdomen: Bowel sounds present in four quadrants, nontender to palpation, negative hepatosplenomegaly or masses.

Spine: Mild kyphosis of dorsal spine, no tenderness to palpation.

Extremities: Warm, without edema, varicosities or stasis changes.

Neurologic: Mental status: alert; well groomed; mild slurring of "s"-sounding words; oriented to person, place, and time; serial 7s and calculations intact; recent and remote memory intact. Cranial nerves: I, not tested; II, visual acuity intact; full visual fields (III, IV, and VI); monocular diplopia is present in the six directions of gaze in the left eye (V, VII, VIII, IX, and X), intact XI; slight weakness on right compared with left XII, tongue with slight deviation to right. Motor: no muscle atrophy, strength 5/5 throughout with the exception of mild weakness 3/5 with right elbow extension. Cerebellar tests intact. Gait steady without ataxia. Romberg negative with no pronator drift. Sensory: slightly decreased sensation to sharp and dull across dorsal aspect of right foot, otherwise normal response to sharp, dull, position, and vibration. Reflexes: 2+ and symmetric, plantar reflexes downgoing.

9. What diagnostics are necessary for the patient at this time?

Maria does not need diagnostic testing in the office at this time. The history and physical examination is suggestive of the diagnosis of TIA. TIA is considered a neurologic emergency, and urgent evaluation in the emergency department is necessary. Diagnostics such as brain imaging, neurovascular imaging, and cardiovascular evaluation will be performed in the emergency department. Laboratory analysis for metabolic and hematologic causes will also be performed.

10. What are your next steps?

Primary care providers along with the emergency medical services team are in a position to reduce delays and improve treatment potential for stroke.[10] Maria's examination findings of mild speech

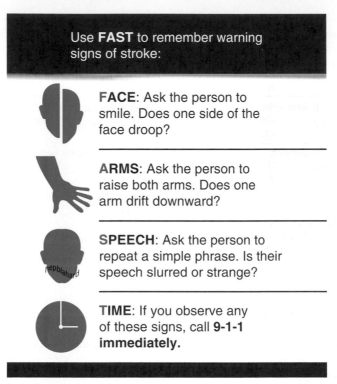

Use FAST to remember warning signs of stroke:

FACE: Ask the person to smile. Does one side of the face droop?

ARMS: Ask the person to raise both arms. Does one arm drift downward?

SPEECH: Ask the person to repeat a simple phrase. Is their speech slurred or strange?

TIME: If you observe any of these signs, call **9-1-1 immediately.**

Fig. 1.1 Face, arm, and speech test (FAST). (From the National Stroke Association. *Act FAST wallet card.* [2015]. http://www.stroke.org/stroke-resources/resource-library/act-fast-wallet-card.)

disturbance with tongue deviation and motor weakness in her right upper extremity are often present in patients with TIA or minor (nondisabling) ischemic strokes. These patients have a higher risk for stroke and recurrent stroke. Her symptoms meet two of the Newcastle face, arm, and speech test (FAST) assessment criteria (Fig. 1.1) and one symptom of the Cincinnati Prehospital Stroke Scale (Fig. 1.2) for a possible stroke diagnosis.[11,12] This places her at higher risk. She needs urgent evaluation in the emergency department. Rapid assessment, emergency transportation, and receipt of appropriate treatment will help confirm the diagnosis, stratify risk, and reduce risk of further deterioration in situations in which a more serious life-threatening diagnosis of acute ischemic stroke is occurring or may occur. The provider activates the emergency medical system for rapid transport to the closest emergency department.

Communication from the primary care office to the emergency medical services team and the emergency department is essential. Details of the patient's chief complaint and HPI need to be communicated. On arrival to the emergency room (ER), nursing and provider staff will determine appropriate care for the patient. It will be helpful for these providers to know the specific history such as Maria's age, time of symptom onset, symptom duration, persistence, and improvement. Important past medical history to relay includes her diagnosis of CAD and DM II. The ER will also want to know whether the patient has any history of coagulopathies, cardiac dysrhythmias, seizures/epilepsy, and prior TIA or stroke. Maria's medication and allergy history should also be communicated.

Cincinnati Prehospital Stroke Scale	
Facial Droop	
Normal:	Both sides of face move equally
Abnormal:	One side of face does not move at all
Arm Drift	
Normal:	Both arms move equally or not at all
Abnormal:	One arm drifts compared to the other
Speech	
Normal:	Patient uses correct words with no slurring
Abnormal:	Slurred or inappropriate words or mute

Fig. 1.2 Cincinnati Prehospital Stroke Scale. (From Walls, R. M., Hockberger, R. S., & Gausche-Hill, M. (2018). Rosen's emergency medicine: Concepts and clinical practice (9th ed.). Philadelphia: Elsevier; adapted from Kothari, R. U., Pancioli, A., Liu, T., Brott, T., Broderick, J. (1999). Cincinnati prehospital stroke scale: Reproducibility and validity. *Annals of Emergency Medicine,* 33[4], 373–378.)

Case Study, Continued

One week has passed since your urgent visit with Maria. She is scheduled today for a hospital follow-up visit. Notes in the medical record indicate that she was called by your medical assistant 2 days after her 36-hour hospital stay to check up on her status. She was well at that time with no new neurologic symptoms. She was not prescribed any new medications. She was then scheduled for follow-up with you today as indicated by your clinic's transitional care management (TCM) protocol. The electronic medical record (EMR) documents that she was evaluated for an acute ischemic stroke and was discharged with a diagnosis of TIA.

11. What is transitional care management and what are your responsibilities as a primary care provider?

TCM services evolved as a mechanism to assist with the high incidence of 30-day readmission rates in patients with complex medical and psychosocial needs.[13] The TCM service strategy is to support the complex patient with the handoffs involved in discharge from an inpatient setting to an outpatient setting. Transitions in care for complex patients are challenging and time-consuming. TCM services involve communication with discharged patients through both face-to-face and non–face-to-face interactions and are reimbursable from the Centers for Medicare and Medicaid (CMS). To receive this reimbursement, provider offices bill for the services and must show documented evidence of their care. TCM services require that providers reach out to the patient within 2 days of their inpatient discharge via telephone, email, EMR portal, or in person. This communication needs to involve more than appointment scheduling. It should seek to gather information on the patient's disposition, discharge diagnoses, procedures performed, and any required follow-up services. Other provider responsibilities associated with TCM services include reconciliation of medications and determination of whether new medications were prescribed. Face-to-face communication must occur within 7 to 14 days after discharge.

Case Study, Continued

Brief Hospital Summary: Maria was evaluated in the ER. It was determined that she required a short inpatient admission given her presentation of acute and prolonged symptoms and examination findings.

Her brain and neurovascular imaging were negative. Her cardiovascular evaluation was negative. She did not require tissue plasminogen activator (TPA) during this recent hospitalization. She continued to have mild elevations in her BP. Her discharge BP was 156/92. Her lipid profile obtained while in the hospital revealed total cholesterol of 230, triglycerides 160, high-density lipoprotein (HDL) 32, and low-density lipoprotein (LDL) 150. The hemoglobin A1C result was 8.8. A carotid duplex study was to be scheduled after her discharge from the observation unit. There were no medication changes during this admission.

12. What are your priorities for this type of follow-up visit today?

Prevention planning to deter future strokes should be the priority for this hospital follow-up visit. Evidence supports the reduction of stroke risk through modification for the following five risk factors: HTN, current smoking, obesity, unhealthy diet, and physical activity.[14] Maria has not smoked cigarettes for many years. However, there are several essential priority areas to address stroke risk reduction for this patient. Maria's prior visits show evidence of BP elevations. Maria's physical examination reveals obesity. Her health history suggests minimal physical activity. Maria also has DM II, hyperlipidemia, and a history of peripheral vascular disease.

13. So where do you begin in regards to implementing medical interventions for these risk factors?

The provider often prioritizes the planning of interventions with a strategy that considers the health care disorders associated with the greatest risk for the patient (e.g., HTN as a risk factor for stroke and TIA has a 2.64 odds ratio of cerebral ischemia compared with 1.35 for the risk factor, unhealthy diet).[14] The best strategy for determining where to center efforts is to research evidence-based practice recommendations for best evidence and work from there. As an example, the clinical recommendation for managing HTN after a TIA receives an A evidence rating,[14] whereas the clinical recommendation for managing physical activity concerns after a TIA receives a C evidence rating.

Initial management to reduce risk of stroke after a TIA should involve the early initiation of appropriate medical and surgical interventions. Ten to twenty percent of strokes following a TIA occur within 90 days of the event.[14] Diagnostic evaluation for Maria during her hospital stay did not identify the presence of cerebral or carotid clot formation. She did not require administration of TPA. She did, however, have elevations in her BP greater than the recommended values of 140 mm Hg systolic and 90 mm Hg diastolic, both of which persisted at the time of hospital discharge.[15] The priority should be placed on improving her BP control. Maria is taking the antiplatelet agent, clopidogrel bisulfate, for her history of PAD in her lower extremities. This medication is also recommended for the prevention of subsequent stroke for patients with a history of TIA.[14] Supplemental antiplatelet therapy with aspirin (ASA) will need to be considered because both are indicated for stroke prevention after a TIA.

Maria's lipid results were elevated when she was hospitalized. She is currently on simvastatin 20 milligrams daily. Prevention planning should include changes to her lipid management. Maria has a history of PAD. A key etiology of embolic stroke is carotid artery atherosclerosis or stenosis. Patients with a history of TIA or stroke are presumed to have disease.[14] Assessment of her carotid arteries should be performed.

14. How can all of this be managed in one visit?

There is no one best way to manage all of Maria's needs. Simplifying care for patients with multiple comorbidities remains extremely challenging.[16] Despite this, it is recommended that providers have a patient-centered approach to managing the complex needs of patients. The provider should begin with adequate assessment of the concerns. This would include collaboration with the patient to involve them more fully in their care.[17,18] An important strategy here is to be sure that the concerns addressed as a priority are in fact prioritized similarly by the patient. Engaged patients who are educated often demonstrate more positive health-producing behaviors.[17,18] When patients are educated about their medical problems, they are more likely to improve their health outcomes. Improvements in patient health outcomes are also associated with interventions that incorporate clinician education and nurse care management.[19] The health care provider may need to involve other individuals in Maria's care and use team-based interventions. All of this will not be accomplished in a day. The majority of the work will be performed over a period of time. Maria will need to return to the office at regular intervals and possibly more often when significant changes are made to her plan of care.

Case Study, Continued

Maria presents for her second hospital follow-up visit and for follow-up of her BP. At the last visit you modified her HTN medications, educated her again on the Dietary Approaches to Stop Hypertension (DASH) diet, and asked her to try walking for 30 minutes every day. There was no change to the isosorbide mononitrate ER. It was continued at 30 milligrams, one tablet po daily. There was no change to the valsartan; it was maintained at 80 milligrams, one tablet po each day. There was a new antihypertensive medication prescribed. Hydrochlorothiazide was added to her medication regimen. The prescribed dose was 12.5 milligrams, one tablet po, also to be taken each day. You reinforced a diet low in saturated fat, low in sodium, and high in vegetable intake.

Review of Systems
Cardiovascular: Her BP at an RN visit 1 week ago is recorded as 152/96. Maria reports no new side effects of the hydrochlorothiazide. She notes no lower extremity swelling.
Respiratory: She denies shortness of breath, cough, or wheeze.
Endocrine: A log of her home blood glucose readings show twice daily glucose levels no higher than 130.
Diet/exercise: Maria reports that she did not use added salt to her diet as recommended at her last visit. She reports having dramatically reduced her usual rice intake. She states that she tried walking 1 day last week but her knees were painful at night so she didn't continue.

Physical Examination
General: Well appearing older female in no apparent distress.
Vital signs: BP sitting 154/92 in the right arm and 154/94 in the left arm, standing in the right arm 152/92 and 150/92 in the left arm.
Cardiac: Regular rate and rhythm, normal S1, S2, no murmurs, no bruits or thrills over the precordium, no carotid bruits or thrills.
Respiratory: Respirations smooth without effort, slightly diminished breath sounds at bases, no adventitious sounds.
Extremities: Warm, without edema, varicosities, or stasis changes
Musculoskeletal: Bilateral knees without effusion, no joint laxity, moderate crepitus present.
Diagnostics: Results of carotid duplex scan reveal 70% stenosis of the right carotid artery and 80% stenosis of the left carotid artery.

15. What is the most efficient method to organize the problems and plan of care?

Many primary providers have adopted the problem-oriented medical record (POMR) as a structure for organizing a patient's medical problems. This approach to organizing and documenting patient problems and diagnoses was introduced to physicians and nurses in the early 1970s.[20] Maria's diagnoses and those areas of concern that were previously identified can be documented in her medical record on the problem list. These problems can be ordered according to the priority placed on them at her initial follow-up visit. The POMR approach involves review and documentation of each problem using a format that includes subjective data, objective data, assessment, and plan. It is common practice for primary care providers who care for patients with multiple medical, health, or social problems to merge the supporting subjective and objective data for all problems addressed at a visit into one description. This is then followed with an assessment and plan for each of the problems addressed at the visit.

Patient Problems

1. Hypertension

Assessment. Maria's BP remains elevated above the recommended range of less than 140 mm Hg systolic and less than 90 mm Hg diastolic for patients with a history of TIA. Her current BP readings show continued high risk for stroke in the post-TIA period. The addition of 12.5 milligrams daily of hydrochlorothiazide did not reduce her BP during a 2-week follow-up interval. She requires more aggressive HTN management.

Plan. Increasing the dose of the hydrochlorothiazide to 25 milligrams daily would not be considered an aggressive change. Doses of 12.5 to 25 milligrams of hydrochlorothiazide are considered in the low range. Evidence reveals no efficacy for hydrochlorothiazide dosing above 25 milligrams a day. A dose increase to 50 milligrams a day may prove to be more harmful in the end given the potential for electrolyte disturbances (e.g., hypokalemia, hyponatremia). It may be more prudent to increase the valsartan dose to 160 milligrams daily. Maria should follow-up in 2 weeks to assess her BP.

2. Peripheral Arterial Disease

Assessment. Maria's arterial disease has advanced and now involves her carotid arteries. Maria's carotid duplex scan results show significant stenosis of 70% and 80%. Maria has been on long-term antiplatelet therapy with clopidogrel since the initial diagnosis of PAD in her lower extremities. Maria is at higher risk for cardiovascular disease. Concomitant therapy with ASA is a consideration for her given the worsening arterial disease. Bleeding risk should be taken into consideration if ASA is to be initiated. Maria has a history of GERD, but has not required maintenance therapy with histamine (H2) receptor blockers or proton pump inhibitors (PPIs).

Plan. Maria should be referred for vascular surgical consult. Communicating her results to vascular surgery will aid in the scheduling of a prompt appointment. Carotid endarterectomy is a recommended intervention for patients with recent TIA (within the past 6 months) and when stenosis is greater than 70%.[14] She is relatively healthy and will likely meet the preoperative requirements for carotid endarterectomy. Maria should remain on the clopidogrel at the dose of 75 milligrams a day. Maria should begin ASA therapy (i.e., 325 milligrams po once a day). Maria should be prescribed the PPI pantoprazole 20 milligrams po daily and monitored closely for ASA side effects given the increased bleeding risk in older adults.[18]

3. Hyperlipidemia

Assessment. Maria's lipid management is not satisfactory despite taking 20 milligrams of simvastatin daily. She was discharged from the hospital with elevated total cholesterol of 230, an elevated triglyceride level of 160, a decreased HDL of 32, and an increased LDL of 160. Evidence supports lipid-lowering therapy to be based on predictive risk for cardiovascular events.[14,15] Maria's atherosclerotic cardiovascular disease (ASCVD) 10-year risk of heart disease or stroke is 40.5% (see http://tools.acc.org/ASCVD-Risk-Estimator-Plus/#!/calculate/estimate/). She is currently on moderate intensity statin therapy. American College of Cardiology (ACC)/American Heart Association (AHA) guidelines suggest that her lipid-lowering therapy move to high intensity.

Plan. Maria's simvastatin 20 milligrams should be discontinued. She should be prescribed atorvastatin 40 milligrams po each day with an aggressive follow-up plan.

4. Lifestyle Management

Assessment. Maria's physical activity is minimal. Maria is obese. Her DJD may be the cause of the knee discomfort she experienced after walking. Physical inactivity contributes to her stroke risk. Regular exercise and weight loss is essential to improving the deconditioning and pain associated with osteoarthritis of the knees. Avoidance of a sedentary lifestyle is beneficial to health. Maintenance of physical activity can improve cardiovascular health and reduce blood glucose levels. Incorporating strategies to support Maria toward a more active lifestyle remain essential to preventing stroke risk.

Plan. Addressing her pain is important to improving her potential to ambulate more often. The addition to her medication list of "as needed acetaminophen 1000 milligrams po twice daily" is an appropriate action. Studies suggest that incorporating resistance exercise is beneficial and effective in reducing pain and improving physical function and self-efficacy in patients with osteoarthritis.[21] Although Maria is less likely to join a fitness facility and begin strength training on her own, she might benefit from a referral to physical therapy to learn foundational level activities for balance, muscle strength, conditioning, and function.

5. Diabetes Mellitus

Assessment. Maria's most recent hemoglobin A1C percentage was 8.8. Hemoglobin A1C percentages between 8 and 9 have corresponding average blood glucose levels of 183 to 212 milligrams/dL. The A1C target for patients who had experienced a TIA is less than 7%. Maria reports that her twice-daily home blood glucose readings are no higher than 130 milligrams/dL. Average blood glucose levels of 126 to 154 milligrams/dL correspond with A1C percentages of 6 and 7. This would suggest that if Maria continues with her current diabetes self-management strategy, her next A1C percentage result is likely to be at the target risk reduction goal.

Plan. No change in her diabetes management is required for today. She should continue to work toward improving her mobility and exercising regularly.

Case Study, Continued

Two weeks have passed and Maria returns to your office for a scheduled follow-up visit. During this period of time she has been seen by the registered nurse (RN) in your office and evaluated by the vascular surgeon. She has been well and without any new symptoms. Her medical record shows a BP result 1 week prior to the nursing visit of 156/94 in her right arm. There was no recorded BP result of the left arm. The consultation report from the vascular surgeon reveals a recommendation for proceeding with a carotid endarterectomy on the left, and then 6 weeks later a repeat procedure on the right. The report notes that to proceed with the vascular surgery, Maria's BP needs to be below 140/90 consistently for at least 1 week before the surgery. Her BP at the time of the vascular consultation appointment was 156/92 in her right arm and 154/94 in her left arm. At Maria's prior visit you recommended that she take two tablets daily of her valsartan 80 milligrams. Her BP reading today is 156/94 in the right arm and 154/94 in the left arm.

16.   What actions for reducing her blood pressure do you take at the visit today?

Over the past few visits, Maria's BP has remained elevated despite the addition of a diuretic agent and an increase in the valsartan. Before making further changes in her medication management, it is important to consider other factors that may be influencing her BP findings. A number of factors contribute to the ineffective response of treatment in patients with HTN.[22] One in particular is adherence to medication treatment regimens. The provider is unaware of Maria having difficulties managing her medications in the past. There have been no concerns regarding adherence to past medication treatment regimens. The recent change in poor control of her HTN suggests a need to assess for medication adherence concerns.

Case Study, Continued

Maria responds to your question as to whether she is having any challenges with taking her daily antihypertensive medications. She replies to you that she is not having trouble taking her medications. However, she reveals that for the past 6 months she has not been able to regularly obtain her medications because of financial concerns. With more questioning, you learned that she has had to make challenging budgetary decisions because of an increase in Medicare drug plan costs. She tells you that she does not have enough money to meet all her spending needs. She reports that over the past 6 months she has had to make the choice to spend money on purchasing her BP medications or buying food and necessary medical treatment for her cat.

17.   What is your response to this information?

Medication adherence in elders with chronic disease is a significant issue in health care. The different factors contributing to medication adherence problems include patient factors, medication factors, socioeconomic factors, health care system factors, and health care provider factors.[22-24] Cost-related medication nonadherence is a serious concern for many older adult patients. Evidence suggests that nearly 34% of older adults alter their medication regimens because of finances. Limited income is identified as a major contributor to reduction in required medication use by patients.[22-24] Patients are often unaware of the impact that reducing medication use can have on their disease treatment and overall health. In Maria's case, it would be most helpful to assist her with referrals to social services and financial counseling. It is important to determine whether her Social Security Income benefits and Medicare prescription drug plans are appropriate and adequate. Medication adherence often improves when a team-based collaborative care approach is considered.[2,23,24] Involving other practice team members such as social workers or community outreach workers to assist would be beneficial.

Case Study, Continued

It has been 6 months since your last visit with Maria. Her prior visit was focused on HTN management, adherence, and financial barriers. She notes lack of recent follow-up because she felt fine and was tired from going to too many medical visits. She reports having had a headache now for several hours. She says she felt somewhat dizzy earlier in the morning and while getting herself dressed. She notes the headache as unilateral and very painful. She states that she does not recall having had a headache like this before. On a scale of 0 to 10 she reports the pain as 8. She reports the pain to be on the right side of her head with some radiation of pain to the back of her head. She tells you the pain feels constant and it worsens when she changes positions or stands up from lying or sitting.

Medications Reconciled by the Triage Nurse
   Clopidogrel bisulfate 75 milligrams, 1 tablet po daily
   ASA 325 milligrams, 1 tablet po daily
   Gabapentin 100 milligrams, 1 capsule po at bedtime

Isosorbide mononitrate ER 30 milligrams, 1 tablet po daily
Levothyroxine sodium 75 micrograms, 1 tablet po daily
Metformin 500 milligrams, 1 tablet po twice daily with food
Atorvastatin 40 milligrams, 1 tablet po at bedtime
Hydrochlorothiazide 12.5 milligrams, 1 tablet po daily
Valsartan 80 milligrams, 1 tablet po daily
Nitrostat 0.4 milligrams, sublingual tablet prn chest discomfort
Cetirizine 10 milligrams, 1 tablet po daily prn

Past Medical History. Past medical history: HTN, DM II, DJD, chronic allergic rhinitis, peripheral neuropathy, GERD, hypothyroidism, PAD, hyperlipidemia, allergy to PCN, TIA.

Review of Systems

General: She has felt well up until earlier today. She denies recent illness or fever.

HEENT: She denies visual disturbance or acuity. She denies diplopia. She denies changes to hearing.

Cardiovascular: She denies chest pain. She denies pressure or palpitations.

Respiratory: She denies shortness of breath, cough, or wheeze.

Gastrointestinal: She denies abdominal or changes in bowel movements.

Genitourinary: She denies dysuria, hematuria, or pelvic pain.

Endocrine: A log of her home blood glucose readings show twice daily glucose levels no higher than 140.

Neurologic: She denies any paresthesias, weakness, or ongoing dizziness. She denies visual disturbances. She denies recent falls or trauma.

Musculoskeletal: She continues to have bilateral knee pain with ambulation. She denies other significant joint pain or swelling.

Diet/exercise: Maria states that she has not walked in the past month. She remarks that the pain in her knees is keeping her from wanting to walk. She reports her diet to be good, and she continues with less rice per serving.

Physical Examination

General: Slightly fatigued–appearing older female, but in no apparent distress.

Vital signs: BP 148/90 in the right arm and 150/90 in the left arm.

Cardiac: Regular rate and rhythm, normal S1, S2, no murmurs, no bruits or thrills over the precordium, no carotid bruits or thrills.

Respiratory: Respirations smooth without effort, slightly diminished breath sounds at bases, no rales, wheezes, or rhonchi.

Extremities: Warm, without edema, varicosities, or stasis changes.

Musculoskeletal: Bilateral knees without effusion, no joint laxity, continued + moderate crepitus.

Neurologic: Mental status: alert; well groomed; speech clear; oriented to person, place, and time; serial 7s and calculations intact; recent and remote memory intact. Cranial Nerves: I, not tested; II, visual acuity intact, full visual fields (III, IV, VI), no diplopia is present in the six directions of gaze in the left eye (V, VII, VIII, IX, X), intact XI, intact XII, tongue with slight deviation to right. Motor: no muscle atrophy, strength 4/5 throughout with the exception of mild weakness 3/5 with left hand grasp. Cerebellar tests intact. Gait slightly ataxic with deviation toward left. Romberg negative with no pronator drift. Sensory: slightly decreased sensation to sharp and dull across dorsal aspect of left foot; otherwise, normal response to sharp, dull, position, and vibration. Reflexes: 2+ and symmetric, plantar reflexes downgoing.

Diagnostics: None at this time.

TABLE 1.1■ ABCD2 Score

Age 60 or older	1 point
Blood pressure ≥140/90	1 point
Clinical:	
Unilateral weakness	2 points
Speech impairment	1 point
Duration:	
60 minutes or more	2 points
<60 minutes	1 point
Diabetes mellitus	1 point

From Daroff, R. B., Jankovic, J., Mazziotta, J. C., & Pomeroy, S. L. (2016). *Bradley's neurology in clinical practice* (7th ed.). St. Louis: Elsevier.

18. What is your assessment?

Maria is a 72-year-old female presenting 6 months after a TIA event with new-onset headache and weakness on physical examination. Headache and weakness are often TIA mimic symptoms.[14] It is essential at this time to determine whether these symptoms represent a mimic or true TIA and ischemia. It is also essential to determine nonischemic etiologies. For example, her unilateral headache might be related to migraines or brain tumor. These symptoms might also be related to anemia from gastrointestinal bleeding given her antiplatelet medications. She has a high-risk status for recurring TIA and ischemic stroke given persistent elevations in BP and severe carotid artery stenosis; therefore her assessment should include stroke risk stratification. The provider should determine Maria's ABCD score to assess stroke risk. This score is based on patient's age, BP, clinical presentation, DM history, and duration of symptoms. The ABCD2 score (Table 1.1) is considered highly predictive for stroke severity, disability, and hospitalization.[25] Maria's ABCD2 stroke risk score is 7. She is considered high risk. High-risk scores of 6 to 7 suggest 2-day stroke risk at 8.1%, 7-day stroke risk at 11.7%, and 90-day stroke risk at 17.8%.[25]

19. What is your plan?

Maria has symptoms suggestive of an active stroke. She should be transported to the nearest emergency facility. She should have urgent neurologic consultation, neuroimaging, cardiac assessment, and laboratory testing. She should be admitted to the hospital for ongoing assessment.

References

1. Dains, J. E., Baumann, L. C., & Scheibel, P. (2016). *Advanced health assessment and clinical diagnosis in primary care* (5th ed.). St. Louis, MO: Elsevier Mosby.
2. Cooper, L. A., & Powe, N. R. (2004). *Disparities in patient experiences, health care processes, and outcomes: the role of patient-provider racial, ethnic, and language concordance* (pp. 1–7). New York: Commonwealth Fund.
3. Østbye, T., Yarnall, K. S., Krause, K. M., Pollak, K. I., Gradison, M., & Michener, J. L. (2005). Is there time for management of patients with chronic diseases in primary care? *The Annals of Family Medicine*, *3*(3), 209–214.
4. Barrows, H. S., & Feltovich, P. J. (1987). The clinical reasoning process. *Medical Education*, *21*(2), 86–91.
5. Bickley, L. S. (2003). *Bates' guide to physical examination and history taking*. Philadelphia: Lippincott Williams & Wilkins.
6. Marewski, J. N., & Gigerenzer, G. (2012). Heuristic decision making in medicine. *Dialogues in Clinical Neuroscience*, *14*(1), 77.
7. LoCurto, J., & Berg, G. M. (2016). Trust in healthcare settings: Scale development, methods, and preliminary determinants. *SAGE Open Medicine*, 4, 2050312116664224.

8. Ilgen, J. S., Bowen, J. L., & Eva, K. W. (2014). Reflecting upon reflection in diagnostic reasoning. *Academic Medicine*, *89*(9), 1195–1196.

9. Simmons, B. B., Cirignano, B., & Gadegbeku, A. B. (2014). Transient ischemic attack: Part I. Diagnosis and evaluation. *Indian Journal of Clinical Practice*, *25*(5), 407–411.

10. Moser, D. K., Kimble, L. P., Alberts, M. J., Alonzo, A., Croft, J. B., Dracup, K., et al. (2006). Reducing delay in seeking treatment by patients with acute coronary syndrome and stroke. *Circulation*, *114*(2), 168–182.

11. Harbison, J., Hossain, O., Jenkinson, D., Davis, J., Louw, S. J., & Ford, G. A. (2003). Diagnostic accuracy of stroke referrals from primary care, emergency room physicians, and ambulance staff using the face arm speech test. *Stroke: a Journal of Cerebral Circulation*, *34*(1), 71–76.

12. Frendl, D. M., Strauss, D. G., Underhill, B. K., & Goldstein, L. B. (2009). Lack of impact of paramedic training and use of the Cincinnati prehospital stroke scale on stroke patient identification and on-scene time. *Stroke; a Journal of Cerebral Circulation*, *40*(3), 754–756.

13. Bindman, A. B., Blum, J. D., & Kronick, R. (2013). Medicare's transitional care payment—a step toward the medical home. *New England Journal of Medicine*, *368*(8), 692–694.

14. Simmons, B. B., Gadegbeku, A. B., & Cirignano, B. (2012). Transient ischemic attack: Part II. Risk factor modification and treatment. *American Family Physician*, *86*(6), 527–532.

15. American Heart Association (AHA). Retrieved from http://www.strokeassociation.org/STROKEORG/Professionals/AHAASA-Acute-Ischemic-Stroke-Initiative_UCM_485512_SubHomePage.jsp.

16. Loeb, D. F., Bayliss, E. A., Candrian, C., & Binswanger, I. A. (2016). Primary care providers' experiences caring for complex patients in primary care: A qualitative study. *BMC Family Practice*, *17*(1), 34.

17. Lin, E. H., Von Korff, M., Ciechanowski, P., Peterson, D., Ludman, E. J., Rutter, C. M., et al. (2012). Treatment adjustment and medication adherence for complex patients with diabetes, heart disease, and depression: A randomized controlled trial. *The Annals of Family Medicine*, *10*(1), 6–14.

18. Li, L., Geraghty, O., Mehta, Z., & Rothwell, P. (2017). Age-specific risks, severity, time course, and outcome of bleeding on long-term antiplatelet treatment after vascular events: A population-based cohort study. *Lancet*, *390*(10093), 490–499.

19. Gruman, J., Rovner, M. H., French, M. E., Jeffress, D., Sofaer, S., Shaller, D., et al. (2010). From patient education to patient engagement: Implications for the field of patient education. *Patient Education and Counseling*, *78*(3), 350–356.

20. Weed, L. L. (2014). Medical records that guide and teach. *Clinical Problem Lists in the Electronic Health Record*, 19.

21. Vincent, K. R., & Vincent, H. K. (2012). Resistance exercise for knee osteoarthritis. *PM & R: The Journal of Injury, Function, and Rehabilitation*, *4*(5), S45–S52.

22. Peacock, E., & Krousel-Wood, M. (2017). Adherence to antihypertensive therapy. *Medical Clinics of North America*, *101*(1), 229–245.

23. Briesacher, B. A., Gurwitz, J. H., & Soumerai, S. B. (2007). Patients at-risk for cost-related medication nonadherence: A review of the literature. *Journal of General Internal Medicine*, *22*(6), 864–871.

24. Yap, A. F., Thirumoorthy, T., & Kwan, Y. H. (2016). Medication adherence in the elderly. *Journal of Clinical Gerontology and Geriatrics*, *7*(2), 64–67.

25. Sanders, L. M., Srikanth, V. K., Blacker, D. J., Jolley, D. J., Cooper, K. A., & Phan, T. G. (2012). Performance of the ABCD2 score for stroke risk post TIA Meta-analysis and probability modeling. *Neurology*, *79*(10), 971–980.

Agitation

Karen L. Dick

Case Study Scenario/History of Present Illness

A 78-year-old man is brought to your primary care clinic by his daughters because they are greatly concerned about his mental status and safety, and they believe him to be confused. His wife passed away 6 months ago, and since that time, they believe him to be more distracted and mixed up about dates. He has been interacting less with family. He does not invite them to his house, and when they do drop by to see him, they find him disheveled, with pots and pans scattered in the kitchen and piled-up newspapers, and lit cigarettes burning in ashtrays left unattended. He has been involved recently in several interactions with his neighbors in which he has been observed to be yelling, and one episode involved a physical altercation. They have brought him here today against his wishes. He has not been seen in your practice in 2 years. Information is obtained from the patient, his daughters, and the medical record.

Medications: Hydrochlorothiazide 25 milligrams/day, lisinopril 20 milligrams/day, aspirin 81 milligrams/day, allopurinol 100 milligrams/day, ranitidine 150 milligrams/day, ES acetaminophen 500 milligrams 1 to 2 tablets/day as needed (prn), albuterol inhaler prn.

Allergies: None.

Habits: Previously smoked 1 pack per day × 40 year. Quit 5 years ago, but has resumed since his wife's death. Ethanol (ETOH) use is rare.

Past medical history: Hypertension (HTN), chronic obstructive lung disease (COPD), history of prostate cancer (status post radiation treatment), depression, gout, spinal stenosis, gastroesophageal reflux disease (GERD), peptic ulcer disease (gastrointestinal [GI] bleed 10 years ago, transfused 2 units packed red blood cells [PRBCs]), and status post–transient ischemic attack (TIA) 2 years ago.

Past surgical history: None.

Family history: Father died age 80 of coronary artery disease (CAD), HTN, and COPD. Mother died age 84 of HTN, depression, and cerebrovascular accident (CVA).

Personal and social history: Retired auto mechanic, widow, 6 months. Lives alone.

Review of Systems

General: Does not feel well, + fatigue, feels tired "all the time." Denies fever, chills, recent injury, or falls.

Skin: Denies rashes or lesions.

Head, eyes, ears, nose and throat (HEENT): No allergies, denies rhinitis, denies head injury, headache, sinus pain, or dizziness, + impaired hearing that is getting worse.

Neck: Denies swollen glands or lumps.

Respiratory: Denies cough, wheeze, or shortness of breath.

Cardiac: Denies chest pain, palpitations, and dyspnea on exertion (DOE).

Gastrointestinal: + heartburn on most days, not eating well, + weight loss. Denies constipation, diarrhea, nausea, vomiting, and blood in stool.

Urinary: Denies frequency, dysuria, and hematuria.

Peripheral vascular: Denies swollen legs and calf pain.

Musculoskeletal: + intermittent back pain described as dull, no radiation, and getting worse over last few weeks. It makes walking difficult. No pain medication and no other joint pain.

Psychiatric: Sleeping poorly, frequent awakenings, misses his wife. "She did everything." Denies seeing/hearing things that are not there. Denies feeling anxious. Unable to say if he is depressed or sad.

Neurologic: Memory getting worse. "It's no good, I was never good with dates." Denies seizures, tremor, arm/leg weakness, difficulty speaking, or swallowing.

Hematologic: Denies bruising. Has had blood transfusions in the past.

Endocrine: Denies temperature intolerance, sweating, and thirst.

Physical Examination

General: Pale, frail-appearing male, sitting between his two adult daughters, avoiding eye contact.

Vital signs: Height 70 inches (177.8 cm). Weight 168 pounds (76.2 kg) (previous recorded weight 3 years earlier 184 pounds [83.4 kg]). Blood pressure (BP) 178/90, heart rate 92, O_2 saturation 94%.

Skin: No lesions.

Eyes: Clear, no drainage.

Ears: Tympanic membranes obscured with cerumen bilaterally.

Mouth: Dry mucous membranes, multiple fillings.

Neck: Supple, no lymphadenopathy, thyroid nonpalpable.

Respiratory: Scattered wheezes throughout, no rales or rhonchi.

Cardiac: Regular rate with multiple dropped beats. No murmurs, rubs, or gallops.

Back: Positive paravertebral tenderness bilaterally, limited flexion, negative straight leg raise, no lesions or bruising.

Abdomen: Soft, nondistended, occasional bowel sounds.

Extremities: No edema.

Musculoskeletal: Gait slightly unsteady.

Neurologic: Speech fluent, cranial nerves (CNs) II to XII grossly intact. Romberg negative. Answers questions with "I don't know." Able to recall two of five objects, oriented to name and place only. No tremor. 4/5 strengths upper and lower extremities. Perseverates throughout the physical examination about neighbor's dog coming into his yard, and is getting more agitated as the visit goes on.

Assessment and Plan

1. Based on the history and physical examination results, what are the possible causes (differential diagnosis) for the patient's current condition?

This patient presents with what is reported to be a decline in overall functioning, with some increase in agitation, decreased memory, malaise, poor sleep, and back pain. It is possible that some of these symptoms are related to grieving and depressed mood. It may have been that he has had existing cognitive deficits that were not obvious while his wife was alive because they may have been hidden. His past history of prostate cancer raises concern for recurrence, with the possibility of central nervous system (CNS) or bony involvement, as well as anemia. A previous TIA may suggest progression of underlying white matter disease. Poor appetite and weight loss may have contributed to metabolic or nutritional imbalances. His long smoking history and current weight loss might suggest a lung carcinoma. Complaints of heartburn, malaise, and weight loss may indicate an underlying GI process. What is clear is that much more information is needed regarding his previous state of cognition before his wife's passing, and more detailed information needs to be obtained from his daughters regarding their observations about his memory and behavior.

2. What components of the physical examination are missing?

Because of the recent death of his wife and change in behavior, an assessment of his cognition and mood is important to evaluate at this time. The patient's daughters could complete the Informant Questionnaire on Cognitive Decline in the Elderly (IQCODE) to help establish his premorbid cognitive functioning and to better understand the trajectory of decline.[1] It also would be important to use a more detailed cognitive screen using the Montreal Cognitive Assessment Test (MoCA) or the St. Louis University Mental Status (SLUMS) test, if he can cooperate, to evaluate his current level of functioning.[2,3] Older adults with depression often have subjective reports of memory loss. Assessment of his mood could be done using the short-form Geriatric Depression Scale (GDS).[4] A review of his record can be done to see if there are any previous cognitive/mood screens to be used for comparison.

3. What diagnostics are necessary for this patient at this time?

Additional laboratory work including a complete blood count (CBC), full metabolic panel, thyroid-stimulating hormone (TSH) with reflexive T_4, and vitamin B_{12}, as well as a noncontrast head computed tomography (CT) or magnetic resonance imaging (MRI), would be ordered at this point to rule out any underlying physiologic imbalances that may be contributing to his change in cognition and behavior.[5] Imaging is done to look for the presence of cerebrovascular disease, stroke, tumor, or subdural hematomas. A prostate-specific antigen (PSA) level is appropriate at this time to evaluate his prostate cancer status. Stool for occult blood × 3 or a guaiac in the office is appropriate to determine whether there is any possible GI bleeding. An electrocardiogram (ECG) and chest x-ray (CXR) would be appropriate as well to rule out arrhythmia, acute myocardial infarction (MI), heart failure, or pulmonary infection. It would also be necessary to obtain more information regarding his use of medications by calling his pharmacy to obtain his prescription refill history and to see if there are other outside providers. His daughters can also collect his current medication bottles to check dates/provider name/quantities. They will also look for any over-the-counter medications (OTCs) that he may be taking. It is also important to do a functional screen by using a tool such as the Timed Up and Go (TUG) to evaluate his gait impairment.[6]

4. What treatments would you recommend for this patient?

The patient's safety is the priority while waiting for diagnostic results because of his confusion and decline in the ability to care for himself. The provider speaks to the patient's daughters who offer to do twice-daily check-ins, grocery shopping, and meal preparation. They will also arrange for help with house cleaning. Aside from the patient's safety, they are most concerned about the status of his bills, and they hope to address that with him over the next few days during one of their visits. The daughters note that one of the sons-in-law has a good relationship with him and has offered to help with that conversation. The daughters will also work to get his medication regimen established using a medication box and will monitor the patient's adherence. The patient's elevated BP is of concern so he should return to the office within 7 to 10 days for a repeat check and to review laboratory and the other completed test results. His ears could be reexamined and cleaned at that time to improve hearing.

Case Study, Continued

The patient returns to the office 10 days later to check his BP and to review his laboratory results and the results of other testing. These include hematocrit (Hct) 38, mean corpuscular volume (MCV) 91, platelets (plts) 168,000, TSH 3.3, T_4 1.6. Liver function tests (LFTs), glucose, and electrolytes are within normal limits. Vitamin B_{12} level is 220 pg/mL. The PSA level is 3.2 ng/mL. The ECG shows normal sinus rhythm (NSR) with occasional premature ventricular contractions (PVCs). A head CT was negative for masses, midline shift, or enlarged ventricles. A CXR was negative for masses and fluid, but it does show some overinflation and basilar atelectasis. A stool guaiac done in the office was negative. His score on the GDS was 7. The MoCA was scored at 22/30. The patient has been accepting of help in the home, and he is eating better. His BP is 148/80, and both his ears are irrigated and large amounts of cerumen removed.

5. What are your next steps?

At this point, it is appropriate to begin vitamin B_{12} replacement. Current practice for older adults is to replace for levels <400 pg/mL with the hopes of improving cognition.[7] Physiologic explanations for his cognitive dysfunction have been ruled out as evidenced by his blood work and imaging results. His BP is 144/86, so there are no changes to his BP medications at that reading because it is within an acceptable range. His score on the TUG test today in the office is 15 seconds (normal is ≤12 seconds), which indicates an increased risk of falling. A referral to the local Visiting Nurse Association (VNA) for a physical therapy (PT) evaluation is an important next step to evaluate and treat his gait disorder. In addition, more assessment is needed related to his complaint of back pain. His daughters agree with the plan for him to have neuropsychiatric testing to further evaluate his cognitive status and to better understand if and how depression is contributing to his current state. Given that his behavior and GDS screen indicated depression, it is reasonable to consider beginning a trial of antidepressants now. A selective serotonin reuptake inhibitor (SSRI) such as citalopram 10 milligrams is a good choice for older adults because of its safety profile and demonstrated efficacy in treating depression. A follow-up of a basal metabolic panel to monitor for hyponatremia, a potential side effect, can be done within 2 to 4 weeks of initiation. If the patient is amenable, a social work consult through the same VNA providing the PT for possible counseling to support him with his wife's death could be beneficial. It is important to evaluate his smoking habit and to provide smoking cessation counseling, out of concern not only for his pulmonary and cardiovascular status, but most importantly, his safety related to leaving lit cigarettes in the home. It is important to counsel his family to begin the work of reviewing his health care proxy status, and to continue to help him manage his finances and independent activities of daily living (IADLs). An evaluation of his driving ability is also critical to consider given his cognitive impairment.

Case Study, Continued

One month later, the patient undergoes a full neuropsychiatric evaluation at a memory disorders clinic in an academic teaching center about an hour from his home per request of his family. Both he and his daughters were interviewed. He is diagnosed with Alzheimer's, disease moderate stage, with depression. The team of clinicians at the memory center recommend increasing the citalopram to 20 milligrams/day and starting him on medications for his Alzheimer's disease, but his daughters want to think about this some more. He is scheduled to return to the clinic to see you in 1 month. In the meantime, his back pain has improved and he has been accepting of PT, which comes to his home two to three times a week for gait training and strengthening of core muscle groups. His daughters have also been putting extra-strength acetaminophen is his weekly medication box for twice daily dosing, which seems to have helped his back pain. The family has removed his car from his driveway telling him it is in the shop for repair. They are conflicted about having to talk to him about giving up driving and are not ready to begin that process yet.

6. What are your priorities for the next visit?

It is important to continue to monitor the patient's general functioning and safety, mood, mobility, back pain, and weight. He will be seen monthly for monthly vitamin B_{12} injections, which will allow for close monitoring. A rescreen using the GDS could be done to evaluate for improvement on the citalopram. A repeat MoCA could be done to establish a new baseline of cognitive functioning and be done at established intervals going forward or during periods of decline. A vitamin B$_{12}$ level could be checked after 6 months to evaluate for improvement. Counseling with the patient and his daughters can focus on maximizing cognitive and social engagement, and exercise. The issue of starting medications for his memory can be revisited. At this time, treatment with one of the cholinesterase inhibitors such as donepezil, galantamine, or rivastigmine could be started. These medications work by increasing the amount of circulating acetylcholine by preventing the action of acetylcholinesterase, which is the enzyme that normally breaks it down. Providing information to his daughters about community-based resources is an important step in the event they need to look for additional help in the home. They had received information from the social worker in the VNA about the programs in their community for individuals with dementia, and continuing that discussion would be important during subsequent office visits. Discussion regarding any outstanding screenings and immunization history should be addressed at this visit.

Case Study, Continued

The patient returns to the office for his monthly check. He has received two doses of vitamin B$_{12}$ by injection. He is now taking citalopram 20 milligrams and tolerating the drug well. He has been seen by PT who continues to work with him to improve balance and muscle strength. They have also completed a home safety evaluation with recommendations to remove scatter rugs, hide cords, and improve lighting in hallways and rooms. His daughters accompany him today and would like to discuss starting donepezil (Aricept) for his memory loss. He is given a prescription for an initial dose of 5 milligrams daily, and is to return to the clinic in 4 weeks for follow-up and dose adjustment.

One-month follow-up visit: The patient is brought to the clinic by his daughter who reports that overall, they think he is doing pretty well. He is staying with his daughter and her family while his house is being cleaned in anticipation of putting it on the market eventually, although not everyone in his extended family is in favor of selling the home. They have been exploring options for care but are still having difficulty getting clarification of his financial status. His oldest daughter has become his health care proxy. He did start the donepezil (Aricept), but during the first 10 days or so of starting it, he had loose stool and they noticed that he was not eating as much, but those symptoms seemed to have improved. His main issue is that he has been bothered by very vivid dreams, which often leave him distressed in the morning. He had been sleeping better throughout the night before the start of the donepezil.

Medications: Hydrochlorothiazide 25 milligrams/day, lisinopril 20 milligrams/day, aspirin 81 milligrams/day, allopurinol 100 milligrams/day, ranitidine 150 milligrams/day, ES acetaminophen 500 milligrams two tablets twice daily scheduled, citalopram (Celexa) 20 milligrams/day, cyanocobalamin 1000 micrograms intramuscularly (IM) monthly, donepezil (Aricept)5 milligrams at bedtime.

Review of Systems
General: Feels "pretty good" no fever, chills, and no falls. Appetite was better before starting donepezil.
Skin: Denies rashes or lesions.
HEENT: No headache or dizziness.
Respiratory: Denies cough, wheeze, and shortness of breath, no sputum production.
Cardiac: Denies chest pain, palpitations, or DOE.
Gastrointestinal: Bowels moving "ok," had diarrhea for about 2 weeks, better now, but still has some nausea after he goes to bed.
Urinary: Denies frequency, dysuria, or hematuria.
Musculoskeletal: Has transient back pain, not every day. He knows he takes medications put in his medication box that help. Uses a cane when he goes outside the home, although

reports less discomfort when using a walker because he can lean forward, which helps the discomfort in his back.

Psychiatric: Reports having vivid dreams, some are nightmares, wakes up frequently during the night, and sleepy during the day. Daughter reports that if the patient does not sleep well the night before, he is "out of sorts" the next day.

Neurologic: Reports continued difficulty with remembering names, and has a system for writing notes to himself.

Physical Examination

General: Well-dressed older male, calm and conversant.

Vital signs: Height 70 inches (177.8 cm). Weight 178 pounds (80.73 kg). BP 146/82, heart rate 78, and O_2 saturation 96%.

Skin: No lesions.

Neck: No lymphadenopathy.

Respiratory: Clear to auscultation.

Cardiac: Normal S1, S2, no murmurs, rubs, or gallops.

Back: Negative paravertebral tenderness.

Abdomen: Soft, nondistended, with occasional bowel sounds.

Extremities: No edema.

Musculoskeletal: Gait wide based, but steady with a cane.

Neurologic: Speech fluent, CNs II to XII grossly intact. Able to recall three of five objects. No tremor.

Cyanocobalamin 1000 micrograms IM given in right deltoid without incident.

Assessment and Plan

Alzheimer's dementia: No safety or behavioral concerns. Will switch donepezil 5 milligrams to the morning to minimize vivid dreaming. Reevaluate function/sleep next visit. Continue support of caregivers, and update advance directives. Will check MoCA next visit.

Depression: Responding well to SSRI. Continue citalopram at current dose, check Na^+ in 4 weeks. Check GDS next visit.

Spinal stenosis: Pain controlled with twice daily ES acetaminophen, continue.

Vitamin B_{12} deficiency: Check B_{12} level in 4 weeks, continue monthly injections.

Hypertension: Controlled, continue lisinopril and hydrochlorothiazide. Check basic metabolic panel (BMP) in 4 weeks.

COPD: Patient is currently asymptomatic and not using albuterol inhaler. Will hold off on changing therapy at this time.

GERD: Asymptomatic, consider stopping ranitidine, and reevaluate symptoms because of risk of polypharmacy.

Gout: Unclear when last flare was. Consider stopping allopurinol.

Health maintenance: Due for PCV13 (Prevnar), PPSV23 (Pneumovax) 8 years ago.

History of TIA: A daily low-dose aspirin.

History of prostate cancer: Obtain urology records.

Case Study, Continued

The provider reviews the subsequent plan of care with the patient and his daughter who agree with the provider's assessment. His daughter asks about whether the donepezil should be discontinued because it seems to be interfering with her father's sleep, which makes nighttime challenging because everyone in the house is awakened if her father is awake during the night. The provider tells the patient and his daughter that case reports regarding dosing of donepezil describe cases of restless sleep, vivid dreaming, and GI problems such as nausea and diarrhea when the drug is given at bedtime.[8] The provider goes on to say that these symptoms can be minimized if the drug dosing is changed to after breakfast. The patient and his daughter agree to try switching the medication to the morning and will let the provider know his response before the next scheduled visit.

References

1. Jorm, A., Scott, R., & Jacobs, P. (1989). Assessment of cognitive decline in dementia by informant question-naire. *International Journal of Geriatric Psychiatry, 4*, 35–39.
2. Nasreddine, Z., Phillps, N., Bedirian, V., Charbonneau, S., Whitehead, V., Colin, I., et al. (2005). The Montreal cognitive assessment MoCA: A brief screening tool for mild cognitive impairment. *Journal of the American Geriatrics Society, 53*(4), 695–699.
3. Tariq, S., Tumosa, N., Chibnall, H., & Morley, J. (2006). The Saint Louis University Mental Status (SLUMS) Examination for detecting mild cognitive impairment and dementia is more sensitive than the Mini-Mental Status Examination (MMSE): A pilot study. *American Journal of Geriatric Psychiatry, 14*, 900–910.
4. Yesavage, J., Brink, T., Rose, T., & Leirer, V. (1982). Development and validation of a geriatric depression screening scale: A preliminary report. *Journal of Psychiatric Research, 17*(1), 37–49.
5. Knopman, D., DeKosky, S., Cummings, J., … Stevens, J. (2001). Practice parameter: Diagnosis of dementia (an evidenced based review). *Neurology, 56*(9), 1143–1153.
6. Mathias, S., Kayak, U., & Isaacs, B. (1986). Balance in elderly patients: The "get up and go" test. *Archives of Physical Medicine & Rehabilitation, 67*, 387–389.
7. Spence, J. (2015). Metabolic vitamin B12 deficiency: A missed opportunity to prevent dementia and stroke. *Nutrition Research, 36*(2), 109–116.
8. Doty, L., & Heilman, K. (2013). Recommendations for the safe administration of donepezil. *Neurology Clinical Practice, 3*(6), 458–459.

Shortness of Breath With Activity

Evelyn G. Duffy ■ Katharine Chapman ■ Terry Mahan Buttaro

Case Study Scenario/History of Present Illness

Ms. Clay, an 80-year-old single female, presents to your primary care clinic complaining of shortness of breath (SOB). She explains that she lives alone in a condominium, no longer drives a car, and depends on public transportation to get to her appointments. She attends a local senior center 1 day a week for lunch and socialization. She is an active member of her congregation and serves on the usher board. She attends services on Sunday morning and bible study on Wednesday night. She has one son who lives in town, but he is unreliably available to help with shopping and transportation. Her two other children live over 500 miles away. Her friends from church provide her primary support.

Over the past 3 weeks she has noticed increasing SOB when walking around her condo. Because of her difficulty with breathing she has felt tired and unable to attend the senior center or church for the past 2 weeks. For the past two nights she has wakened after falling asleep with SOB and sat up in her recliner where she could breathe more easily and be able to sleep through the night.

Medications

Atenolol 50 milligrams once a day by mouth (po)
Atorvastatin 40 milligrams po once a day
Hydrochlorothiazide 25 milligrams po once a day
Ibuprofen 600 milligrams po twice a day as needed (prn) for pain
Levothyroxine 112 micrograms po once a day
Lisinopril 20 milligrams po once a day
Pioglitazone 30 milligrams po once a day
Omeprazole 20 milligrams po once a day
Warfarin 7.5 milligrams po once a day

Allergies: Cephalexin, hives; Levaquin, muscle pain.

Habits: Occasional glass of wine. Denies previous history of smoking.

Past medical history: Atrial fibrillation, cardiomyopathy, coronary artery disease, diabetes mellitus type 2, gastroesophageal reflux disease, hyperlipidemia, hypertension (HTN), hypothyroidism, non-ST elevation myocardial infarction (NSTEMI), obesity (body mass index [BMI] = 52 kg/m^2).

Past surgical history: Cholecystectomy at age 64; colonic polyps removed 3 years ago, benign.

Family history: Father died at age 30, gunshot wound. Mother died at 80 with past medical history of hyperlipidemia, cardiovascular disease, HTN, and heart failure.

Personal/social history: Completed high school, worked on the line at the Ford Motor plant. Now retired. Divorced and ex-husband is now deceased. Two daughters, married and live out of state. One son never married and is presently unemployed. Seven grandchildren and two great grandchildren.

Review of Systems

General: + fatigue, denies fever, chills.

Skin: Denies rashes or lesions.

Head, eyes, ears, nose, and throat (HEENT): + intermittent headaches. Denies nasal congestion, runny nose, or sore throat.

Neck: Denies neck pain, swollen glands, and lumps.

Respiratory: + SOB. Denies cough and wheezes.

Cardiac: + Dyspnea on exertion, + palpitations. Denies chest pain or heaviness.

Gastrointestinal: Denies constipation, diarrhea, nausea, vomiting, and blood in stool.

Urinary: Denies frequency, dysuria, and hematuria.

Peripheral vascular: + swelling of lower extremities. Denies calf pain.

Musculoskeletal: + dull joint pain in knees and back, worse over last few weeks and taking ibuprofen twice a day prn for pain. Denies pain radiation.

Psychiatric: Difficulty sleeping because it is difficult to breathe. Denies anxiety, depression.

Neurologic: Denies memory loss, seizures, and tremors.

Hematologic: Denies unusual bruising and nose bleeds.

Endocrine: Denies temperature intolerance, sweating, polydipsia, and polyuria.

Physical Examination

General: Well-groomed, older female. Mood appropriate. No acute distress.

Vitals: Height, 60 inches; weight, 262 pounds (up 6 pounds in 1 month). BMI 51.16. Blood pressure (BP), 159/104; pulse, 126; respirations, 18; temperature, 98.6°F oral.

Skin: Warm, dry, and intact.

HEENT: Normocephalic, sclera clear, pupils equal, round, reactive to light and accommodation (PERRLA), extraocular movements (EOMs) intact. Ears: scant cerumen bilateral auditory canals. Tympanic membranes (TMs): pearly gray, landmarks visible.

Neck: Supple, no cervical adenopathy, thyroid nonpalpable.

Respiratory: Breath sounds diminished in bilateral lower lobes, crackles present.

Cardiovascular: Irregular rate and rhythm, S1, S2, S3. No S4 or murmur.

Neurologic: cranial nerves (CNs) II to XII intact. Alert and oriented.

Musculoskeletal: Decreased range of motion (ROM) of bilateral knees because of pain. One distal proximal interphalangeal (PIP) joint enlarged with decreased ROM on left hand. Middle finger, two PIP joints on right hand, ring, and pinky finger, also + decreased ROM.

1. Based on the history and physical examination results, what are the "do not miss differential diagnoses" for Ms. C's current complaint? What are the symptoms associated with three likely differentials?

A change in functional status is important information when evaluating an older adult. This patient over the past 3 weeks has had a serious decline in her function. She is no longer attending her church activities or her senior center meal site. She has difficulty walking around her apartment and has had interrupted sleep requiring her to move from her bed to her recliner.

The causes of SOB are numerous and include (although not limited to) anemia, asthma, chronic obstructive pulmonary disease (COPD), pneumonia, and congestive heart failure.

- Symptoms of anemia do include SOB, fatigue, weakness, and a fast heart rate. These are all consistent with Ms. C's concerns and review of symptoms today.
- COPD, cardiovascular disease, and pneumonia are definitely associated with SOB. Symptoms sometimes mimic the common cold but just do not seem to improve, and the cough is sometimes unrelenting. Patients with a COPD exacerbation can experience chest tightness and tachycardia as well. Chest pain, fatigue, fever, chills, diaphoresis, fast heart rate, and

other systemic symptoms (e.g., anorexia, nausea, malaise, weakness) suggest pneumonia. Older adults do not always develop a fever when ill, but Ms. C's symptoms do not seem consistent with pneumonia despite her SOB/dyspnea.

- Waking in the night with SOB and orthopnea suggests that Ms. C had paroxysmal nocturnal dyspnea. She describes feeling short of breath and noting a fast heart rate walking around her condominium, which sounds like dyspnea (i.e., difficulty breathing with exertion). Other symptoms associated with congestive heart failure include chest pain, confusion, coughing, possibly diaphoresis, fatigue (to which she alludes), peripheral edema, and wheezing. Her functional changes combined with her description of her history of present illness (HPI) suggest heart failure. A rapid heart rate, overtreatment of hypothyroidism with levothyroxine, pneumonia or other infection, anemia, myocardial ischemia or infarction, valvular dysfunction, and even medications or stress (e.g., Takotsubo cardiomyopathy) can cause heart failure. Ms. C does have a previous history of a NSTEMI, coronary artery disease, and atrial fibrillation, all of which raise concerns for the development of heart failure. Also of note is her rapid heart rate (her pulse is 126 in the office).

2.   When reviewing Ms. C's history, what further history might aid the health care provider when trying to determine the cause of Ms. C's rapid heart rate and dyspnea?

It is important to carefully review what medications Ms. C has been taking or not taking. If she stopped taking her atenolol, for example, that could explain the increase in heart rate and breathing issues.

She also admits to taking ibuprofen recently. Nonsteroidal antiinflammatory drugs (NSAIDs) such as ibuprofen are associated with cardiovascular events and can affect renal function.[1]

Although ibuprofen might be safer than some NSAIDs, the resultant kidney problems in older adults who already have some renal dysfunction include increased salt and fluid retention. Additionally, the use of NSAIDs and warfarin are also particularly concerning because this combination increases Ms. C's risk for an elevated international normalized ratio (INR) and possible bleeding or anemia and is a potential cause of her tachycardia and possible heart failure.

Pioglitazone (Actos) and some of the other medications in the thiazolidinedione category have been implicated in fluid retention, edema, and resultant heart failure.[2,3] Her elevated BP may actually be a positive sign because it requires the ability of the left ventricle (LV) to generate the BP, which requires myocardial reserve and is associated with lower mortality in heart failure.[4]

3.   What components of the physical examination are important to note for Ms. C, and what aspects of the physical examination are missing for this patient?

The patient has experienced a 6-pound weight gain, and bilateral crackles were heard in the bases of the lungs. She also has an S3 heart sound. Additional physical examination required to support a diagnosis of heart failure would be to examine Ms. C for jugular venous distension, hepatomegaly, hepatojugular reflux, peripheral edema, and decreased peripheral perfusion.[3] Additionally, patients with SOB should have pulse oximetry measured. If pulse oximetry is less than 90%, then oxygen should be initiated.[4,5]

Case Study, Continued

Ms. C's pulse oximetry reading was 92% on room air. On physical examination, the patient had positive jugular venous distention to the jawline at 45°. Hepatomegaly was not apparent and she did not demonstrate a hepatojugular reflux, but she did have 3+ pitting bilateral lower extremity edema.

4. What is the significance of the S3 and S4 as findings in a patient's physical examination?

The S3 ventricular gallop heart sound can be normal in children and young adults, but it is associated with heart failure (more often systolic heart failure) and other disorders (e.g., mitral regurgitation, pregnancy, thyrotoxicosis) in older adults. The S4 is commonly heard in patients with HTN and cardiac conditions (e.g., aortic stenosis, myocardial disorders), but it is not heard in patients who are in atrial fibrillation.

5. What important decision(s) should the health care provider seeing Ms. C consider today?

Older adults frequently attribute symptoms, such as fatigue and a decrease in activity tolerance, to old age rather than identifying it as illness. In this patient, the development of symptoms over 3 weeks makes the etiology less clear. When seeing any patient it is important that the health care provider decide if the patient's problem is acute enough to warrant immediate transfer to an emergency room for treatment or if the patient is stable enough to be treated as an outpatient. Heart failure can be acute or chronic, or even acute on chronic. Ms. C's history, as far as we know, does not suggest a past history of heart failure, so this seems like new-onset heart failure that has occurred over the past few weeks. Thus far, the patient seems to be stable, but more information is necessary (e.g., diagnostics). It is also important to consider Ms. C's age and the fact that she lives alone when considering disposition.

6. What diagnostics (and why) are necessary for this patient at this time?

- An electrocardiogram (ECG) is necessary despite Ms. C's denial about chest discomfort. Additional testing can include point-of-care INR and serum glucose. However, further diagnostics are also indicated requiring that she go to the nearest laboratory service or hospital today.
- **Laboratory evaluation:**
  - Brain natriuretic peptide (BNP) or NT-proBNP to determine presence of heart failure (although this can be elevated with other pathology).
  - Troponin levels are necessary if there are any concerns about myocardial injury.
  - Complete blood count (CBC)/differential to evaluate anemia.
  - Serum electrolytes, blood urea nitrogen (BUN), and creatinine to determine sodium and other electrolyte values and renal status.
  - Liver function tests because elevated liver function can occur with heart failure.
  - Prothrombin time (PT)/INR done to assess possibly that INR is supratherapeutic because patient was taking ibuprofen while on warfarin.
  - Hemoglobin A1C (HgbA1C) should be checked because of Ms. C's diabetes, if not recently obtained.
  - Chest x-ray is a diagnostic evaluation for presence of heart failure versus pneumonia or other abnormality.
  - Echocardiogram, although possibly not urgently indicated for Ms. C today, should be planned for patients with new-onset heart failure to assess heart wall structure, valves, and function and aid in appropriate patient care.[6]

7. How should the health care provider interpret Ms. C's diagnostic results?

Ms. C's diagnostic results include:
1. ECG revealed atrial fibrillation, rate 122.

2. PT/INR in office was "high" according to the office machine. Because the patient needs additional testing and diagnostics, it was decided to send the patient to the emergency room for further evaluation.

8. How should the patient be transported?

The primary care provider needs to decide whether to activate 911, or a private ambulance transport service, or allow her family/friend to drive her. This patient has come to the clinic alone, her son is unreliable, and it will take time to find a friend who can come to pick her up and take her to the hospital. If taken by a family or friend, she will have to go through triage and will end up waiting to be seen. Additionally, it is safer for the patient to be transferred to the hospital by trained health care providers. The best option in this case is to call 911, based on her symptoms and comorbidities. Having medical personnel transport means the patient will have a better handoff because of the direct communication of her history, HPI, and medication list. Her most recent notes, laboratory values, any prior ECG, and today's point-of-care laboratory and ECG results should accompany the patient to improve transition of care. Cowie and colleagues noted the importance of transition of care in achieving the best outcomes in patients with heart failure.[7]

Case Study, Continued

Ms. C is transported to the emergency room and her test results are included:
1. **ECG:** Atrial fibrillation, rate 132, no ischemic changes.
2. **Chest x-ray wet read:** Patient is kyphotic. Heart size is enlarged. Pulmonary vascularity is engorged. Lungs show no clearly defined infiltrate. Impression: Definite congestive failure changes. No evidence for infiltrate.
3. **Troponin:** <0.01 ng/mL (level was normal).
4. **INR:** 8.6.
5. **NT-proBNP:** 3724 pg/mL (5–1800 pg/mL)
6. **Thyroid-stimulating hormone (TSH):** 0.13 μIU/mL (0.27–4.20 μIU/mL)
7. **Hgb A1C:** 8.0 (<5.7)
8. **CBC:**
   - White blood cell (WBC): 9000 (4.0–11 K/mm^3)
   - Red blood cell (RBC): 3.54 (3.80–5.40 (m/mm^3)
   - Hgb: 9.4 (11.0–16.0 g/dL)
   - Hematocrit: 30.1 (35%–48.0%)
   - Mean corpuscular volume (MCV): 83 (80.0–100.0 fL)
   - Mean corpuscular Hgb concentration (MCHC): 31.2 (31.2–36.0 g/dL)
   - Red cell distribution width: 16.7 (11.5%–15.0%)
   - Platelet count: 470 (130–400 K/mm^3)
9. **Chemistry profile:**
   - Sodium: 143 (136–145 mmol/L)
   - Potassium: 4.8 (3.4–5.1 (mmol/L)
   - Chloride: 100 (98–107 mmol/L)
   - Carbon dioxide: 27 (22–32 mmol/L)
   - Glucose: 199 (78–118 milligrams/dL)
   - BUN: 24 (5–23 milligrams/dL)
   - Creatinine: 1.8 (0.4–1.0 milligrams/dL)
   - Estimated glomerular filtration rate (GFR): 26 mL/min/1.73 m^2 (per CKD-EPI Creatinine 2009 equation)
   - Calcium: 8 (8.6–10.2 milligrams/dL)

9. Based on Ms. C's laboratory results, what diagnoses should the health care provider include in the Problem List for this Ms. C's hospitalization? What are the 2018 ICD-10-CM Diagnosis Codes for each of Ms. C's problems?

1. **Atrial fibrillation with rapid ventricular response:** I40.91
2. **Acute heart failure:** I50
   - At this point, the actual cause of Ms. C's heart failure is unknown. Her medical history does not suggest a previous history of heart failure (systolic, diastolic, or even chronic heart failure), so a diagnosis of systolic, diastolic, or acute on chronic heart failure would not be correct at this time. As soon as the cause of her heart failure is known the correct diagnosis code should be updated.
3. **Supratherapeutic INR:** R79.1
4. **Anemia unspecified:** D64.9
5. **Iatrogenic hyperthyroidism:** EO3.2
6. **Type 2 Diabetes mellitus with hyperglycemia:** E11.65
7. **Stage 4 chronic kidney disease (GFR 15–29 mL/min):** N18.4. This ICD-10 code may also need to be updated because her current renal status may be worse than usual, which is a result of her current illness.

10. What are the expected emergency room interventions and the anticipated treatments for each of Ms. C's problems during her hospitalization?

In the emergency room, Ms. C will be reevaluated while diagnostics are done. She will be placed in a 90-degree angle in the bed, oxygen will be started if necessary, and intravenous (IV) access obtained. Insertion of a Foley catheter to monitor urine output is possible. Vital sign assessment will be ongoing.

Atrial Fibrillation With Rapid Ventricular Response. Ms. C is on atenolol (Tenormin), a β_1-selective, hydrophilic beta-blocker. Metoprolol (Lopressor) is a lipophilic beta-blocker that is more often used to control a rapid heart rate in the hospital and is available IV or po. Per the American College of Cardiology (ACC), either medication could be used, but Ms. C needs a small dose of a beta-blocker (e.g., metoprolol 2.5–5 milligrams IV bolus over 2–3 minutes) to slow the heart rate and allow better ventricular filling.[8] Goal heart rate will be less than 110, but greater than 80).[8] An additional dose may or may not be necessary, but in older adults especially, it is best to "start low, go slow."

Acute Heart Failure. Furosemide 20 to 40 milligrams IV will be ordered and administrated. BP and urine output will be monitored and diuretic therapy repeated, if necessary. Higher doses of furosemide may be necessary because of Ms. C's renal dysfunction. Serum electrolytes and renal function will be closely monitored. After she is stabilized, an oral loop diuretic (e.g., furosemide or torsemide) will be added to her regimen. Hydrochlorothiazide, in patients with GFR less than 30 to 50 mL/min/1.73 m², is not helpful in fluid retention and will be discontinued.[9]

An echocardiogram will also be ordered to determine whether Ms. C has wall motion abnormalities, valvular dysfunction, and exclude cardiac tamponade, and to determine the ejection fraction (EF%) to aid in classifying the heart failure as diastolic or systolic.

Supratherapeutic International Normalized Ratio. The patient has been taking an NSAID, which has likely contributed to the elevated INR. In addition, warfarin sensitivity is affected by decompensated heart failure.[10] Warfarin will be held. Oral vitamin K is appropriate, 1 to 5 milligrams when a patient is stable and not bleeding.[11] Orders to have Ms. C's INR checked daily will be entered to ensure that the INR will be monitored, and warfarin will be restarted when appropriate to aid in preventing emboli and stroke.

Anemia. Ms. C is anemic. She will need a rectal examination, fecal immunochemical test (FIT), or stool DNA (Cologuard) test to assess for gastrointestinal (GI) bleeding, even though there is no obvious evidence (e.g., bloody or black tarry stools) of active bleeding at this time. The type of anemia will also need to be discerned. Iron-deficiency anemia (IDA) is the most common anemia in older adults, but other causes of anemia (e.g., anemia of chronic disease) are possible. Ms. C's MCV and MCH are not diminished, but in early stages of anemia, these laboratory tests can still be within the normal parameters and the patient can still have IDA. Further laboratory diagnostics should include a stool guaiac, serum ferritin, serum iron, and total iron-binding capacity. If these are within normal limits, then other causes of anemia will be explored.

Iatrogenic Hyperthyroidism. The levothyroxine dose needs to be decreased to 100 micrograms po daily. A repeat TSH in 4 to 6 weeks will need be obtained to learn if her TSH is then within the recommended range.

Type 2 Diabetes Mellitus. Ms. C's HgbA1C is elevated, but she is also anemic. HgbA1C levels can be erroneously affected (i.e., higher HgbA1C level) by varied anemias and by chronic kidney disease. For this reason, these patients need a different way to monitor blood sugar levels. Fructosamine A1C is one possibility, but there are also variables that affect the results of this test. The best method of monitoring her diabetes while she is in the hospital may be a fasting blood glucose each morning and premeal Accu-Checks. Appropriate sliding-scale coverage with a short-acting insulin is a medication consideration. However, oral antidiabetic agents can also be considered, although renal dysfunction is a significant concern. Linagliptin (Trajenta), a DPP-4, is a possibility because it can be used in patients with chronic kidney disease. However, many other antidiabetic agents (e.g., sulfonylureas, sodium-glucose cotransporter 2 inhibitors, glucagon-like peptide-1 [GLP-1] receptor agonists) are contraindicated in patients with chronic kidney disease as severe as Ms. C's appears to be.[12]

Stage 4 Chronic Kidney Disease (Glomerular Filtration Rate 15–29 mL/min). Stage 4 chronic kidney disease is considered severe. It is possible that Ms. C's renal status has deteriorated because of her heart failure and because she was taking NSAIDs regularly. Her diagnosis would most likely be considered acute on chronic kidney disease, and a consultation with nephrology is initiated.[13]

Case Study, Continued

After stabilization, Ms. C is admitted to the hospital and her health care issues are addressed.

Anemia. A rectal examination revealed guaiac-positive stools and a gastroenterology consult was requested. A colonoscopy and endoscopy were recommended once internal medicine felt she was stable enough for these procedures.
  1. **Endoscopy report:** Ulcerative erosions before the pylorus and at the GI junction.
  2. **Colonoscopy:** Negative

Atrial Fibrillation. Rate control was achieved in the hospital with metoprolol tartrate 12.5 milligrams twice a day. Ms. C is being carefully monitored while hospitalized, and the dose adjusted as needed, but the goal, once it is clear her heart rate is not too low or high, is to change her to metoprolol succinate (Toprol XL), which is extended release and the recommended beta-blocker for patients with heart failure because it has been shown to reduce mortality in heart failure patients.[14]

Anticoagulation. Ms. C's INRs quickly decreased and she was restarted on warfarin when her INR reached 3.0

Heart Failure. Echocardiogram report states: Systolic dysfunction. EF 40% with LV septal hypokinesis. Right ventricle (RV) is mildly enlarged. There is right atrial enlargement. There is borderline pulmonary HTN with a pulmonary artery (PA) pressure of about 40 mm Hg. LV systolic function: estimated LVEF 40%. + septal hypokinesis. LV diastolic function: impaired relaxation with normal left atrial pressure. RV function: appears to be normal, although the RV chamber is mildly dilated.

Acute on Chronic Kidney Disease. The patient was seen by nephrology and recommendations were as follows: Acute on chronic kidney disease most likely the related to NSAIDS and volume overload. Check phosphorus. Discontinue lisinopril for now until renal function improves. Monitor chemistries and renal function. Lisinopril or angiotensin receptor blocker (ARB) can possibly be restarted when renal function stabilizes, but at a small dose.[15]

11. What are the types and causes of heart failure?

Heart failure occurs when heart muscle dysfunction affects the pumping ability of the heart to supply enough blood to meet the body requirements. There are two clinical subtypes of left-sided heart failure: systolic and diastolic. The American Heart Association (AHA) and ACC define systolic heart failure as heart failure with reduced ejection fraction (HFrEF). The inability of the LV to contract efficiently results in a decreased amount of blood ejected out of the LV through the aortic valve into the circulation. Normal LV ejection is 50% to 70%. An EF less than 50% (e.g., 48%) is definitely considered reduced.[3]

Diastolic heart failure, most often referred to as heart failure with preserved ejection fraction (HFpEF), is defined as having normal or near normal LVEF.[3] The pathophysiology of HFpEF differs from HFrEF. In HFpEF, the LV is unable ability to relax enough to enable filling of the LV during diastole.

Right-sided heart failure is usually the sequelae of left-sided heart failure. As the LV weakens, the right side of the heart fails to pump blood adequately and the abdomen, lower extremities, and lungs are affected (e.g., leg edema, pulmonary congestion, ascites).

12. How is heart failure staged and treated?

Chronic heart failure is categorized based on a patient's functional physical ability. The New York Heart Association (NYHA) Functional Classes[3] are used to classify chronic heart failure:

   I. Asymptomatic on ordinary physical activity
  II. Symptomatic on ordinary physical activity
 III. Symptomatic on less than ordinary physical activity
 IV. Symptomatic at rest

The treatments for HFrEF and HFpEF are similar yet different. An angiotensin-converting enzyme (ACE) inhibitor or, if the patient cannot tolerate an ACE inhibitor, an ARB is recommended for patients with both HFrEF and HFpEF. Beta-blockers and loop diuretics are also recommended, although diuretics are used cautiously in patients with HFpEF to preserve preload, renal function, and stroke volume and avoid dehydration. ACE inhibitors, ARBs, and beta-blockers are associated with decreased mortality, whereas diuretics help control the symptoms associated with fluid retention.[16] Digoxin, hydralazine, metolazone, nitrates, and aldosterone antagonists are also used in some circumstances. Patients with heart failure taking any of these medications require careful monitoring to maintain quality of life and avoid hospitalizations. Nonpharmacological treatments are also recommended and should be encouraged. These include the importance of diet and exercise, as well as daily weights, and salt and fluid restriction in some instances.

Case Study, Continued

Ms. C improves over the next few days and one of her daughters comes to visit just before she is ready for discharge home. Ms. C's daughter expresses her concerns for her mother's safety at home but states she plans to stay with her Mom the first week she is home.

The physician assistant working with the hospitalist reviews what has happened with Ms. C and her daughter. He tells them that Ms. C has improved dramatically since the first day of the hospital admission. He reviews with her that some of what caused her symptoms and hospitalization was related to the ibuprofen she was taking. He goes on to recap what is happening now.

Physical Therapy Consultation. *Physical therapy was consulted yesterday and Ms. C is able to get in and out of bed independently and walked in the corridor today with the physical therapist. Physical therapy is not concerned about her ability to ambulate safely and does not think that Ms. C needs to go to a skilled nursing facility for rehabilitation. She will, however, be referred to the local visiting nurse association for posthospital monitoring.*

Vital Signs. *She has dropped 3 pounds in the past 3 days. Her oxygen saturation on room air remained greater than 90 during her hospitalization and is now 94 with exertion but 96 to 97 at rest. Her heart rate has improved and is 76 to 80 with rest and increases to the low 90s with ambulation. Her BP range is 130/66 to 140/80. The weight loss, vital signs, and fact that Ms. C feels better are encouraging.*

Anemia. *Her iron studies were low normal and her blood count has been stable since admission. The gastroenterologist wants her to continue the proton pump inhibitor for 2 months and have a follow-up blood count in 4 weeks.*

Atrial Fibrillation. *Her heart rate is now controlled on metoprolol succinate, and she was restarted on warfarin today but at a lower dose. She will need to have the PT/ INR monitored closely for a short time after discharge and then routinely as in the past.*

Heart Failure. *Her breathing has improved and the proBNP, the blood test that suggests there is fluid in the lungs, is now 2000, which is close to normal and may even be normal for her age. The change in medications has helped, and she will be discharged on the new medications.*

Type 2 Diabetes Mellitus. *Her Accu-Cheks and fasting blood sugars in the hospital have not been out of control. She might be able to go home on an oral medication, but the doctor wants to wait another day to see.*

Renal Status. *Her kidneys improved after the ibuprofen was stopped. When she was admitted to the hospital she had severe renal failure. With all the treatments, her GFR, the measurement we use to monitor kidneys, has improved. Now she has what we label stage 3B chronic kidney disease. This is much better and we think it will improve even more, but kidney function does change as we age, so we will monitor carefully.*

13.   What are the possible concerns for Ms. C after hospital discharge?

The transitions of care are problematic, especially for older adults after a hospitalization.[17] Medication changes and discharge instructions are often not clear, and as a result, medication errors and rehospitalizations are all too common. The reasons are myriad: poor communication among health care providers caring for the patient; culture; language; medication complexity; health literacy; and impaired cognition, hearing, and vision. Health literacy assessment, an understanding of chronic care management, improving patient and family education, and uncomplicated medication instructions are helpful, as is expedient follow-up after hospitalization and promoting coordinated care among health care professionals.[17]

Case Study, Continued

Before discharge home, the physician assistant caring for Ms. C in the hospital reviews the hospital discharge medications and plans.

Admission Medications

Atenolol 50 milligrams po once a day: *discontinued*
Atorvastatin 40 milligrams po once a day
Hydrochlorothiazide 25 milligrams po once a day: *discontinued*
Ibuprofen 600 milligrams po twice a day prn pain: *discontinued*
Levothyroxine 112 micrograms po once a day: *dose changed*
Lisinopril 20 milligrams po once a day: *dose changed*
Pioglitazone 30 milligrams po once a day: *discontinued*
Omeprazole 20 milligrams po once a day
Warfarin 7.5 milligrams po once a day: *dose changed*

Hospital Discharge Medications

Atorvastatin 40 milligrams po once a day
Lisinopril 2.5 milligrams po once a day
Furosemide 20 milligrams po twice a day (8 a.m. and 2 p.m.)
Levothyroxine 100 micrograms po once a day
Omeprazole 20 milligrams po once a day
Warfarin 5 milligrams po once a day
Metoprolol succinate 25 milligrams po once a day
Trajenta 5 milligrams po once a day

Case Study, Continued

Ms. C is discharged from the hospital and a follow-up appointment is scheduled with primary care 6 days after her hospital discharge. A discharge summary was faxed to the local Visiting Nurses Association (VNA) who will see her the day after discharge. A cardiology appointment is also scheduled, although not as soon. Ms. C has her discharge papers from the hospital when she presents for her follow-up appointment at the primary care practice. She states she filled her prescriptions and is taking the new medications. Her daughter accompanies her to the appointment and agrees, and tells the health care provider that the discontinued medications were disposed of at the local pharmacy.

14.   What are important considerations for the health care provider today?

It is estimated that up to 20% of patients go through transitions from hospital to home that are complicated and are frequently rehospitalized within 30 days.[18] There can be problems with information exchange and collaboration at the time of the hospital discharge. Primary care practices report receiving either incomplete, late, or no discharge summaries at all.[18] Patients and their families also report problems with their discharge, such as the lack of clear information and the lack of an understanding of what the follow-up entails. The goals of the follow-up appointment today in the primary care practice are to help the patient effectively transition from inpatient management to self-management at home. To facilitate this transition, it is important to be able to access and review the hospital records, reconcile the patient's medications, and establish a plan with the patient for care at home. The transition of care and coordination of that transition constitute an important piece of primary care. In heart failure, hospital readmission rates have been shown to be reduced if there is close and coordinated follow-up from hospitalization to home. Before the patient's appointment, obtaining and reviewing the hospital admission records and discharge summary is ideal. Primary care providers should receive these at the time of patient discharge, but some institutions require a signed records release form from the patient to release records.

While reviewing the discharge paperwork, it is important that the health care provider note the laboratory values (especially the last ones), as well as any diagnostic imaging and other tests, as well as the discharge summary and instructions. These should summarize the plan formulated by the hospitalist and any specialists seen by the patient while in the hospital.

During the office visit, it is important to review the hospital stay with Ms. C to make sure she understands what happened. Carefully reviewing her medication list and reconciling it with the discharge summary notes received from the hospital is essential. The patient's status, how she is feeling and doing since discharge, verification of vital signs, and a thorough physical examination are necessary. Verifying that she has an appointment with the cardiologist scheduled and stressing the importance of follow-up are also important.

After a hospitalization for heart failure and atrial fibrillation, it is important to make sure Ms. C has the appropriate follow-up care in place, especially because her daughter will be returning home. The provider contacts the VNA and discusses the case with the visiting nurse, who tells the provider that the patient has been enrolled in their telehealth program, which will provide close monitoring and data collection related to the patient's weight, heart rate, BP, and cardiopulmonary examination. The program also provides in-depth teaching related to diet, medications, and exercise. The provider learns from this conversation that the agency has a nurse practitioner (NP) who coordinates the telehealth program and works closely with the nursing staff.

Follow-up in primary care will be often until the patient is more stable and comfortable with her new diagnosis and regimens.

References

1. Murray, M., & Brater, D. (1990). Adverse effects of nonsteroidal anti-inflammatory drugs on renal function. *Annals of Internal Medicine, 112*, 559–560.
2. Paneni, F., & Luscher, T. F. (2017). Cardiovascular protection in the treatment of type 2 diabetes: A review of clinical trial results across drug classes. *American Journal of Cardiology, 120*(Suppl.), S17–S27.
3. Ismail-Beigi, F., Moghissi, E., Kosilborod, M., & Inzucchi, S. E. (2017). Shifting paradigms in the medical management of type 2 diabetes reflections on recent cardiovascular outcome trials. *Journal of General Internal Medicine, 32*(9), 1041–1055.
4. O'Brien, J. F., & Hunter, C. L. (2018). Heart failure. In R. M. Walls, R. S. Hockberger, & M. Gausche-Hill (Eds.), *Rosen's emergency medicine: Concepts and clinical practice* (9th ed., pp. 971–986). Philadelphia, PA: Elsevier.
5. Mace, S. E. (2012). Shortness of breath in adults. In S. V. Mahadevan & G. M. Garmel (Eds.), *Clinical emergency medicine* (2nd ed., p. 518). New York, NY: Cambridge University Press.
6. Marmick, T. (2015). The role of echocardiography in heart failure. *The Journal of Nuclear Medicine, 56*(4), 31S–38S.
7. Cowie, M., Ankerm, S., Cleland, J., Felker, G., Fillppatos, G., Jaarsma, T., et al. (2014). Improving care for patients with acute heart failure: Before, during and after hospitalization. *European Society of Cardiology Heart Failure, 1*(2), 110–145.

8. American College of Cardiology Foundation (ACCF), American Heart Association (AHA), and Heart Rhythm Society (HRS) (2011). *ACCF/AHA/HRS Focused updates incorporated into the ACC/AHA/ESC 2006 guidelines for the management of patients with atrial fibrillation.* Washington, DC: American College of Cardiology Foundation. Retrieved from http://content.onlinejacc.org/cgi/content/full/57/11/e101.

9. KDIGO (2012). KDIGO Clinical practice guideline for the management of blood pressure in chronic kidney disease. Retrieved from http://www.kdigo.org/clinical_practice_guidelines/pdf/KDIGO_BP _GL.pdf.

10. del Campo, M., & Roberts, G. (2015). Changes in warfarin sensitivity during decompensated heart failure and chronic obstructive pulmonary disease. *Annals of Pharmacology, 49*(9), 962–968.

11. Ansell, J., Hirsh, J., Hylek, E., Jacobsen, A., Crowther, M., & Palareti, G. (2008). Pharmacology and management of the vitamin K agonists. *American College of Chest Physicians Evidence-Based Clinical Practice Guidelines, 133*(6), 160S–198S. 8th ed.

12. Prasad-Reddy, L., & Isaacs, D. (2015). A clinical review of GLP-1 receptor agonists: Efficacy and safety in diabetes and beyond. *Drugs in Context, 4*, 212283.

13. Palazzuoli, A., Lombardi, C., Ruocco, G., Padeletti, M., Nuti, R., Metra, M., et al. (2016). Chronic kidney disease and worsening renal function in acute heart failure: Different phenotypes with similar prognostic impact? *European Heart Journal: Acute Cardiovascular Care, 5*(8), 534–548.

14. Cadrin-Tourigny, J., Shohoudi, A., Roy, D., Talajic, M., Tadros, R., Mondésert, B., et al. (2017). Decreased mortality with beta-blockers in patients with heart failure and coexisting atrial fibrillation: An AF-CHF Substudy. *Journal of the American College of Cardiology: Heart Failure, 5*(2), 99–106.

15. Chawla, L., Bellomo, R., Bihorac, A., Goldstein, S., Siew, E., Bagshaw, S., et al. (2017). Acute kidney disease and renal recovery: Consensus report of the acute disease quality initiative (ADQI) 16 Workgroup. *Nature Reviews. Nephrology, 13*, 241–257.

16. American Heart Association. (2017). ACC/AHA/HFSA Focused update of the 2013 ACCF/AHA guideline for the management of heart failure: A report of the American College of Cardiology/American Heart Association task force on clinical practice guidelines and the Heart Failure Society of America. Retrieved from http://www.heart.org/HEARTORG/Conditions/HeartFailure/Heart-Failure-Guidelines-Toolkit_UCM_491412_SubHomePage.jsp.

17. Buttaro, T. (2016). Transitional care. In T. Buttaro, J. Trybulski, P. Bailey, & J. Sandberg-Cook (Eds.), *Primary care: A collaborative practice* (5th ed., pp. 3–6). St. Louis, MO: Elsevier.

18. LeBerre, M., Maimon, G., Sourial, N., Gueriton, M., & Vedel, I. (2017). Impact of transitional care services for chronically ill older patients: A systematic evidence review. *Journal of the American Geriatrics Society, 65*, 1597–1608.

Wheezing

Terry Mahan Buttaro

Case Study Scenario/History of Present Illness

Mr. Michaels, a 68-year-old male, presents to the office complaining of a 3- to 5-day history of shortness of breath (SOB), difficulty breathing lying down, wheezing, dyspnea on exertion (DOE), and increased cough. He describes some chest discomfort that occurs in the center of the chest while coughing. The chest discomfort only occurs with cough; does not linger; and is not radiating, pleuritic, or associated with diaphoresis or nausea. He has been using his albuterol inhaler, but it does not seem to be helping like it usually does. He has not smoked for the past day or two, and that has not helped either. He denies recent infection.

Medications: Albuterol (Proventil HFA) inhaler every 4 to 6 hours used as needed (prn), lisinopril (Zestril) 10 milligrams po each day.

Allergies: Environmental.

Habits: Smoker 1 pack per day (PPD) × 30 years. Has stopped in the past periodically, but just for short periods of time. Occasional beer 1 to 2 times per month.

Past medical history: Obesity, asthma, COPD, impaired fasting glucose, hypertension, gastroesophageal reflux disease (GERD), Barrett esophagus, sleep apnea, posttraumatic stress disorder (PTSD), depression, pneumonia/hospitalized 2 years ago.

Past surgical history: Fundoplication.

Personal and social history: Engineer, divorced. No children.

Family history: Father died in the war. Mother died age 62 of heart attack. Grandparents died of "natural causes." No siblings.

Review of Systems

General: Denies fever, chills, weakness.

Skin: Denies rashes or lesions.

Head, eyes, ears, nose, and throat (HEENT): + history allergies and sinus infections. Denies headache, dizziness, sinus pain.

Neck: Denies neck pain, lumps.

Respiratory: + SOB, cough, wheezing. Denies recent respiratory infection, hemoptysis.

Cardiac: + orthopnea, chest pain. Denies palpitation.

Gastrointestinal: Denies difficulty swallowing, heartburn, nausea, vomiting, diarrhea.

Urinary: Denies urinary burning, frequency, flank pain.

Musculoskeletal: Denies back pain, leg pain, joint pain.

Peripheral vascular: Denies swollen legs, calf pain.

Neurovascular: Denies fainting, numbness, tingling.

Hematologic: Denies easy bruising, bleeding gums, history of anemia.

Endocrine: Denies temperature intolerance, sweating, thirst.

Psychiatric: + history depression.

Physical Examination

General: Obese male sitting on examination table with frequent bronchospastic cough. Mild distress.

Vital signs: Height 6 feet, weight 260 pounds. Temperature 97, blood pressure (BP) 150/88. Heart rate (HR) 110 regular. Respiratory rate (RR) 26 at rest, O_2 sat on room air 92% at rest; 88% with ambulation.

Skin: Warm/dry. No rash or acute lesions.

Eyes: Sclera clear; conjunctiva, no injection.

Ears: Tympanic membranes (TMs) no erythema, bulging/retraction.

Nose: No rhinitis or sinus tenderness.

Mouth: Membranes moist, teeth fair repair with some brown staining, no postpharyngeal cobblestoning or erythema. No lesions of tongue or buccal mucosa.

Neck: Supple: no masses, lymphadenopathy, thyroid enlargement or tenderness.

Cardiac: Rapid regular S1, S2. No S3, S4, murmurs, or rubs. Electrocardiogram (ECG): sinus tachycardia with no T wave changes.

Respiratory: Tight with diffuse inspiratory and expiratory wheezes.

Abdomen: Obese, soft, bowel sounds positive, although diminished. No tenderness or organomegaly.

Extremities: Pedal pulses present bilaterally, no edema or calf tenderness.

1. Based on the history and physical examination, what are the possible causes (Differential Diagnosis) of this patient's discomfort?

This gentleman presents with a 3- to 5-day history of cough, SOB; DOE; difficulty lying down; and some chest discomfort that is nonradiating, not accompanied by fever and chills, or nausea, vomiting, or diarrhea. He has a past medical history of asthma, COPD, and is a smoker, so it is possible that his symptoms are related to asthma or an exacerbation of COPD. Asthma classification is based on severity and forced expiratory volume in 1 second (FEV_1).[1] Symptoms of COPD, especially with chronic bronchitis, include chronic cough, chronic sputum production, and dyspnea. Other differentials should also be considered. For example, SOB, wheezing, and cough are commonly associated with respiratory tree obstruction, reactive airway disease, infection, cardiovascular disease, heart failure, or pericarditis. SOB and cough in an obese patient also should raise concerns about a possible pulmonary embolus.[2] Further considerations include a cough related to angiotensin-converting enzyme (ACE) inhibitors (e.g., lisinopril), but an ACE cough would not be commonly associated with wheezing or this patient's other symptoms. Costochondritis is another possible cause of the chest discomfort induced by coughing.

2. What are the criteria for a diagnosis of chronic obstructive pulmonary disease or asthma?

Asthma classification is based on FEV_1.[1] Symptoms of COPD, especially with chronic bronchitis, include chronic cough, chronic sputum production, and dyspnea. Diagnosis and severity of COPD is also based on FEV_1. There are four classifications of COPD: stage 1 or mild COPD, $FEV_1 \geq$ 80% normal; stage II or moderate COPD, FEV_1 50% to 79% normal; stage III or severe COPD, FEV_1 30% to 49% normal; and stage IV or very severe COPD, $FEV_1 <$ 30% normal, or <50% associated with chronic respiratory failure.[2]

3. What other environmental precipitants or causes of his symptoms should be explored?

Additional history is needed to determine whether there are pets at home, if there are possible environmental triggers at work, or if there have been other exposures. These include recent travel or known exposure to people with a respiratory illness.

4. What components of the physical examination are missing?

In the primary care office, the patient's chest wall would be palpated for tenderness to determine whether costochondritis was the cause of the patient's pain. Orthostatic vital signs would be checked to aid in determining whether the patient is hypovolemic. He would have spirometry or peak flow testing and receive nebulizer treatments. A normal peak flow for a male, age 68, height 183 cm, is approximately 529 L/min. Unfortunately, there is no previous documentation of his baseline peak flow and/or spirometry results, but previous peak flow documentation of the patient's baseline would allow comparison and assist in determining any change from baseline.

5. What diagnostics and treatments are necessary for this patient at this time?

Appropriate diagnostics in the office setting include an ECG to look for ischemic changes or signs of pericarditis and nebulizer therapy to see if the patient's breathing and oxygen saturation improves. Other diagnostics necessary may require referral to the local hospital for laboratory imaging studies. These include a complete blood count (CBC) and differential, D-dimer, and chemistry panel (i.e., to determine fluid, electrolyte, and renal status). A chest x-ray is an important consideration to determine the presence of infection, although it is possible for older patients to have a negative x-ray even when pneumonia is the cause of the patient's symptoms.[3,4]

A patient with diffuse wheezing, below-normal peak flows, and oxygen desaturation requires a series of three nebulizer treatments with 2.5 to 5 milligrams of albuterol every 20 minutes × 3 treatments in the office.[5] A combination anticholinergic/β_2-agonist (i.e., ipratropium 0.5 milligrams/albuterol 2.5 milligrams) is an alternative therapy. Either of these treatments will determine whether there is a decrease in wheezing, as well as improved oxygenation and peak flows/spirometry. Patients who do not respond to nebulizer treatments require hospitalization for more aggressive therapy.

The patient's ECG reveals sinus tachycardia without acute changes (Fig. 4.1). The ECG results are reassuring, but after three nebulizer treatments, the wheezing has not abated and the patient's peak flow is noted to be unchanged at 300 L/min. Normal for this gentleman should be at least 530 L/min. The patient's symptoms and failure to improve with nebulizer treatments in combination with a low oxygen saturation with exertion are concerning. The patient is admitted from the office to the hospital.

The admitting diagnosis is reactive bronchitis, which is also known as bronchospasm. Often this diagnosis is used when the exact cause of the illness is unclear. In this case the patient's bronchospasm is thought to be related to an inflammatory cause, but the chest x-ray obtained did not identify pneumonia. The D-dimer is 269 ng/mL (normal is less than 250 ng/mL). Admitting labs: white blood cell (WBC) 13, hemoglobin (Hgb) 14, hematocrit (Hct) 44, platelets (plt) 252, lymphocytes 11.8, neutrophils % 77.5, neutrophil # slightly elevated at 10.1. Basic metabolic panel (BMP): Na 140, K 3.8, Cl 102, glucose 105, blood urea nitrogen (BUN) 18, creatinine (Cr) 1.0, Ca 8.9, glomerular filtration rate (GFR) 83.4. ProBNP 99 (5–900 nl).

6 What further admitting orders and diagnostics are indicated for the patient at this time?

The elevated D-dimer indicates the need for a spiral computed tomography (CT) to determine whether a pulmonary embolus is present. The spiral CT will also help determine whether pneumonia

Sinus Tachycardia

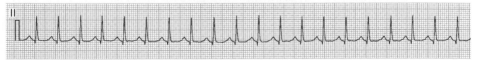

Fig. 4.1 Sinus tachycardia. (From Goldberger, A. L., Goldberger, Z .D., & Shvilkin, A. [2017]. *Goldberger's clinical electrocardiography.* [9th ed.]. Philadelphia: Elsevier.)

is present because a CT scan is often more adept at identifying pneumonia than a chest x-ray[3]. The patient should be checked for influenza and, if not determined previously, an α_1-antitrypsin to assess for the presence of a genetic disorder that affects the lungs and liver should also be obtained.[6] Arterial blood gases are also indicated. Additionally, the Gold guidelines should be reviewed for management of a COPD exacerbation.[7]

If the arterial blood gases are within normal limits, supplemental oxygen 1 to 2 L can be ordered if the oxygen level falls below 90%. Caution is needed to not increase oxygen saturation too much because some COPD patients can be O_2 retainers and too much oxygen will decrease a CO_2 retainer's respiratory drive.

Intravenous (IV) steroids consisting of methylprednisolone 60 milligrams every 6 hours and ipratropium bromide (0.5 milligrams/albuterol 2.5 milligrams [DuoNeb]) treatments every 4 to 6 hours are ordered to decrease inflammation, bronchospasm and, if present, hypoxemia. Torpin and Ottis reviewed the role of steroid therapy to decrease inflammation, bronchospasm, and possible hypoxemia in COPD exacerbations determining that the use of steroids in COPD exacerbations is variable and that often oral steroids for as little as 5 days can be effective therapy for most patients.[7] Patients requiring intensive care are likely to benefit from IV steroid therapy.[7]

Antibiotics (e.g., levofloxacin or ceftriaxone and azithromycin) are indicated for hospitalized patients with a severe exacerbation of COPD and should target those pathogens most commonly associated with pneumonia or a COPD exacerbation (e.g., *Haemophilus influenza, Moraxella catarrhalis, Pseudomonas aeruginosa,* or *Streptococcus pneumoniae*).

Case Study, Continued

Mr. Michaels is started on levofloxacin 500 milligrams IV daily. Although there are no strong studies suggesting that cough medicine is helpful for patients with COPD, it is reasonable to try guaifenesin (Robitussin) 5 mL po every 6 hours as necessary to help relieve this patient's cough. A transdermal nicotine patch (21 milligrams/day) is started, and smoking cessation patient education is initiated. Smoking cessation aids in decreasing COPD exacerbations and slowing the progression of this chronic respiratory disorder. Heparin 5000 IU subcutaneously every 8 hours is additionally ordered to prevent deep vein thrombosis (DVT). Mr. Michaels is ill and overweight increasing his risk for a DVT.

7. The patient has not improved with steroids, DuoNeb treatments, antibiotics, and Robitussin as of hospital day 2. What other therapies are indicated?

The lung CT is negative for pulmonary emboli and does not identify pneumonia. Knowing that triple therapy with inhaled corticosteroids, a long-acting β-agonist, and a long-acting muscarinic antagonist are indicated to decrease inflammation and promote bronchodilation, the provider orders a combination inhaled corticosteroid and long-acting β-agonist (fluticasone 250 micrograms/salmeterol 50 micrograms (Advair 500/50), 1 inhalation twice a day), plus a long-acting anticholinergic (tiotropium [Spiriva Respimat]) 2.5 micrograms per actuation, 2 inhalations once daily). Concerned about the patient's slow response to treatments thus far, the provider requests consultation with a pulmonologist to learn if there are other recommendations that will improve the patient's breathing. A consultation with case management also occurs to verify the need for hospitalization of this patient and begin discussions about possible patient needs after this hospitalization.[8]

Case Study, Continued

Hospital Day 3. Mr. Michaels feels better and is eating. His vital signs are normal and, on examination, the wheezing has significantly diminished. The provider checks orthostatic vital signs and determines that there is no change in BP or HR when the patient changes from a sitting to standing position. This reassures the provider that Mr. Michaels can now be evaluated by physical therapy and begin treatment to decrease the functional decline associated with hospitalizations. Pulmonary consultation recommends decreasing the methylprednisolone to 40 milligrams IV every 6 hours and suggests changing to an oral prednisone taper in 24 to 48 hours if the patient continues to improve.[9]

Short-term glucocorticoid therapy reduces the risk of adverse effects and the REDUCE Randomized Clinical Trial determined that even 5-day steroid treatment regimens were beneficial for mild to moderate COPD exacerbations.[9] The pulmonologist agrees with current treatment and suggests a sleep evaluation after hospital discharge for possible benefit with positive airway pressure therapy. A physical therapy evaluation reveals that Mr. Michaels has continued oxygen desaturation to 89% to 90% on room air and weakness with ambulation. The provider is aware that Mr. Michaels has no close family members to assist him at home.

8. What are criteria for patient discharge from the hospital?

Knowing Mr. Michaels lives alone, the provider calls his primary care provider and learns that Mr. Michaels does not often present for his regularly scheduled follow-up, often does not take his medications, and continues to suffer from PTSD. The nurse practitioner reviews the Hospital Discharge Screening Criteria for High Risk Older Adults and learns that Mr. Michaels, even though he is not 80-plus years, has a history of depression and PTSD, an inadequate support system, and at time of discharge will be prescribed at least six medicines.[10] This information, plus this hospitalization, fulfills the criteria for consulting with case management to determine Mr. Michaels' transitional care needs.[10]

The American Thoracic Society criteria for discharge are simply that the problem causing the hospitalization has resolved or improved. When considering discharge for a patient with COPD, the following should be considered:

- The patient's breathing status and oxygen saturation are baseline or close to it.
- The patient has been stable hemodynamically (e.g., normal BP and pulse and 48 hours without fever).
- The patient is sleeping well (e.g., not waking during night dyspneic).
- The patient is tolerating oral fluids/food and parenteral fluid resuscitation was not required in the previous 12- to 24-hour time period.
- The patient is able to ambulate safely.
- The patient requires less frequent β-agonist therapy.
- The patient and/or caregiver are able to teach back the discharge medication instructions.
- Arrangements for skilled nursing care, visiting nurses, and follow-up are complete and documented.[11]

9. What preparations for hospital discharge are necessary?

Discharge planning should begin when the patient is first admitted to the hospital to prepare the patient and family for this transition in care and also inform case management of a possible need for rehabilitation.[12] Knowing if the patient has a caregiver at home and learning how many stairs lead into the house and to the bedroom or bath is important when considering the patient's needs and goals at discharge.

The provider discusses the concerns about patient safety with the hospital case manager. These include the continued decrease in oxygen saturation with ambulation, the fact that the patient lives alone, and the patient's previous history of nonperseverance with medications. The provider and case manager then discuss with the patient the different options for continued care after hospital discharge. These include rehabilitation in a skilled nursing facility or home with visiting nurses.

Case Study, Continued

Hospital Day 4. Mr. Michaels continues to feel better. His vital signs are stable: temperature: 98.4°F, BP 134/78 sitting and 140/80 standing without any HR changes, HR 78, RR 18, O_2 saturation on room air at rest is 96 and today with ambulation the O_2 saturation with exercise is 90. His lungs have cleared and he agrees to go to a rehabilitation facility for a few days [13]

10. What discharge orders are necessary for Mr. Michaels' discharge home?

Mr. Michaels will need a follow-up with the primary care provider within 7 days of discharge.

Transfer for Short-Term Rehabilitation

1. Problem list
   a. Reactive bronchitis
   b. COPD
   c. Asthma
   d. Hypertension
   e. Smoker
   f. Obesity
   g. Impaired fasting glucose
   h. GERD
   i. Barrett esophagus
   j. Depression
   k. PTSD
   l. Sleep apnea
2. Discharge medications
   a. Lisinopril (Zestril) 10 milligrams per mouth (po) daily
   b. Levofloxacin (Levaquin) 500 milligrams po daily for 3 days
   c. Albuterol (Proventil HFA) metered-dose inhaler, 90 micrograms per actuation, 1 to 2 puffs 4 times a day prn
   d. Fluticasone 500 micrograms/salmeterol 50 micrograms (Advair 500/50), 1 inhalation twice a day
   e. Tiotropium (Spiriva Respimat) 1.25 micrograms per actuation, 2 inhalations once a day
   f. Nicotine patch (NicoDerm) 21 milligrams/day × 6 weeks, then 14 milligrams/day × 2 weeks, then 7 milligrams/day × 2 weeks
   g. Prednisone 40 milligrams po daily × 5 days
3. Nursing home orders
   a. A 2000-calorie American Diabetes Association (ADA) diet.
   b. Blood sugars twice daily before breakfast and lunch. Notify physician if blood sugar greater than 200.
   c. Monitor BP daily.
   d. Monitor oxygen saturation when ambulating.
   e. Nasal oxygen 2 L if O_2 saturation is less than 88% at rest or with ambulation.
   f. Physical therapy/occupational therapy evaluation and treatment.

Case Study, Continued

Mr. Michaels is admitted to the rehabilitation center by the medical director of the rehabilitation facility. No new orders are added to his regimen. The patient continues to improve on days 1 and 2 of his rehabilitation stay. He is able to participate in therapy and on day 2 no longer has an oxygen saturation less than

90% at rest or with ambulation. On rehab day 3, Mr. Michaels complains of a funny feeling in his throat and feels like his throat is sore when the nurse brings him his morning medications. The nurse examines his throat and notices scattered white lesions on the back of his throat. The provider working with the medical director is asked to evaluate the patient.

11. What are the potential causes of Mr. Michaels' complaint?

There are varied reasons for patients to have sore throats. Pharyngitis is commonly caused by bacteria, viruses, postnasal drip, thrush, gastroesophageal reflux, and even smoking. Other causes are also possible. Determining the cause of each patient's complaint requires that the provider obtain a careful history, a focused examination, and then consider the possible and probable diagnoses.

Mr. Michaels reports that the soreness started in his throat yesterday and has been gradually getting worse. He admits to a cough but states his cough is actually better over the past few days. He denies signs and symptoms of an upper respiratory infection, fever, chills, rhinitis, heartburn, or difficulty swallowing. On examination, his vital signs are all within normal limits: BP 130/70 sitting and standing, HR 78, RR 16, temperature 97.6°F. There is no sinus discharge or sinus tenderness. He does have both upper and lower dentures. His posterior pharynx and tongue are erythematous and there are scattered white patches on the tongue and posterior pharynx. His neck is supple without lymphadenopathy or masses; HR regular S1 S2 without S3, S4, murmur, or rub; lung sounds clear without rales, wheezes, or rhonchi; and extremities without edema or calf tenderness.

The provider considers possible causes for the patient's sore throat. He has several risk factors for an oral *Candida* infection: a history of smoking and hyperglycemia, recent antibiotic and steroid therapy, and dentures. The physical examination also suggests oral *Candida* (Fig. 4.2).

12. What treatment is indicated for Mr. Michaels?

Mr. Michaels is diagnosed with oral candidiasis, which is a common complication of steroid therapy, particularly in patients who are immunocompromised, using inhaled steroids, or diabetic. The patient is started on a twice-daily regimen of oral care that includes brushing the tongue; removing the dentures and cleaning them as well; a 12% chlorhexidine oral mouth rinse and denture soaking; and Nystatin suspension, 400,000 to 600,000 units swish and swallow 4 times a day for 7 days.

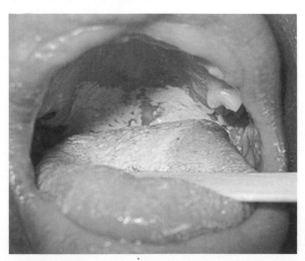

Fig. 4.2 Oral candidiasis. (From Auerbach, P. S., Cushing, T. A., & Harris, N.S. (2017). *Auerbach's wilderness medicine*. [7th ed.]. Philadelphia: Elsevier.)

The provider also reviews Mr. Michaels' records and notes his blood sugars are averaging 180 milligrams/dL. The provider is aware that steroids can increase blood sugars but, concerned about the patient's risk factors for diabetes (i.e., obesity, hypertension, age, sedentary lifestyle, and impaired glucose tolerance), orders the following laboratory tests: Hb A1C, lipid profile, liver function tests (LFTs), and thyroid stimulating hormone (TSH). These diagnostics are important to determine whether the patient has a thyroid disorder, hypercholesterolemia, or liver dysfunction. Thyroid dysfunction can be associated with hyperglycemia; assessing hypercholesterolemia is necessary in assessing cardiovascular risk in a patient with diabetes; and liver function is tested in anticipation of the need for statin therapy.

Rehabilitation Day 7. Mr. Michaels' laboratory results:

- Chem 8: Na 140 mEq/L, K 4.0 mEq/L, Cl 98 mEq/L, HCO_3 28 mEq/L, BUN 20, Cr 1.8 milligrams/dL
- Hb A1C: 6.5
- TSH: 4.0
- Liver functions tests: within normal limits
- Lipids: Total cholesterol 240, high-density lipoprotein (HDL) 45, low-density lipoprotein (LDL) 169 milligrams/dL

The provider is aware that an Hb A1C of 6.5 % or higher is diagnostic for diabetes and that lifestyle changes are recommended initially for patients with type 2 diabetes.[14] The patient's 10-year risk for a cardiovascular event is calculated to be 76%, and the patient is started on high-intensity statin therapy (atorvastatin 40 milligrams po daily).[15]

Rehabilitation Day 8. *Mr. Michaels has met with the skilled nursing facility dietician and learned more about the importance of diet to control his blood sugar. The skilled nursing facility team also meets with Mr. Michaels and determines that Mr. Michaels is ready for discharge home. He is discharged home 48 hours later with the following medications and will follow up with his primary care provider within 7 days. The provider completes the discharge paperwork and sends a copy of the discharge summary to Mr. Michael's primary care provider.*

1. Discharge medications:
   a. Lisinopril (Zestril) 10 milligrams po daily
   b. Albuterol (Proventil HFA) metered-dose inhaler, 90 micrograms per actuation, 1 to 2 puffs 4 times a day prn
   c. Fluticasone 500 micrograms/salmeterol 50 micrograms (Advair 500/50, 1 inhalation twice a day); rinse mouth and spit after using
   d. Tiotropium (Spiriva) 1.25 micrograms per actuation, 2 inhalations once a day
   e. Nicotine patch (NicoDerm) 21 milligrams/day × 5 weeks, then 14 milligrams/day × 2 weeks, then 7 milligrams/day × 2 weeks
   f. Atorvastatin (Lipitor) 40 milligrams po daily

Primary Care Visit
   Chief complaint: Follow-up hospitalization reactive bronchitis.

History of Present Illness. Patient returns to primary care for follow-up after hospitalization and rehabilitation for COPD exacerbation. He feels well, breathing is better, but still has some SOB and cough on occasion. Wants to return to work.
   Medications:
   Lisinopril (Zestril) 10 milligrams po daily
   Albuterol (Proventil HFA) inhaler 1 to 2 puffs 4 times a day prn
   Fluticasone 500 micrograms/salmeterol 50 micrograms (Advair 500/50, 1 inhalation twice a day)
   Tiotropium (Spiriva) 1.25 micrograms per actuation, 2 inhalations once a day

Nicotine patch (NicoDerm) 21 milligrams/day × 5 weeks, then 14 milligrams/day × 2 weeks, then 7 milligrams/day × 2 weeks

Atorvastatin (Lipitor) 40 milligrams po daily

Allergies: Environmental.

Review of Systems
General: Denies falls, fever, chills, weakness.
Skin: Denies rashes or lesions.
HEENT: Denies headache, dizziness, sinus pain.
Neck: Denies neck pain, lumps.
Respiratory: Still some SOB if he exerts himself, but much better per patient; occasional nonproductive cough, but better.
Cardiac: Denies chest pain or pressure, orthopnea, palpitations.
Gastrointestinal: Denies difficulty swallowing, constipation, black stools, diarrhea.
Urinary: Denies urinary burning or frequency.
Musculoskeletal: Denies pain.
Peripheral vascular: Denies edema, calf pain.
Neurovascular: Denies fainting, numbness, tingling.
Hematologic: Denies bleeding, easy bruising.
Endocrine: Denies sweating, thirst.
Psychiatric: Denies depression, anxiety.

Physical Examination
General: Alert, appropriate, overweight male in no acute distress.
Vital signs: Weight 230 pounds; BP 136/82 sitting, 138/78 standing; HR: 72; RR 18; O_2 sat: 93% on room air.
Skin: Warm, dry. No rashes.
Eyes: Sclera clear, conjunctiva within normal limits.
Ears: Canals: clear. TMs: no erythema, bulging or retraction.
Mouth: Membranes moist, no lesions or exudate.
Neck: Supple, no masses or lymphadenopathy.
Cardiac: S1, S2 regular. No S3, S4, murmur, or rub.
Lungs: Somewhat diminished at bases. No rales, wheezes, rhonchi.
Abdomen: Soft, bowel sounds throughout. No organomegaly or tenderness.
Extremities: No edema or calf tenderness.

13. What should be the priorities for this visit?

Mr. Michaels continues to improve, and the primary care physician reinforces the patient's diet and gives him information about a community tobacco control program for people wanting to stop smoking. The primary care provider explains that the laboratory test in the hospital checking for α_1-antitrypsin deficiency did not identify this genetic disorder. An appointment is made for the patient to follow up with pulmonology for the sleep study and pulmonary function tests. Liver function tests should be checked 6 weeks after a patient is started on statin therapy, and these are also requested. A follow-up appointment and laboratory diagnostics to monitor his diabetes (Hg A1C), renal status (Chem 8), liver function (LFTs), and hypercholesterolemia (lipid panel) are planned in 3 months.

References
1. Global Initiative for Asthma. (2018). Asthma Clinical Guidelines. Retrieved from http://www.2018-pocket-guide-for-asthma-management-and-prevention/www.ginasthma.com.
2. GOLD Guidelines. Retrieved from www.goldcopd.com/.

3. Maughan, B. C., Asselin, N., Carey, J. L., Sucov, A., & Valente, J. H. (2014). False-negative chest radiographs in emergency department diagnosis of pneumonia. *Rhode Island Medical Journal, 97*(8), 20–23. Retrieved from https://www.rimed.org/rimedicaljournal/2014/08/2014-08-20-cont-maughan.pdf.

4. Gupta, P., Anupam, K., Mehrotra, K., Khublani, S., & Soni, A. (2015). Value of past clinical history in differentiating bronchial asthma from COPD in make smokers presenting with SOB and fixed airway obstruction. *Lung India, 32*(1), 20 23

5. Aldrich, J., & Soroken, L. (2013). Acute bronchospasm. In T. M. Buttaro, J. Trybulski, P. Polgar-Baily, & J. Sandberg-Cook (Eds.), *Primary care: A collaborative practice* (4th ed.). St. Louis. Elsevier

6. Yang, P., Sun, Z., Krwoka, M. J., Aubrry, M.-C., et al. (2008). Alpha 1 antitrypsin deficiency carriers, tobacco smoke, chronic obstructive pulmonary disease and lung cancer risk. *Archives of Internal Medicine, 168*(10), 1097–1103.

7. Torpin, J., & Ottis, E. (2014). Review article: Determining the optimal steroid treatment regimen for COPD exacerbations: A review of the literature. *Journal of Academic Hospital Medicine, 6*(3). Retrieved from http://medicine.missouri.edu/jahm/review-article-determining-optimal-steroid-treatment-regimen-copd -exacerbations-review-literature.

8. Case Management Society of America (CMSA) (2010). Standards of practice for case management. Retrieved from http://www.cmsa.org/portals/0/pdf/memberonly/StandardsOfPractice.pdf.

9. Leuppi, J. D., Schuetz, P., Bingisser, R., et al. (2013). Short-term vs conventional glucocorticoid therapy in acute exacerbations of chronic obstructive pulmonary disease: The REDUCE randomized clinical trial. *JAMA: The Journal of the American Medical Association, 309*(21), 2223–2231.

10. Bixby, M. B., & Naylor, M. D. (2010). The Transitional Care Model (TCM): Hospital discharge screening criteria for high risk older adults. *Medsurg Nursing, 19*(1), 62–63.

11. American Thoracic Society. (2015). Criteria for Hospital Discharge. Retrieved from http://www.thoracic.org/ copd-guidelines/for-health-professionals/exacerbation/definition-evaluation-and-treatment/inpatient/ criteria-for-hospital-discharge.php.

12. Department of Health and Human Services. (2014). Discharge Planning. Retrieved from https:// www.cms.gov/Outreach-and-Education/Medicare-Learning-Network-MLN/MLNProducts/Downloads/ Discharge-Planning-Booklet-ICN908184.pdf.

13. Kripalani, S., Theobald, C. N., Anctil, B., & Vasilevskis, E. E. (2014). Reducing hospital readmission: Current strategies and future directions. *Annual Review of Medicine, 65*, 471–485.

14. American Diabetes Association. (2016). *Standards of Medical Care in Diabetes, 39*(suppl 1), S1–S106. Retrieved from http://care.diabetesjournals.org/site/misc/2016-Standards-of-Care.pdf.

15. Stone, N. J., Robinson, J. G., Lichtenstein, A. H., et al. (2014). 2013 ACC/AHA guideline on the treatment of blood cholesterol to reduce atherosclerotic cardiovascular risk in adults: A report of the American College of Cardiology/American Heart Association Task Force on Practice Guidelines. *Journal of the American College of Cardiology, 63*(25_PA), 2889–2934.

Homelessness

Terri LaCoursiere-Zucchero ▪ Carolyn Abbanat

Case Study Scenario/History of Present Illness

After years of refusing services, a 55-year-old African American male, Mr. C, who has been living at an abandoned building near the park, is brought into the homeless shelter by an outreach worker. The outreach worker developed a relationship with him over the past 8 months and convinced him to get out of the cold for the night. During the shelter intake process, Mr. C complains of a headache and asks for some medicine. The outreach worker escorts him over to the on-site clinic operated by a local Health Care for the Homeless (HCH) program. Mr. C is malodorous, disheveled, and wearing multiple layers of clothing. He is carrying one large bag. He has poor eye contact, disorganized speech, and his thoughts are generally focused on the government. His breath smells of alcohol. This evening, the clinic is staffed by a nurse practitioner (NP) who has been working with the homeless population for 3 years. After a brief history from the outreach worker, the NP determines that the goal of this initial visit with Mr. C may be to simply begin to earn his trust if there are no urgent needs. The patient's vital signs are not measured and a traditional, formal history and physical (H&P) are not performed.

Instead, Mr. C is offered a foot soak as a nonthreatening way to establish a relationship and introduce contact. He accepts the soak and the NP notices his extremely long toe nails and scaly, erythematous feet, which are characteristic of tinea pedis. The NP learns that Mr. C is a US veteran but has not received care by the Department of Veterans Affairs (VA) in years. He was diagnosed with schizophrenia in his 40s and states, "That's when I knew they were after me." He reports that his headache "is not too bad, comes and goes" and will not elaborate except to acknowledge that it is not new. Mr. C requests Tylenol stating, "It works every time." The NP confirms he has no allergies and gives him a single-dose packet of two tablets of acetaminophen 325 milligrams and a cup of water. Mr. C declines to have his toe nails trimmed, but he allows the NP to apply clotrimazole cream 1% to his feet and accepts a clean pair of socks. The NP states she has enjoyed meeting him and would like to check on his headache and feet again soon. She provides her clinic schedule and recommends a 1-week follow-up unless he would like to be seen sooner.

Three weeks pass and Mr. C returns to the clinic presenting similarly as before. He complains of another headache and requests to see the NP for a foot soak. The NP learns more information about Mr. C during the soak. Other than occasional emergency department (ED) visits for minor injuries and illnesses, he has not had any regular medical care since he left the VA years ago. He was hospitalized at the VA for what sounds like acute psychosis and was discharged on medications, which he never took. Again, Mr. C declines to have his toe nails trimmed, but he allows clotrimazole cream 1% be applied to his feet and takes a new pair of socks. He requests Tylenol and the NP explains she needs to ask a few questions about his headache. "Ok, but not too many," he states.

Mr. C has felt a dull, squeezing pain around his head for the last few hours. It occurs "every now and then over the past 20 years." The headache typically lasts "a couple hours, I don't really know." He rates the pain as 3/10 and denies any increase in frequency or severity. Tylenol was effective a week ago. Mr. C denies fever, stiff neck, or rash and has had no visual changes or photophobia. He attributes the headache to increased stress. "The FBI is closing in. I feel it." The NP asks to do a set of vital signs. Mr. C agrees only to a temperature, which is 98.8°F. The NP provides a sample packet of two 325-milligram tablets of acetaminophen and a cup of water. She explains she would like to see him next week for a follow-up and include a blood pressure (BP) check and a basic physical examination, if he is willing.

Two weeks pass and the patient has not returned. The NP talks with the outreach worker who states that Mr. C is back at the park. The NP and outreach worker arrange to do a visit at the park the next day. They find Mr. C sitting on a bench and offer him a blanket and some gloves, which he accepts. He explains that he had to leave the shelter because "the FBI had found me." There is an empty beer can on the bench. The NP asks him about his alcohol use and he admits to drinking "just a little" every day. "It helps my pain." The outreach worker invites Mr. C back to the shelter, but he declines. A plan is made for the NP and outreach worker to visit him every 1 to 2 weeks as their schedules permit. Over the next 2 months, the NP and outreach worker establish more trust with Mr. C and small details are learned about his life. For example, he loves baseball and enjoyed being a cook in the Army. The NP encourages him to return to the shelter and clinic when he is comfortable and reminds him of the need for a more thorough check-up.

The next day, with temperatures below freezing, Mr. C comes to the shelter and requests to see the NP. At the clinic, he declines a foot soak and states he has another headache and does not feel too well. The headache is described as a dull pain, "the same as usual, a pressure around my head" and rated 4/10. It is not aggravated by movement. He is uneasy because his backpack and money were stolen while he was sleeping last night, and he is convinced an FBI agent is involved. He reports his last drink was about 2 hours ago. The NP asks if today she can obtain a little more history and do a brief examination. Mr. C agrees.

History of Present Illness
Medications: None.
Allergies: None.
Habits: Smokes about $\frac{1}{4}$ to $\frac{1}{2}$ pack per day × 48 years. Daily ethanol (ETOH) use usually 3 to 6 12-ounce cans of beer per day. Denies illicit drug use but reported that the FBI has "drugged my water bottle sometimes."
Past medical history: Schizophrenia, diagnosed about 20 years ago. Never tried medication. "I don't need any meds. I'm doing just fine." Denies cancer, hypertension, diabetes, respiratory illnesses including asthma and chronic obstructive pulmonary disease (COPD), history of head injury or traumatic brain injury (TBI), or any other chronic medical problems.
Past surgical history: Appendectomy age 19.
Family history: Father left during childhood. Mother died in her 70s, cause unknown. Has two sisters and a brother, their health status unknown.
Personal and social history: US veteran, divorced, disconnected from adult son, unemployed, and homeless for last 20 years. Currently uninsured but is eligible for VA health care benefits.

Review of Systems
General: "Surviving." Tired, didn't sleep well last night. "Too cold." Denies fever, chills, weakness, weight loss or gain. Eats two meals a day. "The churches have a good meal most days and I find things to eat at the park."
Skin: Tripped over a bottle at the park last week and scraped right knee. Denies other wounds, lesions, rashes or itching. Denies jaundice.
Head, eyes, ears, nose, and throat (HEENT): Complains of headache as noted previously. No visual changes or photophobia, "but I could use some reading glasses." Denies hearing problems or aversion to loud sounds. No tooth pain or sore throat. No difficulty swallowing. "It's been years since I've seen the dentist."
Neck: Denies stiff neck or swollen glands.
Respiratory: Denies cough, wheezing, or shortness of breath.
Cardiac: Denies chest pain, palpitations, dyspnea with exertion, or swelling.
Gastrointestinal: Occasional reflux 1 to 2× per month. Uses Tums or Rolaids when he can obtain it and that provides relief. Denies abdominal pain, nausea, vomiting, diarrhea, or constipation. Stool is brown, no blood.

Genitourinary: No problems urinating. Denies penile discharge or lesions.

Musculoskeletal: "The usual aches and pains, depends where I sleep and how far I walk that day." Mostly dull low back pain, knee pain, and aching feet. No radiation.

Psychiatric: Believes the FBI is watching him because "I know a lot about how things work in this country." Occasionally hears voices. "They're ok. Nothing bad." Denies depression or excessive worrying. Denies suicidal or homicidal thoughts.

Neurologic: Denies seizures. Occasionally is tremulous "when I'm due for a beer." No problems with memory. "I'm as sharp as a tack. I remember everything."

Hematologic: Denies bruising, anemia, or history of transfusions.

Endocrine: Denies temperature intolerance, hair loss, polydipsia, polyuria, or polyphagia.

Physical Examination

General: Disheveled 55-year-old African American male who looks much older than stated age with poor hygiene and multiple layers of clothing on, which he declined to remove. He declined to sit down. Examination was conducted with Mr. C completely clothed and standing.

Vitals: Height 72 inches (182.9 cm), weight 199 pounds (90.3 kg), body mass index (BMI) 27; temperature 98.5°F; pulse 72; BP 162/98 right arm, declined left arm reading; respiratory 18, O_2 sat: 98%.

Skin: Declined to remove gloves or shoes. Examination deferred.

Head: Declined to remove hat. Examination deferred.

Eyes: Pupils equal, round, react to light and accommodation (PERRLA). Clear, no drainage. Nonicteric.

Ears: No external deformity. Canals normal. Scant amount of cerumen bilaterally. Tympanic membranes pearly gray.

Nose: Patent, no drainage.

Throat: Mucous membranes moist. Pharynx without erythema or exudate. Tonsils 1+ bilaterally. Poor dentition with several broken and missing teeth.

Neck: Supple, no lymphadenopathy.

Respiratory: Respirations even and nonlabored. Posterior lung sounds clear.

Cardiac: Normal S1, S2, regular rate and rhythm. No murmurs appreciated.

Back: Deferred.

Abdomen: Declined.

Genitourinary: Deferred.

Rectal: Deferred.

Extremities: Moves all extremities without problem.

Musculoskeletal: Deferred.

Neurologic: Alert, oriented × 3. Poor eye contact. Blunted affect. Disorganized speech and thought content focused at times on the government. Gait steady.

Assessment and Plan

1. Based on the history and physical examination results, what are the possible causes (differential diagnosis) for Mr. C's current condition?

Mr. C's history of homelessness, schizophrenia, alcohol use, and lack of health care are complicating factors that must be taken into consideration during the assessment and plan. The identified complaint of headache needs further exploration as do the other health problems listed below.

Headache

- Headache is one of the most common physical complaints seen in primary care[1] and is especially prevalent in the adult homeless population because of the physical and emotional stresses of homelessness and its associated problems. Given Mr. C's circumstances, it is not surprising that he complains of a headache. The fact that Mr. C's headaches have been occurring for years suggest that his headaches are most likely a primary headache syndrome versus a secondary headache. In a healthy person with chronic headaches, tension-type headache (TTH), migraine, and cluster are among the top differentials.[1] The other headache characteristics he has (dull squeezing pain across the forehead, mild pain rated at 3/10, and responsiveness to acetaminophen) point to a diagnosis of a TTH. Thankfully, Mr. C does not have any red flag headache signs indicating an infectious or intracranial process such as complaining of the "worst headache of life," headaches dramatically different from past episodes, immunocompromised status, new-onset after age 50 years, or onset with exertion.[1] There are no associated features of migraine, such as nausea, vomiting, photophobia, phonophobia (sensitivity to sound), osmophobia (sensitivity to smells), throbbing, or aggravation with movement.[1] Cluster headaches are unlikely given that the headache is not unilateral, severe, and not associated with ipsilateral lacrimation, nasal congestion, rhinorrhea, miosis, and/or ptosis[1]—at least now that we know of. The headache could also be caused by alcohol consumption and/or dehydration.

Elevated Blood Pressure

- The patient's BP is elevated at 162/98. However, with just one reading and no history of hypertension, a diagnosis of hypertension is not appropriate to make now as the diagnosis of hypertension is made based on the average of two properly taken BP measurements at two or more office visits.[2] BP is affected by a number of factors that may be playing a role for Mr. C, including "white-coat syndrome" (presence of medical staff), stress, pain, and medications including alcohol.[2]

It should be noted that an accurate BP measurement is essential to correctly diagnosing hypertension.[3] The appropriate technique is to allow the patient to sit quietly in a chair with a supported back and feet on the floor for 5 minutes before the measurement. The arm should be elevated to level of the heart. The BP should be measured at least twice, using a calibrated sphygmomanometer and an appropriately sized cuff for the patient.[3] Because Mr. C declined to sit down for the vital signs (and examination), and a second-arm BP reading was not available for comparison, the measurement should be interpreted with due consideration.

The JNC 8 did away with the classification of prehypertension and stages 1 and 2 hypertension to focus in on when pharmacologic therapy should be started.[4] At this time the only assessment that can be made is an isolated elevated BP.

ETOH

- Mr. C reports he drinks 3 to 6 beers daily and may very likely have an alcohol use disorder (AUD).[5] However, without further screening, it is not clear. It is also important to note that many individuals will minimize their amount of alcohol consumption when asked.
- To be diagnosed with an AUD, individuals must meet certain criteria outlined in the Diagnostic and Statistical Manual of Mental Disorders (DSM). Under DSM-5, individuals meeting any 2 of the 11 criteria during the same 12-month period receives a diagnosis of AUD.[5] The severity of an AUD (mild, moderate, or severe) is based on the number of criteria met (see https://online.epocrates.com/diseases/19836/Alcohol-use-disorder/Diagnostic -Criteria).

Schizophrenia

- Mr. C reports a history of schizophrenia × 20 years and presents with features of this disorder including disorganized thoughts and paranoid-type delusions.[6] However, other etiologies of psychotic symptoms could be explored including infectious causes, TBI, medications, nutritional deficiencies, endocrine disorders, dementia, and other central nervous system (CNS) pathology.[6]

2. What components of the history or physical examination are missing?

Given Mr. C's presentation, a limited H&P examination was performed. This was appropriate because many homeless individuals have experienced trauma and thus a gentle, trauma-informed approach must be used.[7] Once engaged with Mr. C, a more comprehensive H&P can be done. If the patient is not ready for a comprehensive H&P, performing sequential, focused examinations over time is an appropriate approach.

Integumentary System
- Skin and foot problems are among the most common reasons that individuals experiencing homelessness seek medical care.[8] Thus a thorough skin assessment,[9] when Mr. C allows for it, would be important in this patient.
- Factors associated with increased risk of skin and foot problems in the homeless include:[8]
    - Living in a shelter or other congregate housing in which scabies, lice, and bed bug infestations are often prevalent;
    - Sporadic opportunities to remove or change socks and shoes;
    - Using public/communal shower facilities;
    - Ambulatory lifestyle and poor-fitting shoes; and
    - Exposure-related skin conditions such as frostbite and immersion ("trench") foot.

Head
- Although Mr. C's headache appears to be an ongoing issue and likely benign, an examination of the head must be conducted. In addition, screening for nonneurologic causes of headache is appropriate, including palpation of the sinuses looking for tenderness consistent with sinusitis, and palpation of the temporal arteries for tenderness or reduced pulsations suggestive of temporal arteritis.[9]

Cardiovascular System
- Because of Mr. C's elevated BP, a comprehensive cardiovascular H&P examination is important. This would include BP measurements in both arms while sitting, a fundoscopic examination for signs of retinopathy; examination of the oropharynx and neck for signs of obstructive sleep apnea; palpation of the thyroid; auscultation for carotid, femoral, and renal bruits; palpation of peripheral pulses; abdominal palpation for signs of aortic aneurysm; and a complete cardiac examination.[9]

Abdomen
- Mr. C admits to taking Tums or Rolaids occasionally for heart burn/reflux 1 to 2× per month. A detailed gastrointestinal history is prudent to adequately determine whether he has typical symptoms of gastroesophageal reflux disease (GERD) versus other differentials, and any complications.[9] An abdominal examination is necessary to assess for organomegaly (particularly liver enlargement given Mr. C's history of alcohol use), pain, and assessment of bruits.[9]

Neurologic System
- Finally, a detailed neurologic assessment is also indicated. This is not only because of Mr. C's complaint of headache but also indicated given his history of psychosis and current mental status.[9]

3. What additional history should the nurse practitioner attempt to obtain when Mr. C is feeling more trusting and comfortable?

Given Mr. C's history of chronic homelessness, there are several additional elements of the history that are important to explore over time to provide the best care.[7]

- Access to shelter; unsheltered locations he stays at
- Access to food and water; nutritional intake, unintended weight loss or gain
- Access to restrooms and showers
- Place to store medications
- How he spends his day; day time locations and activities
- Transportation
- History of trauma
- Incarceration or other legal issues
- Connection to family, friends, and other support

4. What diagnostics are necessary for Mr. C?

- At this time, a conservative diagnostic approach must be taken with Mr. C because of his unwillingness to engage in health care for many years and his mental illness.[7] Although there are no life-threatening problems to attend to currently, being aggressive in the workup (and treatment) may compromise the relationship that has been cultivated and Mr. C may not return.
- Another issue to consider is that Mr. C does not have any health insurance. Although he is eligible to receive care at the VA, and a caseworker could assist him in completing the necessary forms to obtain VA identification, he does not want to receive care there. Alternatively, the caseworker will need to assist him in applying for Medicaid.
- With Mr. C's input, a prioritized list of diagnostics should be made with a time line that he is comfortable with.[7]
- Because there is only one elevated BP reading, a comprehensive hypertension workup is not indicated, but it will be important if a hypertension diagnosis is eventually made.[4]
- As described previously, an ETOH screening is needed. When Mr. C is comfortable to discuss his alcohol use, several validated detailed questionnaires are available including the Alcohol Use Disorders Identification Test (AUDIT) (Fig. 5.1) and the CAGE questionnaire.[10]
- Depression screening using the Patient Health Questionnaire (PHQ)-9 and anxiety screening using the Generalized Anxiety Disorder (GAD)-7 item scale may be reasonable first steps before a formal psychiatric evaluation is scheduled.[9]
- Homelessness is a risk factor for tuberculosis (TB) infection.[11] Therefore TB screening, typically using the Mantoux tuberculin skin test (TST) or purified protein derivative (PPD) is important (and usually required) for all homeless individuals, sheltered or unsheltered. Compared with the overall population, homeless persons have an approximately 10-fold increase in TB incidence and were less likely to complete TB treatment.[11]
- When possible, age-appropriate preventive care and screening should be provided to homeless individuals according to accepted guidelines and the clinical situation.[7] However, aggressively proceeding with health maintenance needs can be overwhelming to patients, especially if they are establishing trust with providers. Partnering with Mr. C to determine the order and priority of pursuing preventive care measures, once more immediate needs are met, is an appropriate strategy.[7] One reasonable approach is to start with noninvasive or minimally invasive labs that can be obtained through point-of-care testing (POCT) in the clinic. These could include a urinalysis (UA), blood glucose, A1C, and lipids, depending on available tests.

1. How often do you have a drink containing alcohol?				
Never	Monthly or less	Two to four times a month	Two to three times a week	Four or more times a week

2. How many drinks containing alcohol do you have on a typical day when you are drinking?				
1 or 2	3 or 4	5 or 6	7 to 9	10 or more

3. How often do you have six or more drinks on one occasion?				
Never	Less than monthly	Monthly	Weekly	Daily or almost daily

4. How often during the last year have you found that you were not able to stop drinking once you had started?				
Never	Less than monthly	Monthly	Weekly	Daily or almost daily

5. How often during the last year have you failed to do what was normally expected from you beacuse of drinking?				
Never	Less than monthly	Monthly	Weekly	Daily or almost daily

6. How often during the last year have you needed a first drink in the morning to get yourself going after a heavy drinking session?				
Never	Less than monthly	Monthly	Weekly	Daily or almost daily

7. How often during the last year have you had a feeling of guilt or remorse after drinking?				
Never	Less than monthly	Monthly	Weekly	Daily or almost daily

8. How often during the last year have you been unable to remember what happened the night before because you had been drinking?				
Never	Less than monthly	Monthly	Weekly	Daily or almost daily

9. Have you or someone else been injured as a result of your drinking?		
No	Yes, but not in the last year	Yes, during the last year

10. Has a relative, friend, doctor or other health worker been concerned about your drinking or suggested you cut down?		
No	Yes, but not in the last ycar	Yes, during the last year

Fig. 5.1 Alcohol Use Disorders Identification Test (AUDIT) Questionnaire. (From Saunders, J. B., Aasland, O. G., Babor, T. F., de la Fuente, J. R., & Grant, M. (1993). Development of the alcohol use disorders identification test (AUDIT): WHO collaborative project on early detection of persons with harmful alcohol consumption–II. *Addiction,* 88(6), 791–804.)

- Additional health maintenance to address when possible include hepatitis screening, vaccinations, eye and dental examinations, and cancer screening such as fecal immunochemical test (FIT) for colorectal cancer.
- Cognitive and functional impairments among the homeless are common and mirror impairments present in much older, housed individuals.[12] Thus the NP should consider screening Mr. C for cognitive impairment and performing an office-based assessment of functioning and mobility when appropriate.

5.   What treatments should be recommended for Mr. C at this time?

- For the individuals experiencing homelessness, health care may not be a priority given the need to obtain basic needs such as food and housing.[13]
- Developing an individualized, realistic plan of care with Mr. C that addresses his basic needs will strengthen the patient–provider relationship, increase his stability, and promote successful treatment.[7]

- First, the NP should carefully assess Mr. C's priorities for his immediate health care needs and the reason for his visit. Later, long-term health care needs can be discussed. The treatments next are ideal, but the NP must approach Mr. C gently with each plan and gauge his comfort level.
  - For his tension headache, simple over-the-counter (OTC) pain relievers are usually the first line of treatment.[1] Although acetaminophen has been effective in this past, this can be an option. However, given Mr. C's daily alcohol use and his unknown liver status, acetaminophen should be used with caution with limits of 2 g/day.[14] Ibuprofen is also an option if Mr. C does not have any nonsteroidal antiinflammatory drug (NSAID) risks (e.g., hypertension, gastrointestinal bleeding, chronic kidney disease, coronary artery disease).
  - Although Mr. C has had only one elevated BP, basic teaching can begin about nonpharmacologic management of hypertension. Specific education should be discussed realistically and sensitively given Mr. C's lifestyle.[15] Although traditional cardiovascular education may include a diet emphasizing vegetables, fruits, and whole grains; limiting sodium intake to less than 2400 milligrams/day; and exercising three or four times per week for an average of 40 minutes per session,[16] many individuals experiencing homelessness will not be able to adhere to these strategies. Nevertheless, the NP can counsel Mr. C on making better food choices, portion control, identifying foods with high salt content, and so forth. Other nonpharmacologic strategies, including tobacco cessation and decreased alcohol consumption are also sensitive topics that should be discussed.
  - During the NP's first encounter with Mr. C, he had tinea pedis; thus foot care and clotrimazole cream 1% can be provided if this problem still exists.
  - Additionally, Mr. C can be gently encouraged to engage with behavioral health services that are available in the shelter and community.
  - The main goal is to continue to engage the client, develop trust, and build rapport.[13]

Case Study, Continued

Mr. C returns to the clinic 1 month later to ask for a new pair of socks and Tylenol for his headache. He has not had a headache for a week, but last night his backpack was stolen again and he did not sleep well. This time he agrees to sit down for vital signs and everything is normal, except his BP is elevated again: right arm 162/94, left arm 160/94.

6.　What are the health care provider's next steps?

These next steps are important for Mr. C, but it is also important to remember that multiple interventions all at once can cause him to feel overwhelmed. Based on Mr. C's comfort level, the NP introduces each step gently and may postpone certain elements of the plan for future visits.

- The health care team continues to build trust and establish rapport with Mr. C.
- The NP discusses the need to do a more comprehensive physical examination as outlined previously.
- A discussion with Mr. C about hypertension including what the diagnosis means, the appropriate evaluation including laboratory tests to rule out secondary causes, and nonpharmacologic versus pharmacologic treatment is initiated.
- Using a harm reduction approach to counseling, the NP begins a discussion about limiting alcohol intake and smoking.
- Mr. C is introduced to the team's licensed independent clinical social worker (LICSW) with hopes that over time, he will agree to meet with her.

Case Study, Continued

During this visit, Mr. C agrees to the cardiopulmonary examination only, which is normal. He declines laboratory tests but will think about returning next week for in-house UA and fasting glucose. He is not ready to cut back his alcohol intake, but he is in a precontemplative stage. He is not ready to quit smoking because it helps him relax. He states he will think about meeting with the social worker in the future.

One month later, Mr. C returns first thing in the morning stating "the FBI knows I'm in the shelter so I had to go off the grid." He allows just a BP check today and the UA and fasting glucose before "going back into hiding again." BP in the right arm is 168/96, and in the left arm is 168/94. UA dipstick is within normal limits (WNL) and fasting glucose is 110.

7. What are the priorities for this visit?

- It is important to remember that when working with individuals experiencing homelessness, especially those with severe mental illness, a priority is to continue to establish trust and build rapport.
- Given the relationship between hypertension and alcohol[17] and alcohol withdrawal,[18] it is important to assess Mr. C's alcohol use. What are the number of drinks he has had and when was his last drink? Is he willing to consider treatment?
- At this point, the NP may consider starting a single regimen antihypertensive treatment per JNC 8. For primary treatment of hypertension in African American patients, thiazide diuretics or calcium channel blockers are the recommended first-line therapy with a BP goal of <140/90.[4] If Mr. C is willing, laboratory work is indicated as previously discussed.
- Connecting Mr. C to behavioral health also remains a priority

Case Study, Continued

During this visit, the NP learns that Mr. C's last drink was 1 hour ago and thus it is unlikely that he is experiencing alcohol withdrawal. Mr. C declines antihypertensive medication but is willing to try lifestyle modification. He agrees to "one laboratory test only" and a comprehensive metabolic panel (CMP) is ordered. Mr. C is still reluctant to meet with a behavioral health clinician and states, "They might be colluding with the FBI."

8. Although Mr. C declined to start an antihypertensive, what should health care providers be aware of in terms of prescribing medications to individuals experiencing homelessness?

Understanding that individuals experiencing homelessness face several challenges related to taking medications is important.[7] Using a realistic patient-centered approach to care and self-management can improve adherence.

Issues	Solutions
- Patients may need to carry medications on their person because of limited space to store belongings - Medications are often lost or stolen - Multidose regimens can be challenging - If meals are irregular, taking medications that have to be taken with food can be difficult - Lack of access to a bathroom - Poor water intake complicates the use of diuretics and medications with gastrointestinal side effects	- Using clinical guidelines, prescribe the simplest medical regimen warranted by standard clinical guidelines, to facilitate treatment adherence - Decide on the amount of medications to dispense at a given time based on clinical indications, patient wishes, and other factors - Dispensing small amounts of medications may provide an incentive to return for follow-up if transportation to and from the clinic is available - Educate about safe storage of prescribed medications

Case Study, Continued

Mr. C's laboratory results are reviewed by the NP (see subsequent list) and reveal a mildly elevated blood urea nitrogen (BUN), normal creatinine, and mildly elevated aspartate transaminase (AST)/alanine transaminase (ALT). The remaining diagnostic tests are unremarkable. The NP tries, but is unable to reach Mr. C to review the laboratory results.

    Albumin: 3.6 (3.4–5.4 g/dL)
    Alkaline phosphatase: 50 (44–147 IU/L)
    ALT: 45 (10–40 IU/L)
    AST: 37 (10–34 IU/L)
    BUN: 22 (6–20 milligrams/dL)
    Calcium: 9.0 (8.5–10.2 milligrams/dL)
    Chloride: 98 (96–106 mEq/L)
    CO_2: 25 (23–29 mEq/L)
    Creatinine: 1.0 (0.6–1.3 milligrams/dL)
    Glucose: 84 (70–100 milligrams/dL)
    Potassium: 4.1 (3.7–5.2 mEq/L)
    Sodium: 138 (135–145 mEq/L)
    Total bilirubin: 0.9 (0.3–1.9 milligrams/dL)
    Total protein: 6.8 (6.0–8.3 g/dL)

Two months go by and Mr. C has not returned for follow-up. Outreach workers look for him each week at the park and other locations around the city, but he is not found. Then another month passes and the medical respite associated with the HCH clinic gets a call from a nearby ED requesting admission for this Mr. C.

9.   What is a medical respite?

According to the National Health Care for the Homeless Council, medical respite is "acute and postacute medical care for homeless persons who are too ill or frail to recover from a physical illness or injury on the streets but are not ill enough to be in a hospital."[19] Often operated by nonprofit organizations, medical respites exist in a variety of settings including shelters, transitional housing, and freestanding facilities and allow patients to rest and recover in a safe environment. Respite care is useful after discharges from the ED and hospital and has been demonstrated to reduce both total hospital days in subsequent 12 months[20] and 90-day readmission rates.[21] Although patients are receiving respite care, it is often an ideal time to address health maintenance needs, as well as coordinate care among health care and social services providers.

Case Study, Continued

According to the ED discharge summary given to the medical respite, Mr. C had been brought to the emergency room after being found intoxicated lying in a puddle. In the ED, acute trauma was ruled out with negative physical examination (PE), normal c-spine x-ray, and head computed tomography (CT). BP was elevated at 170/101. His electrocardiogram (ECG) showed sinus tachycardia but was otherwise normal. The complete blood count (CBC) showed a macrocytic anemia. Mr. C also had signs of alcohol withdrawal and was given Ativan 2 milligrams with a repeat dose in 4 hours along with a liter of intravenous (IV) fluids. He expressed paranoid thoughts, and a psychiatric consultation was completed with a diagnosis of schizophrenia.

    Given that Mr. C is stable in the ED, the HCH's medical respite agrees to admit him and he is transferred. On admission, the benefits coordinator assists Mr. C with completing the paperwork for enrollment in Medicaid.

10. What should the medical respite treatment plan include? (Associated results/outcome are provided.)

Use admission to obtain important diagnostics and complete age-appropriate preventative measures while Mr. C is maintained in a supportive environment.

- Orient Mr. C to the medical respite including physical layout and policies/procedures.
- Monitor vital signs q4h × 48 hours, then twice daily.
- TB screening (negative).
- Laboratory tests:
  - CMP (mildly elevated liver function tests [LFTs], otherwise WNL)
  - Thyroid-stimulating hormone (TSH) (normal)
  - Rapid plasmin reagin (RPR) (negative)
  - HIV (negative)
  - Vitamin D (17 ng/mL)
  - Hepatitis panel (needs Hep A and Hep B vaccines; hepatitis C virus [HCV] is negative)
- Continue alcohol detoxification with Ativan 1 to 2 milligrams by mouth (po) q4h as needed (prn) according to the Clinical Institute Withdrawal Assessment of Alcohol Scale, Revised (CIWA-Ar)[22] × 48 hours then plan for tapering must be considered (Fig. 5.2).
- Start folic acid for macrocytic anemia per CBC results at ED (declined).
- Start 1000 IU of vitamin D_3 po daily (declined).
- Start multivitamin (accepted).
- Monitor BP, and once ETOH detox is completed consider if antihypertensive regimen is indicated.
- Connect to Mr. C to behavioral health team including LICSW and psychiatric NP (meet with each provider to make plans for Mr. C's follow-up appointments).
- Invite to support groups (declined).
- Offer nicotine replacement therapy (NRT) (declined).
- Offer therapeutic recreational and spiritual supports (enjoyed petting therapy dog).
- Connect to case manager to coordinate care including (1) follow-up regarding interest in VA services (declined), (2) referral to Department of Mental Health for evaluation to determine eligibility for services (declined), and (3) housing application (completed).
- Offer referral to dental (declined).
- Offer referral to optometry (accepted and received new glasses).

Case Study, Continued

Three days into his respite admission, Mr. C leaves against medical advice (AMA). Per policy, he cannot continue on the benzodiazepine ETOH detox or taper independently, but the team provides him with the multivitamin. His last three BPs averaged approximately 130/88.

He presents at the shelter clinic 1 week later. He complains of left foot pain and allows examination of his foot. Last drink was 2 hours ago. BP is 150/70.

11. What should the focus of this clinic visit be?

The NP determines that the focus of this visit will be on the left foot pain and BP. During the examination, an object is noted to be stored in his sock. It is a plastic phone charger that Mr. C kept there for safekeeping because many of his belongings have been lost or stolen. The charger's prong has been lodged under the plantar surface of the last three toe digits. "The FBI must have placed this in my shoe when I was sleeping. I told you they spy on me!" The NP notes a small superficial wound, with mild surrounding erythema and a scant amount of serous sanguineous

Patient: _____   Date: _____   Time: _____:_____

Pulse or heart rate, taken for one minute: _____   Blood pressure: ____/____

Nausea and vomiting. Ask "Do you feel sick to your stomach? Have you vomited?"

Observation:
0—No nausea and no vomiting
1—Mild nausea with no vomiting
2—
3—
4—Intermittent nausea with dry heaves
5—
6—
7—Constant nausea, frequent dry heaves, and vomiting

Tremor. Ask patient to extend arms and spread fingers apart.

Observation:
0—No tremor
1—Tremor not visible but can be felt, fingertip to fingertip
2—
3—
4—Moderate tremor with arms extended
5—
6—
7—Severe tremor, even with arms not extended

Paroxysmal sweats

Observation:
0—No sweat visible
1—Barely perceptible sweating: palms moist
2—
3—
4—Beads of sweat obvious on forehead
5—
6—
7—Drenching sweats

Anxiety. Ask "Do you feel nervous?"

Observation:
0—No anxiety (at ease)
1—Mildly anxious
2—
3—
4—Moderately anxious or guarded, so anxiety is inferred
5—
6—
7—Equivalent to acute panic states as occur in severe delirium or acute schizophrenic reactions

Agitation

Observation:
0—Normal activity
1—Somewhat more than normal activity
2—
3—
4—Moderately fidgety and restless
5—
6—
7—Paces back and forth during most of the interview or constantly thrashes about

Tactile disturbances. Ask "Do you have any itching, pins-and-needles sensations, burning, or numbness, or do you feel like bugs are crawling on or under your skin?"

Observation:
0—None
1—Very mild itching, pins-and-needles sensation, burning, or numbness
2—Mild itching, pins-and-needles sensation, burning, or numbness
3—Moderate itching, pins-and-needles sensation, burning, or numbness
4—Moderately severe hallucinations
5—Severe hallucinations
6—Extremely severe hallucinations
7—Continuous hallucinations

Auditory disturbances. Ask "Are you more aware of sounds around you? Are they harsh? Do they frighten you? Are you hearing anything that is disturbing to you? Are you hearing things you know are not there?"

Observation:
0—Not present
1—Very mild harshness or ability to frighten
2—Mild harshness or ability to frighten
3—Moderate harshness or ability to frighten
4—Moderately severe hallucinations
5—Severe hallucinations
6—Extremely severe hallucinations
7—Continuous hallucinations

Visual disturbances. Ask "Does the light appear to be too bright? is its color different? Does it hurt your eyes? Are you seeing anything that is disturbing to you? Are you seeing things you know are not there?"

Observation:
0—Not present
1—Very mild sensitivity
2—Mild sensitivity
3—Moderate sensitivity
4—Moderately severe hallucinations
5—Severe hallucinations
6—Extremely severe hallucinations
7—Continuous hallucinations

Headache, fullness in head. Ask "Does your head feel different? Does it feel like there is a band around you head?"

Do not rate for dizziness or lightheadness; otherwise, rate severity
0—Not present
1—Very mild
2—Mild
3—Moderate
4—Moderately severe
5—Severe
6—Very severe
7—Extremely severe

Orientation and clouding of sensorium. Ask "What day is this? Where are you? Who am I?"

Observation:
0—Orientated and can do serial additions
1—Cannot do serial additions or is uncertain about date
2—Date disorientation by no more than two calendar days
3—Date disorientation by more than two calendar days
4—Disorientated for place and/or person

Total score: _____ (maximum - 67)   Rater's initials _____

Fig. 5.2 Revised Clinical Institute for Withdrawal Assessment for Alcohol (CIWA-Ar) scale. (Adapted from Sullivan, J. T., Sykora, K., Schneiderman, J., Naranjo, C. A., & Sellers, E. M. (1989). Assessment of alcohol withdrawal: the revised clinical institute withdrawal assessment for alcohol scale (CIWA-Ar). *British Journal of Addiction,* 84(11), 1353–1357. This scale is not copyrighted and may be used freely.)

drainage. The area is mildly tender to palpation. Mr. C allows the NP to clean the area and apply Bacitracin and a dressing. He accepts a new pair of socks. He declines a Tdap booster. Although the NP is discussing a plan to connect Mr. C with the behavioral health team, Mr. C stands up and says he has to leave. The NP encourages him to follow up soon.

Case Study, Continued

Over the next year, Mr. C presents at the clinic with various conditions, such as headache, tinea pedis, paranoid thoughts, elevated BP, and early signs of withdrawal. The team continues to collaborate on best ways to address his immediate needs while keeping Mr. C's personal goals and individual concerns in mind. It remains a challenge to significantly improve his BP and sobriety status given that his complex psychosocial situation and lack of housing continues to create barriers to achieving optimal health and wellness. However, the NP notes that there are more frequent and longer periods of improvement, and over time he demonstrates increased engagement with the clinic and shelter staff. He also uses medical respite care periodically for episodic conditions and he has had fewer ED visits than he did the previous year. His case manager has assisted him with receiving Department of Mental Health services.

After 2½ years, Mr. C is housed through Department of Mental Health in a group home facility and continues to engage with a number of supportive community resources including HCH.

12. Homeless health care seems very different than traditional primary care. What are the features of this service model?

- It is important to understand that although homelessness poses unique health risks, the pathophysiology of disorders and treatments mirrors other populations.
- Homeless health care is similar to the concept of patient-centered care. Homeless health care strives to provide care that is "respectful of, and responsive to, individual patient preferences, needs and values, and ensuring that patient values guide all clinical decisions"[23] and aims to address the unique medical and psychosocial comorbidities that individuals without housing may have.
- Features of homeless health care model include:[13,24]
  - Community collaborations
  - Comprehensive case management services
  - Consumer advisory board
  - Harm reduction approaches
  - Low barrier, flexible service system
  - Medical respite care
  - Multidisciplinary collaboration
  - Outreach and engagement
  - Team-based care
  - Trauma-informed care

13. In this case Mr. C, a veteran, was only 55 years of age, but the NP thought Mr. C looked and seemed to be older. Is this common? What is known about the relationship between homelessness and veteran status, and what about homelessness, age, and mortality?

- Homelessness is a major public health problem that disproportionally affects veterans.[25] Older veterans are twice as likely to be homeless than older nonveterans. Almost half of homeless veterans are over the age of 51 (41% are 51–61 years; 8.6% are 62+ years).[26] Veterans have high rates of chronic disease, psychiatric disorders, and substance abuse and tend to use limited preventative/primary care services, often seek care in EDs, and require acute hospitalization.[27]

- Recently there has been increasing concern that the homeless population is aging.[28] The median age of homeless single adults increased from 35 years in 1990 to 50 years in 2010.[29] In 2010 there were roughly 44,000 older homeless adults, and it is estimated that this population will increase by 33% in 2020, and by 2050 more than double to 95,000.[28]
- The limited research suggests there are unique differences between older and younger homeless adults.[12] Although homelessness at every age is associated with increased health vulnerabilities, older homeless adults face additional risks. Starting at around age 50, homeless persons have chronic conditions equal to or higher than housed peers 15 to 20 years older, including geriatric conditions typically limited to the elderly.[12] Furthermore, older homeless adults have three to four times the mortality rate of the general population because of unmet physical, mental health, and substance abuse treatment needs.[30] Age 50 has been used to define older age among the homeless.[12,29]
- Older homeless adults, including veterans, represent a growing vulnerable population that will rely on NPs and other health professionals to provide specialized care.

14. What is it like to work with the homeless? What are some things I should consider if I want to provide care to this population?

Although each person may experience working with the homeless differently, there are some common themes worth noting. Health and social service providers who work with the homeless typically face demanding circumstances and bear witness to incredible human suffering.[13] Despite the nature of this work, it can be very inspiring because health care providers and others working on the front lines of homelessness have the privilege of entering into relationships with society's most vulnerable, watching how resilient the human spirit can be, and observing or participating in seemingly small but significant victories.[31] In addition, because of the medical and psychosocial complexity of homelessness, work is seldom dull and regularly provides opportunities to expand knowledge and increase clinical skills. It is not unusual to feel weighed down by the challenges of providing care to the homeless in the context of inadequate resources and structural supports. Collegial support and seeking work/life balance and self-care are essential to addressing and preventing compassion fatigue.[32]

References

1. Aminoff, M. J., & Douglas, V. C. (2017). Nervous system disorders. In M. A. Papadakis, S. J. McPhee, M. W. Rabow, M. A. Papadakis, S. J. McPhee, & M. W. Rabow (Eds.), *Current medical diagnosis & treatment*. New York, NY: McGraw-Hill. http://accessmedicine.mhmedical.com.ezproxy.umassmed.edu/content.aspx?bookid = 1843&sectionid = 135716257.
2. Siu, A. L. (2015). Screening for high blood pressure in adults: US Preventive Services Task Force recommendation statement screening for high blood pressure in adults. *Annals of Internal Medicine*, *163*(10), 778–786.
3. O'Gara, P. T., & Loscalzo, J. (2014). Physical examination of the cardiovascular system. In D. Kasper, A. Fauci, S. Hauser, D. Longo, J. Jameson, J. Loscalzo, et al. (Eds.), *Harrison's principles of internal medicine* (19th ed.). New York, NY: McGraw-Hill. http://accessmedicine.mhmedical.com.e zproxy.umassmed.edu/content.aspx?bookid=1130&sectionid=79741626.
4. James, P. A., Oparil, S., Carter, B. L., Cushman, W. C., Dennison-Himmelfarb, C., Handler, J., et al. (2014). 2014 evidence-based guideline for the management of high blood pr essure in adults: Report from the panel members appointed to the Eighth Joint National Committee (JNC 8). *JAMA: The Journal of the American Medical Association*, *311*(5), 507–520.
5. American Psychiatric Association. (2013). *Diagnostic and statistical manual of mental disorders* (5th ed.) DSM-5. Arlington, VA: American Psychiatric Association.
6. Reus, V. I. (2014). Mental disorders. In D. Kasper, A. Fauci, S. Hauser, D. Longo, J. Jameson, J. Loscalzo, et al. (Eds.), *Harrison's principles of internal medicine* (19th ed.). New York, NY: McGraw-Hill. http://accessmedicine.mhmedical.com.ezproxy.umassmed.edu/content.aspx?bookid=1130&sectionid=79757166.

7. Bonin, E., Brehove, T., Carlson, C., Downing, M., Hoeft, J., Kalinowski, A., et al. (2010). *Adapting your practice: General recommendations for the care of homeless.* Health Care for the Homeless Clinicians' Network, National Health Care for the Homeless Council, Inc.

8. Contag, C., Lowenstein, S. E., Jain, S., & Amerson, E. H. (2017). Survey of symptomatic dermatologic disease in homeless patients at a shelter-based clinic. *Our Dermatology Online, 8*(2), 133–137.

9. LeBlond, R. F., Brown, D. D., Suneja, M., Szot, J. F., LeBlond, R. F., Brown, D. D., et al. (Eds.), (2014). *DeGowin's diagnostic examination* (10th ed.). New York, NY: McGraw-Hill. Retrieved from http://accessmedicine.mhmedical.com.ezproxy.umassmed.edu/content.aspx?bookid=1192&sectionid=68670445.

10. Pignone, M., & Salazar, R. (*2017*). Disease prevention & health promotion. In M. A. Papadakis, S. J. McPhee, M. W. Rabow, M. A. Papadakis, S. J. McPhee, & M. W. Rabow (Eds.), *Current medical diagnosis & treatment.* New York, NY: McGraw-Hill. http://accessmedicine.mhmedical.com.ezproxy.umassmed.edu/content.aspx?bookid=1843&sectionid=135697501.

11. Bamrah, S., Yelk Woodruff, R. S., Powell, K., Ghosh, S., Kammerer, J. S., & Haddad, M. B. (2013). Tuberculosis among the homeless, United States, 1994–2010. *The International Journal of Tuberculosis and Lung Disease, 17*(11), 1414–1419.

12. Brown, R. T., Kiely, D. K., Bharel, M., & Mitchell, S. L. (2012). Geriatric syndromes in older homeless adults. *Journal of General Internal Medicine, 27*(1), 16–22.

13. Schiff, J. (2015). *Working with homeless and vulnerable people: Basic skills and practices.* New York, NY: Oxford University Press.

14. Imani, F., Motavaf, M., Safari, S., & Alavian, S. M. (2014). The therapeutic use of analgesics in patients with liver cirrhosis: A literature review and evidence-based recommendations. *Hepatitis Monthly, 14*(10).

15. Strehlow, A., Robertshaw, D., Louison, A., Lopez, M., Colangelo, B., Silver, K., et al. (2009). *Adapting your practice: Treatment and recommendations for homeless patients with hypertension, hyperlipidemia & heart failure.* Nashville, TN: Health Care for the Homeless Clinicians' Network, National Health Care for the Homeless Council, Inc.

16. Sutters, M. (2017). Systemic hypertension. In M. A. Papadakis, S. J. McPhee, M. W. Rabow, M. A. Papadakis, S. J. McPhee, & M. W. Rabow (Eds.), *Current medical diagnosis & treatment.* New York, NY: McGraw-Hill. http://accessmedicine.mhmedical.com.ezproxy.umassmed.edu/content.aspx?bookid=1843&sectionid=135707761.

17. Husain, K., Ansari, R. A., & Ferder, L. (2014). Alcohol-induced hypertension: Mechanism and prevention. *World Journal of Cardiology, 6*(5), 245.

18. Williams, N., & DeBattista, C. (2017). Psychiatric disorders. In M. A. Papadakis, S. J. McPhee, M. W. Rabow, M. A. Papadakis, S. J. McPhee, & M. W. Rabow (Eds.), *Current medical diagnosis & treatment.* New York, NY: McGraw-Hill. http://accessmedicine.mhmedical.com.ezproxy.umassmed.edu/content.aspx?bookid=1843&sectionid=135717475.

19. National Health Care for the Homeless Council. (2017). Medical respite. Retrieved from http://www.nhchc.org/resources/clinical/medical-respite/.

20. Buchanan, D., Doblin, B., Sai, T., & Garcia, P. (2006). The effects of respite care for homeless patients: A cohort study. *American Journal of Public Health, 96*(7), 1278–1281.

21. Kertesz, S. G., Posner, M. A., O'Connell, J. J., Swain, S., Mullins, A. N., Shwartz, M., et al. (2009). Post-hospital medical respite care and hospital readmission of homeless persons. *Journal of Prevention & Intervention in the Community, 37*(2), 129–142.

22. Williams, N., & DeBattista, C. (*2017*). Psychiatric disorders. In M. A. Papadakis, S. J. McPhee, M. W. Rabow, M. A. Papadakis, S. J. McPhee, & M. W. Rabow (Eds.), *Current medical diagnosis & treatment.* New York, NY: McGraw-Hill. http://accessmedicine.mhmedical.com.ezproxy.umassmed.edu/content.aspx?bookid=1843&sectionid=135717475.

23. Institute of Medicine. (2001). *Crossing the quality chasm: A new health system for the twenty-first century.* Washington, DC: National Academy Press.

24. Zlotnick, C., Zerger, S., & Wolfe, P. B. (2013). Health care for the homeless: What we have learned in the past 30 years and what's next. *American Journal of Public Health, 103*(S2), S199–S205.

25. Perl, L. (2013). *Veterans and homelessness.* Washington, DC: Congressional Research Service.

26. US Department of Veteran Affairs. (2009). *Veteran homelessness. A supplemental report to the 2009 annual homeless assessment.* Washington, DC: US Department of Veteran Affairs and US Department of Housing and Urban Development.

27. O'Toole, T. P., Conde-Martel, A., Gibbon, J. L., Hanusa, B. H., & Fine, M. J. (2003). Health care of homeless veterans. *Journal of General Internal Medicine, 18*(11), 929–933.

28. Sermons, M. W., & Henry, M. (2010). *Demographics of homelessness series: The rising elderly population.* Washington, DC: National Alliance to End Homelessness.

29. Culhane, D. P., Metraux, S., Byrne, T., Stino, M., & Bainbridge, J. (2013). The age structure of contemporary homelessness: Evidence and implications for public policy. *Analyses of Social Issues and Public Policy, 13*(1), 228–244.

30. O'Connell, J. J. (2005). *Premature mortality in homeless populations: A review of the literature.* Nashville, TN: National Health Care for the Homeless Council.

31. Seiler, A. J., & Moss, V. A. (2012). The experiences of nurse practitioners providing health care to the homeless. *Journal of the American Academy of Nurse Practitioners, 24*(5), 303–312.

32. Apostoleris, N. (January 8, 2013). Self-Care Basics in HCH Settings. National Health Care for the Homeless Program. https://www.nhchc.org/2012/12/self-care-for-hch-providers/.

Initial Primary Care Encounter

Susan Feeney

Case Study Scenario/History of Present Illness

Mr. Aaron Simons, a 66-year-old African American male, comes to your primary care practice today to have a routine physical examination and to establish care. He is accompanied by his partner of 20 years who is a patient in your practice. Mr. Simons retired 4 months ago from the banking industry.

Mr. Simons has not been seen for routine health maintenance for 2 years because he "was very busy at work" and states, "basically I am pretty healthy." He last saw his previous primary care provider (PCP) 6 months ago for a sinus infection and had his prescriptions renewed at that time. He has recently run out of his medications.

His partner, Matthew, tells you, "Aaron had a stent placed about 5 years ago due to severe chest pain and shortness of breath when he walked. His cardiologist left the practice 3 years ago and Aaron has not followed up with cardiology since then. Now that he has retired he needs to start taking care of himself." Mr. Simons states he is ready to start focusing on staying healthy. He states his only concern today is that he seems to be "gaining weight." He has gained 10 pounds over the past 6 months. Information is obtained from the patient, his partner Matthew, and from his medical record, which has been obtained from his previous PCP.

Medications: Lisinopril/hydrochlorothiazide (HCTZ) 10 milligrams/12.5 milligrams daily; tamsulosin 0.4 milligrams daily; pravastatin 40 milligrams daily; aspirin (ASA) 81 milligrams daily; fluticasone nasal spray 2 sprays each nostril daily (uses in spring through summer); fish oil 1000 milligrams twice daily; acetaminophen 500 milligrams two tablets one to two times daily as needed (prn) for arthritis pain typically three to four times per week. The last dose was yesterday afternoon.

Allergies: No known drug allergies. No food or latex allergies. + environmental allergies (pollen and pet dander).

Habits: Remote smoking history, quit 5 years ago after stent placed, 30 pack-year history. Drinks 1 gin martini 5 to 6 evenings per week. Denies illicit drug use. Denies routine exercise.

Past medical history: Essential hypertension (HTN), atherosclerotic cardiovascular disease (ASCVD), osteoarthritis (OA) bilateral knees and LS spine, hyperlipidemia, and benign prostatic hypertrophy (BPH).

Past surgical history: Percutaneous drug eluding stent (DES) placement in left anterior descending artery (LAD) approximately 5 years ago and appendectomy at age 25.

Family history: Father died age 78 from Alzheimer's disease, had HTN and hyperlipidemia. Mother died at age 82 of cerebrovascular accident (CVA). Had diabetes mellitus type 2 (DM II) and HTN. Brother age 62 has HTN and BPH. Another brother age 68 has ASCVD, HTN, and DM II). Two children, son age 32, daughter age 28, both alive and well.

Personal and social: Banker, retired 3 months ago. Divorced 25 years ago. Has two grown children. Lives with longtime partner Matthew. Drafted at age 20 into Army, deployed to

Vietnam for two tours of duty (combat) and honorably discharged after 5 years of service. Has a BA in business and an MBA.

Review of Systems

General: + weight gain of 10 pounds over past 6 months. Denies fatigue, appetite changes, fever, chills, and injury. Feels rested in morning.

Skin: Denies lesions and rashes.

HEENT: + seasonal allergies (spring, summer). Hearing loss right ear x40 years after combat duty. Dentist cleaning every 6 months. Last eye examination 3 years ago. Denies vision changes, sinus pain, rhinitis, sore throat, dysphagia, and ear pain or pressure.

Neck: Denies pain, stiffness, and swollen glands.

Respiratory: + snoring most nights per partner. Denies cough, wheeze, and shortness of breath.

Cardiac: Denies chest pain, palpitations, dyspnea on exertion (DOE), and dizziness.

Gastrointestinal: Denies heartburn, nausea/vomiting, constipation, hemorrhoids, black tarry stools, and rectal bleeding.

Genitourinary (GU): + hesitancy, + nocturia (two to three times per night), and intermittent erectile dysfunction (ED). Mutually monogamous relationship. Denies frequency, urgency, burning, hematuria; dribbling/incontinence, and penile discharge. Denies history of sexually transmitted infection (STI).

Peripheral vascular: Denies swollen legs, calf pain, and ulcers.

Musculoskeletal: + intermittent bilateral knee pain along lateral and medial joint lines, aching in knee joint, and + intermittent low back ache and muscle tightness. Denies radiation of pain, numbness, tingling, and leg weakness. Denies joint swelling, redness, instability, popping, and locking.

Neurologic: Denies headache, vertigo, forgetfulness, numbness, and tingling.

Psychiatric: Denies insomnia, moodiness, and anxiety. Denies lack of interest or feeling depressed or sad.

Hematologic: Denies bruising and history of blood transfusions in past.

Endocrine: Denies heat or cold intolerance, excessive thirst or urination, or increased appetite, and sweating.

Physical Examination

General: Well-groomed, attentive African American male in no apparent distress. Affect and responses appropriate.

Vitals: Height 73 inches. Weight 245 pounds (111.13 kg). Basal metabolic index (BMI): 30.6. Blood pressure (BP) (left arm) 138/92, pulse 88 regular, respiratory rate (RR) 18, O_2 saturation 98% room air (RA).

Skin: No lesions, ulcers, or rashes.

Head: Normocephalic, atraumatic.

Eyes: Without redness or discharge.

Nose, sinuses: Nares clear, mucosa pink, moist without lesions, and sinuses nontender to percussion and palpation.

Mouth: Moist without lesions or discoloration. Posterior pharynx without injection or exudate.

Ears: Bilateral ears without cerumen. Left tympanic membrane (TM) gray with cone of light at 7 o'clock. Right TM dull with scarring.

Neck: Supple, without lymphadenopathy. Thyroid smooth and nonenlarged.

Cardiac: Apical rate 88, regular rate, rhythm without murmurs, rubs, or gallops.

Respiratory: RR 18 even, lungs clear to auscultation in all fields.

Abdomen: Soft, nondistended, bowel sounds normal, nontender, without hepatosplenomegaly.

Musculoskeletal: Full range of motion of all joints with crepitus noted bilateral knees with active flexion. Joints are smooth without redness or swelling, and nontender to palpation. Some stiffness of knees noted when moving from sitting to standing.

Extremities: Skin warm, dry, uniform color. Trace pretibial edema bilaterally (minimal pitting) with indentation noted from socks. Skin lower legs smooth with no hair noted. Bilateral anterior lower legs inferior to sock indentation, no varicosities.

Neurologic: Alert, oriented ×3. Gait normal. Movements are smooth and coordinated.

Assessment and Plan

1. Based on the history and physical examination results, what are the possible causes (differential diagnosis) for the patient's current condition?

Mr. Simons states the reason for his visit today is to reestablish primary health care. His last health maintenance visit was 2 years ago. His only complaint today is a 10-pound unintentional weight gain over the past 6 months. Of significance is his history of ASCVD status post DES placement, HTN, hyperlipidemia, degenerative joint disease, BPH, and recent retirement. His BP today is not at goal with an elevated diastolic blood pressure (DBP) of 92, and he is obese. His history reveals that he snores most nights and experiences nocturia.

It is possible that Mr. Simon's weight gain could be a result of fluid retention from congestive heart failure (CHF) based on his history of ASCVD, hyperlipidemia, and HTN. Renal failure can also cause fluid retention resulting in weight gain. Cardiovascular disease and BPH are risk factors for renal failure. Poor diet (excessive caloric intake and high-fat diets) with lack of exercise will result in weight gain. Mr. Simons has several risk factors associated with obstructive sleep apnea (OSA) including male gender, age (>55 years), snoring, and obesity (elevated increased BMI).[1] OSA is associated with HTN and weight gain.[1] It is important to ask Mr. Simons' about the presence of daytime drowsiness, which in another important indicator of OSA.[2] The practitioner can use OSA screening tools to determine his level of daytime drowsiness, such as the Epworth Sleepiness Scale (epworthsleepinessscale.com) and the STOP BANG questionnaire, as well as other validated tools (Fig. 6.1).[2] Changes in daily dietary and activity patterns associated with retirement may be associated with weight gain. Both depression and anxiety can affect appetite and physical activity, which can result in changes in weight. Thyroid dysfunction, specifically underactive thyroid function, can cause weight gain and elevate BP.

The elevation in Mr. Simons' DBP may be directly related to his weight gain, as discussed previously. Most of the causes for unintentional weight gain can also cause increased BP such as CVD, renal disease, OSA, hypothyroidism, sedentary lifestyle, and high-fats diets.[3] Other causes for poorly controlled HTN may be the result of poor compliance with the medication regimen and/or use of over-the-counter (OTC) medications, such as nonsteroidal antiinflammatory drugs (NSAIDs) or α-adrenergic agonist decongestants.[2]

Nocturia may be the result of an enlarging prostate, as well as OSA. Frequent awakenings to void during the night often result in inadequate, poor restorative sleep and can cause weight gain and increase BP, independent of OSA.

What is clear is that more information is needed to determine the cause of his weight gain. A 24-hour dietary recall is helpful in determining food choices and eating patterns. An assessment of the usual daily physical activity can give the provider a better understanding of activity during the day and to help with developing a realistic and reasonable exercise plan for the individual. A thorough discussion regarding OTC medications and supplements is required to assess possible contributing factors. Finally, a thorough review of past medical records to assess previous laboratory tests, imaging, screenings, and vital sign trends is essential.

1. *Snoring*
   Do you snore loudly (louder than talking or loud enough to be heard through closed doors)?
       Yes   No

2. *Tired*
   Do you often feel tired, fatigued, or sleepy during daytime?
       Yes   No

3. *Observed*
   Has anyone observed you stop breathing during your sleep?
       Yes   No

4. Blood *pressure*
   Do you have or are you being treated for high blood *pressure*?
       Yes   No

5. *BMI*
   BMI more than 35 kg/m^2?
       Yes   No

6. *Age*
   Age over 50 yr old?
       Yes   No

7. *Neck* circumference
   Neck circumference greater than 40 cm?
       Yes   No

8. *Gender*
   Gender male?
       Yes   No

High risk of OSA: answering yes to three or more items
Low risk of OSA: answering yes to less than three items

Fig. 6.1 STOP-Bang Scoring Model. (From Chung, F., Yegneswaran, B., Liao, P., Chung, S. A., Vairavanathan, S., Islam, S., Khajehdehi, A., & Shapiro, C. M. (2008). STOP questionnaire: A tool to screen patients for obstructive sleep apnea. *Anesthesiology, 108*, 812–821.)

2. What components of the history or physical examination are missing?

Mr. Simons has documented ASCVD. A thorough assessment of all components of the cardiovascular system is required. Starting with eyes, a thorough funduscopic examination is required to look for signs of hypertensive retinopathy (narrowing and straightening of terminal vessels, arteriovenous [AV] nicking, etc.). Also, Mr. Simons has a family history of DM II. The provider should be on the lookout for diabetic retinopathy (proliferative changes, white patches, etc.) because he is at increased risk for DM II. Visual acuity (Snellen test) should be assessed at this visit unless there is documentation of a thorough visual examination within the past 12 months.

A thorough assessment of the cardiovascular system, including the arterial system, is essential for this gentleman. Auscultation of all five cardiac landmarks should be performed and documented. Auscultation of the heart should be performed sitting and supine, because murmurs may be appreciated in one but not the other position. Palpation of the point of maximal impulse (PMI) is necessary because a downward and/or laterally displaced PMI may indicate left ventricular hypertrophy (LVH), which is associated with poorly controlled HTN.[4] Palpation should be performed bilaterally on all peripheral arteries for symmetry and quality of pulsation. Temporal, carotids, aortic, renal, iliac, and femoral arteries should be auscultated for presence of bruits. In light of a complaint of weight gain in the context of CVD, Mr. Simons should have an assessment of jugular vein distention (JVD). The abdominal aorta should be assessed for location of pulsation and approximate width. Mr. Simons' age, history of HTN, and smoking put him at risk for an abdominal aortic aneurysm.[4]

Due to the report of snoring, a measurement of neck circumference is appropriate. Men with neck circumferences >17 inches have a significant risk of OSA.[2] A thorough evaluation of Mr. Simons' oropharynx, specifically the clearance between the palate (hard and soft) and the outstretched tongue, is recommneded.[2] Diminished clearance to no visual opening between these structures when the mouth is opened wide and tongue protruding can indicate a risk for OSA.[1] As described previously, The Epworth Sleepiness and the STOP BANG questionnaires are validated tools to help screen for the signs and symptoms of OSA.[2]

Mr. Simons has BPH and is symptomatic with hesitancy, dribbling, and nocturia. A rectal examination is indicated to assess the size of the prostate and the presence of any nodules or irregularities. Mr. Simons' race and age increase his risk for prostate cancer.[5]

3.   What diagnostics are necessary for this patient at this time?

Mr. Simons has several chronic conditions that need monitoring, has a complaint of unintentional weight gain that needs investigation, and it is time for the secondary prevention screenings he needs. Many of these diagnostic tests will overlap.

Regarding his ASCVD, hyperlipidemia, HTN, and frequent acetaminophen use (which can cause liver inflammation), Mr. Simons should have a complete metabolic panel (CMP) and lipid profile drawn. Recent evidence indicates that fasting status may not be necessary for an accurate lipid panel, which aids in obtaining these laboratory tests.[6] To further investigate his increased BP and unintentional weight gain, a thyroid-stimulating hormone (TSH) with reflexive free T_4 and thyroid antibodies is indicated. Because of age, obesity, hyperlipidemia, ASCVD, and family history, Mr. Simons should be screened for prediabetes and DM II by checking a hemoglobin (Hb) A1C.[6]

Obtaining a serum prostatic-specific antigen (PSA) may be considered; however, the risk of a false-positive or an elevated result in the absence of cancer is a real possibility because BPH can cause an elevated PSA. A frank discussion with Mr. Simons regarding the sensitivity and specificity of the PSA is necessary before ordering this screening test. A validated screening tool called the International Prostate Symptom Score/American Urologic Association Symptom Index (IPSS/AUA-SI) measures quality of life and can assist with determining which men would benefit from medical management, and who might benefit from invasive procedures and/or surgical treatment.[5] If the score of the IPSS-AUA-SI is ≥8 while on medical management and/or if his prostate is significantly enlarged, a referral to a urologist may be warranted based on severity of symptoms, risk of obstruction, and his risk factors for prostate cancer.[5]

Because it has been reported that Mr. Simons snores, the Epworth Daytime Sleepiness and STOP BANG questionnaires should be administered. If findings indicate OSA, then a sleep study should be considered. According to the United States Preventative Services Task Force (USPSTF), all individuals 50 years and older should have a screening colonoscopy.[7] It is necessary to review his previous health records to determine when and if he had a colonoscopy. If he has never had one or his last was >10 years ago, one should be ordered for him. He should have an electrocardiogram (ECG) today as part of his ASCVD monitoring. It is important to compare today's ECG with any previous strips to determine the presence of any changes.

If Mr. Simons had any evidence of fluid retention, such as complaint of wheezing, cough, or shortness of breath, or presence of adventitious lung sounds (rales), JVD, or significant pitting edema, additional laboratory tests and imaging would need to be considered to determine the presence of CHF. If any of these history or physical examination findings were present, then a serum brain natriuretic peptide (BNP) and a chest x-ray (anteroposterior [AP] and lateral) would be recommended.

Mr. Simons' knee pain needs to be thoroughly evaluated through history and physical examination. Bilateral x-rays of his knees to determine the degree of joint degeneration may be considered, especially if the discomfort is interfering with his ability to exercise or if it is disturbing his sleep.

It is important to determine Mr. Simons' secondary prevention screening needs. The USPSTF recommends screening all individuals born between 1945 to 1965 for hepatitis C,[8] as well as screening for HIV for those at risk.[7] A decision to test for syphilis, gonorrhea, and chlamydia should be based on individual risk factors and the presence of signs/symptoms of infection.[7] If risk factors are present or appropriate screening has not been done previously, offer explanation and education and recommend appropriate screening tests.

4.   What treatments would you recommend for this patient?

Mr. Simons' DBP is not at the recommended goal set by the Eighth Joint National Committee (JNC 8) of the National Heart, Lung, Blood Institute of the National Institutes of Health (NIH) evidenced-based guidelines.[3] The recommended goal for Mr. Simon, based on his age, DM or chronic kidney disease (CKD), is systolic blood pressure (SBP) < 150 and DBP < 90.[3] If it is determined that he has been compliant with his current regimen, it can be assumed that the current regimen is inadequate to keep the BP within goal. The recommendations of the JNC 8 reflect evidence indicating that African Americans with HTN benefit more from calcium channel blockers (CCBs) and diuretics than an angiotensin-converting enzyme (ACE) inhibitor. The provider may want to consider switching him from lisinopril, which is an ACE inhibitor, to a CCB such as amlodipine. The provider could consider switching his current medication of lisinopril 10 milligrams/HCTZ 12.5 milligrams daily to amlodipine 5 milligrams with HCTZ 12.5 milligrams daily. CCB can be therapeutic within 1 week, so a recheck of his BP in 1 to 2 weeks would be reasonable. Both of these medications are generic.

The American College of Cardiology/American Heart Association (ACC/AHA) guideline for prevention and treatment of ASCVD has classified four statin benefit categories in an effort to reduce CVD events through primary and secondary prevention.[8] The recommendations indicate that treatment should be based on the individual's risk and expected benefit from statin therapy. The assessment to prescribe a stain and the intensity of the statin (based on expected percent reduction of low-density lipoprotein [LDL]) is based on the expected benefit, and specific target treatment goals are no longer recommended. High-intensity statins should reduce LDL by 50% or more, medium-intensity statins by 30% to 50%, and low-intensity statins reduce by 30% or more.[9] According to the ACC/AHA guideline, individuals with known clinical ASCVD should be prescribed a high-intensity statin unless there is a concern for patient tolerance.[8] In Mr. Simons' case, a high-intensity stain would be appropriate. Mr. Simons is currently on pravastatin 40 milligrams daily. Pravastatin when dosed between 40 and 80 milligrams daily is considered a medium-intensity statin. Atorvastatin 40 to 80 milligrams daily and rosuvastatin 20 to 40 milligrams daily are both considered high intensity. They are both generic, are efficacious, and have similar side effect profiles. Rosuvastatin has less interaction in the CP450, which is a 3A4 pathway, and has better efficacy improving high-density lipoprotein (HDL) and triglyceride values.

Lifestyle changes (diet and exercise) and achieving ideal weight are highly recommended for treatment of ASCVD. The JNC 8 Dietary Approaches to Stop Hypertension (DASH) diet includes low saturated fats (fats from animal sources) and complex carbohydrates, limiting simple carbohydrates.[3] Recommendations for exercise are for 30 minutes of sustained aerobic exercise (brisk walk or more) five or more days per week. A total of 150 minutes of weekly exercise is suggested, and there is evidence that achieving this goal over several days is superior to doing more exercise on fewer days for reducing risk and improving cardiovascular status. Before starting exercise, Mr. Simons should have an ECG to determine whether there have been any changes to his cardiovascular status since his last evaluation. Weight loss (oftentimes as little as a 10% loss) is associated with improved BP and lipid profile.[3,8] Therefore a weight loss of 24 to 25 pounds could very well result in demonstrable improvement in Mr. Simons' conditions. Plant sterols and viscous fiber have shown efficacy in reducing LDL; however, their impact on cardiovascular outcomes has not been determined.[8] Including these recommendations into dietary changes is reasonable. A referral to a nutritionist can be helpful if it is determined that there are knowledge gaps and/or difficulty in applying the dietary changes into his daily routine.

It also needs to be said that Mr. Simons has been lost to follow-up regarding his ASCVD. He was under the care of a cardiologist for his ASCVD and previous DES. It is very important that he reestablish care with a cardiologist in the very near future. Laboratory tests and ECG can be done through the primary care office while an appointment is made for Mr. Simons with a cardiologist. He is currently on ASA 81 milligrams daily, which he should continue. He was most likely on clopidogrel initially after his stent was placed. Obtaining copies of medical records from his previous PCP and other specialists, especially cardiology, is essential to providing comprehensive, coordinated care.

Mr. Simons' bilateral knee OA bothers him enough for him to take acetaminophen several times per week. The provider needs to determine the extent of discomfort affecting his activity level. He may have better relief with an NSAID; however, there is some concern of this class of medication increasing BP- and ASCVD-related events.[9] Before instituting this option, a CMP needs to be evaluated. In the meantime, weight loss strategies and daily walking can be started, which may be beneficial. If there is evidence of joint narrowing on x-ray, treatment with injectable artificial synovial fluid replacement may be an option. A referral to orthopedics based on the level of joint degeneration seen on x-ray is a reasonable plan. If the x-rays are normal, then a referral to physical therapy (PT) may be considered for advice on strengthening exercises for joint support and to reverse any deconditioning that may be present.

Mr. Simons is currently taking an α_1-receptor blocker (tamsulosin) for BPH, and he remains symptomatic. It should be determined whether the medication is being taken consistently and appropriately before determining whether it is ineffective. He is currently on the recommended starting dose (0.4 milligrams daily); however, he could benefit by increasing the dose to the maximum dose of 0.8 milligrams daily. As mentioned previously, a referral to urology should be considered if screening indicates his symptoms affect his quality of life and/or increase prostate cancer risk. Another class of medication, 5 α-reductase inhibitors (5ARIs), reduces prostate size hormonally. They are efficacious and can be taken with the α_1-receptor blockers. This medication may be a good option for Mr. Simons at this time. The current recommendations are to evaluate for the presence of prostate cancer before starting any treatment.[5] In light of this, a referral to urology for Mr. Simons is very reasonable.

5.   What are your next steps?

There are many wide and varying concerns that have come to light at today's visit. Establishing a trusting and open relationship with Mr. Simons is essential to determining his priorities, communicating concerns and priorities for his health, and determining a realistic plan going forward. Developing a treatment plan with mutual goals are meaningless if the patient does not return for follow-up because he feels distrustful or marginalized. The conscious development of a therapeutic relationship is considered essential to meeting patient goals and health needs.[10] This framework is often referred to as relationship-centered care. Management of Mr. Simon's chronic disease has been lost to follow-up. The cause for this gap in care should be considered regarding any barriers to care that might exist for Mr. Simons. Individuals from diverse backgrounds (race, ethnicity, sexual orientation, religion, and socioeconomic levels) often feel marginalized and encounter barriers to adequate, quality care.[11] Health disparities are well documented within the US health care system,[11] and it is imperative that the provider be cognizant of these barriers to provide quality care to all individuals. It can be surmised from the information at hand that Mr. Simons appears to be vested in his health and has a supportive and knowledgeable partner. He seems concerned about his weight gain, and his partner is concerned about Mr. Simons' lack of follow-up with cardiology. Important priorities for Mr. Simons are to safeguard and improve his cardiovascular health and should be at the top of the management plan.

Next steps should include ordering labs (metabolic profile, lipids, TSH with reflex, Hgb A1C, and hepatitis C, if needed), obtaining an ECG, and scheduling a visit with cardiology. These are priorities, and treatment decisions will be based on these results. Because there does not appear to be an acute cause of weight gain (such as CHF or thyrotoxicosis), the provider can wait until the lab results are back to refine the treatment plan. Discontinuing the ACE inhibitors and switching to a CCB, such as amlodipine, is a good idea. Making multiple changes to treatment plans at one time can be overwhelming and often can impair compliance. With this in mind, waiting until the lipid profile and CMP values are back to switch to a high-intensity statin may be a good approach. The provider can discuss exercise recommendations, stressing brisk walking as choice of exercise. There are few contraindications to walking, however, his knee pain, potentially related to OA, may affect his ability to walk briskly. More vigorous aerobic exercise can begin if Mr. Simon's stress test indicates no contraindication and cardiology gives clearance. Referral to nutritionist is a good option. Also, increasing Mr. Simons' dose of tamsulosin to 0.8 milligrams daily today may help with his current BPH symptoms.

Scheduling a follow-up visit is an essential part of the plan for Mr. Simons. A follow-up in 2 to 4 weeks would allow for evaluation of the efficacy of both the antihypertensive medication (amlodipine) on his BP and increased α_1-receptor blocker on his BPH symptoms. At this follow-up the provider can review laboratory results and refine treatments, such as changing statins and monitoring lifestyle changes, as well as offering encouragement. It has been shown that self-monitoring of biophysical parameters, such as BP, may be associated with improved adherence to plans of care and better outcomes.[12] Encouraging monitoring BP at home a couple times per week with a home BP monitor and weekly weigh-ins is an easy and efficacious method to improve Mr. Simons' BP and weight loss.

Case Study, Continued

Fasting laboratory studies (CMP, lipids, TSH with reflex, Hgb A1C, Hep C, HIV, rapid plasma reagin [RPR]) were drawn the day of the visit. Mr. Simmons' ECG was within normal limits, without signs of ischemia, previous injury, or LVH. He returns for a follow-up visit 1 month after his initial appointment. He consulted a nutritionist and has begun a low saturated-fat, low simple-carbohydrate, 2000-calorie diet, which he states has been "easy" to maintain. He was seen by cardiology and a stress echocardiogram has been scheduled for next week. Cardiology encouraged exercise to include brisk walking and some resistance training.

Both he and his partner feel they have been "accepted and included" in the planning of the care, and this has encouraged him to follow through with recommendations. Mr. Simons shares that he stopped going to the cardiologist 3 years ago because his new provider and others in the office had made him feel guilty about his "heart condition." He has felt this type of judgment before because of his "color" and his "lifestyle." Mr. Simons states that he has felt comfortable with his care at both this office and at the cardiology office. His comfort with the providers at this office and at his new cardiology office has encouraged him to take an active role in his health and reassured him.

Mr. Simons purchased a pedometer and has been getting between 7000 to 10,000 steps per day without chest pain, shortness of breath, or worsening knee pain. Mr. Simons' BP today is 138/84 and his weight is down 3 pounds (now 242 pounds). He sees no changes in his BPH symptoms with the increase in his tamsulosin dose. His knees are slightly better during the day since walking daily; however, he is still quite stiff and painful when getting out of bed in the morning.

His laboratory results are as follows: CMP, normal fasting glucose 98; Hgb A1C 5.9 (normal ≤5.6); lipids, LDL 154 (<100); triglycerides 165 (<150); HDL 38 (>40); non-HDL 116 (<130); ratio 4.05

(<4.0); TSH 2.5 (0.5–4.0); HIV negative; Hep C negative. His results indicate that he has prediabetes (Hgb A1C 5.7–6.4), which means he has insulin resistance and is at increased risk of developing DM II. His lipids remain out of range even on a medium-intensity statin. This particular pattern of lipid abnormality is consistent with metabolic syndrome, which is highly atherosclerotic.[8] In light of his known ASCVD, it is imperative that he start a high-intensity stain now. If Mr. Simons has evidence of metabolic syndrome (increased abdominal fat, apple shape, low HDL, and elevated triglycerides, all evidence of insulin resistance), then rosuvastatin may be a better choice than atorvastatin. However, both of these medications are efficacious in lowering LDL, triglycerides, and reducing risk of ASCVD events. For primary prevention, the ACC/AHA guidelines for prevention recommend that adults age 40 to 75 years who do not have ASCVD but have one or more risk factors (dyslipidemia, HTN, diabetes, smoking) and who have a 10% or greater risk of having a cardiovascular event within next 10 years, should be started on a low- to medium-intensity statin.[8] The 10-year risk can be determined by using the pooled cohort equations developed by the ACC/AHA.[8]

6. What are your priorities for the next visit?

Mr. Simons should return in approximately 3 months because good progress was seen at his initial follow-up. Ordering repeat lipids at this time is recommended to assess for response to the high-intensity statin. If values were not at goal, consideration of increasing the dose would be appropriate. A new class of cholesterol-lowering medication has recently been approved by the US Federal Drug Association (FDA). Proprotein convertase subtilisin/kexin type 9 (PCSK9) inhibitors are monoclonal antibodies that target LDL.[13] The indications for use are in individuals with primary hypercholesterolemia (nonfamilial or heterozygous familial) mixed dyslipidemia (including those with DM II and metabolic syndrome), and those with suboptimal response to or who are intolerant to statins. They have been shown to be effective in significant reduction in LDL levels; however, their impact on CVD outcomes has not been established.[14] They are expensive and would require prior authorization by insurers. This could be an option for Mr. Simons if he became intolerant to statins or his response was less than optimal on standard therapy. Once his lipids are within range and are well tolerated, lipids should be assessed once a year.

Continued monitoring of Mr. Simons' BP, BPH, and OA symptoms, and response to treatment should be evaluated at every visit. Revisiting sleep adequacy, snoring, and possible OSA should be addressed as well. If unchanged, then a referral for a sleep study should be initiated if not done at an earlier visit. The provider needs to assess for tolerance of all medications. A review of notes from specialty providers (cardiology and urology) is essential to ensure that their recommendations (medication changes, diagnostic studies) have been incorporated into Mr. Simons' care. Discussion regarding any outstanding screening, such as a colonoscopy, which has not been ordered in previous appointments should be addressed at this visit. Follow up of bilateral OA of the knees should occur. As always, the provider should ensure that Mr. Simons' concerns are assessed and addressed. Fostering a trusting relationship with Mr. Simons is essential to the foundation of his health and wellness.

References

1. Drager, L. F., Togeiro, S. M., Polotsky, V. Y., & Lorenzi-Filho, G. (2013). Obstructive sleep apnea: A cardiometabolic risk in obesity and metabolic syndrome. *Journal of the American College of Cardiology*, *62*(7), 569–576.
2. Chung, F., Abdullah, H. R., & Liao, P. (2016). STOP-BANG questionnaire: A practical approach to screen for obstructive sleep apnea. *Chest*, *149*(3), 631–638.
3. James, P. A., Oparil, S., Carter, B. L., Cushman, W. C., Dennison-Himmelfarb, C., Handler, J., et al. (2014). Evidence-based guideline for the management of high blood pressure in adults: Report from the panel members appointed to the eighth Joint National Committee (JNC 8). *JAMA: The Journal of the American Medical Association*, *311*(5), 507–520.

4. Bickley, L., & Szilagyi, P. G. (2016). *Bates' guide to physical assessment and history* (12th ed.). Philadelphia, PA: Lippincott Williams & Wilkins.

5. American Urological Association Guideline: Management of Benign Prostatic Hypertrophy (BPH). 2010 (reviewed and validity confirmed 2014). https://www.auanet.org/common/pdf/education/clinical-guidance/Benign-Prostatic-Hyperplasia.pdf.

6. Mora, S. (2016). Nonfasting for routine lipid testing: From evidence to action *JAMA Internal Medicine*, *176*(7), 1005–1006. http://jamanetwork.com/journals/jamainternalmedicine/article-abstract/2518766.

7. United States Preventative Services Task Force Published Recommendations. 2016. https://www.uspreventiveservicestaskforce.org/BrowseRec/Index/browse-recommendations.

8. American College of Cardiology/American Heart Association (ACC/AHA). (2013). Guideline on the treatment of blood cholesterol to reduce atherosclerotic cardiovascular risk in adults. *Circulation*. Retrieved from https://doi.org/10.1161/01.cir.0000437738.63853.7a.

9. U.S. Food and Drug Administration Drug safety and Availability. FDA Drug Safety Communication: FDA strengthens warning that non-aspirin nonsteroidal anti-inflammatory drugs (NSAIDs) can cause heart attacks or strokes. 1/16/2016. https://www.fda.gov/Drugs/DrugSafety/ucm451800.htm.

10. Beach, M. C., & Inui, T. (2006). Relationship-centered care: A constructive reframing. *Journal of General Internal Medicine*, *21*, S3–S8.

11. Foglia, M. B., & Fredriksen-Goldsen, K. I. (2014). Health disparities among LGBT older adults and the role of nonconscious bias. *The Hastings Center Report*, *44*(0 4), S40–S44.

12. Uhlig, K., Balk, E. M., Patel, K., et al. (2012). *Self-measured blood pressure monitoring: Comparative effectiveness [Internet]*. Rockville, MD: Agency for Healthcare Research and Quality. (Comparative Effectiveness Reviews, No. 45). Retrieved from https://www.ncbi.nlm.nih.gov/books/NBK84604/.

13. Shah, P., Glucek, G., Goldenberg, N., Min, S., Mahida, C., Schlam, I., et al. (2017). Efficacy, safety, low density lipoprotein cholesterol lowering, and calculated 10- year cardiovascular risk reduction of alirocumab and evolocumab in addition to maximal tolerated cholesterol lowering therapy: A post-commercialization study. *Lipids in Health and Disease*, *16*, 19.

14. Everett, B. M., Smith, R. J., & Hiatt, W. R. (2015). Reducing LDL with PCSK9 inhibitors: The clinical benefit of lipid drugs. *The New England Journal of Medicine*, *373*(17), 1588–1591.

Rash

JoAnn Lepke

Case Study Scenario/History of Present Illness

Mrs. Ramos, a 67-year-old female, presents to the office with complaints of an increasing number of itchy blisters on the skin, mostly on her lower abdomen and in the creases of her elbows, but now presenting in the groin and upper thighs. She states that a rash started about 6 months earlier, "just after a very bad wind storm," with intensely itchy patches she thought could have been hives or possibly a heat rash. However, over the last month, blisters have appeared. Originally, she applied lotion, which was purchased in the Philippines about a year ago, but it has not helped. She also reports showering with very hot water, "gently" scrubbing with a Japanese towel, and using "white soap" that was also obtained from the Philippines. She states that no one else in her household is having any skin problems. Mrs. Ramos has eliminated eggs from her diet for over a month; she is wondering why her skin has not improved since she has changed her diet.

Medications: Atorvastatin (Lipitor) 20 milligrams by mouth (po) at bedtime, metformin 500 milligrams po twice daily (patient reports taking "as needed").

Allergies: No known drug allergies (NKDA).

Habits: Nonsmoker, no alcohol use.

Past medical history: Type 2 diabetes, hypercholesterolemia, peripheral neuropathy, and peripheral edema.

Past surgical history: None.

Personal and social history: Checkout clerk. Married with 3 children and has 5 grandchildren.

Family history: Lives with her 68-year-old husband, 40-year-old daughter, and 16-year-old grandson. Mother alive, lives in the Philippines, currently age 85, with type 2 diabetes and arthritis. Father died at age 75 from "alcoholism." Younger brother died at age 65 from "heart problems." Has three younger sisters and one older brother, one sister with type 2 diabetes. Children and grandchildren healthy.

Review of Systems

General: Reports fatigue. Denies fever, chills, and weakness.

Skin: Blistering, itchy rash "all over." Some of the blisters have "popped, but they seem to be pretty strong." States that they heal quickly after "popping." Denies previous history of sensitive skin, eczema, psoriasis, or other skin disorders.

Head, eyes, ears, nose, and throat (HEENT): Denies sores in mouth, headache, dizziness, or nasal discomfort.

Neck: Denies neck discomfort or lumps.

Respiratory: Denies shortness of breath, cough, and wheezing.

Cardiac: Denies chest pain, pressure, and palpitations.

Gastrointestinal: Denies nausea, vomiting, diarrhea, difficulty swallowing, and change in appetite.

Urinary: Denies frequency, burning, flank pain, and discomfort.

Musculoskeletal: Denies back, leg, arm, and joint pain.

Peripheral vascular: Reports swollen legs about 3 months ago, given an oral "water pill," which helped.

Neurovascular: Denies fainting, numbness, and tingling.

Hematologic: Denies easily bruising, bleeding gums, and history of anemia.

Endocrine: Reports increased thirst since blisters developed. Denies temperature intolerance or excessive sweating.

Psychiatric: Denies history of depression or other psychiatric problems.

Physical Examination

General: Obese female sitting on examination table. Well dressed, well groomed. No distress.

Vital signs: Height 5 feet 3 inches, weight 170 pounds, temperature 98°F, blood pressure 138/85, heart rate 92 regular, respiratory rate 18, O_2 saturation on room air 95%.

Skin: Numerous large, tense, straw-colored blisters in bilateral antecubital spaces, lower abdomen, and groin. Some present on erythematous, urticarial plaques. Few on back and scattered throughout body. Scattered areas of erosion.

Eyes: Sclera clear, no conjunctival injection, extraocular movements (EOMs) normal.

Ears: Bilateral tympanic membranes (TMs) normal.

Nose: No congestion or rhinorrhea.

Mouth: Moist, intact mucous membranes. Good dentition. No lesions present on tongue, mucous membranes, soft palate, or pharynx.

Neck: Supple, no masses, lymphadenopathy, thyroid enlargement, or tenderness.

Cardiac: Regular rate and rhythm, normal S1, S2. No S3, S4, murmurs, or rubs.

Respiratory: Clear bilaterally.

Abdomen: See skin. Obese, soft. Normal bowel sounds in all four quadrants. No tenderness, nodules, or organomegaly.

Extremities: 1+ bilateral ankle edema. Pedal pulses present bilaterally. No calf tenderness.

1. Based on the history and physical examination results, what are the possible causes (differential diagnoses) of this patient's blistering?

This woman presents with a 6-month history of an itchy rash that now has tense, pruritic blisters present primarily in the creases of the skin. She reports generally feeling well. Her past medical history includes type 2 diabetes and hypercholesterolemia. She is also using skin care products with unknown ingredients, washing her body with hot water, and scrubbing her skin with a Japanese towel. Blisters may be caused by any of the blistering diseases, irritant contact dermatitis, eczema/atopic dermatitis, or infection.

Mrs. Ramos' rash is not likely caused by contact with irritating materials because of the locations of the blisters and lesions, which is primarily in skinfolds. The patient's use of soaps, lotions, and scrubs covers all of the skin, and is not confined to particular areas. Contact dermatitis typically presents in specific locations related to where the offending irritant comes in contact with the skin.[1] Although contact dermatitis is not the source of Mrs. Ramos' rash, the use of her personal care products along with hot water significantly contributes to her discomfort. Irritant contact dermatitis has eczematous properties such as dry skin, erythema, inflammation, and itchiness; it is commonly caused by strong soaps or other chemical exposures.[2]

Eczematous dermatitis and atopic dermatitis commonly occur in skinfolds, such as antecubital and popliteal areas, but can be present anywhere on the body. Atopic dermatitis is usually present from an early age, with over 60% initially occurring before the age of 1 year.[3] Other associated comorbidities include asthma and allergic rhinitis.[4] There are three stages of eczematous inflammation: acute, subacute, and chronic. The acute phase typically presents with itchy vesicles, blisters, and intense erythema. The subacute phase involves some itching, pain, and burning, along with redness, scale, fissures, and dryness. Chronic eczematous inflammation is itchy and usually with the presence of some areas of thickened skin, excoriations, and sometimes fissuring.[2] Mrs. Ramos has reported no history of "sensitive skin," eczema, atopic dermatitis, asthma, or allergic rhinitis. Although eczematous dermatitis and atopic dermatitis are on the list of differentials, they are not causing Mrs. Ramos' symptoms.

Narrowing down the numerous possibilities of blistering diseases is the next step in specifying a working list of differential diagnoses. A good way to begin is to determine the distribution of lesions: Are they localized or generalized? Are mucous membranes involved? Localized lesions are considered to include dependent areas, hands/feet, and areas that are photodistributed, dermatomal, or linear.[5] Next, the blister itself should be categorized. Is it flaccid with sloughing skin, or tense, or vesicular? Do the blisters itch? Have there been any recent illnesses? What medications and supplements is the patient taking systemically or applying topically?

Mrs. Ramos' blisters are primarily present in the skinfolds, which is considered a generalized distribution, with no mucous membrane involvement. Mrs. Ramos' blisters are specifically categorized as generalized, tense, and itchy. The differential diagnoses that should be considered with these symptoms include bullous pemphigoid (BP), linear IgA bullous dermatosis, epidermolysis bullosa acquisita (EBA), dermatitis herpetiformis, paraneoplastic pemphigus, and bullous systemic lupus erythematosus (Fig. 7.1).

2. What are the clinical presentations of the various blistering disorders in the differential diagnosis?

See Table 7.1.

3. What components of the initial physical examination are missing?

In the primary care office, the body surface area (BSA) involved should be noted. The "rule of nines" (Fig. 7.2) can be used where each leg represents 18% of total BSA, each arm 9%, and each side of the trunk 18%. The palm method may prove to be better for smaller, more patchy areas. The palm of the hand, including the fingers, is approximately 1% of total BSA.

Mrs. Ramos' BSA involved is estimated to be 7% using the palm method.

4. What diagnostics and treatment are necessary for the patient at this time?

The patient should be reassured that eggs are not likely the source of her skin condition because food allergy symptoms usually appear within 2 hours of ingesting the food.[11] Further tests will be needed to determine the cause of her symptoms.

A wound culture is necessary to rule out a secondary bacterial infection. Laboratory diagnostic tests should be reviewed to evaluate the overall health status of the patient before the consideration of systemic treatment. These include a complete blood count with differential (CBC with differential), comprehensive metabolic panel (CMP), glycated hemoglobin (A1C), spot urine albumin-to-creatinine ratio, lipid panel, 25-hydroxy vitamin D, and thyroid-stimulating hormone (TSH).

The blood tests and urinalysis are particularly pertinent for this patient because she has significant known comorbidities that include a blistering disease, type 2 diabetes, and hyperlipidemia. Mrs. Ramos reports fatigue on her initial office visit. An evaluation of the CBC with differential will help determine whether she has any underlying conditions that may be a cause of fatigue including anemia, infection, or other abnormalities. Hypothyroidism and/or decreased vitamin D levels can also cause fatigue and weight gain. Although Mrs. Ramos has not complained of weight gain, she is considered obese with a body mass index (BMI) of 30.1. Evaluating TSH would be appropriate given her complaint of fatigue and elevated BMI. The CMP is indicated to determine fluid and electrolyte imbalances that may be present due to poorly managed diabetes and the presence of a blistering disease. Kidney and liver functions, also included with the CMP, should

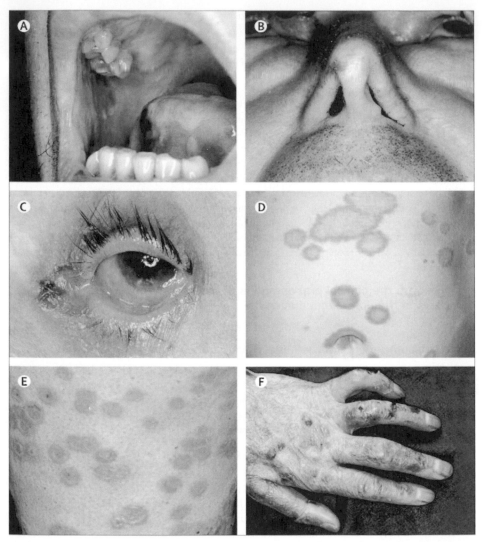

Fig. 7.1 Clinical characteristics of other pemphigoid diseases. (A) Erosions and fibrinous plaques in the oral cavity. (B) Hemorrhagic crusts on and scar-related miniaturization of nasal orifices. (C) Conjunctival injection, symblepharon, erosions, and yellow crusts in a patient with mucous membrane pemphigoid. (D) Wheel-like plaques on the abdomen (D) of a patient with pemphigoid gestationis. (E) Annular erythematous plaques with blistering along the edges (the so-called string-of-pearls sign) in a patient with linear IgA disease. (F) Vesicles, erosions, atrophic erythematous plaques, and milia on the extensor surfaces of the left hand of a patient with epidermolysis bullosa acquisita. (From Schmidt, E. & Zillikens, D. [2013]. Pemphigoid diseases. *Lancet*, 381[9863], 320–332.)

be assessed in the presence of diabetes and periodically during use of statins in controlling hyperlipidemia. According to the American Diabetes Association, a hemoglobin (Hgb) A1C should be checked every 3 months in patients with poor glycemic control, and the following tests should be checked at least yearly: fasting lipid profile (total, low-density lipoprotein [LDL], high-density lipoprotein [HDL], and triglycerides), liver function tests, spot urinary albumin-to-creatinine ratio, serum creatinine, and estimated glomerular filtration rate (GFR).[12]

TABLE 7.1 ■ Clinical Presentation of Various Blistering Disorders in the Differential Diagnoses

	Typical Age of Onset (Years)	Race, Gender, Other Preference	Affected Sites	Presentation	Additional Information
Bullous pemphigoid	>60	None	Inner thighs, groin, axillae, neck, palms and soles, <25% mucous membranes	Moderate to severe itch, urticarial, erythematous plaques with 1- to 7-cm tense bullae that rupture within a week	May be self-limited, low mortality
Linear IgA bullous dermatosis	Typically <5 years old or >60 years old, but may occur at any age	Rare in Asians and blacks	Symmetric on face, elbows, knees, scalp, nape of neck, shoulders, buttocks; common on mucous membranes	Start as itchy papules, evolve into severely itching/burning, urticarial papules, vesicles, and sometimes bullae	Appear as "cluster of jewels" or "string of beads"
Epidermolysis bullosa acquisita	All ages, most common in middle age	None	Trunk, knees, elbows, soles, palms	Blisters on noninflammatory base, itchy, sometimes surrounded by urticarial and inflamed skin	Common on trauma-prone areas; may heal with milia and dense scars
Dermatitis herpetiformis	30–40	Most common in Northern-European heritage, males > females (2:1), >80% have celiac or subclinical gluten sensitivity	Symmetrically grouped on elbows, knees, shoulders, nape of neck, sacral area, buttocks, scalp	Intense burning, itchy, papulovesicular over urticarial base, often excoriated	Lifelong
Paraneoplastic pemphigus	45–79	Males > females, usually seen in patients with lymphoma	Eye and mucosal involvement progressing to trunk and extremities	Skin ulcerations leading to blisters; similar to bullous pemphigoid, pemphigus, erythema multiforme, graft versus host disease, or lichen planus	—
Bullous systemic lupus erythematosus	20–40	Most common in African Americans, females	Sun-exposed areas, upper trunk, face, neck, arms	Itchy, tense vesicles and bullae with some erythematous macules and papules	—

From Calonje, E., Brenn T., & Lazar, A. (2012). Inherited and autoimmune subepidermal blistering diseases. In P. H. McKee (Ed.), *McKee's pathology of the skin* (4th ed., pp. 99–150). Philadelphia: Saunders Elsevier.

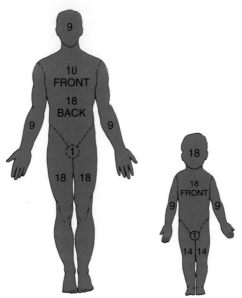

Fig. 7.2 Rule of nines.

Referral to dermatology is appropriate for further workup. If the primary care provider (PCP) is adept at performing biopsies, two 4-mm punch biopsies are recommended. The first is for evaluation via light microscopy (routine hematoxylin and eosin [H&E] staining). This biopsy needs to contain lesional tissue. If blisters are smaller than the punch size, a complete, intact lesion/blister is preferred. For larger blisters and bullae, a sample from the edge of a blister containing both lesional and normal skin is required. This biopsy specimen is placed in a container with formalin. Analysis of this tissue sample identifies the layer of skin that contains the blister, narrowing down the list of differential diagnoses.

The second biopsy is for analysis with direct immunofluorescence (DIF). This is a type of immunohistochemical testing that highlights the presence of tissue-bound antibodies and complement using fluorescent dye.[2] DIF determines the type and location of autoantibodies that are bound to the tissue.[13] The punch biopsy site should be perilesional skin, located 2 to 3 mm from the affected area, and normal in appearance (contains no part of the blister). This specimen is placed in a container with Michel's or Zeus transport medium, which is critical in preserving the presence of antigens within the tissue.[5]

Treatment modalities to be started at today's visit include topical corticosteroids to decrease inflammation. Systemic corticosteroids can be considered depending on the amount of body surface involved and how much discomfort the patient is experiencing. However, systemic corticosteroids induce postprandial hyperglycemia.[14] For this reason, caution is prudent in this case because the patient has not been adherent with the health care provider's recommendations regarding oral diabetes medication.

A topical antibiotic ointment such as mupirocin should be considered if a bacterial infection is suspected. It can be combined with the topical corticosteroid in a 50/50 mixture and applied to affected areas in a thin film. Silver sulfadiazine may be considered, but risk of silver toxicity exists and caution is recommended in its use.[15] Sensitive skin care needs to be reviewed with the patient (Table 7.2) in an attempt to minimize supplemental inflammation from personal care practices.

The biopsies are performed and sent to a dermatopathologist for review. Mrs. Ramos has no recent laboratory results on file, so the following tests were ordered: CBC with differential, CMP, A1C, lipid panel, TSH, spot urine albumin-to-creatinine ratio, and 25-hydroxy vitamin D.

TABLE 7.2 ■ **Sensitive Skin Care**

Bathing	• Gentle, fragrance-free cleanser • Minimize quantity of cleanser used (only apply to underarms, groin area, soiled areas) • Hands to wash body (no washcloths, buff puffs, Japanese towels, brushes, etc.) • Warm or cool water temperature • Limit duration to 5–10 minutes • Gently pat dry with towel, do not rub
Moisturize	• Twice daily is preferable, avoid areas with open wounds, blisters, and so forth. • Immediately after bathing (pat dry and apply within 3–5 minutes of bathing) • Gentle, fragrance-free moisturizers (CeraVe, Cetaphil, Aveeno, etc.)
Laundry	• Fragrance- and dye-free detergents (hypoallergenic) • No fabric softeners or dryer sheets
Sun Protection	• Sunscreen with SPF 30 or greater, do not apply to lesional areas • Long sleeves/pants (clothing with SPF preferred) • Wide-brimmed hats • Avoid sun between 10 a.m. and 4 p.m.

Data from Dermatologists' top tips for relieving dry skin. (2018). <https://www.aad.org/public/skin-hair-nails/skin-care/dry-skin>.

Mrs. Ramos is prescribed clobetasol propionate 0.05% cream and mupirocin 2% cream to be mixed (50/50) and applied sparingly to affected areas twice daily. Clobetasol propionate is a very-high-potency topical corticosteroid (Group I, also called a superpotent topical corticosteroid). Topical corticosteroids induce vasoconstriction in the upper dermis, resulting in decreased inflammation.[2] Mupirocin is a topical antibiotic. Mixing these two topical creams will decrease inflammation and potentially treat a secondary bacterial infection, if present. Systemic corticosteroids are avoided at the present time because the BSA involved is 7%, and topical treatment should be considered even in those with extensive involvement.[7] It has been demonstrated that overall survival in very-high-potency topical steroid treated BP exceeded those treated with oral prednisone, and had better clinical outcomes. Clinical response was faster with clobetasol than systemic prednisone, and resulted in fewer serious complications.[17] Additionally, the use of systemic corticosteroids could further increase Mrs. Ramos' elevated blood glucose levels.

Chronic use of topical corticosteroids may result in skin atrophy, striae, and folliculitis. Adrenal suppression can occur with application of liberal amounts of very-high-potency topical corticosteroids, but its incidence is thought to be small.[18,19]

A follow-up appointment is scheduled in 2 weeks.

Case Study, Continued

Mrs. Ramos presents to the office 2 weeks later to discuss biopsy and laboratory results. She reports less itching with use of prescribed creams.

Vital signs at time of visit: Weight 170 pounds, temperature 98.2°F, blood pressure 145/80, heart rate 88 regular, respiratory rate 18, O$_2$ saturation on room air 96%.

Pertinent laboratory results:

Serum testing:

LDL: 82 milligrams/dL

HDL: 39 milligrams/dL

Triglycerides: 163 milligrams/dL

25-hydroxy vitamin D: 32 ng/mL

TSH: 2.3 µIU/mL
Fasting glucose: 120 milligrams/dL
A1C: 8.4%
Blood urea nitrogen (BUN): 22 mmol/L
Creatinine: 1.1 milligrams/dL
Estimated GFR (eGFR): 50 milligrams/dL
Eosinophils: 10%
Urinalysis:
    Protein: trace
    Glucose: trace
    Albumin-to-creatinine ratio: 109 milligrams/g
Biopsy results:
Light microscopy: Subepidermal blister with numerous eosinophils and neutrophils present.
DIF: Presence of linear IgG and C3 staining along the basement membrane zone. Differential diagnoses include BP and EBA. It is suggested that a serum pemphigoid panel be performed.

5. What is the underlying pathology involved in bullous pemphigoid and epidermolysis bullosa acquisita? How do these two diagnoses differ?

BP is an autoimmune blistering skin disease that typically begins in people aged 60 years or older, with a mean age of onset at 80 years. In many cases BP is self-limiting, resolving in months to years. It is associated with increased mortality, although overall the mortality rate is low.[2]

Most cases of BP occur spontaneously without any clear cause. However, in a small number of cases, certain drugs may precipitate BP. These include penicillin, ibuprofen, captopril, fluoxetine, β-adrenergic blockers, terbinafine, gabapentin, etanercept, sulfasalazine, loop diuretics, neuroleptics, and spironolactone.[20,21,22] Other causes may include ultraviolet light therapy and radiation therapy for cancer.[20]

Pruritus and erythema usually precede blistering by months, and many times a diagnosis of urticaria is made. The most common areas of involvement include the lower abdomen, groin, and antecubital and popliteal spaces. Oral mucosa blisters are present in approximately 20% of those with BP. Sometimes BP may occur in areas of trauma.[2] In rare cases, the eyes may also be involved (Fig. 7.3).[7]

In BP, the body's immune system creates antibodies (anti-BP180 and anti-BP230) against the basement membrane, which connects the epidermis to the dermis. The presence of these antibodies results in neutrophil proliferation and the release of proteinases and reactive oxygen species. These neutrophils, along with the presence of mast cells and complement activation, break down cell adhesion between the epidermis and dermis, causing damage to the basement membrane zone, resulting in tense blisters and bullae.[7,20,23] BP is the most common subepidermal blistering disease.[24]

EBA is rare, accounting for only 5% of blistering diseases. It can occur at any age, but is most common in middle age. EBA is classified into two subtypes: mechanobullous (noninflammatory) and inflammatory. People affected by EBA may exhibit either or both subtypes, and it may vary throughout the duration of the disease.[25] Irritable bowel disease is frequently present among those with EBA.[26]

The tense blisters in noninflammatory EBA are typically induced by mild frictional trauma, and they are commonly found on trauma-prone areas such as palms, soles, elbows, and knees. Nail dystrophy, mucosal involvement, and postinflammatory pigmentation changes occur frequently. Itching is common, skin is fragile, and healing occurs with milia formation and scarring.[2,25,27]

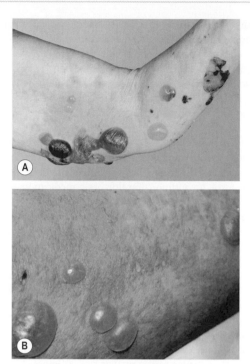

Fig. 7.3 (A and B) Bullous pemphigoid, classic presentation. (From Bolognia, J. L., Schaeffer, J. V., & Lorenzo, C. [2018]. Dermatology [4th ed.]. London: Elsevier.)

Inflammatory EBA (sometimes called BP-like subtype) clinically resembles other autoimmune blistering conditions such as BP and linear IgA disease (LAD). Skin fragility, milia, and significant scarring are not typically present. Urticaria and inflammation usually surround the bullae. Tense bullae usually occur in the trunk, arms, legs, and skinfolds.[2,25]

The exact cause of EBA is unknown. Evidence indicates that antibody formation against critical building blocks of the dermal–epidermal junction (DEJ) may occur after trauma to the skin. It is believed that the body's immune system creates antibodies that target type VII collagen, which is an important ingredient necessary to anchor the dermis to the basement membrane via fibrils. In patients with EBA, fewer anchoring fibrils are present in the DEJ and antibodies against type VII collagen are present in serum. Animal studies have shown that these antibodies result in skin fragility, tense bullae and blisters, milia, and scarring.[26]

6. What further diagnostics and treatment are necessary for the patient at this visit?

A serum pemphigoid panel was ordered for the patient, per the recommendation of the dermatopathologist. This blood test measures the levels of autoantibodies to BP180 and BP230 (also called BPAG1 and BPAG2). The combination of these two tests yields a sensitivity of 66% and a specificity of 89%. Therefore a positive result is most helpful in making the diagnosis of BP.[28] This diagnostic can also be used to measure the progress of the disease.

Mrs. Ramos' diabetes is poorly controlled, with an A1C of 8.4. The skin barrier is compromised in this patient, making her more susceptible to infection and further complications. It is well known that patients with diabetes have more difficulty healing wounds than those without diabetes. Those with poorly controlled diabetes are at further risk of impaired healing.[29] Specific education regarding the importance of managing diabetes is required. Stressing the fundamentals of lifestyle modification (e g, Dietary Approaches to Stop Hypertension [DASH] diet, exercise, reduced sodium intake, weight loss) and medications to manage her condition is crucial to the continued health and well-being of Mrs. Ramos. This is initiated in the primary care setting along with a referral to a diabetes educator to assist the patient in understanding and making important lifestyle changes.

Metformin is restarted at 500 milligrams daily, increasing to twice daily in one or 2 weeks if well-tolerated. Monitoring of kidney function is important because her metformin dose may need to be lowered or eliminated if GFR drops below 45 mL/min/1.73 m^2. Depending on kidney function and glycemic control, an additional antidiabetic medication may be added or another agent(s) considered.

Mrs. Ramos' blood pressure at this encounter is 145/80, which is greater than the recommended target of less than 140/90 in those with diabetes and chronic kidney disease.[30] According to the JNC 8, the target blood pressure control in those with diabetes and chronic kidney disease is less than 140/90 mm Hg.[30] The provider should consider recommending home blood pressure monitoring with semiautomated devices available at local pharmacies or big box stores. Self-monitoring of blood pressure has been shown to improve blood pressure control and give clinicians a better idea of readings outside of the office visit.[31] The American Diabetes Association[12] recommends an ace inhibitor or angiotensin receptor blocker for renal protection. Mrs. Ramos is at increased risk for atherosclerotic cardiovascular disease given her diagnosis of hyperlipidemia, albuminuria, and likely diagnosis of hypertension. Low-dose aspirin therapy (75–162 milligrams/day) should also be considered to decrease the patient's cardiovascular risk.[12] Before initiating these medications, the PCP should determine whether the patient can tolerate a lower blood pressure safely, and if any increased risk of bleeding exists.

Mrs. Ramos' GFR of 50 milligrams/dL correlates with Stage 3a chronic kidney disease, but decreased renal function must be present for three or more months for this diagnosis to be validated.[32] The provider may consider referring the patient to nephrology after repeated laboratory tests in 3 months. Microalbuminuria is present with the patient's albumin/creatinine ratio of 109 milligrams/g. Microalbuminuria is an indicator of cardiovascular mortality and morbidity, and its persistence indicates diabetic nephropathy.[33]

A CMP is ordered to be drawn before her next office visit. Additionally, a referral is initiated to ophthalmology because Mrs. Ramos indicated she has not seen the eye doctor in over 5 years. A thorough eye examination including dilation to assess for retinopathy and macular edema is recommended on initial diagnosis of type 2 diabetes. If no evidence of retinopathy exists at one or more annual examinations, comprehensive ophthalmic examinations are recommended every 2 years; otherwise, these examinations should occur at least annually.[12]

A referral to dermatology was initiated to assume ongoing care regarding Mrs. Ramos' skin condition. Included in the referral to dermatology are the biopsy reports and all recent laboratory work, including the pending results of serum pemphigoid panel.

Low-dose noncoated aspirin therapy, 81 milligrams, and 10 milligrams of lisinopril po daily have been prescribed to Mrs. Ramos. A follow-up appointment is scheduled in 2 weeks with primary care.

Case Study, Continued

Mrs. Ramos presents to the office for her appointment with the PCP 2 weeks later. She reports new, itchy blisters on her trunk and back, and just saw the dermatologist earlier today and was "given a shot," pointing to her left flank. She states the dermatologist talked about pills to take for her blisters, and he ordered more blood tests. She is scheduled to see him again in 1 month.

The patient reports taking all her medications as previously prescribed, including metformin once in the evening with dinner. She states that her bowel movements are loose but not problematic, and she is scheduled to meet with a diabetes educator immediately after this appointment. Mrs. Ramos expresses frustration about the number of "pills, doctors' visits, and blood tests" she has and asks when she can just go back to the way her life was before she had blisters.

Vital signs at time of visit: Weight 169 pounds, temperature 98°F, blood pressure 130/78, heart rate 85 regular, respiratory rate 18, O_2 saturation on room air 95%.

BSA involvement: 6%

Results of serum pemphigoid testing (enzyme-linked immunosorbent assay):

IgG BP180 antibodies: 32 units (reference range, negative <9 units, positive ≥9 units)

IgG BP230 antibodies: 19 units (reference range, negative <9 units, positive ≥9 units)

Comment on laboratory report: Consistent with pemphigoid.

Other pertinent laboratory results:

BUN: 21 mmol/L

Creatinine: 1 milligrams/dL

eGFR: 56 milligrams/dL

7. What are the next steps for Mrs. Ramos?

The biopsies and serum pemphigoid results indicate a diagnosis of BP. The patient saw the dermatologist again today and was likely administered an intramuscular injection of triamcinolone acetonide (Kenalog), based on her recount of the appointment. The notes from Mrs. Ramos' dermatology encounter are typically received within a week of the appointment.

Several treatment options for BP include topical and/or systemic glucocorticoids, mycophenolate mofetil, azathioprine, methotrexate, tetracyclines, nicotinamide, and dapsone.[18] The immunosuppressive medications have significant associated adverse effects, and careful monitoring by medical providers familiar with the risks associated with them is imperative. Baseline laboratory tests need to be reviewed before initiation of any of these medications to evaluate the status of the individual being prescribed an immunosuppressive medication. Topical treatment with clobetasol propionate 0.05% (a very-high-potency topical corticosteroid) is preferred as a first-line therapy, with better overall survival and clinical outcomes than systemic steroid treatment.[17] Systemic doxycycline has been shown to be noninferior to oral prednisolone, and has a much better safety profile in long-term use.[34]

The health care provider discussed Mrs. Ramos' diabetes with her and offered encouragement regarding her scheduled appointment with the diabetes educator. Mrs. Ramos stated she had a glucometer "somewhere at home" but does not think she will be able to find it. She also expressed that "I really don't like poking myself and checking my blood."

The PCP validates Mrs. Ramos' frustration and also describes the positive actions that the patient has completed. These include reliably attending her scheduled appointments, getting all her blood drawn for laboratory tests, taking her diabetes medication as directed, and having realistic expectations that improvement in her skin problem will take time.

It is necessary for Mrs. Ramos to continue to follow up with primary care to ensure adequate monitoring of Mrs. Ramos' comorbidities including diabetes, decreased renal function, blood pressure concerns, and overall health. Mrs. Ramos has an established relationship with her PCP and may be more likely to disclose concerns regarding the ongoing management of her new skin condition.

Somewhat appeased by her conversation with the health care provider, Mrs. Ramos agrees to a follow-up appointment in 1 month.

Case Study, Continued

One week later, the encounter notes and laboratory results from dermatology are received in the primary care office before Mrs. Ramos' follow-up appointment. It is noted that an intramuscular injection of Kenalog, 40 milligrams, was administered at the time of Mrs. Ramos' initial appointment. The dermatology provider notes that systemic treatment with doxycycline is initiated at 100 milligrams po twice daily. Mrs. Ramos is to continue topical treatment with clobetasol dipropionate cream, 0.05%. The provider's notes reflect concern with the patient's poorly controlled diabetes, and the provider reports that long-term use of oral prednisone is not recommended.

Significant side effects in most body systems are associated with glucocorticoid therapy. These include hypothalamic pituitary axis suppression, psychosis, hair thinning, hirsutism, acne, flushed cheeks, cataracts, moon face, peptic ulcer, compression fracture, hypertension, hyperglycemia, obesity, osteoporosis, thinning of skin, muscle weakness, poor wound healing, higher tendency for infections, and bruising.[35] The use of steroids such as prednisone in people with diabetes typically results in increased blood glucose throughout the day but normal to below-normal fasting blood sugar levels. In diabetics, the presence of systemic steroids causes the liver to release more glucose than under normal conditions. Additionally, steroids adversely affect the storage of glucose in adipose tissue.[36]

8. What are cultural considerations that need to be considered in the care of Mrs. Ramos?

Understanding the cultural values and integrating culturally appropriate interactions for all patients will help facilitate a better provider–patient relationship and hopefully facilitate the best possible health outcome. Filipinos are ranked the third-largest Asian group in the United States reported in the 2010 census.[37] In the 2010 Diabetes Study of Northern California (DISTANCE), the estimated prevalence of diabetes in this ethnic group is 16.1%, compared with 7.3% in whites, and 8.9% in all racial/ethnic groups studied. Similarly, the estimated incidence (new cases per 1000 person-years) for each group is 14.7, 6.3, and 7.7, respectively.[39] The prevalence of hypertension in Filipinos is also significantly higher than in other Asian Americans, Hispanics, and non-Hispanic whites.[39,40]

Filipino Americans (FAs) tend to eat steamed, white rice as part of their traditional diet, and it is considered a staple food.[41] Rice is served with breakfast, lunch, and dinner and is a fundamental part of all meals, including both sweet and savory.[42,43] Rice is frequently cooked in large batches so it is available throughout the day.[43] In Hawaii, many families carry their cooked rice in an insulated rice steamer to have available while spending a day at the beach or a family outing. Most daily meals also contain fish or meat, vegetables, fruit, and dessert. Preparations may include stir-fried, roasted, or deep-fried meat and fish; stews; bread; deep-fried egg rolls; pasta; and dessert, which is frequently made from rice. Recipes typically include a large amount of salt, which may come from sources such as fish sauce, shrimp paste, anchovies, anchovy paste, and soy sauce. Some families eat up to six times daily.

Rapid transitions from hot to cold are believed to incite illness, and warmth is considered necessary for maintaining health. Having a layer of fat on the body is considered good because it helps to keep warm and foster optimum health.[44]

The most common language spoken in the Philippines is Tagalog/Pilipino, with English as the second official language. In the United States in 2011, it is estimated that over 60% of Filipinos speak Tagalog in the home.[45] In stressful situations, older Filipino Americans may feel more comfortable speaking their native language. It is quite common for an adult daughter, son, or extended family member to accompany the patient to medical appointments to help facilitate communication. However, an older male of the family is typically the primary decision maker. Family and extended social connections are an integral part of Filipino tradition, and multigenerational households are common.[46] Caring for elders is integrated into family beliefs from childhood and is a strongly embedded value in Filipino culture. The majority (estimated at 80%) of Filipinos are Catholic, and prayer can play an important part in treatment of illness.[46]

Handshakes are welcomed as a greeting. Proper titles (Mr., Mrs., Miss, etc.) should be used when addressing the patient, rather than using first names.[44] Most health care providers will be addressed as "doctor" in conversation, regardless of their actual title. Health care providers are considered authority figures, and personal anecdotes relating to the provider's children, grandchildren, or other family members may result in more open discussions. Providers should sit and maintain eye contact and allow periods of silence. Older patients may not maintain eye contact or look down as a sign of respect. The provider should encourage the patient to ask questions or give opinions because the patient may not want to offend the authority figure by doing so. When assessing the patient's understanding, it is better to ask them to repeat instructions or their understanding of your communication versus asking them outright if they understand. Patient head-nodding may not indicate agreement or understanding.[46] Reviewing risks and possible negative outcomes when obtaining patient consent may cause anxiety and feelings of indifference from the provider.[44] Patients who travel to the Philippines should be asked about what medications and supplements they use from there because many seek health care while visiting.[46] It is essential to ask this of Mrs. Ramos because she was using personal care products from the Philippines. Undisclosed medications and supplements may provide useful information in evaluating abnormal symptoms or diagnostics.

References

1. Nixon, R., & Diepgen, T. (2014). Contact dermatitis. In *Middleton's allergy: Principles and practice* (8th ed., pp. 365–574). Philadelphia: Saunders.
2. Habif, T. (2016). *Clinical dermatology* (6th ed.). St. Louis, MO: Mosby Elsevier.
3. Tofte, S. (2015). Eczematous disorders. In *Dermatology for advanced practice clinicians* (pp. 24–37). Philadelphia: Wolters Kluwer.
4. Kapoor, R., Menon, C., Hoffstad, O., Bilker, W., Leclerc, P., & Margolis, D. J. (2008). The prevalence of atopic triad in children with physician-confirmed atopic dermatitis. *Journal of the American Academy of Dermatology, 58*(1), 68–73.
5. Hull, C., & Zone, J. (2017). Approach to the patient with cutaneous blisters. In Post, T.W., ed. UpToDate. Waltham, MA. Retrieved from https://www.uptodate.com/contents/approach-to-the-patient-with-cutaneous-blisters?search=approach%20to%20the%20patient%20with%20cutaenous%20blisters&source=search_result&selectedTitle=1~150&usage_type=default&display_rank=1.
6. Patterson, J. (2016). The vesiculobullous reaction pattern. In *Weedon's skin pathology* (pp. 176–178). Philadelphia: Elsevier.
7. James, W., Berger, T., & Elston, D. (2016). Chronic blistering dermatoses. In *Andrews' diseases of the skin: Clinical dermatology* (pp. 451–470). Philadelphia: Elsevier.
8. Goldberg, L., & Elston, D. (March 2016). Paraneoplastic pemphigus. [Online]. Retrieved from http://emedicine.medscape.com/article/1064452-overview#a6.
9. Paller, A., & Mancini, A. (2016). Chronic blistering dermatoses. In *Hurwitz clinical pediatric dermatology* (5th ed., pp. 327–333). Philadelphia: Elsevier.
10. Calonje, E., Brenn, T., & Lazar, A. (2012). Inherited and autoimmune subepidermal blistering diseases. In P. H. McKee (Ed.), *McKee's pathology of the skin* (4th ed., pp. 99–150). Philadelphia: Saunders Elsevier.
11. Mayo Clinic Staff. (2017). Diseases and Conditions: Food Allergy Symptoms. [Online]. Retrieved from http://www.mayoclinic.org/diseases-conditions/food-allergy/basics/symptoms/con-20019293.
12. American Diabetes Association. (2017). Standards of medical care in diabetes – 2017. *The Journal of Clinical and Applied Research and Education Diabetes Care, 40*(Suppl. 1), S1–S135.
13. Bobonich, M. A. (2015). Cutaneous manifestations of connective tissue diseases and immune-mediated blistering diseases. In *Dermatology for advanced practice clinicians* (1st ed., pp. 231–248). Philadelphia: Wolders Kluwer.

14. Paauw, D. S. (2000). Case study: A 60-year-old woman with type 2 diabetes and COPD: Worsening hyperglycemia due to prednisone. *Clinical Diabetes, 18*(2), 88–90.
15. Mintz, E. M., George, D. E., & Hsu, S. (2008). Silver sulfadiazine therapy in widespread bullous disorders: Potential for toxicity. *Dermatology Online Journal, UC Davis, 14*(3).
16. Dermatologists' top tips for relieving dry skin. [Online] Retrieved from https://www.aad.org/public/skin-hair-nails/skin-care/dry-skin.
17. Joly, P., Roujeau, J. C., Benichou, J., Picard, C., Dreno, B., Delaporte, E., et al. (2002). A comparison of oral and topical corticosteroids in patients with bullous pemphigoid. *The New England Journal of Medicine, 346*, 321–327.
18. Murrell, D. F., & Ramirez-Quizon, M. (2014). Management and prognosis of bullous pemphigoid. In Post, T.W., ed. UpToDate. Waltham, MA. Retrieved from https://www.uptodate.com/contents/management-and-prognosis-of-bullous-pemphigoid?search=%E2%80%9CManagement%20and%20prognosis%20of%20 bullous%20pemphigoid&source=search_result&selectedTitle=1~150&usage_ type=default&display_rank=1.
19. Aronson, J. (2016). Corticosteroids-glucocorticoids, topical, skin. In *Meyers side effects of drugs* (16th ed., pp. 691–693). Amsterdam: Elsevier.
20. Mayo Clinic Staff. (2017). Bullous Pemphigoid. [Online]. Retrieved from http://www.mayoclinic.org/diseases-conditions/bullous-pemphigoid/symptoms-causes/dxc-20157320?p=1.
21. Lloyd-Lavery, A., Chi, C., Wojnarowska, F., & Taghipour, K. (2013). The associations between bullous pemphigoid and drug use: A UK case-control study. *JAMA Dermatololgy, 149*(1), 58–62.
22. Vassileva, S. (1998). Drug-induced pemphigoid: Bullous and cicatrical. *Clinical Dermatology, 16*, 379–387.
23. Wieslab, A. B. (2010). Guide to autoimmune testing. Clavis Communications AB, Malmo.
24. Bernard, P., Vaillant, L., Labeille, B., Bedane, C., Arbeille, B., Deneux, J., et al. (1995). Incidence and distribution of subepidermal autoimmune bullous skin diseases in three French regions. Bullous Diseases French Study Group. *Archives of Dermatology, 131*(1), 48–52.
25. Ludwig, R. (2013). Clinical presentation, pathogenesis, diagnosis, and treatment of epidermolysis bullosa acquisita. *International Scholarly Research Notices, 2013.*
26. Woodley, D., Chen, M., & Kim, G. (2015). Epidermolysis bullosa acquisita. In Post, T.W., ed. UpToDate. Waltham, MA. Retrieved from https://www.uptodate.com/contents/epidermolysis-bullosa-acquisita.
27. Croom, D. Epidermolysis bullosa acquisita. [Online]. Retrieved from http://emedicine.medscape.com/article/1063083-overview#a6.
28. Keller, J., Kittridge, A., Debanne, S., & Korman, N. (2016). Evaluation of ELISA testing for BP180 and BP230 as a diagnostic modality for bullous pemphigoid: A clinical experience. *Archives of Dermatological Research, 308*(4), 269–272.
29. Weintrob, A. C., & Sexton, D. J. (2016). Susceptibility to infections in persons with diabetes mellitus. In Post, T.W., ed. UpToDate. Waltham, MA. Retrieved from https://www.uptodate.com/contents/susceptibility-to-infections-in-persons-with-diabetes-mellitus?search=A.%20C.%20Weintrob%20and%20 D.%20J.%20Sexton,%20%E2%80%9CSusceptibility%.
30. James, P. A., Oparil, S., Cushman, W. C., Dennison-Himmelfarb, C., Carter, B. L., Handler, J., et al. (2014). 2014 evidence-based guideline for the management of high blood pressure in adults: Report from the panel members appointed to the Eighth Joint National Committee (JNC 8). *JAMA: The Journal of the American Medical Association, 311*(5), 507–520.
31. Staff Writer, AMA Wire. Delivering care: What you need to know aout self-measured blood pressure monitoring. [Online]. Retrieved from https://wire.ama-assn.org/delivering-care/what-you-need-know-about-self-measured-blood-pressure-monitoring.
32. Rosenberg, M. (2016). Overview of the management of chronic kidney disease in adults. *UpToDate.*
33. Rossing, P., Fioretto, P., Feldt-Rasmussen, B., & Parving, H. (2016). Diabetic nephropathy. In *Brenner and Rector's the kidney* (pp. 1283–1321). Philadelphia: Elsevier.
34. Williams, H., Wojnarowska, F., Kirtschig, G., Mason, J., Godec, T., Schmidt, E., et al. (2017). Doxycycline versus prednisolone as an initial treatment strategy for bullous pemphigoid: A pragmatic, non-inferiority, randomised controlled trial. *Lancet, 389*(10079), 1630–1638.
35. Strachan, M., & Newell-Price, J. (2014). Endocrine disease. In *Davidson's principles and practice of medicine* (22nd ed., pp. 733–796). Elsevier Limited.
36. Joslin Communications. Diabetes Day2Day. [Online]. Retrieved from http://blog.joslin.org/2014/02/how-prednisone-affects-blood-sugar.

37. Hoeffel, E. M., Rastogi, S., & Shahid, H. (2012). The Asian Population: 2010. *2010 Census briefs*. Retrieved from http://www.census.gov/prod/cen2010/briefs/c2010br-11.pdf.

38. Karter, A. J., Schillinger, D., Adams, A. S. M. H. H., Liu, J., Adler, N. E., & Kanaya, A. M. (2013). Elevated rates of diabetes in Pacific Islanders and Asian subgroups. *Diabetes Care, 36*(3), 574–579.

39. Ursua, R. A., Islam, N. S., Aguilar, D. E., Wyatt, L. C., Tandon, S. D., Abesamis-Mendoza, N., et al. (2013). Predictors of hypertension among Filipino immigrants in the northeast US. *Journal of Community Health, 38*, 847–855.

40. Dalusong-Angosta, A., & Gutierrez, A. (2013). Prevalence of metabolic syndrome among Filipino-Americans: A cross-sectional study. *Applied Nursing Research, 26*(4), 192–197.

41. Jordan, D. N., & Jordan, J. L. (2010). Self-care behaviors of Filipino-American adults with type 2 diabetes mellitus. *Journal of Diabetes and Its Complications, 24*, 250–258.

42. Fox, M. (2015). Global food practices, cultural competency, and dietetics: Part 3. *Journal of the Academy of Nutrition and Dietetics, 115*(5), 701–705.

43. Johnson-Kozlow, M., Matt, G. E., Rock, C. L., Conway, T. L., & Romero, R. A. (2011). Assessment of dietary intakes of Filipino-Americans: Implications for food frequency questionnaire design. *Journal of Nutrition Education and Behavior, 43*(6), 505–510.

44. Healthcare Chaplaincy. (2013). Handbook of patients spiritual and cultural values for healthcare professionals. *Healthcare Chaplaincy*. Retrieved from http://www.healthcarechaplaincy.org/userimages/Cultural%20Sensitivity%20handbook%20from%20HealthCare%20Chaplaincy%20%20(3-12%202013).pdf.

45. Ryan, C. (2013). Lanuguage use in the United States: 2011. U.S. Census Bureau, 2011 American Community Survey.

46. McBride, M. Health and Healthcare of Filipino Americans. Stanford University School of Medicine.

Dizziness

Terry Mahan Buttaro

Case Study Scenario/History of Present Illness

- *68-year-old Asian male, married lives with wife, one stay-at-home adult child*
- *Primary problem: Dizziness*
- *Comorbidities: Hypertension (HTN), diabetes mellitus type 2 (DM II), obstructive sleep apnea, and benign prostatic hypertrophy (BPH)*
- *Care settings: Emergency room, acute care hospital, primary care*

Wang Li is a 68-year-old married Asian male who presents to the emergency room complaining of feeling dizzy and tired over the past 2 days. He describes the feeling as intermittent, not constant, but he feels worse today, like he might fall. He feels a bit better when he lies down, but the minute he starts to get up he states, he feels "dizzy" again. He did not want to come, but his wife drove him to be sure everything is okay. He denies feeling like the room is spinning, chest pain, shortness of breath, cough, or recent illness.

Medications: Valsartan (Diovan) 80 milligrams by mouth (po) daily; metformin (Glucophage) ER, 1000 milligrams po twice a day; doxazosin (Cardura) 8 milligrams po daily, atorvastatin (Lipitor) 40 milligrams po daily.

Allergies: Sulfa (rash).

Habits: Smoker for many years, 1 to 1½ packs per day, alcohol daily.

Past medical history: HTN, hypercholesterolemia, DM II, BPH, and obstructive sleep apnea.

Past surgical history: Appendectomy.

Personal history: Married, one daughter. He was born and married in China but moved here shortly after marriage.

Family history: Grandparent history: unknown. Father died of "heart problems," age 60. Mother died age 80 of "old age." No sisters or brothers.

Review of Systems

General: Periods of feeling weak. Denies spinning sensation, falls, fever, chills.

Skin: Denies rashes or lesions.

Head, eyes, ears, nose, and throat (HEENT): Denies headache, upper respiratory infection, and sinus pain.

Neck: Denies neck pain.

Respiratory: + smoking cough, especially in morning. Occasional shortness of breath going up stairs. Denies hemoptysis.

Cardiac: Denies chest pressure, pain, and palpitations.

Gastrointestinal: Denies difficulty swallowing, weight loss, constipation, and diarrhea.

Urinary: Denies urinary hesitancy, burning, and frequency.

Musculoskeletal: Denies muscle aches or joint pain.

Peripheral vascular: Occasional leg pain walking. Denies swollen legs and calf pain.

Neurovascular: + neuropathy feet.

Hematologic: + history of iron-deficiency anemia. Denies bruising or bleeding gums.
Endocrine: Denies low blood sugar or thirst.
Psychiatric: Denies anxiety or depression.

Physical Examination
  General: Thin, Asian man who appears older than his years.
  Vital signs: Height 65.5 inches. Weight 128 pounds. Body mass index (BMI) 21.3. Temperature 97.8°F. Blood pressure 114/86. Heart rate 128, ? irregular, Respiratory rate 24 at rest, O_2 saturation on room air 94% at rest.
  Skin: Warm/dry. No jaundice, rash, or acute lesions.
  Eyes: Sclera clear; conjunctiva, no injection.
  Ears: Tympanic membranes (TMs): no erythema, bulging/retraction.
  Nose: No rhinitis or sinus tenderness.
  Mouth: Membranes moist, teeth fair repair, no postpharyngeal erythema or exudate. No lesions of tongue or buccal mucosa.
  Neck: Supple, no masses, lymphadenopathy, thyroid enlargement, or tenderness.
  Cardiac: Rapid, ? irregular S1, S2. No gallop, murmurs, or rubs.
  Respiratory: Diminished at bases but clear without rales, wheezes, or rhonchi.
  Abdomen: Scaphoid, soft, bowel sounds positive. No organomegaly or tenderness.
  Extremities: Pedal pulses present bilaterally, no edema or calf tenderness.
  Neurologic: Alert, oriented to person, place, and time. Thought coherent. No fasciculations or tremors. Cranial nerves II to XII show no focal deficits. Somewhat slow getting out of chair. Gait fairly smooth, coordinated. Romberg negative. No pronator drift. Muscle tone 3/5 upper/lower extremities. Reflexes: biceps 1+ bilaterally, triceps 1+ bilaterally. Knees 2+ bilaterally. Ankles 1+ bilaterally. Plantar down bilaterally.

1. Mr. Li complains of feeling dizzy and tired, vague symptoms that do not help determine the severity of his illness, nor suggest the cause. What questions can help the provider elicit a clearer understanding of this patient's complaints, especially when the patient's cultural background or ethnicity is different from the provider's background?

The history of present illness (HPI), the initial interaction between patient and provider, is the patient's opportunity to explain the reason for seeking care. During this time the patient is encouraged to tell the story in his or her own words. Most often, further exploration and specific questioning to determine the exact cause are necessary. OLD CARTS (onset, location/radiation, duration, character, aggravating factors, reliving factors, timing, and severity) is an easy mnemonic to remember and can help clarify the HPI. It is also important to clarify what the words used by the patient mean. Mr. Li describes feeling "dizzy," but dizzy can have varied meanings to people and culture or language differences can also affect our understanding of a patient's complaints.

    Additional concerns during the patient/provider encounter are the influence of culture, ethnicity, religion, and family dynamics on illness, as well as health and wellness.[1] Culture influences everyone's responses to illness and medical treatment, so cultural awareness and sensitivity are paramount concerns in health care. Chinese, even those who are American born, often nod "yes" when speaking with a health care provider, but the "yes" does not necessarily indicate understanding or agreement; instead, it is a nod of respect for the provider. Respect is important in the Chinese culture, so addressing Mr. and Mrs. Li as "Mr. Li" and "Mrs. Li" courteously and making them feel comfortable in the office is essential. Introducing yourself and encouraging the patient and family to sit and talk with you for a few minutes before starting the interview will help the patient feel more at ease and realize you are genuinely interested in his well-being. Often family members are helpful, and care is improved when family members or friends are present.[1] However, it is always important to skillfully and respectfully ask questions and learn the patient's preferences regarding the involvement of a friend or family member in his care. The provider's primary responsibility is to the patient, so it is necessary to determine the reason others are accompanying the patient to the visit, as well as their relationship with the patient. Once accomplished, it is the patient who should be queried first, then, if the patient agrees, it is appropriate to ask the family member if they have added information or concerns to be addressed.[1] Learning who in the family or group of friends the patient wants help from with decisions about health care treatments is also helpful.

Once the patient and family feel at ease, it is appropriate to ask the patient and family if you can ask some questions to help determine what is causing the patient's symptoms. Assessing the meaning of "dizziness" or "weakness" requires asking the patient what is meant by the term because the terms are not specific enough to help providers understand the physiologic cause for the symptom.[2] Culture, language, and age can also affect how patients describe the symptoms they are experiencing, so it important to not only ask questions in an open-ended manner but also verify what the patient means by a specific term. Many patients use the term "spinning" or "off balance," but the meanings of these terms need to be explored and verified to clarify the experience. It is important when a family member or friend is present to concentrate on what the patient describes. The patient or family member might need to be reminded that it is important for the health care provider to first listen to the patient, but the provider will be willing to listen to the family or friend after the provider talks with the patient. Important questions to consider asking the patient include:

- Did you feel like you were going to faint or pass out?
- When exactly did the patient first notice these feelings?
- Can the patient relate the feeling to any specific incidence or movement (e.g., a fall or head movement)?
- Is the person sitting or standing when lightheaded or weak feeling occur?
- If the patient is in bed, does rolling from one side to another cause the feeling?
- Does the patient feel like he is going to fall or faint?
- Does going from a sitting to standing position precipitate the feeling?
- Where does the patient feel bad when the episodes occur?
- How often do they occur, and how long does each episode last?
- Is there any one thing that stands out about these episodes?
- Does anything make the symptoms better or worse?
- Is the feeling associated with nausea, sweating, or other symptoms?

Case Study, Continued

Further conversation with Mr. Li reveals that he does not remember any one thing that caused his symptoms. He describes just feeling more tired and maybe a little sweaty (like he might pass out) the past couple of days. Sometimes, the feeling of weakness occurs when he gets up, but not always. If he sits down when it happens, he sometimes feels a little better, but he feels weak even sitting. Sometimes he thinks his heart is pounding when this happens, but he is not sure. The feeling does not occur with coughing, urinating, or moving his bowels. It does not last long, but long enough that he feels scared about falling. Nothing he does makes it better or worse. The feeling makes him afraid that he will fall or pass out.

The health care provider asks the family if they have noted anything else that would be important information to know. Mrs. Li complains, "He drinks much and this is the problem." Further questioning reveals Mr. Li drinks vodka several times a day, but quantifying the actual amount with the patient and family is not clear.

2. Based on Mr. Li's history and physical examination, what are the possible differential diagnoses that should be considered?

Differential diagnoses in older adults can be challenging because in older adults the symptoms can be varied. The cause of Mr. Li's symptoms could be related to low blood sugar. Mr. Li does have DM II and is taking metformin, which is an antidiabetic medication. Metformin is not usually associated with hypoglycemia, but other causes of hypoglycemia are possible (e.g., alcohol, illness, postprandial hypoglycemia).[3]

The sensation of almost falling or fainting suggests presyncope, which is a condition that occurs when patients are upright. Presyncope, a syncopal prodrome that may or may not result in syncope, is also often associated with visual changes, sweating, and nausea. Mr. Li relates possible pounding heart, and his physical examination is positive for a rapid, irregular heart rate suggesting a cardiac etiology.

The cause could also be related to a seizure, orthostatic hypotension, or a neurally mediated syncope such as vasovagal syncope, which is particularly common in older adults.[4] Orthostatic hypotension can be related to inadequate intravascular volume (e.g., dehydration), excess alcohol consumption and medications, or it can be postprandial. He is taking two antihypertensives, valsartan and doxazosin, and for patients of all ages a high index of suspicion for any chief complaint should be a drug or drug–drug interaction. If his renal status has diminished, the half-life of these two antihypertensives could be prolonged and cause orthostasis.[5] Neurally mediated syncope, also known as neurocardiogenic syncope or neurogenic orthostatic hypotension, is associated with multiple causes that commonly include stress, swallowing, coughing, carotid massage, urination, and defecation.[4] Neurally mediated syncope can also be related to autonomic dysfunction associated with neurodegenerative disorders such as Parkinson's disease or Shy–Drager syndrome.

3. What diagnostics should be considered?

It would be important to check the blood glucose immediately to help exclude the possibility of hypoglycemia as a cause of his symptoms. Many patients forget that lightheadedness is a sign of low blood sugar, although a random blood sugar might be normal. Orthostatic vital signs (both blood pressure and heart rate) should also be obtained to exclude orthostatic hypotension. Orthostatic hypotension, defined as a 20 mm Hg or greater decrease in systolic blood pressure or a 10 mm Hg decrease in diastolic blood pressure in less than 3 minutes, can have varied causes.[4] It is also necessary to be attentive to the proper way to assess orthostatic changes. Patients should be supine for at least 5 minutes before the blood pressure is assessed. The heart rate should also be determined when the patient's blood pressure is auscultated in the supine, sitting, and standing position. In older adults, the heart rate may not increase substantially, even in the presence of dehydration, so this testing may not be helpful, but orthostatic testing is still important to determine any changes. Blood pressure that decreases more than 30 mm Hg that is not accompanied by an increase in s heart rate of 115 mm Hg or more suggests a neurodegenerative disorder.[6]

An electrocardiogram is necessary to determine whether prolonged QT, an arrhythmia (i.e., bradycardia, tachyarrhythmia), left ventricular hypertrophy, or other cardiac anomaly is present. All health care providers should be familiar with reading an electrocardiogram and should collaborate with physicians skilled in electrocardiogram interpretation because in some circumstances identification of atrial fibrillation can be challenging and misdiagnosed. Necessary laboratory diagnostics would include a complete blood count (CBC) to determine whether an infection or anemia is present; serum electrolytes to assess any abnormalities; a blood, urea, nitrogen (BUN); and creatinine level to establish renal status. Additional testing would include a thyroid-stimulating hormone (TSH) level, if tachycardia or tachyarrhythmia is present, and liver function tests with history of significant alcohol intake. A serum ammonia level should be considered if the patient displays cognitive or neuromuscular changes that would be consistent with hepatic encephalopathy. It is unclear exactly what Mr. Li's alcohol intake is, but he does not appear to be jaundiced and his conversation with the health care provider is fluent and appropriate at this time. Troponins are necessary if acute coronary syndrome is suspected.

4.   Mr. Li's electrocardiogram indicates atrial fibrillation with rapid ventricular response. What is the pathophysiology of atrial fibrillation and how does this knowledge affect a provider's decisions regarding treatment?

In atrial fibrillation, the coordination of electrical impulses that initiate cardiac muscle contraction have for some reason become disorganized (Fig. 8.1). There seems to be a significant genetic predisposition, but sometimes the cause of atrial fibrillation is not identified. Possible precipitants include alcohol, coronary artery disease, diabetes, heart failure, HTN, obesity, thyroid disease, and other illnesses.[7] Instead of the organized electrical impulses initiated by the sinoatrial node, the result is erratic, electric impulses. This causes the cardiac muscle to fibrillate, resulting in the absence of atrial contraction and a rapid, irregular ventricular rate commonly between 120 and 160 beats/min.[8] It is the rapid heart rate that causes Mr. Li's discomfort and presyncopal feelings, but an uncontrolled heart rate can cause cardiac ischemia, heart failure, and/or stroke. These sequelae are related to inefficient cardiac contractions that result in inadequate stroke volume. The blood in the fibrillating heart falls back into the pulmonary veins. Because the heart is pumping inadequately, the blood backs up into the lungs and is not effectively oxygenating the other body tissues.[9] It is this lack of tissue oxygenation that likely caused the "tired" feeling Mr. Li described.[9] It is important, however, to not presume this is the cause of his tired complaint because there are other possibilities that should also be excluded (e.g., anemia, hypothyroidism). The risk of blood clots forming is related to the pooling blood.[9] A clot in the atria can then easily be ejected and with one heart beat ejected into the circulation and cause a stroke.[9]

Treatment of atrial fibrillation is based on determining and treating the underlying pathophysiology, as well as controlling heart rate and decreasing the risk of embolization. Many patients are hospitalized with new-onset atrial fibrillation, but some patients will refuse hospitalization and many can be managed as outpatients. When a patient presents with atrial fibrillation it is first important to determine whether the patient is stable or unstable. Most patients are stable, but a patient with hypotension, chest pain, or pulmonary edema would be considered unstable and require urgent electrical cardioversion and hospitalization for stabilization.

Mr. Li's CHA_2DS_2-VASc (available at https://www.chadsvasc.org/) risk stratification score is calculated to estimate his stroke risk. Using the CHA_2DS_2-VASc calculator aids health care providers in determining which patients with nonvalvular atrial fibrillation should be anticoagulated based on age, sex, and comorbidities.[10] His sex, age, and comorbidities (HTN and diabetes) reveal a risk stratification score of 3, suggesting a 3.2% chance of stroke.[10] If a patient has a score of 2 or greater, anticoagulation is recommended.[10]

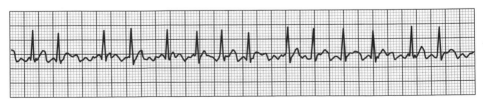

Fig. 8.1   Rhythm strip of atrial fibrillation. (From Cameron, P. Jelinek, G., Kelly, A. M., Brown, A., & Little, M. (2015). *Textbook of adult emergency medicine* [4th ed.]. Edinburgh: Churchhill Livingstone.)

The health care provider considers Mr. Li's disposition knowing that patients can be discharged home on an anticoagulant and rate control medication such as a calcium channel blocker or beta-blocker. An echocardiogram and other diagnostics could be obtained as an outpatient in clinically stable patients. However, Mr. Li's age, comorbidities, rapid heart rate, presyncopal sensations, alcohol ingestion, and the uncertainty about the cause of his atrial fibrillation are concerning, and the health care provider decides that hospitalization is appropriate.

It is also unclear how long Mr. Li has been in atrial fibrillation. Based on his symptoms, the provider suspects at least a couple of days, but many patients can have atrial fibrillation and be completely asymptomatic. The hospital admissions office is called and the patient is admitted to the telemetry unit.

5.   11 a.m.: Mr. Li is admitted to the hospital. What treatment and admitting orders are indicated for Mr. Li?

Hospital Admission Orders
1. Admit to telemetry for cardiac monitoring.
2. Daily weight.
3. Vital signs every shift and as needed (prn).
4. Intake and output.
5. Heparin lock.
6. Intravenous (IV) normal saline (0.9% N/S) with thiamine 100 milligrams at 100 mL/hr × 1 L.
7. Metoprolol 2.5 milligrams IV every 6 hours. Monitor heart rate. Call covering physician for heart rate over 100 beats/min. Hold metoprolol and call covering physician for heart rate less than 70.
8. Nicotine patch, 21 milligrams, applied to dry skin daily.
9. Enoxaparin (Lovenox) 1 milligrams/kg subcutaneously (SQ) twice a day.
10. Valsartan 80 milligrams po daily.
11. Metformin ER, 1000 milligrams po twice a day with food.
12. Doxazosin 8 milligrams po daily at bedtime.
13. Atorvastatin 40 milligrams po daily.
14. Thiamine 100 milligrams intramuscularly (IM) now and then thiamine 100 milligrams po daily × 3 days.
15. Folic acid 1 milligrams po now and then daily × 3 days.
16. Multivitamin 1 po daily.
17. Lorazepam, 0.5 milligrams IV every 4 hours prn for agitation.
18. TSH, free T4, CBC/differential (CBC/diff), serum glucose, serum electrolytes, magnesium, BUN, creatinine, troponin × 3, proBNP, liver function tests, alcohol level, prothrombin time/international normalized ratio (PT/INR), alcohol level, serum B_{12} and folate, amylase, and lipase.
19. Chest x-ray, posteroanterior/lateral.
20. Transthoracic echocardiogram.
21. Cardiology consult.
22. Accu-Chek before meals and at bedtime.
23. Regular diet.
24. Clinical Institute Withdrawal Assessment of Alcohol Scale-Revised (CIWA-AR) every 4 hours (https://www.mdcalc.com/ciwa-ar-alcohol-withdrawal).
25. Alcohol-Benzodiazepine Withdrawal Protocol every 4 hours:
    a. If CIWA-AR scale less than 9, no lorazepam.
    b. If CIWA-AR scale 10 to 19, lorazepam 2 milligrams po or IV.
    c. If CIWA-AR scale 20 to 29, lorazepam 3 milligrams, po or IV.

    d. If CIWA-AR scale 30 or greater, lorazepam 4 milligrams po or IV.

    e. Reassess patient every hour after lorazepam is administered. If patient's symptoms are not controlled, STAT page health care provider.

    f. If patient develops any of the following, contact the on-call physician:

      1) Fever > 101.5°F

      2) Heart rate < 50 or > 120

      3) Blood pressure

        a) Systolic 180 or greater or systolic 110 or less

        b) Diastolic 100 or greater

      4) Urine output < 250 mL in 8 hours

26. Out of bed with assistance for meals and toileting.

Mr. Li is admitted to the telemetry unit so that his heart rate and rhythm can be monitored. He will need a heparin lock to receive metoprolol IV to control his heart rate, and his heart rate will be monitored to determine his response to the beta-blocker. He will also be started on enoxaparin to prevent blood clots and bridged to warfarin (Coumadin). The newer novel oral anticoagulants like the factor Xa inhibitors rivaroxaban (Xarelto), apixaban (Eliquis), and edoxaban (Savaysa), or dabigatran (Pradaxa), a thrombin inhibitor, were considered, but family finances are a possible concern.[8] A nicotine patch is also ordered because Mr. Li is a heavy smoker. His medications at home will also be continued in the hospital.

Both cardiac and noncardiac causes of atrial fibrillation need to be excluded. Noncardiac laboratory diagnostics will include a TSH and free T_4 to determine whether hyperthyroidism is the cause of atrial fibrillation. A CBC/diff will help eliminate the presence of infection or anemia. A CBC is also indicated before warfarin is initiated to assess the hemoglobin (Hgb) and platelet count as well.[11] Electrolyte abnormalities and alcohol toxicity should also be excluded.[11] Laboratory diagnostics should also include a PT/INR before warfarin is started.[11] A chest x-ray will also be necessary to assess if pneumonia or pleural effusion is present. Sleep apnea has also been associated with atrial fibrillation, so it will be important to obtain more information from Mr. Li to learn if he uses a sleep apnea device at night or not.[8]

Varied cardiac causes of atrial fibrillation should be considered. A myocardial infarction is one possibility, so serial cardiac troponin (cTn) levels (on admission, and at hours 3 and 6 after admission) are as important as the electrocardiogram in diagnosing myocardial ischemia or infarction. A proBNP is helpful when heart failure is a consideration, but it is important to remember that age, sex, and renal function can affect proBNP levels, so a patient's baseline proBNP level might be greater than normal.[12,13] An echocardiogram is necessary to evaluate the heart's chamber sizes and the possible presence of valvular heart disease.[14] The health care provider caring for Mr. Li orders a transthoracic echocardiogram to determine the presence of valvular heart disease, as well as thrombi, ventricular heart disease, pulmonary heart disease, and pericardial disease. The possible presence of thrombi necessitates a transesophageal echocardiogram if early cardioversion in planned, but the onset of atrial fibrillation in Mr. Li's case is not clear. The cardiology service is consulted. Mr. Li is not a candidate for cardioversion at this time, but depending on the diagnostic testing, cardioversion might be an option in the future. For some patients, a cardiac stress test is indicated to evaluate for coronary artery disease.

Point-of-care blood glucose testing will be required before meals and at bedtime for the first 24 hours. Because Mr. Li's Hgb A1c was 7.5% 6 weeks ago, an insulin sliding scale was not deemed necessary at this time. It is important in older patients, particularly when they are not feeling well and perhaps not eating regularly, to avoid hypoglycemia. A regular diet is ordered initially because many older diabetics do not eat well and can be malnourished. The nutritionist is also consulted. The liver function tests will determine whether Mr. Li's albumin is below normal, and if so, further diagnostic testing will be considered.

Mr. Li's history of alcohol ingestion is concerning. The physical examination should include determining the presence of spider angiomata, gynecomastia, ascites, and abdominal organomegaly (i.e., hepatomegaly and splenomegaly), as well as cognitive status changes. Liver function tests are necessary as is a PT/INR to assess coagulation. An amylase and lipase could be checked in addition to the other laboratory diagnostics, although they are not necessarily indicated in all patients.

Mr. Li is possibly at risk for delirium tremens (DTs) and alcohol withdrawal, so the health care provider orders IV normal saline to be started at 100 mL/hr. IV glucose is avoided in patients at risk for DTs because thiamine deficiency is common, increasing the risk of triggering Wernicke psychosis.[15] Mr. Li does not exhibit signs of Wernicke psychosis (e.g., confusion, nystagmus, gait ataxia) at the present time, but not all patients have a classical presentation and these signs can be subtle and easily missed. Being proactive in patient care is important and helps avoid injury. For that reason, thiamine (B_1) repletion is indicated at initially 100 milligrams IM, then thiamine 100 milligrams po daily.[16,17] Folic acid will also be started; 1 milligram po on admission, and then one tablet po daily for 3 more days. As alcohol withdrawal is a possibility, the CIWA-AR scale will be initiated to monitor for increasing agitation and other withdrawal symptoms (see Exemplar Case Study 5) and the Alcohol-Benzodiazepine Protocol is ordered.[18,19]

Case Study, Continued

Hospital Day 2: 8 a.m.
Mr. Li had a difficult time sleeping during the night, but his CIWA-AR scale never rose above 4. At most, the nurses described him as somewhat anxious but easily calmed and redirected. His heart rate during the night ranged from 81 to 115, and he remained in atrial fibrillation. His Accu-Chek results have been consistently between 118 and 150.

Mr. Li asks to go home and states he is "much better." He would like a "cigarette." He denies fever, chills, dizziness, weakness, difficulty eating, chest pressure or pain, cough, shortness of breath, abdominal pain, nausea, vomiting, leg pain, or other discomfort. Mr. Li is also asked if he uses a sleep apnea device at home, but Mr. Li replies he tried one but did not like it. He felt like he was smothering and does not want to try it again.

   Objective: Alert, older male sitting in chair eating breakfast. Temperature 97.8°F. Blood pressure 120/74. Heart rate 99, irregular, respiratory rate 22 at rest, O_2 saturation on room air 95% at rest.
   Weight: 130 pounds.
   Intake: IV 2100 mL; po 560 mL.
   Total intake: 2660 mL.
   Output: Urine 1350 mL.

Physical Examination
   Skin: Warm/dry. No rash, jaundice, or acute lesions.
   Eyes: Sclera clear; conjunctiva, no injection.
   Nose: No rhinitis or sinus tenderness.
   Mouth: Membranes moist. No lesions of tongue or buccal mucosa.
   Neck: Supple. No masses, lymphadenopathy, thyroid enlargement, or tenderness.
   Cardiac: Irregular, irregular.
   Respiratory: Clear without rales, wheezes, or rhonchi.
   Abdomen: Soft, bowel sounds positive, nontender, no organomegaly.
   Extremities: Pedal pulses present, no edema or calf tenderness.
   Laboratory diagnostics:
      White blood cell (WBC): 10. 5 (4.0–11.0 K/mm3)
      Hgb: 10.9 (11–16 g/dL)

Hct: 32.6 L (35%–48%)
MCV: 101.4 (80–100 fL)
Platelets: 136 (130–400 K/mm$_3$)
Neutrophils % (Auto): 84.3 H (37.0%–80.0%)
Lymphocyte % (Auto): 8.4 J (23.0%–45.0%)
Neutrophils # (Auto): 8.9 H (1.9–7.5 K/mm$_3$)
Lymphocytes #: 0.9 L (1.2–3.4 K/mm$_3$)
Sodium: 135 (136–145 mmol/L)
Potassium: 3.3 (3.4–5.1 mmol/L)
Chloride: 97 L (98–107 mmol/L)
Carbon dioxide: 26 (22–32 mmol/L)
BUN: 35 H (5–23 milligrams/dL)
Creatinine: 1.6 H (0.4–1.0 md/dL)
Estimated glomerular filtration rate (GFR): 36.8 (mL/min/ m$_2$)
Glucose: 140 H (74–118 milligrams/dL)
Calcium: 9.7 (8.6–10.2 milligrams/dL)
Magnesium: 2.1 (1.6–2.6 milligrams/dL)
Troponin T: <0.03 (<0.03 ng/mL)
TSH: 3.22 (0.27–4.2 µIU/mL)
Free T$_4$: 0.9 (0.8–1.5 ng/dL)
Vitamin B$_{12}$: 202 (200–900 pg/mL)
Folate (>2.5 ng/mL):
PT (10.0–12.3 seconds): 11. 0
PTT/INR range: 1.0 (0.8–1.2)
Blood alcohol level: None detected
Total protein: 7.1 (6.4–8.3 g/dL)
Albumin: 3.2 (3.4–5.2 g/dL)
Globulin: 4.3 (2.3–3.5g/dL)
Bilirubin, total: 1.0 (0.3–1.2 milligrams/dL)
Bilirubin, direct: 0.4 (0.1–0.5 milligrams/dL)
Alkaline phosphatase: (40–129 U/L)
AST (aspartate aminotransferase) (serum glutamic oxaloacetic transaminase [SGOT]): 143 (0.4 U/L)
ALT (alanine aminotransferase) (serum glutamic pyruvic transaminase [SGPT]): 92 (0. 41 U/L)
N-terminal proBNP: 888 (5–900 pg/mL)
B$_{12}$: 316 (>300 pg/mL)
Folate: 9 (>4 ng/mL)

Echocardiogram:
1. Mild concentric left ventricular hypertrophy. Estimated ejection fraction 50% to 55%. No diastolic dysfunction.
2. Mildly thickened aortic valve leaflets without obvious vegetations on aortic valve leaflets. No aortic stenosis. Mild aortic regurgitation. Mildly dilated aortic root at 4.3 cm.
3. Mildly thickened mitral valve leaflets. Positive prolapse posterior mitral valve leaflet. Moderate to severe mitral regurgitation. Mild left atrial enlargement with elevated left atrial pressure.
4. Mild tricuspid regurgitation. No obvious vegetations on tricuspid valve leaflets.
5. Mild pulmonic insufficiency. Pulmonic leaflets not well visualized.

Impression: Mild pulmonic insufficiency.

6. After seeing Mr. Li and reviewing the nursing note and diagnostics results, what are the essential management plans for Mr. Li today? What patient and family education should be initiated to ensure a smooth transition to home?

Mr. Li was seen by cardiology and he is not a candidate for cardioversion at this time, but he will be started on warfarin. His heart rate continues to be higher than the goal heart rate of 60 to 70 beats/min, which is considered reasonable for patients with atrial fibrillation and heart failure.[20] He will be started on Toprol XL 25 milligrams po daily and monitored during sleep and with activity to determine whether his heart rate is too slow when sleeping or too high with activity. The medication dose can then be adjusted to his needs, although he will need monitoring also as an outpatient because of his renal dysfunction. His calculated creatinine clearance based on the Cockcroft–Gault equation is 38.67 mL/min today. This indicates that Mr. Li has Stage 3b chronic kidney disease (GFR 30–44 mL/min), a point where he could have fatigue, fluid retention, and become short of breath.

Mr. Li's serum potassium is 3.3 mmol/L. Historically, the serum potassium goal in hospitalized patients has been 4.0, but a retrospective study of 38,000 patients hospitalized for acute myocardial infarction revealed that a serum potassium between 3.5 and 3.9 mEq/L was associated with the least mortality.[21] These results cannot be extrapolated to all hospitalized patients. Although this study suggests that the ideal serum potassium for hospitalized patients with varied comorbidities is not known, a serum potassium less than 3.0 or greater than 4.0 was associated with greater mortality.[21] Mr. Li's potassium will be repleted, but cautiously. Usually 10 mEq of oral potassium will increase the serum potassium by 0.1 mmol/L. If the health care provider orders 40 mEq of oral potassium, Mr. Li's serum potassium should increase to 3.7 mmol/L, which is a little below 4.0. It is best with a patient who has renal dysfunction to be conservative when ordering medications because as the GFR decreases, serum drug levels can increase raising the risk of drug side effects and toxicity. For that reason Mr. Li will receive 30 mEq of potassium chloride orally × 1 and his serum potassium will be rechecked in the morning to be certain his potassium is not too high or too low.

The estimated glomerular filtration rate (eGFR) on admission for this patient is 36.8 mL/min. The patient is on metformin and regular assessment of GFR is necessary for an older patient taking this medication. For older adults with a GFR this low, continuing metformin is a concern. If the estimated GFR is less than <30 mL/min/1.73 m^2, then the metformin should be discontinued. Mr. Li's estimated GFR is greater than 30 mL/min/1.73 m^2, but it is appropriate to decrease his metformin dose and monitor his eGFR.[22]

The abnormal liver enzymes for this patient do not conclusively indicate alcoholic liver disease. Alcoholic liver disease is suggested when the AST is twice the ALT. Mr. Li's admission alcohol level was normal, so it is possible that the elevated ALT and AST are related to another liver disorder (e.g., drug related, nonalcoholic fatty liver disease, hepatitis, other disorder). The elevations in ALT and AST may also be transient. The liver function tests should be repeated. If the elevations are related to alcohol, the liver enzymes will likely decrease if Mr. Li stops drinking alcohol. If the AST and ALT remain elevated, further diagnostics will be necessary to determine the underlying cause.

Mr. Li is anemic and his MCV appears to be slightly macrocytic. This suggests a macrocytic anemia, which would be consistent with chronic alcohol ingestion, liver disease, or a B_{12} or folate deficiency. There are other more serious considerations with an increased MCV. These include hypothyroidism, a hemolytic anemia, aplastic anemia, or myelodysplastic disorder. His platelets are also somewhat diminished, which may or may not be related to chronic alcohol ingestion. These laboratory results will need to monitored.

Continued anticoagulation is imperative because of the risk of stroke in atrial fibrillation. Mr. Li will be continued on enoxaparin but also started on warfarin 5 milligrams po this day. The PT/INR will be checked daily, but the suspected dose of warfarin tomorrow will be 2.5 milligrams. Usually patients who are started on warfarin receive 5 to 10 milligrams po the first 2 days, then a PT/INR is checked on day 3. Mr. Li, however, is older and has chronic kidney disease putting him at increased risk for an elevated INR, so he will be started on 5 milligrams and, depending on the daily PT/INR results, continued on half that dose on days 2 and 3.[23]

Mr. Li and his family will need considerable education regarding the cause of his symptoms and the treatment. Ideally, the education of the patient and his family should begin at the time of admission to promote understanding and avoid complications, adverse drug events, injuries, and rehospitalizations.[24] The discharge plan should address the transition from hospital to home or skilled nursing facility (SNF); promote understanding of Mr. Li's illness, its causes and treatments; medication safety; and healthy lifestyle changes. For patients with substance use disorder, there are additional management concerns. Patient stabilization in the hospital setting is essential, but discussing the health issues related to substance abuse of any kind must include empathetic guidance for the patient and family, which includes resources, counseling, and the benefits of lifestyle changes in terms of quality of life.[25] Discussion with the patient's primary care doctor is indicated to promote frequent follow-up and patient support. A dietary consult with the patient and family before hospital discharge will also be requested because Mr. Li is underweight and his albumin is slightly lower than normal.

Assessment and Plan

1. **Atrial fibrillation, new onset:** His troponins were negative and seen by cardiology. His IV metoprolol will be discontinued and he will be started on Toprol XL 25 milligrams po daily. He will remain in the hospital and his heart rate monitored for at least one more day.
2. **Anticoagulation:** PT/partial thromboplastin time (PTT)/INR within normal limits. PT/INR daily. Start warfarin. Continue enoxaparin.
3. **ETOH history:** Maintain CIWA-AR and Alcohol-Benzodiazepine Withdrawal Protocol.
4. **Fluid status:** Heparin lock. Discontinue IV fluids and encourage po fluids to 2000 mL/24 hours.
5. **Anemia:** ? etiology. Plan stool occult blood.
6. **Thrombocytopenia:** ? related to ETOH. Plan recheck.
7. **Hypokalemia:** Goal serum K 3.9.
8. Physical therapy consult.
9. **Nutrition consult:** Low BMI in older adult with DM II.
10. Patient education regarding cause of illness and hospitalization, smoking cessation, ETOH ingestion, and medication changes.

Hospital Day 2: Orders

1. Continue CIWA-AR and Alcohol-Benzodiazepine Withdrawal Protocol.
2. PT/INR daily.
3. Warfarin 5 milligrams po today.
4. Potassium chloride 30 mEq po × 1.
5. Discontinue metformin 1000 milligrams po twice a day.
6. Start metformin 500 milligrams po twice a day.
7. Stool for occult blood × 3.
8. CBC/diff, Chem 8 tomorrow morning.
9. Physical therapy evaluation.
10. Nutrition consult shows low BMI in older adult with DM II.
11. Stool for occult blood.

Hospital Day 3

Subjective: Mr. Li is asking to return home and tells the health care provider he feels fine. He has not moved his bowels since hospital admission. He denies fever, chills, difficulty swallowing, heartburn, chest pain, shortness of breath, cough, abdominal pain, urinary frequency, burning, or leg pain. Physical therapy reports he did reasonably well yesterday, but is impulsive. Able to get out of bed with minimal assistance, but rushes, gait a bit unsteady. Nurses report no confusion or agitation.

Objective: Temperature 98°F. Blood pressure 136/78 sitting, standing 130/70 without increase in heart rate. Heart rate 81, irregular, respiratory rate 20 at rest, O_2 saturation on room air 95% at rest.

Weight: 130 pounds.

Intake : 1650 mL po.

Output: Urine 1350 mL.

Physical Examination
Skin: Warm/dry. No rash or acute lesions.

Eyes: Sclera clear; conjunctiva, no injection.

Nose: No rhinitis or sinus tenderness.

Mouth: Membranes moist. No lesions of tongue or buccal mucosa.

Neck: Supple. No masses, lymphadenopathy, thyroid enlargement, or tenderness.

Cardiac: Irregular, irregular.

Respiratory: Clear without rales, wheezes, or rhonchi.

Abdomen: Soft, bowel sounds sluggish/diminished, but nontender throughout and no organomegaly.

Extremities: Pedal pulses present, no edema or calf tenderness.

Laboratory diagnostics:
WBC: 9 (4.0–11.0 K/mm$_3$)

Hgb: 9.9 (11–16 g/dL)

Hct: 30.1 L (35%–48%)

MCV: 101.4 (80–100 fL)

Platelets: 142 (130–400 K/mm$_3$)

Neutrophils % (Auto): 80.1 H (37.0%–80.0%)

Lymphocytes % (Auto): 13.9 L (23.0%–45.0%)

Neutrophils # (Auto): 7.9 H (1.9–7.5 K/mm$_3$)

Lymphocytes #: 1.0 L (1.2–3.4 K/mm$_3$)

Sodium: 138 (136–145 mmol/L)

Potassium: 3.9 (3.4–5.1 mmol/L)

Chloride: 98 L (98–107 mmol/L)

Carbon dioxide: 26 (22–32 mmol/L)

BUN: 22 H (5–23 milligrams/dL)

Creatinine: 1.3 H (0.4–1.0 md/dL)

eGFR: 45.36 (mL/min)

Glucose: 140 H (74–118 milligrams/dL)

PTT/INR: 1.2 (0.8–1.2)

7. What is the appropriate assessment and plan for Mr. Li today?

Mr. Li's heart rate, vital signs, and laboratory values are improved. His potassium is at goal but should be repeated before discharge. Additionally, his Hgb and Hct have decreased a bit, which may be related to improved fluid volume.

Assessment and Plan
1. **Atrial fibrillation:** Heart rate stable.
2. **Anticoagulation:** PT/INR daily. Warfarin 2.5 milligrams po today. Continue enoxaparin.
3. **ETOH history:** DC CIWA-AR and Alcohol-Benzodiazepine Withdrawal Protocol,
4. Chem 8 in a.m.

   5. **Fluid status:** Monitor, encourage po fluids to 1800 to 2000 mL/day.
   6. **Constipation:** Add linaclotide (Linzess) 145 micrograms po daily.
   7. **Discharge plans:** ? discharge home versus SNF tomorrow. Discuss with family and case management.

Case Study, Continued

Health care provider hospital note: Discussed with Mr. Li the possibility of discharge tomorrow and options for home or skilled nursing care. The health care team expressed concerns about the effects of alcohol and smoking on Mr. Li's health and suggested that a few days of skilled nursing might be helpful if Mr. Li and his family agree. The new medicines and reason for them will also be discussed. Mr. Li was asked if it is okay for the health care provider to talk with his wife and daughter and he agreed. Mr. Li's family is called to update them on his progress.

   Phone conversation with Mr. Li's daughter: Explained her father is stable and improving, but will need to take some new medications each day and have regular blood tests. Mr. Li's daughter is concerned about her mother's ability to care for her father. She works every day and her mother will be home with her father. She is not sure her mother can stop him from drinking and thinks a nursing home would be helpful for a few days, but she is not sure her father will agree. She agrees to come in later to visit her father and will talk with her mother and father then.

Hospital Day 3: Orders
   1. Warfarin 2.5 milligrams. po today. Continue enoxaparin.
   2. DC CIWA-AR and Alcohol-Benzodiazepine Withdrawal Protocol.
   3. Chem 8 in a.m.
   4. PT/INR in a.m.
   5. Linaclotide (Linzess) 145 micrograms po daily.
   6. Consult Case Management for possible discharge tomorrow. ? home versus skilled nursing care.

Mr. Li's primary nurse calls Mrs. Li to ask when she will be in to see her husband. The nurse explains she would like to teach Mrs. Li how to give her husband his Lovenox injection. Mrs. Li tells the nurse she cannot give injections, so the nurse decides that Mr. Li might really be the better person to learn how to give his own Lovenox and explains to Mr. Li that she will show him how to give the medication today and he will be able to give himself the medicine at home for the few days it might be needed.

8. What are the criteria for admission to a skilled nursing facility (SNF), and how is the decision made regarding discharge home versus admission to a skilled nursing facility?

Admission to an SNF is often initiated by the hospital case manager after discussion with the health care provider. Some SNFs have screeners who will come to the hospital. Often, case management will discuss the available facilities and communicate with those facilities to see if there is a bed available. The health care provider needs to be able to determine patient needs to aid families and case management in choosing the best facility for the patient's needs.

   There are specific criteria for admission to an SNF unit, and the patient's health insurance can affect the decision. In general, admission to a SNF subacute unit requires that the patient needs 4 to 6 hours of skilled nursing care daily or is able to fulfill the minimum daily rehabilitation (e.g., physical or occupational therapy requirements).

Hospital Day 4
   Subjective: Mr. Li feels well and asks again about discharge home. He talked with his family and wants to go home. He tells the primary care provider that his family agrees and he will

let the visiting nurses visit him at home. He also tells the health care provider that he knows he should not drink or smoke and he can "cut down." He did move his bowels after the linaclotide (Linzess) yesterday. Today he denies fever, chills, sweats, headache, dizziness, feeling like he will fall, difficulty swallowing, heartburn, chest discomfort, shortness of breath, abdominal pain, constipation, diarrhea, urinary pain or frequency, muscle pain, or calf pain. The dietician did see Mr. Li and reviewed his daily dietary choices at home. The recommendation was that Mr. Li continue his regular dietary regimen at home, monitor his blood sugars in the morning and before dinner, and discuss elevated blood sugars greater than 150 milligrams/dL with his family doctor. The dietician's note suggested that Mr. Li's diet at home did consist of alcohol each day and that alcohol cessation would aid blood sugar control, but the importance of not drinking alcohol and avoiding concentrated sweets was stressed.

Objective: Temperature 97.6°F. Blood pressure 128/76 sitting, standing 132/74 without increase in heart rate. Heart rate 75, irregular, respiratory rate 18 at rest, O_2 saturation on room air 95% at rest.

Weight: 132 pounds (60 kg).

Intake: 1850 mL po.

Output: Urine 1550 mL.

Physical Examination

Skin: Warm/dry. No rash or acute lesions.

Eyes: Sclera clear; conjunctiva, no injection.

Nose: No rhinitis or sinus tenderness.

Mouth: Membranes moist. No lesions of tongue or buccal mucosa.

Neck: Supple. No masses, lymphadenopathy, thyroid enlargement, or tenderness.

Cardiac: Irregular, irregular rate 75 to 80.

Respiratory: Clear without rales, wheezes, or rhonchi.

Abdomen: Soft, + bowel sounds, no organomegaly or tenderness.

Extremities: Pedal pulses present, no edema or calf tenderness.

Laboratory diagnostics:

Stool for occult blood: Negative

Sodium: 137 (136–145 mmol/L)

Potassium: 3.9 (3.4–5.1 mmol/L)

Chloride: 98 L (98–107 mmol/L)

Carbon dioxide: 26 (22–32 mmol/L)

BUN: 21 H (5–23 milligrams/dL)

Creatinine: 1.1 H (0.4–1.0 md/dL)

eGFR: 54 (mL/min)

Glucose: 122 H (74–118 milligrams/dL)

PTT/INR: 1.6 (0.8–1.2)

The health care provider decides that Mr. Li can return home with visiting nurses to check the PT/INR each day and a visit to the primary care provider within 72 hours. The health care provider calls the primary care provider to discuss the discharge plans and an early posthospital appointment.

9. What discharge orders can aid Mr. Li in a smooth transition from hospital to home? How should these orders be written?

Hospital Day 4: Orders

1. Discharge home with visiting nurses for daily PT/INR and Lovenox teaching.
   a. Goal INR 2.5 (2–3).

2. Warfarin 2.5 milligrams po today. Goal INR 2 to 3. Call patient's primary care provider with daily PT/INR.
3. Nicotine patch, 21 milligrams, applied to dry skin daily × 6 weeks, then 14 milligrams/day × 2 weeks, then 7 milligrams/day × 2 weeks.
4. Enoxaparin 1 milligrams/kg (60 milligrams) SQ twice a day.
5. Valsartan 80 milligrams po daily.
6. Discontinue metformin 1000 milligrams po twice a day. Start metformin ER, 500 milligrams po twice a day with food.
7. Doxazosin 8 milligrams po daily at bedtime.
8. Atorvastatin 40 milligrams po daily.
9. Multivitamin 1 a day po.
10. Toprol XL 25 milligrams po daily.

Mr. Li's INR needs to be between 2.0 and 3.0 for two consecutive days for the Lovenox to be discontinued.[26] His nurse continues trying to teach Mr. Li how to give himself the Lovenox injections, but he seems inattentive, disinterested, and gets confused easily. Discouraged, the nurse calls Mr. Li's daughter and explains how important it is for Mr. Li to have the Lovenox twice a day. If Mr. Li's daughter could come to the hospital in the late afternoon, they can hold his discharge until later and the nurse can teach Mr. Li's daughter how to do it for the few days he will need it.

The daughter does come with her mother to pick up her father around 6 p.m. and is able to learn how to give the Lovenox without difficulty. In addition to the discharge and medication instructions, Mr. Li's daughter is able to teach back what her father needs to do at home.

Home Day 1

Mr Li. arrives home after dinner and has an uneventful night.

10. What are the responsibilities of the visiting nurse at the initial home visit after patient discharge from an acute care facility?

The visiting nurse first calls the Li household and asks if Mr. Li had his Lovenox injection that morning. Mrs. Li explains that her daughter did give him the injection before she went to work. Relieved that he did get his first Lovenox injection today, the visiting nurse explains she will be at their home around 2 p.m. to see Mr. Li. She also quickly explains to Mrs. Li that when she comes to their home, she will need to see the discharge paperwork from the hospital, check Mr. Li's blood for the new medication (warfarin) he is taking, and do a home safety evaluation to assure Mr. Li's safety after his hospitalization.

When the visiting nurse arrives that afternoon, she senses tension in the home and takes the time to sit for a few moments with Mrs. Li who answered the door. After introducing herself to Mrs. Li, she asks how Mr. Li is doing. Mrs. Li is worried about her husband drinking again, but explains that she threw all the alcohol and cigarettes in the house away, so now Mr. Li will not talk with her. Not certain exactly what to say, the visiting nurse explains that she has many questions to ask during the first visit and needs to check Mr. Li's blood and call the doctor, so they will be able to know what warfarin dose Mr. Li will need tonight.

Mr. Li is sitting watching television when Mrs. Li brings the visiting nurse to him. He turns off the television at the nurse's request. The nurse explains the visit process for today: first, the many questions, then an examination, and then the blood test. The new medication prescriptions were filled and the new metformin pills, warfarin, and Toprol are on the table next to Mr. Li's chair. The nurse asks if Mr. Li uses a pill box, but he replies that he does not need a pill box, he knows when to take his meds. The visiting nurse first goes through Mr. Li's discharge papers, reconciles his medications with the discharge summary, and reiterates to both Mr. and Mrs. Li the change in the metformin dose. The remainder of the interview process takes some time and Mr. Li is restless, so the nurse does a review of systems to which Mr. Li responds "fine, fine, no problem."

Physical Examination

General: There is no scale to weigh Mr. Li, but the visiting nurse notes that he is frail and appears deconditioned. His appearance, age, and current medications (beta-blocker and anticoagulant) raise her concerns about his fall risk. She first asks Mr. Li to get up out of his chair and walk to the kitchen, which she thinks might be 20 feet away from where he sits. Mr. Li has difficulty getting up out of the chair by himself and his wife rushes to help him and helps him start the walk to the kitchen, but he turns around earlier and returns to his chair.

Vital signs: Blood pressure sitting 134/86, 144/90 standing. Heart rate irregular, irregular rate 89, respiratory rate 20, O_2 saturation 94%.

Skin: Warm/dry, no lesions.

Eyes: Sclera clear, no icterus, conjunctiva pale.

Nose: No rhinitis or sinus tenderness.

Mouth: Membranes moist, no lesions.

Neck: Supple, no masses.

Cardiac: Irregular irregular, no murmurs or rubs.

Lungs: Diminished at bases, but clear without wheezes or crackles.

Abdomen: Soft, bowel sounds possible, nontender.

Extremities: No calf tenderness or edema.

Concerned about the possibility of falls, the visiting nurse explains to Mr. and Mrs. Li the concern about falls when patients are taking warfarin and asks Mr. and Mrs. Li if she can now do a quick home safety evaluation. She explains that when a home safety evaluation is done, it can help point out areas that can cause falls, for example, a slippery rug on a floor. Mr. Li tells the nurse that he never falls, but both agree that the nurse can look and Mrs. Li and the visiting nurse together start the home safety evaluation looking to be certain all hallways and rooms had working lights and that there were no slippery rugs that could cause falls. The nurse shows Mrs. Li that checklist as they walk through the house together (available at http://www.agis.com/Document/13/home-safety-and-security-checklist.aspx).

The home safety evaluation goes well, and there are minimal recommendations: primarily keeping the stairs clear and adding a safety rail to the bathtub.

The nurse checks Mr. Li's PT/INR and the result is 1.9. The nurse knows that the effect of Mr. Li's warfarin dose is not yet fully realized and calls the patient's primary care provider who then orders a 2.5-milligrams tablet of warfarin tonight and requests that the visiting nurse return tomorrow to check Mr. Li's PT/INR again.

Home Day 2

The visiting nurse returns to check Mr. Li's PT/INR. Mr. Li tells her he had his injection this morning and that he has an appointment with his doctor in two more days. Today his INR is 2.6 and his warfarin dose is 2.5 milligrams.

11.   The visiting nurse calls Mr. Li's primary care provider to determine what dose of warfarin is appropriate for Mr. Li today. Mr. Li has now been taking warfarin for several days and his INR is now within the therapeutic range for a patient who has atrial fibrillation. What should his primary care provider order now for his warfarin dose today and when could Mr. Li's Lovenox be discontinued?

The visiting nurse reports today's PT/INR (2.6) to Mr. Li's health care provider who requests the nurse to report his recent warfarin doses and daily PT/INR results:

Hospital day 2: INR: 1.0, warfarin 5 milligrams

Hospital day 3: INR: 1.2, warfarin 2.5 milligrams

Hospital day 4: INR: 1.6, warfarin 2.5 milligrams
Home day 1: INR 1.9, warfarin 2.5 milligrams
Home day 2 (today): INR 2.6, warfarin ?

Older patients are usually started on low-dose warfarin (2.5–5 milligrams) because aging changes (e.g., pharmacodynamic, pharmacokinetic, organ changes, medications) can make bleeding on any anticoagulant or antiplatelet a potential concern. The risk is heightened in frail elders who are at increased risk for falls. The goal INR (i.e., 2–3 for atrial fibrillation), however, remains the same despite aging and risk management (e.g., falls, bleeding) concerns.

The primary care provider is aware that for a patient on day 5 of warfarin therapy and an INR of 2.0 to 3.0, no change in the dose is necessary. Warfarin 2.5 milligrams po today is ordered and a repeat INR will be necessary tomorrow. If the INR remains within goal, the Lovenox can then be discontinued.[27]

The visiting nurse explains the warfarin dose to Mr. and Mrs. Li and together the dose is put with Mr. Li's afternoon medications. Mr. Li tells the nurse he is doing fine and he will see her tomorrow. He wants to play mahjong with his friend and does not want to be late. Mrs. Li explains that the nurse does not have to come tomorrow because he has an appointment with the doctor.

Home Day 3

Mr. Li's daughter takes time off from work to drive her parents to her father's hospital follow-up appointment. Hospital follow-up within 1 week is recommended to review medication changes, the reason behind the need for hospitalization, and prevent rehospitalizations. Often, it is challenging to arrange an appointment so quickly in primary care, but Mr. Li's health care provider is particularly troubled about the alcohol concern in the hospital and wanted to see Mr. Li as soon as possible. "Mr. Li, nice to see you. I was sorry to learn you were in the hospital and I am glad you are here to tell me how you are doing." Mr. Li is very quiet and the review of systems is negative. The health care provider then tells Mr. Li that the hospitalist doctor was very concerned about Mr. Li's smoking and drinking and thought that alcohol might have played a role in Mr. Li's illness. Mr. Li says little, but Mrs. Li explains to the health care provider that there is no alcohol and no cigarettes anymore as Mr. Li nods in agreement. The health care provider explains to the Li family that many Chinese are born with low amounts of acetaldehyde dehydrogenase, an enzyme in the liver that breaks down alcohol. When that happens, the liver can stop working well. Mr. Li nods his head, but says little. The health care provider nods his head also and tells Mr. Li, "I care about your health, Mr. Li, so please let me know if I can help you at any time. I'll check you out and check your blood today, but maybe you could come back in a couple of weeks."

Mr. Li's physical examination is within normal limits, his blood pressure and heart rate are within goal, and his INR is 2.7. The health care provider tells Mr. Li, he is doing well. The Lovenox is discontinued, and the warfarin dose is continued at 2.5 milligrams per day, but his INR will be checked again in 2 days to be certain it is between 2.0 and 3.0.

12.   What other information would be helpful for Mr. Li today?

It would be important to ask Mr. Li about his diet and if he is taking any Chinese herbal medicines and to talk about his prescribed medicines. Explaining the medicines and how other medicines and foods can affect his medicines is important. Asking too about socialization with other elders helps determine whether the Li's feel isolated or lonely in any way. Knowing community resources that can offer support and socialization to elders can help improve quality of life and provide support when necessary.

References

1. Omole, F. S., Sow, C. M., Fresh, E., Babalola, D., & Strothers, H. (2011). Interacting with patients' family members during the office visit. *American Family Physician, 84*(7), 780–784.

2. Lanska, D. J. (2013). Dizziness: Step-by-step through the workup. *Consultant, 360*(53), 3. Retrieved from http://www.consultant360.com/article/dizziness-step-step-through-workup.

3. Cryer, P. E., & Davis, S. N. (2015). Hypoglycemia. In D. Kasper, A. Fauci, S. Hauser, D. Longo, J. Jameson, & J. Loscalzo (Eds.), *Harrison's principles of internal medicine* (19th ed.). Retrieved from http://accessmedicine.mhmedical.com.ezproxy.simmons.edu:2048/content.aspx?bookid=1130&Sectio nid=79753191.

4. Freeman, R. (2015). Syncope. In D. Kasper, A. Fauci, S. Hauser, D. Longo, J. Jameson, & J. Loscalzo (Eds.), *Harrison's principles of internal medicine* (19th ed.). Retrieved from http://accessmedicine.mhmedical .com.ezproxy.simmons.edu:2048/content.aspx?bookid=1130&Sectionid=7972461.

5. Katsung, B. G. (2015). Special aspects of geriatric pharmacology. In B. G. Katzung & A. J. Trevor (Eds.), *Basic & clinical pharmacology* (13th ed.). Retrieved from http://accessmedicine.mhmedical.com .ezproxy.simmons.edu:2048/content.aspx?bookid=1193&Sectionid=69114333.

6. Shibao, C., Lipsitz, L. A., & Biaggianoi, I. (2013). ASH position paper evaluation and treatment of orthostatic hypotension. *Journal of the American Society of Hypertension, 7*(4), 147–153.

7. Kapur, S., & MacRae, C. A. (2014). Atrial fibrillation. In M. F. Murray, M. W. Babyatsky, M. A. Giovanni, F. S. Alkuraya, & D. R. Stewart (Eds.), *Clinical genomics: Practical applications in adult patient care* (1st ed.). Retrieved from http://accessmedicine.mhmedical.com.ezproxy.simmons.edu:2048/content.aspx?booki d=1094&Sectionid=61900120.

8. Michaud, G. F., & Stevenson, W. G. (2015). Supraventricular tachyarrhythmias. In D. Kasper, A. Fauci, S. Hauser, D. Longo, J. Jameson, & J. Loscalzo (Eds.), *Harrison's principles of internal medicine* (19th ed.). Retrieved from http://accessmedicine.mhmedical.com.ezproxy.simmons.edu:2048/content.aspx?bookid= 1130&Sectionid=79742251.

9. American Heart Association. Why atrial fibrillation (AF or Afib) matters. Retrieved from http:// www.heart.org/HEARTORG/Conditions/Arrhythmia/AboutArrhythmia/Why-Atrial-Fibrillation-AF-or-AFib-Matters_UCM_423776_Article.jsp#.V5gFojWM7VI.

10. CHA$_2$DS$_2$-VASc Score for atrial fibrillation stroke risk. Retrieved from http://www.mdcalc.com/ cha2ds2-vasc-score-for-atrial-fibrillation-stroke-risk/.

11. Ezekowitz, M. D., Aikens, T. H., & Nagarakanti, R. (2011). Atrial fibrillation: Outpatient presentation and management. *Circulation, 121*, 1. Retrieved from http://circ.ahajournals.org/content/124/1/95.

12. Takase, H., & Dohi, Y. (2014). Kidney function crucially affects B-type natriuretic peptide (BNP), N-terminal pro BNP, and their relationship. *European Journal of Clinical Investigation, 44*(3), 303–308.

13. Srisawasdi, P., Vanavanan, S., Charoenpanichkit, C., & Kroll, M. H. (2010). The effect of renal dysfunction on BNP, NT-proBNP, and their ratio. *American Journal of Clinical Pathology, 133*(1), 14–23.

14. Prystowsky, E. N., Padanilam, B. J., & Waldo, A. L. (2011). Atrial fibrillation, atrial flutter, and atrial tachycardia. In V. Fuster, R. A. Walsh, & R. A. Harrington (Eds.), *Hurst's the heart* (13th ed.). Retrieved from http://accessmedicine.mhmedical.com.ezproxy.simmons.edu:2048/content.aspx?bookid=376&Sect ionid=40279769.

15. Ropper, A. H., Samuels, M. A., & Klein, J. P. (2014). Alcohol and alcoholism. In A. H. Ropper, M. A. Samuels, & J. P. Klein (Eds.), *Adams & Victor's principles of neurology* (10th ed.). Retrieved from http:// accessmedicine.mhmedical.com.ezproxy.simmons.edu:2048/content.aspx?bookid=690&Sectionid=50910893.

16. Aminoff, M. J., Greenberg, D. A., & Simon, R. P. (2015). Confusional states. In M. J. Aminoff, D. A. Greenberg, & R. P. Simon (Eds.), *Clinical neurology* (9th ed.). Retrieved from http://accessmedicine.mhmedical .com.ezproxy.simmons.edu:2048/content.aspx?bookid=1194&Sectionid=78426447.

17. Schuckit, M. A. (2015). Alcohol and alcoholism. In D. Kasper, A. Fauci, S. Hauser, D. Longo, J. Jameson, & J. Loscalzo (Eds.), *Harrison's principles of internal medicine* (19th ed.). Retrieved from http:// accessmedicine.mhmedical.com.ezproxy.simmons.edu:2048/content.aspx?bookid=1130&Sectio nid=79757307.

18. Clinical Institute Withdrawal Assessment of Alcohol Scale-Revised. Retrieved from http://my.ireta.org/ sites/ireta.sitesquad.net/files/CIWA-Ar.pdf.

19. Leahy, L. G., & Rosof-Williams, J. (2012). Psychosocial health problems. In J. G. Whetstone Foster & S. S. Prevost (Eds.), *Advanced practice nursing of adults in acute care*. Philadelphia: F.A. Davis Co.

20. Heist, K. E., Mansour, M., & Ruskin, J. N. (2011). Rate control in atrial fibrillation. *Circulation, 124*, 2746–2755.

21. Al-Quthami, A. H., & Udelson, J. E. (2012). What is the "goal" serum potassium level in acute myocardial infarction? *American Journal of Kidney Diseases, 60*(4), 517–520.

22. Lipska, K. J., Bailey, C. J., & Inzucchi, S. E. (2011). Use of metformin in the setting of mild-to-moderate renal insufficiency. *Diabetes Care, 34*(6), 1431–1437.
23. Ansell, J., Hirsh, J., Hylek, E., Jacobson, A., Crowther, M., & Palareti, G. (2008). Pharmacology and management of the vitamin k antagonists: American college of chest physicians evidence-based clinical practice guidelines (8th edition). *Chest, 133*(6 Suppl.), 160S–198S.
24. Buttaro, T. M. (2016). Transitional care. In T. M. Buttaro, J. Trybulski, P. Polgar-Bailey, & J. Sandberg-Cook (Eds.), *Primary care: A collaborative practice* (5th ed.). St. Louis, MO: Elsevier.
25. Wagley, J. N. (2016). Substance use disorders. In T. M. Buttaro, J. Trybulski, P. Polgar-Bailey, & J. Sandberg-Cook (Eds.), *Primary care: A collaborative practice* (5th ed.). St. Louis, MO: Elsevier.
26. Wigle, P., Hein, B., Bloomfield, H. E., Tubb, M., & Doherty, M. (2013). Updated guidelines on outpatient anticoagulation. *American Family Physician, 87*(8), 556–566.
27. Cushman, M., Lim, W., & Zakai, N. A. (2014). Clinical practice guide on antithrombotic drug dosing and management of antithrombotic drug associated bleeding complications in adults. *American Society of Hematology.* Retrieved from http://www.hematology.org/Clinicians/Guidelines-Quality/Quick-Reference.aspx.

Fatigue

Bethany Gentleman

Case Study Scenario/History of Present Illness

An 82-year-old female comes to the office today with complaints of increasing shortness of breath (SOB). She is new to this practice and today's visit is in advance of her scheduled initial comprehensive visit. She did not want to further postpone an evaluation for this complaint. She first noticed this several weeks ago when she needed to rest while making her bed. She then observed feeling short of breath while getting dressed and reaching for items. She is no longer able to transfer into the shower, so she must sponge bathe. This has been accompanied by easy fatigue. Self-imposed rest periods during such activities have resulted in complete resolution of the shortness of breath. She denies associated cough, wheezing, or tightness in chest. She does not experience SOB when lying flat. She describes generalized weakness. Information is gathered from direct patient interview.

Medications: Lisinopril 20 milligrams once daily, omeprazole 20 milligrams once daily, aspirin 81 milligrams once daily, ibuprofen 400 milligrams twice daily, and q6h as needed (prn), Advair Diskus 100/50 one inhalation twice daily, tiotropium 18 micrograms two inhalations once daily, and albuterol 90 micrograms one inhalation q4h prn.

Allergies: Penicillin.

Habits: 50 pack-year smoking; quit 3 years ago. ETOH: Never used.

Past medical history: Hypertension (HTN), chronic diastolic heart failure, gastroesophageal reflux disease (GERD), chronic obstructive pulmonary disease (COPD), chronic kidney disease stage 2 (CKD), and osteoarthritis.

Past surgical history: Appendectomy, age 12; cholecystectomy, age 54.

Family history: Mother died age 78 with breast cancer, cerebrovascular accident (CVA), HTN. Father died age 72 with colon cancer, HTN.

Personal and social history: Retired leather factory worker for 47 years; widowed 5 years, no children, lives alone in elderly housing with elevator access.

Review of Systems

General: Positive for weight loss of 8 pounds in 6 months; denies fever, chills, or sweats.

Skin: Occasional pruritus; denies lesions or rashes; positive for dry skin.

Head, eyes, ears, nose, and throat (HEENT): No dizziness, headache, visual changes, hearing loss, nasal congestion, or sore throat.

Neck: No swollen glands; positive for neck pain with lateral rotation, relieved with ibuprofen, which she has been using for "years."

Breasts: Denies knowledge of changes in appearance; does not perform self-examination.

Respiratory: See history of present illness. Denies SOB at rest, recent infection or sputum production.

Cardiovascular: Positive for occasional palpitations. Denies chest pain, paroxysmal nocturnal dyspnea (PND), or orthopnea.

Gastrointestinal: Has been taking omeprazole for "years." Denies dysphagia, dyspepsia, nausea, or vomiting. Denies melena or black, tarry stools. Appetite has declined in 6 to 8 months,

199

and is now eating two small meals per day with crackers between meals. Moves bowels every other day, normal consistency.

Peripheral vascular: Positive for bilateral leg swelling daily in the late afternoon. Denies calf pain.

Urinary: Nocturia twice a night. Denies frequency, urgency, incontinence, or hematuria;

Genital: Denies vaginal bleeding.

Musculoskeletal: see "Neck." Positive for joint pain in hips, low back, knees, relieved with twice daily ibuprofen and occasional additional prn dose; positive for generalized muscular weakness.

Psychiatric: Denies difficulty falling to or maintaining sleep, feeling anxious, or depressed.

Neurologic: Denies seizures, tremors, poor balance, or concerns with memory; positive for occasional poor concentration and occasional paresthesias in feet.

Hematologic: Denies history of easy bruising, anemia, or blood transfusions.

Endocrine: Denies polydipsia, polyphagia, or polyuria, temperature intolerance, or sweating.

Physical Examination

General: Pale, thin-appearing female. Neatly groomed.

Vital signs: Height 60 inches, weight 98 pounds. Temperature 98.2°F, blood pressure134/72, pulse 88, respiratory rate 18, O_2 saturation 96%.

Skin: Scattered dry thin scales, no lesions.

HEENT: Normocephalic. Eyes: Without exudate or injection, acuity 20/40 without correction. Ears: Tympanic membranes (TMs) pearly, no cerumen or lesions, acuity intact. Nares: Patent, no exudates. Pharynx: Moist, no exudate or injection.

Neck: Limited range of motion (ROM) in all directions; no jugular venous distension, thyromegaly; no palpable lymph nodes.

Back: Kyphosis of thoracic spine; palpable tenderness at lumbosacral spine.

Lungs: Respirations even, relaxed; diminished lung sounds bilaterally; no adventitious sounds.

Cardiac: Regular rate rhythm, S1, S2, grade I/VI holosystolic murmur loudest in second intercostal space.

Breasts: Symmetrical bilaterally. Nipples everted bilaterally. No dimpling, retraction, peud'orange, form lesions, lymphadenopathy or nipple discharge bilaterally.

Abdomen: Nondistended, normoactive bowel sounds, soft, nontender, no hepatosplenomegaly or masses.

Extremities: Mild nonpitting edema bilaterally, pretibial to pedal.

Neurologic: Alert, oriented; speech articulate; three-item recall intact immediately and after 3 minutes; Cranial nerves (CN) II to XII intact; strength 3/5 in all extremities; sensation intact.

Assessment and Plan

1. Based on the history and physical examination results, what are the possible causes (differentials) for the patient's current condition?

Shortness of breath, easy fatigue, and weakness are common, nonspecific complaints among older adults who have multiple chronic comorbid medical conditions. This patient's diagnoses of COPD and chronic diastolic heart failure would raise initial concern for a possible acute exacerbation of either. The absence of additional supporting subjective symptoms and objective examination findings make this unlikely. The etiologies of edema in older adults are multifactorial and alone would not support a diagnosis of acute heart failure.

A decline in appetite and weight over several months points to a possible physiologic response to a potential additional underlying chronic illness, or gastrointestinal (GI) pathology. The patient's long history of tobacco use and occupational exposures, in addition to a strong family history of cancer, raise concern for occult malignant disease. Adverse medication effects on the GI tract in the older adult give rise to consideration for the risk of bleeding with ibuprofen. An increased effect of aspirin caused by its interaction with ibuprofen further increases this risk.[1] Prolonged use of omeprazole, particularly in older adults, may result in diminished vitamin B_{12} absorption with an eventual potential deficiency.[2] The presence of multiple chronic comorbidities supports consideration for coexisting anemia. CKD is associated with anemia of chronic inflammation. Low nutritional intake and paresthesias also point to anemia as high on the differential for the cause of this patient's current presentation.

2.   What components of the physical examination are missing?

Because of self-reported weight loss and decline in appetite, a nutrition screening tool such as the Modified Mini Nutritional Assessment Short Form (MNA) is important.[3] An oral examination to determine the condition of the teeth, gums, and tongue will reveal useful information about the ability to orally manage food, and for evidence of vitamin deficiencies, such as the presence of glossitis or angular cheilitis. Because the patient experiences arthritic pain, easy fatigue, and muscle weakness, a thorough musculoskeletal examination is necessary. To determine the impact of the patient's chronic comorbidities and current symptoms on functioning, the Katz Index of Independence in Activities of Daily Living (Katz ADL Index)[4] and the Timed Up and Go test (TUG) should be used.[5] In the neurologic examination, evaluate proprioception and the Romberg test due to the complaint of parathesias in her feet.

3.   What diagnostics are necessary for the patient at this time?

Initial laboratory evaluations should include a thyroid-stimulating hormone (TSH) and a complete blood count (CBC) to evaluate for anemia and hypothyroidism because of symptoms of SOB, fatigue, and weakness. A comprehensive metabolic panel is necessary. CKD is associated with anemia, and the adverse effects of ibuprofen use on kidney functioning in the older adult highlight the need to evaluate kidney functioning for progression in disease staging. Values will also be useful for appraisal of protein and liver function in the presence of weight loss and low appetite. A chest x-ray (CXR) is indicated because of the patient's subjective symptoms, weight loss, and long history of tobacco use. A family history of colon cancer and the use of ibuprofen and aspirin make the rectal examination essential to detect lesions and masses and to evaluate for fecal occult blood.

4.   What treatments would you recommend for this patient?

Priorities today include prevention of potential instability of the patient's chronic health conditions or functioning. While awaiting laboratory and CXR results, the patient's actual use of ibuprofen should be further evaluated to acquire an accurate appraisal of her total daily use. In the review of systems, she described a long duration of using 400 milligrams twice daily. The provider should inquire about specific use of prn doses and ask how often she is taking additional doses on a typical day and confirm the prn dose. An elaboration on her subjective pain report should be expanded with an in-depth pain assessment. For each site of her pain location, the provider should inquire about the intensity, character, frequency, patterns, aggravating factors, additional alleviating measures used, and the degree of effect on relief. Use of a standardized tool will aide in measuring the patient's pain intensity.[6]

Acetaminophen is recommended as the first-line pharmacologic choice for the management of pain and it is not linked with risks of GI bleeding risk or kidney toxicity.[7] The patient is therefore counseled to stop the ibuprofen and to begin acetaminophen. The recommended starting dose for acetaminophen ranges from 325 to 500 milligrams every 4 hours or 500 to 1000 milligrams every 6 hours. Based on her pain assessment and current chronic daily use of ibuprofen, she is counseled to begin with 500 milligrams twice daily and every 6 hours prn. She should not exceed the maximum daily dose of 4 g. If this patient were to have liver disease or a history of alcohol abuse, the maximum dose should be 50% to 75% lower.[7] Although the recommended daily dose of acetaminophen should not exceed 4 g, the concern for liver toxicity risk prompted the Food and Drug Administration (FDA) advisory committee to recommend that the total daily dose should be reduced to 3250 milligrams.[8] Many over-the-counter and prescribed products contain acetaminophen. It is important to regularly inquire about all medications that she is taking, and to educate her of this. If her total daily dosage reaches 4 g, she must be counseled to avoid all additional medications containing acetaminophen.

It is important to consider the benefit against the risk of preventive aspirin use in this woman over age 80. The US Preventive Services Task Force deems the evidence insufficient for its preventive use in older age.[9] The decision to stop aspirin in all older adults should be individualized according to the indication for its use. Considering this patient's GI bleeding as a potential cause of her symptoms, it would be prudent to advise her to stop the aspirin at this time.

The MNA score today of 7 indicates malnutrition, and the patient's Katz ADL and TUG scores show some mild limitations in functioning and endurance. She agrees to a referral for home health services through the local Visiting Nurse Association (VNA). This should include physical and occupational therapy evaluations, nursing for assessment of symptom changes, and education on today's medication changes. A referral to a dietician is recommended for further nutritional assessment and education. If her local VNA does not have a consulting dietician on staff, a referral will be made to her local hospital outpatient services.

The patient will return to the office in 2 weeks for a reevaluation of symptoms and review of laboratory and CXR results.

Case Study, Continued

Two weeks later the patient returns to the office. She is adhering to the prescribed medication changes, and VNA services have been implemented. She describes symptoms as unchanged from the previous visit. Laboratory and CXR results are reviewed (Table 9.1).

TABLE 9.1 ■ Laboratory and Chest X-Ray Results

Hgb	10.2
Hct	30
MCV	89
Platelets	289,000
RDW-CV	14.9
TSH	2.88
BUN	20
Creatinine	0.9
eGFR	60
Albumin	3.0
Blood pressure sitting	128/72
Blood pressure standing	120/68

BUN, Blood, urea, nitrogen; *eGFR,* estimated glomerular filtration rate; *Hct,* hematocrit; *Hgb,* hemoglobin; *MCV,* mean corpuscular volume; *RDW-CV,* red blood cell distribution width; *TSH,* thyroid-stimulating hormone.
Liver function tests, glucose, and electrolytes are normal.
Chest x-ray: Low, flat diaphragm and mild blunting of costophrenic angles, consistent with chronic obstructive pulmonary disease.
Fecal occult blood: 2 out of 3 samples positive

5.   What are your next steps?

The low hemoglobin (Hgb) and hematocrit (Hct) and normal MCV suggest that the patient has normocytic anemia. The CKD remains stable at stage 2. The albumin of 3.0 coincides with malnutrition. It is now necessary to determine which type of anemia she has and then to consider underlying causes. The evaluation can be challenging, and it is not uncommon for the older adult to have more than one cause in the presence of multiple chronic comorbidities. The lack of microcytosis does not exclude blood loss anemia. If the blood loss is not chronic, cellular changes may not have yet manifested. Additional laboratory evaluations are necessary and should include a serum iron profile, ferritin, vitamin B_{12}, folate levels, and a reticulocyte count. The patient should return in 10 to 14 days for a review of findings (Table 9.2).

The laboratory findings reveal that the patient has an iron-deficiency anemia with a coexisting low vitamin B_{12} level. The low iron, ferritin, and transferrin saturations with a high total iron-biding capacity (TIBC), reflective of low iron stores, and an occult positive stool indicate blood loss anemia.

Although a gold standard evaluation is currently lacking in defining B_{12} deficiency, the patient's low level in the presence of self-reported paresthesias dictates further testing to evaluate for pernicious anemia (PA). At the next visit, her blood will be drawn to test for antiintrinsic factor antibodies (anti-IFAB).[10] A positive result will indicate a high likelihood of PA.

6.   What are your priorities for the next visit?

The goals of anemia treatment are to promote optimal health and functioning while preventing deterioration of the patient's health conditions. Treatment with oral iron and vitamin B_{12} should begin. An iron tablet containing a lower elemental dosage of 15 to 20 milligrams offers similar efficacy and is better tolerated with respect to the potential GI side effects of nausea or constipation than with higher doses. She is advised to take ferrous sulfate 325 milligrams daily. Taking this with a vitamin C source, such as orange juice, will enhance its absorption.

While awaiting results of the anti-IFAB testing, the patient is advised to start oral vitamin B_{12} replacement. An oral daily dose of 1000 micrograms will generally provide adequate vitamin B_{12} absorption. Oral replacement is considered as effective as intramuscular (IM) replacement in this patient with a low vitamin B_{12} level; however, if her level was severely low, or in confirmed PA, initial IM replacement would be necessary.[10] Oral tablets of both ferrous sulfate and vitamin B_{12} are purchased over the counter, and she will begin taking these daily.

It is important to determine the underlying cause of this patient's GI blood loss. A patient-centered discussion should include an overview of individual goals to determine how aggressive the evaluation and subsequent treatments should be. She is enjoying her existing social and functional lifestyle, and given her family and medical history, the patient agrees to a gastroenterology referral for further diagnostic testing. The patient subsequently undergoes an endoscopy and colonoscopy. The endoscopy shows normal findings, and several intestinal adenomatous polyps are removed during the colonoscopy. Mild diverticular disease is also identified.

TABLE 9.2 ■ Additional Laboratory Evaluations, Results

Serum iron	34
Total iron-binding capacity	420
Ferritin	14
Transferrin saturation	20%
Vitamin B_{12}	144
Folate	24.2
Reticulocyte count	0.85%

TABLE 9.3 ■ Three Month Visit Results

Hgb	11.2
Hct	34
MCV	91
Platelets	294,000
RDW-CV	14.0
Reticulocyte count	1.8%
Ferritin	146
B_{12}	300

Hct, Hematocrit; *Hgb,* hemoglobin; *MCV,* mean corpuscular volume; *RDW-CV,* red blood cell distribution width; *TSH,* thyroid-stimulating hormone.
Stool for occult blood in the office is negative.

Omeprazole should be discontinued, based on the absence of symptoms, a normal endoscopy, and its effect on vitamin B_{12} absorption. The patient should remain on acetaminophen for pain management. Ongoing VNA services should continue until individual functional goals are achieved.

An increase in the Hgb should be seen after 2 to 3 weeks of iron initiation, and the Hct improves after several weeks of vitamin B_{12} replacement. A rise is seen in the reticulocyte count in the first week of starting both the iron and the vitamin B_{12}.[10,11] Based on these expected improvements, a CBC, reticulocyte count, ferritin, and B_{12} level will be reevaluated in 1 month.[11,12]

She will return in 3 months for her scheduled initial comprehensive visit.

Case Study, Continued

Ten days later you receive the results of the anti–IFAB testing, which is negative for PA.

You contact the patient by phone to explain the results. She is adhering to the prescribed daily oral vitamin B_{12} and you advise her to continue with this.

Three months later the patient is experiencing improved activity tolerance and her appetite and nutritional intake have improved (Table 9.3).

The patient's Hgb and Hct have improved, and the normal ferritin reflects increased iron stores. She is advised to continue the ferrous sulfate for three more months,[12] at which time a CBC, ferritin, and reticulocyte count will be reevaluated. The vitamin B_{12} value has improved, and she should also continue with daily vitamin B_{12} and have the level reevaluated in 3 months.[10]

The removal of colonic polyps has arrested the source of GI blood loss.

A patient-centered discussion should continue relevant to prevention and future diagnostic testing and management. The presence of multiple chronic comorbidities in older age as they relate to anemia, whether the anemia is of blood loss, chronic inflammation, or chronic disease, or of malnutrition, require that ongoing monitoring of hematologic and renal laboratory values occurs. The patient should be seen at regular intervals for health surveillance. She may require future specialist referrals such as gastroenterology, nephrology, or hematology as part of the comprehensive management plan.

References

1. Lexi-Drugs, Ibuprofen. Lexi-Comp, Inc. Version 2.40, updated August 15, 2016.
2. Drugs for peptic ulcer disease and GERD. (2014). *Treatment Guidelines From the Medical Letter, 12*(140), 25–26.

3. Kaiser, M. J., Bauer, J. M., Uter, W., Donini, L. M., Stange, I., Volkert, D., et al. (2011). Prospective validation of the modified mini nutritional assessment short-forms in the community, nursing home, and rehabilitation setting. *Journal of the American Geriatrics Society, 59*(11), 2124–2128.

4. Kresevic, D. M. (2012). Assessment of physical function. In M. Boltz, E. Capezuti, T. T. Fulmer, & D. Zwicker (Eds.), *Evidence-based geriatric nursing protocols for best practice* (pp. 89–103). New York: Springer Publishing Company.

5. Podsiadlo, D., & Richardson, S. (1991). The "Timed Up and GO": A test of basic functional mobility for frail elderly persons. *Journal of the American Geriatrics Society, 39*(2), 142–148.

6. Flaherty, E. (2012). Pain assessment for older adults. In *Hartford Institute for Geriatric Nursing*. Retrieved from http://consultgerirn.org.

7. American Geriatrics Society Panel on the Pharmacological Management of Persistent Pain in Older Persons. (2009). Pharmacologic management of persistent pain on older persons. *Journal of the American Podiatric Medical Association, 57*(8), 1331–1346.

8. Krenzelok, E., & Royal, M. (2012). Confusion: Acetaminophen dosing changes based on no evidence in adults. *Drugs in R and D, 12*(2), 45–48.

9. Final Update Summary. (2017). Aspirin for the Prevention of Cardiovascular Disease: Preventive Medication. Retrieved from www.uspreventiveservicestaskforce.org.

10. Vinod, D., Hamilton, M. S., & Molloy, N. M. (2014). Guidelines for the diagnosis and treatment of cobalamin and folate disorders. *British Journal of Haematology, 166*, 496–513.

11. Johnson-Wimbley, T. D., & Graham, D. Y. (2011). Diagnosis and management of iron deficiency anemia in the 21st century. *Therapeutic Advances in Gastroenterology, 4*(3), 177–184.

12. Langan, R. C., & Zawistoski, K. J. (2011). Update on vitamin B12 deficiency. *American Family Physician, 83*(12), 1425–1430.

Agoraphobia

Patricia White

Case Study Scenario/History of Present Illness

A call is received from a local home care agency requesting the services of a health care provider who can provide primary care for homebound patients. The patient, Ms. W, is an 82-year-old white female discharged last week from a local hospital in which she was evaluated in the geriatric psychiatric unit for increasing agitation and altered mental status. The local council of aging and the local mental health center are both requesting a home visit because the patient is in need of a provider who makes home visits; otherwise this patient has no access to primary care. The patient has been homebound for the past 5 years because of her agoraphobia and anxiety. It is possible that she has not had any primary care over that time period, and her previous psychiatric provider is no longer available to do home visits. Consideration for a short-term placement in a local rehabilitation setting was rejected by the patient; she was adamant that she wanted to remain at home. She also reiterated that while she had had a challenging life, she was very proud of owning her own home and wanted to remain there as long as possible. The hospital providers decided to make recommendations for a home-based primary care (HBPC) referral and a possible visiting nurse agency (VNA) referral when her hospital discharged was planned. A call is made to the patient who has agreed to have a health care provider do home visit. A one-page discharge summary from the geriatric psychiatric unit is faxed over and reviewed.

The patient was found by a caseworker from the local Council on Aging (COA) after neighbors reported that someone was crying out in the neighborhood. The neighbors then called local police who then contacted the COA to conduct a wellness evaluation. The patient was found by the COA representative to be agitated and confused. The patient was sent to the hospital, admitted, and subsequently treated for chronic anxiety, type 2 diabetes mellitus, panic disorder, and agoraphobia.

- Hospital diagnostics revealed:
  - A computed tomography (CT) of the head and magnetic resonance imaging (MRI) were both negative for masses, intracranial bleeds, or infectious processes. An electroencephalogram (EEG) showed no seizure activity.
  - A full drug screen panel was negative for substances.
  - Chest x-ray was negative for infiltrates, masses, or pleural effusion.
  - An electrocardiogram revealed normal sinus rhythm with no acute changes. Troponins were negative.
  - A complete blood count (CBC), comprehensive metabolic panel (CMP), and thyroid studies were all within normal range. Other relevant laboratory results included an Hgb A1C of 7.5 on her current dose of metformin 1000 milligrams by mouth (po) twice a day. The patient was begun on quetiapine (Seroquel) 300 milligrams po twice a day with good effect.
- Hospital discharge statements:
  - The patient's agitation improved and cognitively she returned to baseline by the end of the admission. She had previously been on as needed (prn) clonazepam (Klonopin) and this medication was continued. On discharge the patient was advised to take Klonopin, 1 milligram po three times a day and quetiapine (Seroquel) 300 milligrams po twice a day.

- Psychiatry recommends a home-based evaluation by a psychiatric nurse practitioner (NP). Additionally, a referral to the Elder Protective Services was made for issues related to self-neglect, and they will see her after discharge.
- Discharge Medications
  - Clonazepam 0.5 milligrams po three times a day
  - Quetiapine 300 milligrams po twice a day
  - Metformin 1000 milligrams po twice a day

Allergies: No known drug allergies (NKDA).The NP calls the patient to schedule a visit and is told by the patient that it could not be this week because the VNA nurse was coming tomorrow and it would be "too much" to have lots of people coming in and out of her home. She does agree to a visit the following week. In the interim, the NP had time to talk to the local Elder Service agency for some additional background information about Ms. W. The NP was able to learn more about Ms. W at the first home visit and was able to illicit the subsequent information.

Past medical history: Hypertension, type 2 diabetes mellitus (DM II), depressive disorder, agoraphobia, and panic disorder.

Surgical history: None.

Immunizations/screenings: Patient has previously refused mammograms, colonoscopy, or any adult immunizations.

Family history: Unknown because of long-term estrangement.

Personal and social history: Patient is a retired office executive assistant who became disabled at the age of 54 because of chronic anxiety, depression, and agoraphobia. She previously reported a long history of childhood physical and sexual abuse and a 10-year marriage also characterized by physical and emotional abuse. She has two adult children of whom she relinquished custody when they were young adolescents. She receives Social Security Disability and a small pension. She does own her own home and is supported by a local church whose members assist with tax payments. She has no mortgage on her property.

Review of Systems

General: Does not feel well, reports overall fatigue and loneliness, but denies fever and chills.

Skin: Denies rashes or lesions.

HEENT: No allergies. Denies rhinitis. Denies previous history of head injury, headache, sinus pain, and dizziness.

Neck: Denies swollen glands, lumps.

Respiratory: Denies cough, wheeze, and shortness of breath.

Cardiac: Denies chest pain, palpitations, and dyspnea on exertion (DOE).

Gastrointestinal: Admits to + weight loss. Denies constipation, diarrhea, nausea, or vomiting.

Urinary: Denies frequency, dysuria, or hematuria.

Peripheral vascular: Denies swollen legs, calf pain.

Musculoskeletal: Denies pain, tenderness, or swelling in joints.

Psychiatric: Anxious, reports difficulty sleeping.

Neurologic: Denies seizures, tremor, arm/leg weakness, difficulty speaking, or swallowing.

Hematologic: Denies bruising, but reports she did have blood transfusions in the past.

Endocrine: Denies temperature intolerance, sweating, or thirst.

Functional Status

Activity: Patient says that she is able to ambulate around her apartment without assistive devices. She states that she has stairs that she climbs to use the only bathroom on the second floor.

Activities of daily living (ADLs): She reports that she is able to manage her hygiene and bathes self in the bathroom once a day. She does note that she gets "winded" at times walking around her apartment.

Nutrition: Patient reports that she eats independently without dysphagia and reports that she is disinterested in meal preparation and gets takeout food from local restaurants. She also reports that her previous case worker bought prepared foods at the local supermarket and brought them to her.

Independent activities of daily living (IADLs): Ms. W reports she is dependent in all IADLs and receives support from the local COA and case worker from the local mental health center for support with bill paying, shopping, and errands. A case worker also assists with negotiating payment plans with local utilities because she often is late with bills. Her current income from social security is adequate for her expenses; however, she admits to being disorganized with recordkeeping and timely bill paying. Also, when taxes were raised last year, she was not able to meet that additional expense and her case worker was able to find a local church organization to provide some supplemental income. She states that keeping her home is very important to her because that has been an important accomplishment in her adult life.

Sleep: She sleeps on her couch every evening. Reports restless sleep and reports that she naps frequently during the day.

Relationships/roles: Patient reports that she has had a long-time estrangement from her children. She says she is still grieving the loss of them in her life and prays for them daily. She describes having work colleagues whose company she enjoyed during her work years; however, she has not maintained those relationships since she left work.

She also reports that her brother also is important to her; however, he lives out of state. She speaks of their stressful childhood in which they were both victimized by their parents. She says that they have not been able to maintain a close bond. She writes letters to him monthly, but he has not responded to her.

She also relates her regret about staying in an abusive marriage and feels she should have protected her children more. In spite of the history of childhood and spousal abuse, she does describe a community of nuns who she speaks to every Sunday evening. She states that they provide spiritual support to her and that they speak to her of "God's mercy and forgiveness," which she feels she needs. She states that this connection, along with the support of case workers from the community, has helped assist her with the challenges of feeling isolated and alone. She reports that she would be grateful for more personal connections with people; however, her anxiety and overall weakness contribute to her fear of being outside and socializing with groups of people.

Physical Examination

Ms. W did allow a brief physical examination and vital signs, although stated she "doesn't like to be touched."

General: Pale, frail-appearing female. + anxious affect, unkempt, clothing in disrepair, urine odor evident.

Vital signs: Height 64 inches, weight 122 pounds (previous recorded weight 3 years earlier 140 pounds). Blood pressure 138/76, heart rate 84, O_2 saturation 98%.

Skin: No obvious lesions.

Eyes: Sclera clear, no drainage.

Ears: Tympanic membranes obscured with scant cerumen bilaterally.

Mouth: Dry mucous membranes, multiple dental caries.

Neck: Supple, no lymphadenopathy. Thyroid nonpalpable.

Respiratory: Lungs clear to auscultation, without rales, wheezes, or rhonchi. Respiratory rate 12, nonlabored.

Cardiac: Regular rate, no murmurs, rubs, or gallops.
Abdomen: Occasional bowel sounds, soft, nondistended.
Extremities: No edema.
Musculoskeletal: Gait slightly unsteady, no use of assistive devices.
Neurologic: Speech fluent, cranial nerves (CNs) II to XII grossly intact, Romberg negative, no pronator drift.

Assessment and Plan

1. What should be the priorities for Ms. W's care at this time?

It is important to establish a rapport with the patient that communicates trust and support to develop a therapeutic relationship. A comprehensive assessment of this long-time homebound woman with chronic mental illness can be performed over time to establish mutually agreed-on goals and priorities as the relationship evolves. Understanding the interplay between her medical and psychiatric conditions will be necessary to identify what interventions, strategies, and supports are necessary.[1]

According to the American Association of Retired Persons (AARP), researchers in the United States estimate that approximately 21.3% of American adults over age 50 are living with mental illness, which ranks within the top five chronic health conditions experienced by this population. This number does not include dementia or substance use disorders. Differences exist across racial and ethnic groups reporting mental illness among adults aged 50 and over, with 23.4% of whites, 16.4% of Hispanics, 14.7% who identify as other, and 12.7% of blacks over 50 reporting mental illness.[2]

Self-harm, anxiety, and substance use disorders are significant mental and behavioral health issues among aging adults, with approximately 25% of deaths in persons over 60 worldwide attributed to self-harm; 3.8% of older adults worldwide reporting anxiety disorders; and approximately 1% of older adults worldwide reporting substance use problems. According to the World Health Organization (WHO), the numbers of older adults living with mental illness in 2016 is higher than what is reflected in this data, taking into account the likelihood of under self-reporting among this group, the tendency of health care providers to fail to recognize these issues among older adults, and the existence of stigma around mental health issues for the elderly.[3]

It is also essential to determine the community supports that have been in place for this patient and learn who is performing specific roles in providing ongoing care to this woman. In particular, it is important to assess the current status of her long-term mental health issue of panic disorder and agoraphobia given how often anxiety and depression are overlooked and undertreated.

Her long history of DM II needs continued follow-up and monitoring of her glycemic status. Plans for her ongoing pharmacologic and dietary management are important, particularly because of her recent weight loss.

The shortness of breath and sleeping problems need further evaluation. Also, continued discussion of appropriate screenings and immunizations as they relate to the patient's goals of care will need to take place.

2. What components of the history or physical examination are missing?

Determining whether Ms. W is taking any herbals or over-the-counter medications is an important component of her history.

Additional components of the physical examination should focus on evaluation of gait and overall strength given her long history of being homebound. The Timed Get Up and Go test (TUG) may be helpful in further assessing the need for assistive devices and home-based exercises for overall strengthening.[4]

A more in-depth cognitive assessment such as the Montreal Cognitive Assessment (MoCA) is an important consideration because of the incident that precipitated her hospitalization. It is unclear if this was conducted during her hospitalization.[5]

Additional screening for depression and anxiety are also indicated given her past history of agoraphobia and trauma. The Geriatric Anxiety Scale (GAS)[6] and the Geriatric Depression Scale (GDS)[7] should be conducted to establish a current baseline now that the patient has returned home.

3. What diagnostics are necessary for this patient at this time?

A review of the discharge summary indicated that no new laboratory diagnostics were needed at this time.

It would also be helpful to obtain more information regarding her medication use/adherence by calling the pharmacy to obtain her prescription refill history and to see if there are other health care providers prescribing medications for Ms. W.

More information is obtained from the local VNA who also made a visit to evaluate Ms. W:

- A home health aide (HHA) referral was made to assist with bathing and assistance with attending to her overall hygiene and dressing.
- Homemaking assistance was secured, and the patient also agreed to medication management.
- A nutritional evaluation was conducted and revealed that the patient relied mostly on takeout delivery from a local fast-food restaurant and ate prepared foods that the previous case worker bought at the local grocery store. Although reimbursement for a Registered Dietician (RD) is not covered by Medicare, the VNA had recently obtained pilot grant funding for RD consultations, so a referral was made.
- A TUG test was conducted. The results revealed that she was deconditioned and at risk for falls and that it took additional time for her to transfer from chair to standing. A physical therapy evaluation was then recommended and was conducted within a week of the referral. Chair exercises with light weights to attempt to enhance her overall strength were discussed as important goals. Gait evaluation revealed that her weakness contributed to balance issues, and it was hoped that chair exercises would assist with balance and coordination. No assistive devices were recommended at this time.
- Her MoCA test revealed a score of 25/30 indicating short-term memory issues. This information was shared with the psychiatric NP who replied that she would perform additional neurologic, psychiatric, and cognitive testing as part of her evaluation. Although the MoCA evaluation identified these issues, her overall mental status evaluation demonstrated remarkable insight into her mental health history and the reasons she is so anxious. Overall evaluation also demonstrates her strong determination to remain at home in spite of her homebound status, inability to manage IADLs, and financial challenges in maintaining and financially affording her home.
- Results of her GDS were greater than 10, indicating depression. Results of her GAS indicated high levels of anxiety, especially in the somatic and affective categories. The HBPC provider communicated these results to the psychiatric NP who is scheduled to see the patient in 2 weeks.

4. What should be considered for this patient's plan of care?

Unless future evaluation of her laboratory results indicates a change in therapy, the subsequent assessment and plan of care will be considered.

- Type 2 DM: Will continue to ensure her adherence to the metformin and do a complete nutritional assessment including review of weekly shopping and food choices.
- Agoraphobia/panic disorder: Will review her current use of Klonopin and Seroquel and the effectiveness of these medications. Given her scores on the GDS and GAS, she may require

further pharmacologic treatment in the future. Ms. W did agree to help with medication management, but consideration will also have to be made about having medications administered by professional staff to ensure medication adherence if this identified as an issue.

5.   What are the advantages of a team model of care?

A recent study by Karlin and Karel (2014) examined HBPC programs that served geriatric patients who received care for mental illness from the Veteran's Administration (VA). This type of care includes comprehensive, long-term services for older adult veterans, generally age 75 and older, who are experiencing a range of physical, mental, and behavioral health conditions. HBPC programs take an interdisciplinary care team approach, which includes nurses, social workers, and other health care professionals who work to develop patient-centered plans for addressing the integrated medical and mental health needs of patients and their family caregivers in the home setting.

Karlin and Karel looked at recent changes to the HBPC model, which included integrating mental health care providers into HBPC sites across the United States. Survey results showed that social workers and nurses requested mental health provider referrals at the highest frequency (social workers at 93%, nurses at 89%, and 67% advanced practice nurses). In addition, social workers and nurse visits with patients included universal or standard screenings for mental health issues including dementia, substance use, depression, posttraumatic stress disorder, caregiver stress, and other mental health concerns. Overall results showed potential for further care integration among mental health needs and services with the routine and specialized care received by older VA adult patients. In addition, researchers believe that integrated HBPC programs could serve as a model for home-based care among other older adult patient populations.[8]

FOLLOW-UP: ONE MONTH

The NP in the HBPC program visits Ms. W at her home in 1 month. The patient has also been seen by the practice's psychiatric NP, who recommended adding fluoxetine (Prozac) 10 milligrams po daily to Ms. W's medication regimen in accordance with the current recommendations for the treatment of her anxiety and depressive disorders.

Today, the patient is quite talkative and goes into great detail when answering questions about her health status.

Nutrition: The patient reports that she is struggling to eat a more nutritious diet; however, she is trying to incorporate foods such as fresh vegetables and fruit. She mentions that she does not really have a taste for fresh food because she has previously relied on fast-food takeout and prefers the taste of fast food. She currently denies any signs/symptoms of hyperglycemia or hypoglycemia. She also reports that she is not certain she is taking her medication for diabetes because there are so many new people in and out of her house. Although she realizes that this additional support will eventually assist her, she is worried that there are too many people involved and wants her privacy.

Agoraphobia/anxiety/depressive disorder/panic: Ms. W states she is grateful for the additional support, but also says, "So many people coming and going." She is still anxious about all the changes in her household. She reports that she is enjoying getting to know the nurse case manager who is working with her. The case manager comes frequently to ensure accurate medication administration and the overall monitoring of both Ms. W's health status and the health care team. Ms. W also reports that even with all the changes of adjusting to the home care team, she feels better. She even reports that she is sleeping more restfully, but she adds she is still nervous. She denies any current panic attacks, worsening anxiety, or suicidal ideation.

Activity/exercise: The patient tells the NP that she is feeling a little stronger with physical therapists coming to the house. She is worried about walking around the house and yard more often but hopes to be more confident as long as someone is with her when she walks. She has not walked in years but knows that this activity will be good for her. She is trying to remember to use a cane when walking around the house, and when she does remember thinks it helps her feel more confident when she walks.

ADLs: Although she does not like having someone help her showering, Ms. W admits that she feels cleaner now that the HHA is with her for showers. She also reports being able to manage her toileting more effectively because she has more strength in getting on and off the toilet.

Relevant Physical Examination

General: Pale, frail-appearing female, no malodorous odors noted. Wearing clean clothes.

Vital signs: Height 125 lbs. Blood pressure 138/72, heart rate 60, O_2 saturation 98%.

Skin: No rash or lesions.

Eyes: Clear, no crusting or discharge.

Ears: Tympanic membranes obscured with scant cerumen bilaterally.

Mouth: Mucous membranes fairly moist, multiple dental caries, but no lesions tongue or mucosa.

Neck: Supple, no lymphadenopathy or thyroid tenderness.

Respiratory: Lungs clear. No rales, wheezes, rhonchi, or obvious distress.

Cardiac: Regular rhythm and rate. No murmurs, rubs, or gallops.

Abdomen: Soft, nondistended, occasional bowel sounds.

Extremities: Pulses present. No edema or calf tenderness.

Musculoskeletal: Gait fairly steady with use of cane.

Neurologic: Alert, appropriate. No fasciculations or tremor.

Psychiatric: Alert, pressured speech, coherent thought processes, thought content related to her new registered nurse case manager and her appreciation for additional assistance with her personal hygiene. No observed agitation, restlessness, or depressive symptoms.

6.   What should the health care provider's assessment and plan be for this patient's current mental health and other problems?

Agoraphobia/anxiety/depressive disorder/panic: In addition to adding Prozac, all of the members of her team are focused on establishing ongoing trusting relationships with the patient who has suffered multiple losses and has been victimized in past relationship violence. A trusting relationship can have a significant impact on homebound patients' well-being and reinforces the importance of maintaining consistency in developing the ongoing relationships with vulnerable patients.[9] Her symptoms of anxiety do seem to be subsiding slightly with the additional home care support. However, the health care team's assessment determined that it was inconsistent medication adherence that contributed to Ms. W's hospitalization. The supervised medication administration will be continued, and her symptoms of anxiety seem to be subsiding slightly with additional home care.

Type 2 DM: The provider will wait 3 months before reevaluating Ms. W's Hgb A1C, electrolytes, and renal status of the Hgb A1C. Efforts to improve Ms. W's nutritional status with the RD's suggestions will be continued.

Functional Status

Activity/exercise: Patient's overall strength has improved with patient performing the recommended physical therapy exercises. She is walking more in her home, and her HHA accompanies her on walks around her yard and neighborhood.

ADLs: Patient's hygiene has improved because she is now able to bathe and shower with HHA assistance in her upstairs bathroom. Three-month follow-up from initial visit: The patient is seen in her home and her Hgb A1C is now 7.2. Her care is now being provided under a Senior Care Option (SCO) program in which she has enrolled. She continues to receive RN, HHA, and homemaker visits.

Type 2 DM: Patient reports that her appetite is improving. She is eating more nutritious foods and feels she is doing better taking her medications. The patient reports the RN case manager manages her medications and she takes them.

Agoraphobia/anxiety/depressive disorder/panic: Ms. W has not had a panic attack for some time now, and she has more "peace of mind" now that the RN is administering her new medications. RN reports that Ms. W is taking her medications with her supervision. Ms. W states she has enjoyed speaking to the psychiatric NP, but wants only to think about the good memories of her life with her children. She states she knows she will probably never see them again, but enjoys thinking about them as children. She requests that the psychiatric NP be available if she needs her but only wants to speak to her home care team and her community of nuns over the phone. She denies worsening anxiety, panic episodes, or agitation.

Sleep: The patient says she is sleeping a bit better.

ADLs and IADLs: The patient reports that her bills are being paid on time with the help of the case worker. The Office of Elder Affairs protective service division is involved and is speaking to the case worker regularly about Ms. W's ongoing needs and support. The household is less cluttered and there are no extension cords on the floors.

Relevant Physical Examination

Vital signs: Weight 125 lbs. Blood pressure 112/68, heart rate 70.
Cardiac: S1, S2, regular rate and rhythm.
Lungs: Clear to auscultation and percussion, respiratory rate 12, nonlabored.
Musculoskeletal: Gait steady with use of walker.
Psychiatric: Alert, conversant, thought content related to her children and the new HHA that is assisting her daily. No observed agitation, restlessness.

Assessment/Plan

Type 2 DM: Small improvements in nutritional status and more consistent medication administration of metformin are resulting in improved glycemic control. Will continue metformin at 1000 milligrams po twice daily and encourage lifestyle efforts with the support of the HHA and home care team. Her HgbA1C and renal function will be checked every three months along with a yearly microalbumin.

Agoraphobia/anxiety/depressive disorder/panic: Patient's affect is less anxious with the addition of fluoxetine. Patient is also responding to the supportive home care team and consistent medication administration.

Functional Status: Overall functional status continues to improve with noted increased activity, steadier gait, and improved sleep. Will continue to encourage home-based exercise regimen and increased walking.

Six-month evaluation: The HBPC provider receives a call from the RN case manager who reports that Ms. W had a fall last evening and refused to go the emergency room. The nurse reports that the patient states she tripped over a cord on the floor, fell on her left arm, and there is an ecchymotic area over her olecranon process. The patient has full range of motion (ROM) in that joint; otherwise the patient seems fine with no other reported area of injury.

7. Based on the previously mentioned phone call, what should the priorities be in planning for Ms. W's ongoing evaluation? What additional physical examination is needed?

A home visit is planned for a post-fall assessment and includes a review of the fall history and a review of systems and physical examination that emphasizes evaluation of the skin and musculoskeletal function. Except for the contusion described during the phone call, the health care provider determines that Ms. W's examination is without significant findings and her overall functional status is at baseline.

8. What other diagnostics could the health care provider consider in the evaluation of this patient after a fall?

Diagnostics would depend on the patient's review of systems and the provider's examination. Postural vital signs should be done. If weakness, dizziness, or presyncope was the cause of the fall, a CBC, chemistry profile, and/or urinalysis could be considered, because anemia, an electrolyte abnormality (e.g., hyponatremia), dehydration, or urinary tract infection could be a potential cause of the fall. If the physical examination suggested a fracture, an x-ray would be appropriate.

9. What should the health care provider's plan of care be now that that Ms. W suffered a community-based fall?

A 2014 article by Marks highlights the current evidence that supports a comprehensive approach to preventing falls in older adults. Removal of Ms. W's psychiatric medications is not clinically appropriate although understandable because clonazepam is associated with falls. It is important to continue to individualize her overall care and continue with home-based exercises, careful attention to her environment with taping of cords that cannot be removed, and continued management of her current chronic health problems.[10]

ONE-YEAR FOLLOW-UP

Type 2 DM: Patient reports that she has acquired more taste for fresh foods and is eating more fruits and vegetables. States she is consistently taking metformin. Denies any symptoms of hypoglycemia.

Agoraphobia/anxiety/depressive disorder/panic disorder: Doing well and continues with the same medication regimen. Medications continue to be administered by the RN home-based case manager. No reports of any episodes of panic in the past 11 months.

Functional status/exercise/activity: She continues to work with physical therapy with chair exercises for strength. Still nervous at times. Denies falls.

Nutrition: Feeling more energetic. Uses microwave more to heat prepared foods. Snacking more on vegetables and selected fruits. She reports great pride in her current weight of 132 pounds and states she feels more comfortable at that weight.

IADLs: Home-based care with daily RN medication administration and monitoring of her overall health status with stabilization of her chronic mental illness. She also reports that twice weekly HHA support and homemaking has helped her. Her hygiene is improved and her home is less cluttered.

Sleep: Continued anxiety at times. Sleep patterns have improved. She now sleeps in her upstairs bedroom and is more comfortable. She is napping less frequently and reports less fatigue over the past year.

Roles/relationships: Patient still longs for more family connection, but is considering going to a local day program for older adults. Enjoys her ongoing Sunday evening calls from the nuns and has arranged to speak to them more during the week. She continues to write to her brother, which still brings her comfort, but is realistic about the chance of reconnecting. She prays with the nuns weekly to come to more peaceful acceptance of this relationship. She knows that the psychiatric NP is available for counseling; however, she feels that her current coping mechanisms with her supportive care team and the prayers with the nuns are sufficient for the present time.

Relevant Physical Examination
Vital signs: Weight 132 pounds, blood pressure 118/72, O_2 saturation 98%.
The remainder of the physical examination is unremarkable.
HgbA1C 5.7
Sodium: 138 (136–145 mmol/L)
Potassium: 3.7 (3.4–5.1 mmol/L)
Chloride: 98 (98–107 mmol/L)
Carbon dioxide: 25 (22–32 mmol/L)
BUN: 32 H (5–23 milligrams/dL)
Creatinine: 1.1 H (0.4–1.0 md/dL)
Glucose: 115 (74–118 milligrams/dL)

Assessment/Plan
Functional Status: Ongoing physical therapy for chair exercises for strength and overall conditioning have resulted in her being able to transfer with more balance and confidence. She also feels less fatigued and is able to participate with her HHA for assistance in bathing and showering.

DM II: A1C is now at 5.7, suggesting that her glycemic control is improving with consistent medication administration of metformin, weight loss, and improved nutritional status.

Hypertension: Patient remains normotensive and refuses antihypertensive medication at this time. There will be an ongoing recommendation for an angiotensin-converting enzyme inhibitor given her DM II; however, we will respect her choice at present. Will continue lifestyle efforts and congratulated her on her successes for improved nutrition, weight loss, and general increased activity.

Agoraphobia/anxiety: Since the addition of fluoxetine to her regimen, her panic attacks have decreased and she is better able to engage with her RN case manager and HHA. She is also responding to the consistency of the care team and is able to participate more in decisions about her overall self-care and plans for the future now that her anxiety disorder has been stabilized. Although she reports ongoing longing for her children and brother, she is open to the support of her care team and community supports and identifies her gratitude for everyone's assistance in maintaining her home and enhancing the quality of her life. The psychiatric NP continues to consult with the primary care NP to assess medication efficacy and is available for ongoing home visiting as needed.

In summary, intensive home-based care with daily RN medication administration and monitoring of her overall health status has resulted in the stabilization of her chronic mental illness and improved overall health and functional status. This patient continues to remain at home without any hospitalizations for the past year.

In addition, the patient has been able to review goals of care with a signed Massachusetts Medical Orders for Life Sustaining Treatment (MOLST) form on her refrigerator door. Ongoing HBPC in coordination with the case worker and support from community agencies continues.

The patient also has worked with an attorney from the COA to have the proceeds from her home sale go to a local women's shelter after her death, which she is very pleased about. She highlights that without this coordinated care and the stabilization of her chronic illnesses, she may not have been able to consider such a gesture. She remains grateful for the ongoing efforts of the integrated primary care and community-based approach to her well-being.

Ongoing coordination with the NP and RN case manager is an essential component of her care, which will continue to include at least monthly case management telephone calls, the securing of one pharmacy in which the pharmacist works collaboratively with the NP and RN, and NP home visits every 2 to 3 months or more frequently as needed. Ongoing psychiatric medication review by the psychiatric Advanced Practice Nurse and NP is done on at least a quarterly basis Elder Protective Services continue to remain involved and may consider discharging her as her home situation has stabilized with the appropriate services and support.

References

1. Antai-Otong, D. (2016). Caring for the patient with an anxiety disorder. *Nursing Clinics of North America*, 51(2), 173–183.
2. Lind, K. D., & Noel-Miller, C. (2011). Fact sheet 245. Chronic condition prevalence in the 50+ U.S. population. AARP Public Policy Institute. Retrieved from http://www.aarp.org/content/dam/aarp/research/public_policy_institute/health/chronic-conditionprevalence-50-plus-fact-sheet-AARP-ppi-health.pdf.
3. World Health Organization. (2016). Mental health and older adults fact sheet. Retrieved from http://www.who.int/mediacentre/factsheets/fs381/en/.
4. Mathias, S., Kayak, U., & Isaacs, B. (1986). Balance in elderly patients: The "get up and go" test. *Archives of Physical Medicine & Rehabilitation*, 67, 387–389.
5. Nasreddine, Z., Phillips, N., Bedirian, V., Charbonneau, S., Whitehead, V., Colin, I., et al. (2015). The Montreal cognitive assessment MoCA: A brief screening tool for mild cognitive impairment. *Journal of the American Geriatrics Society*, 53(4), 695–699.
6. Segal, D. L., June, A., Payne, M., Coolidge, F. L., & Yochim, B. (2010). Development and initial validation of a self-report assessment tool for anxiety among older adults: The geriatric anxiety scale. *Journal of Anxiety Disorders*, 24, 709–714.
7. Sheikh, J., & Yesavage, J. (1986). Geriatric Depression Scale (GDS): Recent evidence and development of a shorter version. *Clinical Gerontology*, 5, 165–173.
8. Karlin, B. E., & Karel, M. J. (2014). National integration of mental health providers in VA home-based primary care: An innovative model for mental health care delivery with older adults. *The Gerontologist*, 54(5), 868–879.
9. Haugan, G., Innstrand, S., & Moksnes, U. (2013). The effect of nurse–patient interaction on anxiety and depression in cognitively intact home patients. *Journal of Clinical Nursing*, 22, 2192–2205.
10. Marks, R. (2014). Falls among the elderly: Multi-factorial community-based falls prevention programs. *Journal of Aging Science*, 2(1): e109.

Joint Pain

Terry Mahan Buttaro

Case Study Scenario/History of Present Illness

A 67-year-old female presents to the office complaining of joint pain over the past week. She first noted a discomfort in her left arm and shoulder, but then in her right hip, quickly followed by pain in her left hip. Now the pain is constant and she cannot seem to get comfortable no matter what she does. She hurts so much that even at night she cannot get comfortable even though she tried "Tylenol and ibuprofen." She describes the pain as an aching that is worse with movement. When queried about how much pain she has on a scale of 1 to 10, she exclaims: "It is more than 20. I can barely move it hurts so much." She also describes feeling cold all the time but denies fever, chills, anyone else sick at home, recent travel, or known injury or illness. She has been taking ibuprofen 2 tablets by mouth every 4 to 6 hours, but the pain is not relieved.

Medications: Lisinopril 10 milligrams by mouth (po) daily, vitamin D 2000 IU po daily, calcium 600 milligrams po daily, and albuterol inhaler prn.

Allergies: No known drug allergies (NKDA).

Habits: Coffee 2 cups daily. Rare alcohol. Smokes five cigarettes a day and has for more than 30 years. Seatbelt always. Sunscreen always.

Past medical history: Asthma with any respiratory illness. Hospitalized with pneumonia × 3. Last hospitalization 2013. Hypertension. Osteopenia. A 30-pound unintended weight loss over past year. Did see a gastroenterologist and had a negative workup.

Past surgical history: C-section.

Personal history: Married, one son. Social worker at local high school, part-time.

Family history: Paternal grandfather died of stomach cancer, not certain of age. Paternal grandmother died of dementia, age 99. Maternal grandfather died of pneumonia, renal failure, age 62. Maternal grandmother died in her sleep, age 72. Two sisters both died in their 60s from accidents.

Review of Systems

General: Feeling cold and somewhat weak but denies chills, feeling faint, or lightheaded.

Skin: Denies rashes or lesions.

HEENT: Denies headache, recent upper respiratory infection, or sinus pain.

Neck: Denies neck pain.

Respiratory: Denies cough, shortness of breath.

Cardiac: Denies chest pressure, pain, or palpitations.

Gastrointestinal: Occasional problems with constipation, although not currently. Denies difficulty swallowing, heartburn, or diarrhea.

Urinary: Denies urinary hesitancy, burning, or frequency.

Musculoskeletal: + muscle aches or joint pain. Denies trauma.

Peripheral vascular: Occasional leg pain walking.

Endocrine: Denies low blood sugar, thirst.

Psychiatric: Denies anxiety, depression.

217

Physical Examination

> **General:** Pleasant female in no acute distress, but obviously uncomfortable moving from the sitting to standing position.
>
> **Vital signs:** Height; 65.5 inches, weight 126.6 pounds. Body mass index (BMI) 21.07. Temperature 100°F, blood pressure 138/90.
>
> **Skin:** Warm, dry, no rashes, or acute lesions.
>
> **Eyes:** Sclera clear, no icterus. Conjunctiva: no injection.
>
> **Ears:** External auditory canals clear. Tympanic membranes (TMs): Landmarks visible, no erythema, bulging, or retraction.
>
> **Nose:** No rhinitis or sinus tenderness.
>
> **Mouth:** Teeth in good repair. Mucous membranes moist, no lesions. Slight postpharyngeal but no exudate.
>
> **Neck:** Supple with shoddy posterior cervical nodes; soft. Mobile, nontender. No masses or thyroid tenderness.
>
> **Cardiac:** S1, S2 regular. No S3, S4, murmur, or rub.
>
> **Lungs:** Clear to auscultation. No rales, wheezes, or rhonchi.
>
> **Abdomen:** Soft, bowel sounds +, no organomegaly or tenderness.
>
> **Musculoskeletal:** + tenderness left shoulder with limited abduction secondary to pain, but no edema or erythema. Bilateral hip pain with internal/external rotation, but no edema or erythema. Muscle strength upper and lower extremities: 5+ bilaterally.
>
> **Extremities:** Left hand: + erythema, slight edema, and tenderness of the thumb. Other joints: Bilateral hands and feet, no edema or tenderness. Pedal pulses present bilaterally, no edema or calf tenderness.
>
> **Neurologic:** Alert, oriented to person, place, and time. Thoughts coherent. No fasciculations or tremors.

Case Study, Continued

The health care provider caring for Mrs. Carroll codes the visit as M25.50, pain in unspecified joint, and notes in the plan, "This may be viral because she does have a temperature, but it seems unusual that three joints are involved rather than all or most of them."

1. Based on this patient's presentation and the health care provider's assessment, what would be the best plan of care for this patient today? Are there other diagnoses that would be appropriate to consider for this patient, or are there other issues that the provider should address at this visit?

It is common for a patient to present to primary care or even urgent care complaining of joint pain. The causes of joint pain are varied, but with a low-grade temperature it would not be unusual for this patient to have a viral illness. Still, it is always important to think in terms of differential diagnoses when caring for patients and try to avoid cognitive bias.[1] Choosing the correct diagnosis and treatment requires careful analysis. Accurately summarizing the patient's history and asking the patient if his or her understanding of the problem is correct validates the patient and helps avoid misunderstanding. The patient's past medical and family history, the review of symptoms, and physical examination determine abnormalities and, combined with knowledge of the patient's history of present illness, allow the provider to develop the differential diagnoses. Mrs. Carroll has polyarticular joint pain, which she describes as aching. If she described the pain as numbness or burning, the cause would seem to be neuropathic. The aching quality she describes is more consistent with an inflammatory etiology, and a viral illness is a possible consideration. The low-grade temperature suggests a systemic disease, although the physical examination did not reveal a hot, tender, edematous joint or joints, so a bacterial infection seems less likely. Other possibilities include (but are not limited to) Lyme disease, crystal-induced synovitis (e.g., gout), spondyloarthropathy, or a systemic rheumatic or vasculitic disease.

Additional issues to be considered are Mrs. Carroll's blood pressure and that she is taking ibuprofen, an over-the-counter nonsteroidal antiinflammatory drug (NSAID), which is a concerning medication in an older adult. Knowing exactly what dose of ibuprofen and how many and how often she is taking the ibuprofen, and determining whether she has experienced any stomach discomfort since starting the medicine are important. A repeat blood pressure both sitting and standing should be assessed. If Mrs. Carroll's blood pressure remains elevated (i.e., greater than 150 mm Hg systolic or 90 mm Hg diastolic), even when standing, the hypertension should be addressed. It is possible the increased blood pressure is related to the NSAID, and simply stopping the NSAID will result in a lowering of the blood pressure. It is also possible that Mrs. Carroll will have orthostatic hypotension, suggesting the possibility of dehydration as part of her illness, and then requiring further diagnostics (e.g., electrolyte panel; blood, urea, nitrogen [BUN]; creatinine).

The third issue that should be addressed by the health care provider is smoking cessation. Mrs. Carroll is a smoker, and it is possible that the health care provider has discussed smoking cessation in the past. However, every encounter with a patient who smokes should include asking the patient the 5A's (Table 11.1).[2] Counseling patients to stop smoking at every encounter and offering information about available methods that can be helpful is important. The counseling and encouragement to stop smoking should also be documented on the medical record.

2. Because the diagnosis is not clear at this point in the patient's illness, it may be premature to order laboratory or imaging tests. If the provider did choose to order diagnostics, which laboratory tests should be considered? What information would be learned from these diagnostics?

The patient's skin examination did not reveal presence of erythema migrans, which would enable a clinical diagnosis of Lyme disease and immediate treatment. Mrs. Carroll lives in an area that is endemic for Lyme diseases, so a Lyme antibody with Western blot (i.e., enzyme-linked immunosorbent assay [ELISA] followed by a Western blot) is thus indicated. A complete blood count (CBC) and an erythrocyte sedimentation rate (ESR) and C-reactive protein (CRP) will aid in determining the presence of infection and/or inflammation. A rheumatoid factor (RF) is also appropriate, but can be negative despite a clinical presentation consistent with rheumatoid arthritis. Antibody tests may not be specific, but they can eliminate some disorders, so an antinuclear

TABLE 11.1 ■ The Five As

Ask	Identify and document tobacco use status for every patient at every visit (you may wish to develop your own vital signs sticker, based on the sample in the text)
Advise	In a clear, strong, and personalized manner, urge every tobacco user to quit
Assess	Is the tobacco user willing to make a quit attempt at this time?
Assist	For the patient willing to make a quit attempt, use counseling and pharmacotherapy to help him or her quit
Arrange	Schedule follow-up contact, in person or by telephone, preferably within the first week after the quit date

From Agency for Healthcare Research and Quality (AHRQ). Five Major Steps to Intervention (The "5 A's"). (2012). http://www.ahrq.gov/professionals/clinicians-providers/guidelines-recommendations/tobacco/5steps.html.

antibody and anti-double-stranded (ds) DNA antibodies can be helpful diagnostics in diagnosing systemic lupus erythematosus, which can have a similar clinical presentation to Mrs. Carroll's presentation.

Case Study, Continued

The provider caring for Mrs. Carroll decided to have her stop the ibuprofen to see if her blood pressure would decrease and asked her to take two acetaminophen (Tylenol) 500 milligrams tablets twice a day for the joint discomfort. The patient was asked to go home and rest and was encouraged to call if she was not improving or getting worse. A follow-up appointment in 7 to 10 days was made to be certain Mrs. Carroll had improved.

SECOND OFFICE VISIT

Five days later Mrs. Carroll presents to the practice today as an urgent visit stating she thinks she has "a terrible case of the flu." She describes chills alternating with sweats and even more pain than at her last visit. She cannot even roll over in bed, let alone sleep because of the pain, plus she has trouble getting out of bed, getting up from a chair, walking, or doing any work. "The Tylenol does nothing for my pain." She has been taking her temperature and it has not been higher than 100°F.

Review of Systems

General: + chills, + sweats, + body aches, and + joint pain.

Skin: Denies rashes or lesions

Head, eyes, ears, nose, and throat (HEENT): + dull headache in back of her head. Denies rhinitis, upper respiratory symptoms, sinus pain, vision changes, earaches, or sore throat.

Neck: Denies neck pain.

Respiratory: Denies cough, shortness of breath.

Cardiac: Denies chest pressure, pain, or palpitations.

Gastrointestinal: Denies difficulty swallowing, heartburn, constipation, diarrhea, or abdominal pain.

Urinary: Denies urinary hesitancy, burning, or frequency.

Musculoskeletal: + muscle aches, + joint pain, + pain walking or with any movement.

Peripheral vascular: Denies numbness, tingling.

Endocrine: Denies low blood sugar, thirst.

Psychiatric: "Anxious that something is really wrong."

Physical Examination

General: Alert female who is obviously uncomfortable with any movement. Blood pressure recheck 136/80, no orthostatic changes.

Vital signs: Height: 65.5 inches, weight 122.3 pounds. BMI 21.07, temperature 99.2°F, blood pressure 132/78, pulse 89, respiratory rate 18, O_2 saturation 95%.

Skin: warm, dry, no rashes, or acute lesions.

Eyes: Sclera clear, no icterus. Conjunctiva: No injection.

Ears: External auditory canals clear. Tympanic membranes (TMs): Landmarks visible, no erythema, bulging, or retraction.

Nose: Hyperemic, but no rhinitis or sinus tenderness.

Mouth: Teeth in good repair. Mucous membranes moist, no lesions or exudate. Posterior pharynx shows no undue erythema. No exudate.

Neck: Supple. No nuchal rigidity. Some faint posterior cervical lymphadenopathy, smooth, slippery nontender. No supraclavicular or subclavicular lymphadenopathy.

Cardiac: S1, S2 regular. No S3, S4, murmur, or rub.

Lungs: Clear to auscultation. No rales, wheezes, or rhonchi.

Abdomen: Soft, bowel sounds +, no organomegaly or tenderness.

Musculoskeletal: Every movement seems to cause discomfort. No joint erythema or edema.

Extremities: Pedal pulses present bilaterally. No edema or calf tenderness.

Neurologic: Alert, oriented to person, place, and time. Pupils equal reactive to light and accommodation (PERLA), extraocular movements (EOMs) intact. Funduscopic: No papilledema. Cranial nerves (CNs) II to XII, no deficits. Romberg negative, no pronator drift. Reflexes symmetric 2+ bilaterally. Thoughts coherent. No fasciculations or tremors.

Lymph nodes: There is no other lymphadenopathy other than previously noted.

Assessment: Fever and chills: R50.00; Myalgia: M79.1.

Plan: Fever, chills, and myalgias. Plan laboratory testing: CBC and differential, serum glucose, serum electrolytes, BUN, creatinine, urinalysis with culture and sensitivity, ESR, CRP, Lyme screen with Western blot reflex, RF screen, anticitrullinated peptide antibodies (anti-CCP), antinuclear antibody, anti-dsDNA antibodies, and liver function tests (LFTs).

3. What treatment is indicated for the patient today? Are there other diagnostics that should be ordered?

Because the cause of Mrs. Carroll's symptoms is not yet known, the treatment continues to be supportive. There is no clear physical evidence of a bacterial infection, and there is no significant joint edema suggesting septic arthritis. Some of the diagnostic testing results will be quickly available (ordered STAT), whereas other tests results may not be available for several days. Further diagnostics will be determined whether deemed necessary after the results of the initial laboratory results are available.

Initial Laboratory Results
RF screen: negative
CRP: 3.0 (<0.5 milligrams/dL)
ESR: 1 (0–20 mm/hr)
CBC
    White blood count (WBC): 14.0 (4.0–11.0 K/mm^3)
    Red blood cell count (RBC): 4.6 (3.8–5.0 M/mm^3)
    Hemoglobin: 11.7 (11.0–16 g/dL)
    Hematocrit: 35.0 (35.0%–48%)
    Mean cell volume: 98.6 (80–100 fL)
    Mean corpuscular hemoglobin: 32.9 (27.0–34.0 pg)
    Platelet count: 264 (130–400 K/mm^3)
    Neutrophils %: 81.2 (37%–80.0%)
    Lymphocytes %: 13.1 (23.0%–45.0%)
    Monocytes %: 2.7 (2.5%–14.0%)
    Eosinophils %: 1.8 (0.5%–4.0%)
    Basophils %: 0.3 (0.0%–2.0%)
    Neutrophils #: 12 (1.9–7.5 K/mm^3)
    Lymphocytes #: 1.9 (1.2–3.4 K/mm^3)
    Monocytes #: 0.4 (0.0–0.7 Kmm^3)

Eosinophils #: 0.27 (0.0–0.7 K/mm³)
Basophils #: 0.0 (0.0–0.05 K/mm³)
Chem 8
    Sodium: 142 (136–145 mmol/L)
    Potassium: 4.3 (3.4–5.1 mmol/L)
    Chloride: 105 (98–107 mmol/L)
    Carbon dioxide: 27 (22–32 mmol/L)
    Glucose: 96 (74–118 mmol/L)
    BUN: 15 (5–23 milligrams/dL)
    Creatinine: 0.7 (0.4–1.0 milligrams/dL)
    Estimated glomerular filtration rate (eGFR): 92.7 mL/min
    Calcium: 9.5 (8.6–10.2 milligrams/dL)
Urine microscopic
    Renal epithelial cells: None per high-powered field (hpf)
    Squamous epithelial cells: 1 to 4/hpf
    Transitional epithelial cells: None per high-powered field
    Urine bacteria: 1+(none)
    Urine casts: None
    Urine crystals: Calcium oxalate
    Urine RBC: 1 to 4 (1–4/hpf)
    Urine WBC: 1 to 4 (1–4/hpf)
Urinalysis
    Urine color: Yellow
    Urine appearance: Clear
    Urine glucose: Negative
    Urine bilirubin: Negative
    Urine ketone: Negative
    Specific gravity: 1.025 (1.005–1.030)
    Urine blood: negative (negative)
    pH urine: 5.5 (5.0–8.0)
    Urine protein: Negative
    Urine urobilinogen: 0.2 (0.2–1.0 EU/dL)
    Urine nitrate: Negative
    Urine Leukocyte esterase: Negative

4. When reviewing Mrs. Carroll's diagnostics, what abnormalities should the provider be concerned about? What treatment should the provider initiate this visit?

Not all the laboratory results are available, but the provider recognizes that the elevated CRP is consistent with inflammation. It is interesting that the ESR is normal, although not surprising because CRP is more sensitive and accurate, particularly if inflammation is present.[3] Mrs. Carroll's WBC count is elevated, as are the percentage and number of neutrophils. Although leukocytosis is associated with infectious processes, these elevations also are consistent with inflammatory processes. Her urinalysis does not suggest that she has a urinary tract infection, although there are calcium oxalate crystals that could cause renal calculi. However, there is no blood in her urine and even though kidney stones are not always associated with pain, renal calculi seem inconsistent with her presentation.

A chest x-ray (CXR) posterior/anterior and lateral and blood cultures will be also ordered because Mrs. Carroll does have both a fever and leukocytosis.

5. Acetaminophen has not helped decrease Mrs. Carroll's pain. Her blood pressure did decrease when she stopped taking ibuprofen, and the ibuprofen was not controlling her pain, so restarting the nonsteroidal antiinflammatory drugs is not an option. What other pain control options should the health care provider consider for Mrs. Carroll? What consultations and/or follow-up should be considered for this patient?

At this point in time, Mrs. Carroll's pain would be classified as acute pain. Her pain is new in onset and the etiology of her discomfort is not yet clear. Acute pain is often associated with injury and frequently resolves within 3 months, although sometimes the discomfort can take up to 6 months to resolve. After that, continued pain is considered chronic or persistant. The management is not necessarily different, although the hope always is patient comfort, continued quality of life, and as few medications as possible. Nonpharmacologic approaches are always indicated and include alternating hot and cold therapy and capsaicin cream, acupuncture, massage, physical therapy, and other pain management strategies. For providers caring for older adults, choosing the right medication for the patient can be challenging because of physiologic aging changes, multiple comorbidities, and often numerous medications. The provider considers several pharmacologic categories and tries to weigh the risks and benefits of each for Mrs. Carroll. The potential considerations are listed below. As the various options are considered, it is important to remember that it is possible that there is no one perfect choice. Health care providers try to choose the best option for each patient, but when prescribing medications for a patient it is important to understand that no medication is risk free. An adverse drug reaction is always a possibility. Explaining the risks and benefits of each medication and being certain that the patient knows when to call and documenting the conversation is an important risk management consideration.

HEALTH CARE PROVIDER TREATMENT CONSIDERATIONS

Celecoxib (Celebrex) is an NSAID, specifically a cyclooxygenase-2 (COX-2) inhibitor. COX-2 inhibitors are different than cyclooxygenase-1 (COX-1) inhibitors in that there is a *decreased* chance of gastrointestinal (GI) affects, especially less GI bleeding. There remains a concern about hypertension and other adverse effects, however, with both COX-1 and COX-2 inhibitors. Both these categories of NSAIDs have been associated with heart attacks and strokes in older adults and potential GI and renal complications. The risks of these medications often outweigh the benefits, so NSAIDS are frequently avoided in this population.[4,5] A more recent study determined that celecoxib posed no greater risk than Cox-1 inhibitors (i.e., ibuprofen and naproxen); however, that study did not negate the concern about the potential effects of both these NSAID classes.[6]

Often, when acetaminophen is not helpful and NSAIDS cannot be used, corticosteroids are used for pain relief in inflammatory conditions. Steroids are prescribed cautiously, however, because the side effects of steroid therapy can be serious, particularly if used long term. Mrs. Carroll may require steroid therapy, but until the cause of her discomfort is known, steroids should be avoided, if possible.

Opioids, although helpful in pain management, have potentially serious side effects that include constipation, cognitive changes, falls, increased hospitalizations, and death.[7] Prescribers need to be wary when considering opioid therapy in older adults, and when used, the dosage is always started at the lowest possible dose. Tramadol (Ultram) is an opioid agonist and is sometimes used for a limited amount of time for acute pain in older adults. Unfortunately, tramadol is not safer than other opioids, nor less addicting. Concerning side effects in elders include hypoglycemia, hypotension, cognitive changes, gait abnormalities, and, if used with medications that are serotonergic, possibly serotonin syndrome.[8]

For some patients, an antidepressant is prescribed for patients with chronic muscle pain. Duloxetine (Cymbalta), a selective serotonin and norepinephrine reuptake inhibitor, is an antidepressant used for patients with chronic muscle pain, fibromyalgia, osteoarthritis, neuropathy, and other pain-related disorders. However, there is a risk of orthostatic hypotension and falls in older adults.[9] Still, duloxetine is possibly safer than most tricyclic antidepressants. One tricyclic that could be considered is doxepin (Silenor). Low-dose doxepin (1–3 milligrams) can be used for older adults who are having difficulty sleeping,[10] but it is not clear if this dose would be efficacious in terms of pain control.

After consultation with colleagues in the primary care office, the provider decides that Mrs. Carroll is so uncomfortable that something needs to be tried to control her discomfort. Because the pain is so disabling and interfering even with sleep, tramadol hydrochloride (37.5 milligrams) and acetaminophen (325 milligrams) (Ultracet), 1 tablet every 8 hours, is prescribed. The patient is advised that this medicine can cause confusion, weakness, dizziness, and constipation among other side effects and to stop the medication and call the office if experiencing any adverse feelings.

It is possible that Mrs. Carroll's symptoms are related to a virus. If her symptoms continue or worsen, the differential diagnoses considered should include other infectious processes and cancer. A consultation appointment with rheumatology can be made for the patient and a follow-up appointment in primary care. If Mrs. Carroll's fever and symptoms continue, more laboratory diagnostics and an infectious disease consult could be considered.

RHEUMATOLOGY EVALUATION

Mrs. Carroll is a 67-year-old female referred from her primary care provider for evaluation of myalgias and muscle weakness in her shoulders and hips. The onset was abrupt. She awoke one morning with pain in her right hip. The pain increased over the next few days so much so that she "felt like every bone in her body hurt" and "could not move" the pain was so disabling. She continues to have significant pain with malaise and low-grade fever up to 100.2°F. Today the pain is across her upper chest, shoulders, fingers, hips, knees, and feet. Her feet are sometimes swollen, but she denies swelling in any other joints. She initially took Tylenol and Ibuprofen with no effect and then was started on Tramadol again without relief.

She did have some leukocytosis and an increase in one inflammatory marker (i.e., CRP 3.0). However, other laboratory diagnostics were negative: ESR 1, RF negative, ANA 1:40, anti-CCP < 20 u/mL, anti-ds deoxyribonucleic acid (dsDNA) negative, LFTs normal, CXR negative, blood cultures negative, Lyme and other tickborne disease testing negative.

Physical Examination

General: Conversant, appropriate female with an antalgic gate. Appears somewhat uncomfortable but is in no acute distress.

Vital signs: Weight 120 pounds. Temperature 99°F, blood pressure 118/86, heart rate 96, respiratory rate 22.

Skin: Warm, dry without rash or plaques.

Eyes: Sclera anicteric, conjunctiva pink without hemorrhages.

Oral cavity: Membranes moist, clear without lesions. Dentition, tongue normal.

Neck: Supple. No edema, palpable masses, or tenderness.

Cardiac: Regular rhythm, rate. No S3, S4, murmur, or rub.

Pulmonary: Clear without rales, wheezes, or rhonchi.

Abdomen: Soft, bowel sounds positive. No tenderness or hepatosplenomegaly.

Musculoskeletal: Able to sit and get up from chair without assistance or difficulty. Able to lift arms overhead, but with pain and not fully. Back examination negative. No spinal processes tenderness. No ischial tuberosity tenderness. No radiculopathy. Hands, fingers are normal. There is no edema or tenderness of the proximal interphalangeal or metacarpophalangeal joints. No pain with passive or active range of motion. Knees are normal. No edema. No pain with active or active range of motion. Feet: No edema or tenderness of metatarsophalangeal joints. No synovitis of any joint.

Extremities: No edema or calf tenderness.

Neurologic: Alert, conversant. Speech fluent. No apparent deficits.

Assessment/plan: M79.1: Unspecified myalgia; M60.9: Unspecified myositis; D72.829: Unspecified leukocytosis. Other than mild leukocytosis and the CRP 3.0, all diagnostics are negative. This does not seem to be an infectious process. Her examination today is not consistent with rheumatoid arthritis, although presentations can be atypical. An aldolase and creatine kinase (CK) may be helpful and will check that and repeat CBC/differential.

6. Why does the rheumatologist think that Mrs. Carroll's presentation is not consistent with rheumatoid arthritis? What examination or diagnostic criteria is needed to confirm a diagnosis of rheumatoid arthritis? What information does the rheumatologist think will be learned by ordering an aldolase and creatine kinase level? Are there other diagnostics that should also be ordered at this time?

Rheumatoid arthritis can be insidious and the diagnosis challenging. The RF is not always positive in early stages of this autoimmune disorder, but specific clinical criteria are necessary for diagnosis. Joint involvement, a positive RF, or anti-CCP, abnormal ESR or CRP, and symptoms longer than 6 weeks are the clinical and diagnostic requirements necessary for diagnosis.[11]

Aldolase and CK are both enzymes found in muscle and other body tissues. These laboratory diagnostics can be elevated in patients with muscle disease or disorders. A thyroid-stimulating hormone (TSH) is indicated to exclude hypothyroidism, which is a potential cause of muscle pain.

Third Office Visit

Before Mrs. Carroll's office visit, the primary care provider caring for Mrs. Carroll reviews the office and specialist notes and diagnostics, and then considers the differential diagnoses for the patient's symptoms (Table 11.2). After careful deliberation of the differentials and reviewing the most recent laboratory tests (aldolase, TSH, and CK are normal), the provider decides that crystalline arthritis could be a possibility, but an x-ray or joint aspiration has not yet been obtained. However, even though Mrs. Carroll complained of joint pain, the recent physical examinations have not really identified a specific joint or joints that are inflamed. Additionally, Mrs. Carroll's systemic symptoms make pseudogout less likely.

Mrs. Carroll's signs and symptoms are consistent with an inflammatory disorder (i.e., systemic symptoms [fever, fatigue] and an elevated CRP.[12] Other symptoms of inflammation include edema, erythema, rash, warmth, weight loss, anemia of chronic disease, low albumin, increased ESR, and thrombocytosis.[12] Viral polyarthritis, polymyalgia rheumatica (PMR), paraneoplastic disease, or one of the spondyloarthropathies also seem possible, but the other differentials could be excluded based on Mrs. Carroll's clinical presentations and diagnostic results. When Mrs. Carroll arrives, the provider again asks Mrs. Carroll about her symptoms.

Mrs. Carroll: "It has been more than 5 weeks now. I just remember waking up one morning with pain in my left shoulder. Then it seemed the pain was in my hips, but it just got worse and was everywhere. I felt feverish and tired. I still feel like that. It is worse in the morning, so bad that I can barely move. The pain pill helps me sleep better, but I don't feel better. I ache all over."

TABLE 11.2 ■ Rheumatoid Arthritis Differential Diagnoses

Disorder	
Crystalline arthritis (pseudogout)	One or more painful, stiff, edematous joints X-ray or joint fluid analysis
Dermatomyositis	Fever, rash, muscle pain, proximal muscle weakness Aldolase, creatine kinase, CRP, ESR, TSH
Fibromyalgia	Generalized MS pain, fatigue Fibromyalgia diagnostic criteria • Presence of generalized pain, in a minimum of four of five regions • Consistent degree of symptoms for 3 months at least • WPI ≥ 7 and SSS score ≥ 5 or WPI of 4–6 and SSS score ≥ 9 • The fibromyalgia diagnosis is legitimate regardless of other diagnoses; a diagnosis of fibromyalgia does not eliminate the possibility of other serious illnesses
Infectious arthritis	Painful onset erythematous, warm, usually single + tender joint; pain is constant at rest and with movement, + fever CBC/differential, CRP, ESR, blood cultures, joint aspiration fluid analysis
Lyme disease	Arthralgia, fever, headache, joint pain, lymphadenopathy, myalgia, polyarthritis Lyme ELISA Western blot
Osteoarthritis	Pain and stiffness affecting one joint or more, worse on arising, after long periods of activity, but alleviated with rest; + Heberden and Bouchard nodes may be present; can affect DIPs, spine, hips, and knees; no systemic symptoms X-rays primary diagnostic; laboratory tests/joint fluid examination exclude other disorders
Paraneoplastic disease	Muscle/joint pain and inflammation can be associated with systemic lupus erythematous, scleroderma, solid organ tumors, acute leukemia, myelomas, and other malignancies; anorexia, dysgeusia, and fever common Routine laboratory diagnostics, paraneoplastic antibody screening, serum and CSF protein electrophoresis, lumbar puncture, electrophysiology, and neuroimaging
Polymyalgia rheumatica	Stiffness, aching shoulders/hips, synovitis/bursitis, low-grade fever, decreased range of motion (particularly shoulder abduction) ESR/CRP usually, but not always elevated; possible normochromic, normocytic anemia LFTs maybe abnormal, other laboratory tests are usually normal
Spondyloarthropathies (inflammatory arthritides: ankylosing spondylitis, enteropathic arthritis, psoriatic arthritis, reactive arthritis, undifferentiated spondyloarthritis)	Can be asymmetric inflammation spine/joints/ligaments/tendons, dactylitis, uveitis, skin and other systemic manifestations (e.g., heart, lungs, bowels) Fatigue, low-grade fever, weight loss X-ray, MRI, ANA, CBC/differential, CRP, ESR, HLA-B27, RF, and uric acid
Systemic vasculitis	Fatigue, fever, rash (palpable purpura), systemic pain (depending on area affected) Biopsy is definitive diagnosis
Viral polyarthritis	Usually symmetric joint pain and edema and fever; usually self-limiting Laboratory diagnostics indicated if symptoms continue

ANA, Antinuclear antibody; CBC, complete blood count; CRP, C-reactive protein; CSF, cerebrospinal fluid; DIP, distal interphalangeal; ELISA, enzyme-linked immunosorbent assay; ESR, erythrocyte sedimentation rate; HLA, human leukocyte antigen; LFT, liver function test; MRI, magnetic resonance imaging; MS, musculoskeletal; RF, rheumatoid factor; SSS, symptom severity scale; TSH, thyroid-stimulating hormone; WPI, Widespread Pain Index.

Review of Symptoms. Not able to work. Not feeling well. Feels sick, weak, "so tired, it is hard to get up, to move, and to get dressed." + trouble sleeping. Denies trauma, previous similar pain. Denies falls, fever now, chills, headache, difficulty swallowing, chest pain, palpitations, cough, shortness of breath, abdominal pain, constipation, nausea, vomiting, diarrhea, urinary burning or frequency, and depression.

Physical Examination

General: Alert, older female.

Vital signs: Weight 119 pounds. Temperature 98.8°F. Heart rate 100, respiratory rate 22, blood pressure 142/80.

HEENT: No temporal tenderness. Eyes: Sclera clear, no icterus. Nose: No erythema or sinus tenderness.

Neck: + discomfort with range of motion. No masses or lymphs.

Mouth: Membranes moist, no lesions.

Cardiac: S1, S2 regular. No S3, S4, or murmur.

Lungs: Clear. No rales, wheezes, or rhonchi.

Abdomen: Soft, bowel sounds +, nontender.

Extremities: + tenderness in both upper arms, bilateral thighs. + discomfort shoulder abduction, abduction less than expected because of discomfort. No extremity edema.

Musculoskeletal: No edema, warmth, or joint tenderness.

Case Study, Continued

Other providers in the office also are asked to evaluate Mrs. Carroll today, and the collaborative decision is to treat Mrs. Carroll with prednisone. The rationale for this treatment is that PMR is a strong possible diagnosis and treatment with prednisone should markedly decrease her symptoms in the next 3 to 4 days. If she does not improve, the prednisone can be stopped.

7.   What components of Mrs. Carroll's history and physical examination(s) suggest that polymyalgia rheumatica might be the cause of her discomfort? What further diagnostics are indicated and why? What dose prednisone is appropriate for Mrs. Carroll at this time? When should she be seen again in follow-up? What other medications are indicated for a patient with polymyalgia rheumatica? What patient education is necessary for this patient?

PMR is an interesting disorder. It affects primarily older adults (i.e., patients over age 50), more women than men, and has an unclear etiology.[13] The discomfort associated with PMR is referred to as both neck and limb girdle discomfort related to muscle edema and inflammation of the synovial membranes, bursa, tendons, and the tendon sheaths.[13] Other common signs and symptoms include a low-grade temperature, stiffness and swelling, fatigue, weight loss, and presence of an inflammatory marker (e.g., elevated CRP or ESR).[13] The requirements for diagnosis include age 50 or older (usually), elevated ESR or CRP, aching of both shoulders, morning stiffness greater than 45 minutes, hip pain, lack of other joint pain, and negative RF or anti-CCP antibody.[14]

No further diagnostics are indicated. A trial of oral prednisone 20 milligrams/day will be ordered for Mrs. Carroll. If she has PMR, her symptoms should improve dramatically within a few days.[13] Mrs. Carroll will return to the office within a week to be certain her symptoms have resolved. If she does improve, Mrs. Carroll will continue on this dose of prednisone for 4 weeks, and then be slowly tapered. The usual taper is 2.5 milligrams every 4 weeks or if tolerated every 2 weeks until the dosage reaches 10 milligrams/day.[13] After that the prednisone taper is decreased by 1 milligrams a month.[13] Often health care providers monitor the ESR each month, but the taper should continue as long as the symptoms are abating. If the patient's symptoms increase during the taper, the prednisone should be increased[13] (e.g., 2.5 milligrams more than the current dose).

All patients with PMR should be seen regularly (e.g., monthly) to assess symptoms and determine whether giant cell arteritis has developed.[10] Additionally, patients taking prednisone should understand the importance of taking prednisone with food and can be started on a proton pump inhibitor for gastric protection, if necessary. A bisphosphonate is also indicated for patients taking prednisone for an extended length of time.[13]

Fourth Office Visit

Six days later, Mrs. Carroll returns for follow-up. Her pain has resolved and she feels like herself again. She is able to sleep and even feels like eating. She states she is taking the prednisone daily with food and denies any gastric discomfort. The provider notes that Mrs. Carroll looks better and moves today with agility. Her weight is up almost a pound, her vital signs are stable, and her physical examination reveals less discomfort, especially with range of motion. The improvement with prednisone strongly suggests that PMR is the likely cause of Mrs. Carroll's illness.

The provider reiterates the importance of taking the prednisone with food and plans follow-up in 3 weeks. Mrs. Carroll will have a repeat CRP, a vitamin D-25 OH level, and bone density before the follow-up appointment. The necessity of immediate follow-up is stressed if Mrs. Carroll develops a headache, jaw discomfort or pain, vision loss, or if the viral-like symptoms (e.g., fever, malaise) she had initially return. The provider explains that these symptoms are associated with giant cell arteritis, a serious complication of PMR that can result in blindness. The provider also explains that at the next visit, Mrs. Carroll will likely be started on alendronate (Fosamax), but the provider wants to wait until then before starting another medication. Mrs. Carroll is encouraged to have 1200 milligrams of calcium daily and start Vitamin D3, 800 IU orally every day. She is given a food diary to record what she eats for 1 week, so that the health care provider can decide if she actually eats enough calcium daily when they meet in 3 weeks. The provider will also address the issue of smoking cessation and Mrs. Carroll's readiness to quit smoking.

References

1. Croskerry, P. (2013). From mindless to mindful practice — cognitive bias and clinical decision making. *New England Journal of Medicine, 368*, 2445–2448.
2. Agency for Healthcare Research and Quality. Five major steps to intervention (The "5 A's"). Retrieved from https://www.ahrq.gov/professionals/clinicians-providers/guidelines-recommendations/tobacco/5steps.html.
3. Harrison, M. (2015). Erythrocyte sedimentation rate and C-reactive protein. *Australian Prescriber, 38*(3), 93–94.
4. Liantonio, J. J., & Simmons, B. B. (2013). NSAIDS and the geriatric patient: a cautionary tale. *Clinical Geriatrics, 21*(5). Retrieved from http://www.consultant360.com/articles/nsaids-and-geriatric-patient-cautionary-tale.
5. Dowell, D., Hagearith, T. M., & Chou, R. (2016). CDC guideline for prescribing opioids for chronic pain—United States, 2016. *New England Journal of Medicine, 315*(15), 1624–1645.
6. Nissen, S. E., Yeomans, N. D., Solomon, D. H., Lüscher, T. F., et al. (2016). Cardiovascular safety of celecoxib, naproxen, or ibuprofen for arthritis. *New England Journal of Medicine*, 2519–2529.
7. Teater, D. (2015). The psychological and physical side effects of pain medications. Retrieved from http://www.theherrenproject.org/wp-content/uploads/2015/09/Side-Effects-WhitePaper.pdf.
8. Volpi-Abadie, J., Kaye, A. M., & Kaye, A. D. (2013). Serotonin syndrome. *The Ochsner Journal, 13*(4), 533–540.
9. U.S. Food and Drug Administration. (2014). Cymbalta. Retrieved from http://www.fda.gov/Safety/MedWatch/SafetyInformation/ucm319241.htm.

10. Krystal, A. D., Durrence, H. H., Scharf, M., Jochelson, P., Rogowski, R., Ludington, E., et al. (2010). Efficacy and safety of doxepin 1 milligrams and 3 milligrams in a 12-week sleep laboratory and outpatient trial of elderly subjects with chronic primary insomnia. *Sleep, 33*(11), 1553–1561.

11. Aletaha, D., Neogi, T., Silman, A. J., Funovits, J., et al. (2010). 2010 Rheumatoid arthritis classification criteria. *Arthritis and Rheumatism, 62*(9), 2569–2581. Retrieved from http://www.rheumatology.org/Portals/0/Files/2010_revised_criteria_classification_ra.pdf.

12. Cush, J. J. (2015). Approach to articular and musculoskeletal disorders. In D. Kasper, A. Fauci, S. Hauser, D. Longo, J. Jameson, & J. Loscalzo (Eds.), *Harrison's principles of internal medicine* (19th ed.). New York: McGraw-Hill. Retrieved from http://accessmedicine.mhmedical.com.ezproxy.simmons.edu:2048/content.aspx?bookid=1130&Sectionid=79750978.

13. O'Rourke, K. S. (2016). Myopathies, polymyalgia rheumatica, and giant cell arteritis. In J. B. Halter, J. G. Ouslander, S. Studenski, K. P. High, S. Asthana, M. A. Supiano, et al. (Eds.), *Hazzard's geriatric medicine and gerontology* (7th ed.). New York: McGraw-Hill. Retrieved from http://accessmedicine.mhmedical.com.ezproxy.simmons.edu:2048/content.aspx?bookid=1923&Sectionid=144562869.

14. Dasgupta, B., Cimmino, M. A., Kremers, H. M., et al. (2012). Provisional classification criteria for polymyalgia rheumatica: A European League Against Rheumatism/American College of Rheumatology collaborative initiative. *Arthritis & Rheumatism, 64*, 943–954.

Urinary Frequency

Ruth Palan Lopez ■ Teresa L. Hagan

Case Study Scenario/History of Present Illness

Ms. Camila A., a 71-year-old, white Hispanic woman comes to the primary care clinic with her daughter for a follow-up visit for her hypertension and hypercholesterolemia. She has not been to the primary care office in over 3 years, when the provider in the office referred her to a gynecologic oncologist on suspicion of ovarian cancer. Initially, she reports feeling well and denies new complaints. However, with her daughter's encouragement, she admits to feeling generally run down, tired, and lacking interest in participating in church activities, which she had previously enjoyed. Over the last 2 weeks, she suddenly developed urinary frequency including the need to void many times during the day and voiding only small amounts. She denies irritation, urgency, dysuria, or hematuria. She denies fever, flank, or groin pain. She also reports abdominal pain that she describes as the worst pain she has ever experienced. As a result, she has been reluctant to leave the house.

Past medical history: Ovarian cancer, hypertension, high cholesterol, arthritis, and hypothyroidism.

Medications: Levothyroxine sodium 0.075 milligrams one tablet daily without food, lisinopril 20 milligrams one tablet daily, ezetimibe 10 milligrams one tablet daily, fenofibrate 145 milligrams one tablet daily, and celecoxib 100 milligrams one capsule twice daily as needed for pain.

Allergies: Penicillin and cephalosporins caused hives.

Habits: Nonsmoker, two drinks a week socially, no recreational drug use.

Past surgical history: Tonsillectomy and appendectomy as a child; hysterectomy with bilateral salpingo-oophorectomy.

Family history: Mother died of breast cancer at age 60. Father died from stroke at age 85. She has two siblings. Her older sister died of ovarian cancer at age 50. She has four living children. Her younger brother is alive and well at age 69. He has two living children.

Personal + social history: Camila has been married to her husband for 50 years. She is a retired elementary school teacher for an inner-city school district, and her husband is a retired civil engineer. Camila has four children who all live in the area and regularly visit each other and their parents. She has eight grandchildren with whom she is very close. She is a devout Roman Catholic and is extremely involved in her church community's religious services and volunteer activities. In general, she has an active lifestyle, a positive attitude, and a strong family that she supports and who support her.

Review of Systems

General: Reports a 10-pound weight gain in past 3 months. Endorses some fatigue but denies difficulty sleeping, fevers, or chills.

Skin: Denies skin lesions or changing moles. No rashes or itching.

Head, eyes, ears, nose, and throat (HEENT): No complaints of headache, change in vision, nose or ear problems, sore throat, tinnitus, trouble swallowing, or voice change. Negative for photophobia, pain, and visual disturbance.

Neck: Denies swollen glands.

Breasts: Denies breast mass, pain, or discharge.

Respiratory: Denies cough, chest tightness, shortness of breath, or wheezing.

Cardiovascular: Denies chest pain, palpitations, or lower extremity edema.

Peripheral vascular: Denies leg pain when walking.

Gastrointestinal: Admits to new onset of constipation in the past 2 weeks. Complains of early satiety and abdominal bloating, which she attributes to constipation. Mild abdominal distention. Severe abdominal pain described today as 7/10. Reported constipation over 2 weeks with painful bowel movements. Denies complaints of dysphagia, nausea, or vomiting.

Genital/reproductive: Frequency and urgency reported for past month. + history of ovarian cancer. Treated with surgery and chemotherapy per patient report.

Musculoskeletal: Reports long-standing moderate knee pain, right less than left. No complaints of back pain or muscle aches.

Psychiatric: Denies feeling sad or depressed.

Neurologic: Denies weakness, dizziness, numbness, tingling, light-headedness, headaches, or incoordination.

Hematologic: Denies bruising or bleeding easily.

Endocrine: Reports polyuria (see history of present illness). Denies polydipsia, polyphagia.

Physical Examination

General: She appears well developed, well nourished, and well groomed. She is oriented to person, place, and time. She is neatly dressed, appropriate for the weather. She is accompanied by her daughter who is very concerned about the recent decline in her mother's overall health and lack of interest in her usual activities. No acute distress.

Vitals: Weight 192 pounds (unplanned 10-pound weight gain from 3 months ago per patient). Height 5'5," body mass index (BMI) 31.9. Blood pressure (BP) sitting in chair 138/86, orthostatic BP 125/80. Pulse 88 regular, respiration rate 20 unlabored, and temperature 98.4°F.

Skin/lymphatic system: Normal in appearance, texture, and temperature. No rash noted. She is not diaphoretic. No erythema. No pallor. No palpable nodes in the cervical, supraclavicular, axillary, or inguinal areas.

HEENT: Scalp normal. Pupils equal round reactive to light and accommodations. Sclera and conjunctiva normal, visual fields intact. Extraocular movements (EOMs) intact. Outer ears without lesions, normal acuity; tympanic membranes and canals normal. Oropharynx is clear and moist, no erythema or exudate. Tongue and gums normal.

Neck: Supple. Full pain-free range of motion. Trachea midline and thyroid gland without masses. No adenopathy. Carotid artery without bruits.

Cardiovascular: Normal rate, regular rhythm. Examination reveals no gallop and no friction rub. Point of maximal impulse (PMI) is in the fifth intercostal space at the midclavicular line. Split S2 heard best at left sternal border. A grade 2/6 systolic ejection murmur is present. No third or fourth heart sounds or rub are heard.

Lungs: Lungs are clear to auscultation and percussion bilaterally.

Breasts: Symmetric bilaterally. No dimpling, retraction, or peau d'orange. No breast/chest wall masses or nipple discharge is seen. No lesions or axillary adenopathy.

Abdomen: Symmetric with distention, responsive to touch. Bowel sounds are normal in quality and intensity in all areas. No palpable mass. Lower quadrants bilaterally sensitive to touch with 7/10 pain reported by patient. No splenomegaly noted. Liver span is 8 cm by percussion. Low transverse scar from radical hysterectomy.

Genital/rectal: Normal rectal sphincter tone; no rectal masses or tenderness. Stool is brown and guaiac negative. Pelvic examination reveals normal external genitalia, vaginal atrophy. Bimanual examination positive for possible mass on left abdomen.

Extremities. No cyanosis, clubbing, or edema is noted. Peripheral pulses in the femoral, popliteal, brachial, and radial areas are normal. Anterior tibial pulses are diminished.

Musculoskeletal: No spinal costovertebral angle tenderness, no joint tenderness. Full range of motion in upper and lower extremities.

Neurological: She is alert and oriented to person, place, and time. Cranial nerves II to XII are intact. Motor strength 5/5 throughout and no increased tone. Biceps, brachioradialis, triceps, knee, ankle reflexes 2+ bilaterally. Babinski absent. Gait smooth, coordinated. Romberg negative.

Assessment and Plan

1. Based on the history and physical examination results, what are the possible causes (differential diagnosis) for the patient's current condition?

Ms. A presents with complaints of new-onset urinary urgency, bowel pain and constipation, and significant new unplanned weight gain. She has attempted to manage the abdominal pain with constipation remedies at home, although none of these approaches have reduced her pain. Given her previous history of ovarian cancer, it is possible that her abdominal and genitourinary complaints are related to complications from cancer treatments because of the presence of scar tissue and changes in the physical structure. Yet the new and persistent onset of these symptoms within the past 2 weeks is alarming.

In general, the urinary symptoms should alert the primary care provider to the possibility of a urinary tract infection, urinary incontinence, urinary tract calculi, or diabetes mellitus. The lack of other urinary tract infection signs and symptoms (e.g., fevers, chills, dysuria, hematuria) would seemingly make a urinary tract infection unlikely. Urinary frequency and polyuria can also be caused by elevated blood sugars. However, if elevated blood sugars were the cause of Ms. A's frequency, additional symptoms such as polydipsia, polyphagia, or blurred vision would also likely be present.

The lower abdominal symptoms should also concern the health care provider. The differential diagnoses for constipation and abdominal pain must be considered, and the possible causes will need to be excluded.

Loss of interest in usual activities and change in appetite could be signs of depression. However, although depression may coexist with other comorbidities, given her other physical findings, depression alone is unlikely to be causing Ms. A's lack of interest in her usual activities and change in appetite.

The patient's past medical history and recent weight gain are particularly alarming. The health care provider recognizes that most women with ovarian cancer are diagnosed at a late stage (stage III or stage IV) when the 5-year survival is only 44% and the rate of recurrence is over 80%.[1] Although there are rarely gross symptoms related to ovarian cancer, a constellation of symptoms that are new and persistent for 2 weeks are commonly reported by women with ovarian cancer. These include pelvic and abdominal pain, urinary frequency and urgency, early satiety, and bloating. Other symptoms include fatigue, back pain, pain during intercourse, constipation, indigestion, and menstrual irregularities. The health care provider should consider whether the presenting symptoms of urinary frequency and abdominal pain may be related to a recurrence of Ms. A's ovarian cancer.

2. What components of the history or physical examination are missing?

The primary care provider should conduct a more thorough pain assessment to assess the location, intensity, duration, and aggravating or alleviating factors affecting Ms. A's abdominal pain using a validated measurement tool. Because the pathophysiology of pain determines the types of appropriate treatment, such an assessment should be conducted before selecting the proper pharmacologic and/or nonpharmacologic treatments. The provider can ask Ms. A to more fully describe her pain (e.g., stabbing, throbbing, aches, pressure, etc.), if it is constant or intermittent, if it is localized or not, if movement makes it worse, and what helps relieve the pain. The provider can also ask for an estimate of the pain using a numeric rating scale in which 0 indicates no pain, 1 to 3 indicates mild pain, 4 to 6 indicates moderate pain, and 7 to 10 indicates severe pain.[2] For reference, the National Cancer Institute publishes a widely used pain assessment tool.[3] Similarly, the health care provider can assess the details of Ms. A's urinary frequency including number of times a day and night she urinates, pain on urination, and changes in color and smell of her urine.

Although the provider caring for this patient did ask about feeling sad, a formal assessment for depression could be conducted using the Geriatric Depression Scale (GDS). There are two forms of this assessment: a 30-item long form and a 15-item short form. Both are successful in differentiating depressed from nondepressed adults.[4] In addition, a functional assessment including activities of daily living (ADLs) and instrumental activities of daily living (IADLs) would give the provider an objective baseline of Ms. A's level of functioning and provide information helpful in determining the need for assistance in her home.

Ovarian cancer is only the ninth most prevalent cancer among adult women in the United States, but it is the fifth deadliest cancer. Every year is the United States, 22,440 women are newly diagnosed with ovarian cancer and 14,080 women die of the disease.[5] Although the average age of diagnosis is 63 years, younger and older women are regularly diagnosed. Family history is the strongest predictor of a women being diagnosed with ovarian cancer, and there are no known ways to prevent ovarian cancer. The US Preventive Task Force Services does not recommend screening asymptomatic women for ovarian cancer because of the lack of sensitive and specific screening tests, and symptom reports remain the primary way to identify new and recurrent ovarian cancer.[6]

Although Ms. A saw the primary care provider frequently before her ovarian cancer diagnosis 3 years ago, she has not been back to the clinic since she received the referral to see the gynecologic oncologist (who diagnosed her cancer). The primary care office gave this referral based on Ms. A's report of symptoms of abdominal pain, significant fluid-like weight gain in her belly (ascites), and a computed tomography (CT) scan that identified a mass near her left fallopian tube. The provider does not know additional details beyond Ms. A's diagnosis and surgery, which are listed in her medical history.

The patient's previous treatments for her cancer are missing, including the date of primary diagnosis; stage and grade of primary tumor; previous treatments including surgery(ies), chemotherapy regimen(s), and any radiation therapy(ies); any recurrences; and any complications or concerns arising after treatment. Because she is currently posttreatment, the health care provider should attempt to identify if Ms. A has a survivorship care plan summarizing her oncologic history and plans for future care. However, although the Commission on Cancer requires accredited programs to provide survivorship care plans to individuals completing cancer treatment,[7] an overwhelming minority of patients currently receive survivorship care plans and fewer have these plans listed in their electronic medical record. Because many of the guidelines for cancer survivorship focus on breast cancer, there is limited information about best follow-up care planning for women with a history of ovarian cancer and other less prevalent cancers. Therefore primary care providers must consider the unique cancer and health history of an individual while providing them with their ongoing care.

3. What diagnostics are necessary for this patient at this time?

Although there are no imminent signs that Ms. A is experiencing a complication from her ovarian cancer or a cancer recurrence, the primary care provider is primarily focused on assessing and determining whether there is a relationship between Ms. A's presenting symptoms and her oncologic history. For example, the provider can more thoroughly assess Ms. A's symptoms related to ovarian cancer by asking for additional physical and emotional symptoms she has experienced recently, especially within the last 2 weeks. As previously noted, symptoms that are commonly associated with a new or recurrent ovarian cancer diagnosis and therefore should be thoroughly assessed include abdominal bloating/swelling, back pain, changes in urinary or bowel function, early satiety, and difficulty eating.[8]

Importantly, some older adults may not report symptoms because they learn to tolerate symptoms, attribute them to old age, or fear the diagnosis or treatment of an illness. Providing health care to older adults may be complicated by atypical presentation of acute illness, and severe acute or chronic conditions may present with vague, nonspecific symptoms. The provider can encourage Ms. A and her daughter in reviewing the presence and evolution of her symptoms and encouraging honest, timely reporting of new and distressing symptoms.

Because Ms. A's oncology team led her care during the diagnosis and treatment of her ovarian cancer, it is important that this patient is again referred to her gynecologic oncology team and that the new presentation of symptoms is communicated to that oncology team. Currently, there are no screening tests for ovarian cancer (either a primary or recurrent diagnosis). Although the pelvic examination would allow the health care provider to palpate a large mass, most tumors would not be grossly palpated during physical examination. A blood test to determine Ms. A's serum cancer antigen 125 (Ca-125) level is a nonspecific but comparatively useful test for individuals with a personal history of ovarian cancer.[9] Although not recommended as a screening tool for ovarian cancer among asymptomatic women in a primary care setting,[10] Ca-125 levels can be compared with a woman's previous levels to provide a rough estimate of the amount of tumor present. The provider, in consultation with Ms. A's oncology team, can order a complete blood count (CBC) in addition to a Ca-125 test to identify any abnormalities and compare her current Ca-125 levels to her previous levels. Also in conjunction with the oncology team, a CT and/or positron emission tomography (PET) scan to assess for a suspected cancer recurrence is indicated, although the final diagnosis of a recurrence will require a tissue biopsy and pathology. According to the Agency for Healthcare Research and Quality (AHRQ) guideline for the management of a suspicious adnexal mass, a transvaginal ultrasound should be the first modality of choice in patients with a suspicious, isolated ovarian mass.[11] Magnetic resonance imaging (MRI) is the most appropriate test to help clarify the malignant potential in patients in which ultrasound may be unreliable. CT is most useful in cases in which extra ovarian disease is suspected or needs to be excluded as part of the differential diagnosis.

The primary care provider should order a urinalysis and culture and sensitivity to determine whether there is a urinary tract infection. A CBC is necessary to assess the possibility of anemia. The provider should also order a BRAC1 and BRAC2, as well as a TSH, to assess thyroid status and determine whether Ms. A's weight gain is associated with changes in thyroid function. To determine whether the urinary frequency is caused by diabetes mellitus, the provider should also order a fasting blood sugar and hemoglobin A1C. To establish the cause of her abdominal issues, an intense workup for abdominal pain should be considered, focused on the lower quadrants in which the patient reports pain and the physical examination revealed distension. However, the major concerns are her symptoms of early satiety, weight gain, urinary frequency, and the findings of a possible adnexal mass and ascites.

The health care provider should note from Ms. A's family history that her sister died of ovarian cancer at age 50 and her mother died of breast cancer at age 60. This strong history of ovarian and breast cancer among Ms. A's first-degree relatives should raise concerns of possible genetic mutations, namely BRCA1 and BRCA2. These gene mutations raise individuals' risks for ovarian, breast, pancreatic, and prostate cancers.[12] The provider should inquire if she and/or anyone in her family has undergone testing for the BRCA1 and BRCA2 gene mutations because these dominant mutations are passed through men and women. Women with an increased risk because of family history should be considered for genetic counseling to further evaluate their potential risks.[13] Increased risk related to family history generally means having two or more first- or second-degree relatives with a history of ovarian cancer or a combination of breast and ovarian cancer. First-degree relatives of women with ovarian cancer should seek genetic counseling to determine whether genetic testing is warranted. If Ms. A has not undergone testing and meets the guidelines for genetic counseling, she should receive a referral for testing along with a referral to a genetic counselor to evaluate her risk and her children's and grandchildren's risk for cancer.[13,14]

4.   What treatments are recommended for this patient today?

Treatment for the urinary frequency depends on the results of her urinalysis and hemoglobin A1C to determine whether the frequency is caused by an infection, incontinence, stones, or hyperglycemia.

Although Ms. A describes that her over-the-counter and home remedies have not reduced her abdominal pain, it is important to recommend evidence-based treatments for abdominal pain based on the results of the abdominal pain workup and cause of pain. In additional to routine pain management protocols, the health care provider can also consider management strategies proposed by the Oncology Nursing Society to manage abdominal pain.[15] Independent of the etiology of the pain, nonpharmacologic and behavioral treatments for cancer survivors can be used to assist Ms. A in managing the pain until her workup is complete. Because her bowel function has changed in the past weeks, medications for constipation are possibly indicated, but assessing her diet and fluid intake is also necessary. A kidneys, ureter, bladder (KUB) x-ray to determine whether Ms. A is constipated may be indicated initially because arranging an abdominal CT or MRI may take longer.

Based on the assessment of other symptoms, the health care provider can also use the Oncology Nursing Society's Putting Evidence into Practice guidelines to find a synthesized collection of evidence-based treatments for patients with cancer and cancer survivors experiencing cancer-related and treatment-related symptoms.[16] These treatment recommendations are written for a wide audience with citations to support their level of effectiveness, permitting primary care and other nurse specialties to implement these strategies within their care.

The provider caring for Ms. A needs to collaborate with the gynecologic oncologist to review her past pain medications and recommended treatments. Typical treatments for severe pain include morphine, a fentanyl patch, hydromorphone, and methadone. A tapering regimen would be created for when Ms. A's pain improves, which includes using nonsteroidal antiinflammatories such as aspirin, or ibuprofen, or acetaminophen.

The health care provider also should discuss nonpharmaceutical ways to address the patient's pain, including guided imagery, aromatherapy, and massage. Ms. A indicates previous success using massage to address pain, and the provider reviews Ms. A's cultural beliefs about pain and pain medication to determine whether she has any concerns that would affect her willingness to take pain medications. The patient is started on Oxycodone 5 milligrams po to be taken every 4-6 hours as needed for pain. The health care provider works with Ms. A and her daughter to provide pain education including safe use and storage of medicine, side effects of opioids, and limitations to driving.

Case Study, Continued

Ms. A does not report any additional symptoms that require immediate attention, and she assures the provider that she will report any new or distressing symptoms to her oncology team and her in the future.

SECOND PRIMARY CARE VISIT

The next week, the results of Ms. A's abdominal workup (separate from the ovarian cancer workup) are negative, indicating that her pain is not related to other abdominal issues. Ms. A reports that her pain has gone from a 7 to a 3 with medication and massage therapy. The health care provider completes the same pain assessment to determine the intensity, duration, and so forth of the pain and if she is experiencing any breakthrough pain. Then the provider assesses whether or not a long-acting pain medication combined with a short-acting medication for breakthrough pain is warranted or if the pain is resolving. She continues to collaborate with the gynecologic oncologist in case this pain is cancer-related or treatment-related.

The results of her urinalysis show no infection, and the hemoglobin A1C is within normal range, indicating that the frequency of urination is not caused by an infection, incontinence, stones, or diabetes. Ms. A reports tracking the number of times she is voiding per day, which she notes has diminished as her abdominal pain has decreased.

The BRCA testing results indicated that Ms. A does not have a mutation for either BRCA1 or BRCA2, indicating that she is not at increased genetic risk for breast and ovarian cancer. The genetic testing also indicates that her children and grandchildren are less likely to have these cancers, although BRCA mutations are also carried by men.

5.   What are your next steps?

If the primary care provider is not intimately aware of Ms. A's oncologic history, then the provider's priority should be to identify the primary gynecologic oncologist involved in Ms. A's oncologic care. Frequently, patients receiving cancer treatment rely on their gynecologic oncologist for most of their health needs and do not return to their primary care provider until after treatment has ended. Even if patients have no evidence of disease, their ongoing care provider must consider their past treatments and ongoing follow-up needs including new and ongoing long-term side effects, routine surveillance for cancer recurrence, screening for early detection of new cancers, reinforcement of health-promoting behaviors, and issues that patients faced while receiving treatment (e.g., emotional problems, financial issues, spiritual concerns, etc.).

After treatment ends, women with a history of ovarian cancer typically have routine transvaginal ultrasound scans and Ca-125 blood tests every 6 months. It is not uncommon for women to experience recurrences and additional chemotherapy treatment.

Once the primary oncologist is identified, the health care provider can request a meeting or conversation to review her oncology history, identify if a survivorship care plan exists, and collaboratively develop an ongoing plan of care. If a survivorship care plan does not exist, the Society for Gynecologic Oncology offers a basic template[17] that can be tailored to Ms. A's cancer experience and needs. Because the urinary and abdominal tests were negative, the health care provider aims to determine whether the nature of Ms. A's urinary frequency and abdominal pain is related to her cancer history. Even if testing reveals that Ms. A's pain is related to a cancer recurrence or a new malignancy, the health care provider can remain involved in Ms. A's care by collaborating with the oncology team to discuss a co-management model of care to ensure treatment for her comorbidities aligns with the treatment for her cancer. Oncology and primary care can integrate their care models to treat her based on their respective specialties, ensuring that the expertise of each clinician is maximized and each understands the care Ms. A receives from the other clinician.

With respect to Ms. A's health promotion needs, the health care provider should support Ms. A in maintaining a healthy lifestyle as a cancer survivor. The BMI of 31.9 indicates that Ms. A is obese. Before introducing any modifications to her diet and physical activity, the health care provider needs to review the results of Ms. A's CBC to detect nutritional deficiencies. The patient's comorbidities need to be reviewed before starting a new dietary regimen, especially any contra-indications and limitations from her arthritis, high blood pressure, and hyperlipidemia. Evidence-based diet and exercise recommendations from the American Cancer Society[18] for individuals receiving treatment for cancer and cancer survivors should also be considered.

Case Study, Continued

Immediately after the appointment, the primary health care provider calls the gynecologic oncologist Ms. A indicated was her primary oncologist. The oncologist reviews Ms. A's past treatments and health status the last time he saw her 3 months ago for a follow-up scan. Her treatments included a hysterectomy with bilateral salpingo-oophorectomy (previously noted in her surgical history) and six rounds of intravenous carboplatin and Taxol combination chemotherapy. He has a copy of Ms. A's survivorship care plan using the hospital's template, which he offers to send electronically to the primary care office. He notes that it has a summary of her diagnosis, treatment, and suggested follow-up visits. The health care provider reviews Ms. A's urinary frequency and abdominal pain assessment, and the two clinicians collaborate to discuss a plan for diagnosing and treating this pain. They agree that a pelvic ultrasound, Ca-125 blood serum test, and follow-up visit with the gynecologic oncologist is warranted along with additional workups for the urinary and abdominal symptoms.

Ms. A's Ca-125 level is 337, which the provider sends to the gynecologic oncologist for interpretation and comparison with Ms. A's previous levels. The pelvic ultrasound was positive for a mass, which the gynecologic oncology team will review.

Ms. A's CBC indicated no nutritional deficits (e.g., anemia, low white count), and her overall health is strong enough for her to introduce moderate changes to her diet and physical activity. The health care provider consults with Ms. A's other health team members to review recommended physical activity guidelines for individuals who are older and have comorbidities of hypertension, high cholesterol, and arthritis.

At the next appointment, the health care provider asks Ms. A about her dietary and physical activity habits and assesses her level of interest and motivation to making changes. Although Ms. A indicates interest in being healthy, she notes that previous attempts to change her routines have not worked. She also comments that since her cancer diagnosis she is reluctant to attempt to lose weight or overexert herself because of ongoing fatigue. The health care provider emphasizes that cancer survivors improve their quality of life and fitness by engaging in healthy activity. Then the provider reinforces that a healthy, well-balanced diet, rich in whole grains, lean meats, fruits, and vegetables, is recommended for individuals with a history of cancer and that physical activity is safe and feasible during and after cancer treatment. Recommendations are provided for Ms. A to engage in moderate levels of physical activity at least 150 minutes per week, including strength training at least 2 days a week, according to guidelines from the American Cancer Society.[18] The provider works with Ms. A and her daughter to create goals for healthy eating and physical activity that account for her ongoing health comorbidities. They agree on a plan to incorporate walking and water aerobics at their nearby senior center 3 days a week. As a pair, they plan that in the next month they will reduce the amount of fast food they eat and increase fish and fresh vegetables and fruits at least 5 days a week. They strategize specific ways to integrate these goals into their daily living.

The primary care provider asks if Ms. A is aware of advocacy and support groups for individuals with cancer, especially ovarian cancer, in her city. Because Ms. A has primarily relied on her family for her caregiving and support needs, she has not reached out to others with ovarian cancer but is interested in seeing their resources. She is referred to the American Cancer Society local chapter, the National

Ovarian Cancer Coalition, and Facing Our Risk of Cancer Empowered. These advocacy organizations provide trustworthy health information, resources, support groups, and advocacy for patients and family members and have national and local chapters.

6. What are the health care provider's priorities for Ms. A's next visit?

The goal of the next visit will be to, alongside her oncology team, determine whether the cause of the urinary frequency and abdominal pain is related to Ms. A's cancer history, a new recurrence, or a benign process unrelated to her cancer. Depending on the underlying cause, the primary health care provider will either work with the oncology team to treat the cancer and manage her other health care problems or start a robust plan to manage her abdominal pain. In either case, the health care provider should be concerned with ensuring that Ms. A receives an accurate, robust survivorship care plan from the oncology team to ensure comprehensive documentation of Ms. A's cancer history and guidelines for possible and likely long-term consequences relevant to her ongoing primary care. The survivorship care plan should be kept up to date as her treatment and issues evolve over time. Also, the plan should be shared across Ms. A's team of health care providers so that all clinicians are aware of her history and understand their respective role in providing follow-up care. The health care provider is aware that Ms. A will likely need continuing care from her oncology team and that Ms. A may prefer to primarily receive her care with her oncology team[19] that will implement recommendations from the Society of Gynecologic Oncology[20,21] and other national oncology organizations. However, the health care provider recognizes that it is the role of primary care to maintain the overall health and continued support of Ms. A alongside her other care providers.

Because the possibility of a recurrence or a new cancer is likely to illicit fear, anxiety, and stress to both Ms. A and her family members, the primary care provider can also assess how the family caregivers (daughter, husband, and other children) are coping with this process and if they have any concerns. Many patients with a history of cancer experience a fear of recurrence, and once a possible recurrence is detected, they may begin to have clinical symptoms of distress, posttraumatic stress disorder from their original diagnosis, and depression. Moreover, their caregivers may face their own emotional reaction and have concerns about their ability to provide support. The health care provider can assess for these symptoms and if necessary refer the patient and caregiver to a psycho-oncology specialist. Most cancer centers have a psychologist or psychiatrist to whom Ms. A can be referred.

Case Study, Continued

Ms. A's Ca-125 and pelvic ultrasound are determined to not be a cancer recurrence by the oncology team. The palpated mass is expected to be benign. To verify this, Ms. A is scheduled for a biopsy. Ms. A and her daughter are extremely relieved, although they recognize that this type of recurrence situation could happen (and is likely to occur) in the future.

The oncology team continues to update the primary care team on Ms. A's status, demonstrating communication and collaboration across the two clinics. The two treatment teams agree that the primary care team will focus on treating Ms. A's current symptoms in addition to encouraging health promotion, cancer screenings, and management of her comorbidities (in consultation with her additional specialists). They develop an ongoing communication plan because their medical record systems are not unified. They work together to update and expand Ms. A's survivorship care plan as a template to document her ongoing cancer treatment and managing her symptoms, quality-of-life concerns, and other cancer-related issues. A plan is made to taper the patient off Oxycodone and to reevaluate her pain intensity and characteristics. They share this plan with Ms. A and her family, encouraging their input. They also share the survivorship care plan with Ms. A's other health care teams.

Ms. A schedules her cancer screenings accordingly to national guidelines. Although she tested negative for the BRCA mutation, she wishes to continue to have mammograms annually. A colonoscopy will be scheduled after the biopsy because she was due to have it within this calendar year. Planning the timing of subsequent cancer screenings can be determined with conversations between Ms. A, her oncologist, and primary care team. She has not had a Pap smear in the past 10 years because her radical hysterectomy removed her cervix; therefore she does not need screening for cervical cancer. Because she has no smoking history, lung cancer testing is not indicated.

Ms. A continues to engage in more physical activity and healthy eating according to the American Cancer Society guidelines. Although her goals of increasing healthy foods like fish, vegetables, and fruits and working out at the senior center are difficult to integrate into her life, she is committed to staying as healthy as possible and regaining her active lifestyle, which she lost during her cancer treatment. Therefore the provider adjusts her short-term goal to be more attainable for the next month, and plans to adjust her goal as she and her family slowly make changes to their diet and physical activity patterns. The provider again reinforces that safe adjustments to diet and physical activity are recommended for patients with a history of cancer.

Ms. A starts attending events sponsored by her local chapter of the National Ovarian Cancer Coalition including a monthly support group and a monthly educational series. Even though she is not experiencing a cancer recurrence now, she finds it helpful to hear about topics related to survivorship, advocacy, and quality of life. She enjoys meeting women who have gone through the same type of cancer and feels comfortable sharing her story and her concerns with these women. Although her husband, daughter, family, and friends support her, there are certain topics that she does not want to burden her family with, especially concerns about cancer recurring. Nonetheless, Ms. A relies on the strong social and emotional support she receives from her family and with them remains vigilant in maintaining her health and communicating changes in her health as an ovarian cancer survivor.

References

1. Salani, R., Backes, F. J., Fung, M. F. K., Holschneider, C. H., Parker, L. P., Bristow, R. E., et al. (2011). Posttreatment surveillance and diagnosis of recurrence in women with gynecologic malignancies: Society of Gynecologic Oncologists recommendations. *American Journal of Obstetrics and Gynecology, 204*(6), 466–478.
2. Oldenmenger, W. H., Pleun, J., de Klerk, C., & van der Rijt, C. C. (2013). Cut points on 0–10 numeric rating scales for symptoms included in the Edmonton Symptom Assessment Scale in cancer patients: A systematic review. *Journal of Pain and Symptom Management, 45*(6), 1083–1093.
3. National Cancer Institute. (2017). Patient cancer pain. Retrieved from https://www.cancer.gov/about-cancer/treatment/side-effects/pain/pain-hp-pdq.
4. Kurlowicz, L., & Greenberg, S. A. (2007). The Geriatric Depression Scale (GDS). *The American Journal Of Nursing, 107*(10), 67–68.
5. Siegel, R. L., Miller, K. D., & Jemal, A. (2016). Cancer statistics, 2016. *CA: A Cancer Journal for Clinicians, 66*(1), 7–30.
6. U.S. Preventive Services Task Force. (2016). Final Recommendation Statement: Ovarian Cancer: Screening. Retrieved from https://www.uspreventiveservicestaskforce.org/Page/Document/RecommendationStatementFinal/ovarian-cancer-screening.
7. Commission on Cancer. (2016). Cancer Program Standards: Ensuring Patient-Centered Care.
8. Goff, B. A., Mandel, L. S., Drescher, C. W., Urban, N., Gough, S., Schurman, K. M., et al. (2007). Development of an ovarian cancer symptom index. *Cancer, 109*(2), 221–227.
9. Sölétormos, G., Duffy, M. J., Hassan, S. O. A., Verheijen, R. H., Tholander, B., Bast, R. C., Jr., et al. (2016). Clinical use of cancer biomarkers in epithelial ovarian cancer: updated guidelines from the European group on tumor markers. *International Journal of Gynecological Cancer, 26*(1), 43–51.
10. Buys, S. S., Partridge, E., Black, A., Johnson, C. C., Lamerato, L., Isaacs, C., et al. (2011). Effect of screening on ovarian cancer mortality: the Prostate, Lung, Colorectal and Ovarian (PLCO) cancer screening randomized controlled trial. *JAMA: The Journal of the American Medical Association, 305*(22), 2295–2303.

11. Dodge, J. E., Covens, A. L., Lacchetti, C., Elit, L. M., Le, T., Devries–Aboud, M., et al. (2012). Management of a suspicious adnexal mass: A clinical practice guideline. *Current Oncology*, *19*(4), e244–e257.

12. Petrucelli, N., Daly, M. B., & Feldman, G. L. Hereditary breast and ovarian cancer due to mutations in BRCA1 and BRCA2. Genetics in Medicine, 12(5), 245–259.

13. Berliner, J. L., & Fay, A. M. (2007). Risk assessment and genetic counseling for hereditary breast and ovarian cancer: Recommendations of the National Society of Genetic Counselors. *Journal of Genetic Counseling*, *16*(3), 241–260.

14. National Comprehensive Cancer Network. (2016). Genetic/Familial High-Risk Assessment: Breast and Ovarian. Retrieved from https://www.tri-kobe.org/nccn/guideline/gynecological/english/genetic_familial.pdf.

15. Oncology Nursing Society. (2017). Putting Evidence into Practice: Pain. Retrieved from https://www.ons.org/practice-resources/pep/pain.

16. Oncology Nursing Society. (2017). Putting Evidence into Practice. Retrieved from https://www.ons.org/practice-resources/pep.

17. Society for Gynecological Oncology. (n.d.) Survivorship Summary. Retrieved from https://www.sgo.org/wp-content/uploads/2016/08/SGO-Ovarian-cancer-survivorship-care-plan_FINAL_form2.pdf.

18. Rock, C. L., Doyle, C., Demark-Wahnefried, W., Meyerhardt, J., Courneya, K. S., Schwartz, A. L., et al. (2012). Nutrition and physical activity guidelines for cancer survivors. *CA: A Cancer Journal for Clinicians*, *62*(4), 242–274.

19. Hudson, S. V., Miller, S. M., Hemler, J., Ferrante, J. M., Lyle, J., Oeffinger, K. C., et al. (2012). Adult cancer survivors discuss follow-up in primary care: 'NOT what I want, but maybe what I need'. *Annals of Family Medicine*, *10*(5), 418–427.

20. Salani, R., Backes, F. J., Fung, M. F. K., Holschneider, C. H., Parker, L. P., Bristow, R. E., et al. (2011). Posttreatment surveillance and diagnosis of recurrence in women with gynecologic malignancies: Society of Gynecologic Oncologists recommendations. *American Journal of Obstetrics and Gynecology*, *204*(6), 466–478.

21. Salani, R., Khanna, N., Frimer, M., Bristow, R. E., & Chen, L. M. (2017). An update on post-treatment surveillance and diagnosis of recurrence in women with gynecologic malignancies: Society of Gynecologic Oncology (SGO) recommendations. *Gynecologic Oncology*, *146*(1), 3–10.

Hoarseness

Laura J. Thiem

Case Study Scenario/History of Present Illness

Todd Summers is a 62-year-old married Caucasian male who presents to the primary care office complaining of a sore throat, hoarseness, fatigue, and enlarged lymph nodes for the past 7 days. He describes the symptoms as constant, maybe slightly worse than yesterday. He has had similar symptoms three times in the past 6 months. He has been prescribed antibiotics, with improvement in throat pain and lymph nodes becoming smaller, but the sore throat and lymph nodes reappear after a few weeks. He denies fever, headache, shortness of breath, or other recent illnesses.

Medications: Over-the-counter (OTC) ranitidine 150 milligrams by mouth (po) daily, levothyroxine 112 micrograms po daily, and polyethylene glycol (Miralax) 17 grams added to 4 ounces of juice po daily.

Allergies: Cephalexin (rash).

Habits: 1 ounce vodka daily in cocktail. Swims or bikes daily at the local gym where he has a membership. Nonsmoker.

Past medical history: GERD, constipation, and hypothyroidism.

Past surgical history: None.

Personal history: Married since 2008. Has been in monogamous relationship with wife since 1983. He is employed by the state as a case worker. He has a high school education and some college coursework but did not complete a degree.

Family history: Maternal grandfather + coronary artery disease (CAD), died with myocardial infarction (MI). Maternal grandmother type 2 diabetes mellitus (DM II), chronic kidney disease (CKD), hypertension. Paternal grandfather chronic obstructive pulmonary disease (COPD). Maternal grandmother died from head trauma. Father deceased, age 90, atrial fibrillation, hypertension. Mother deceased, age 88, atrial fibrillation, CAD, pulmonary hypertension. Four sisters living "well as far as I know."

Review of Systems

General: Admits fatigue. Denies fever or chills.

Skin: Denies rashes or lesions, changes in texture in hair or skin.

Head, eyes, ears, nose, and throat (HEENT): Denies headache, rhinorrhea, or changes in vision.

Neck: Denies pain beyond tender lymph nodes, denies stiffness.

Respiratory: Denies cough, shortness of breath, or sputum production.

Cardiac: Denies chest pressure, pain, palpitations.

Gastrointestinal: Denies nausea, vomiting, weight loss, diarrhea. + constipation.

Urinary: Denies urinary hesitancy, burning, and frequency.

Musculoskeletal: Denies muscle aches or joint pain.

Peripheral vascular: Denies swollen legs, calf pain, or cramps.

Neurovascular: Denies numbness, tingling, or burning in extremities.

Hematologic: Denies bruising, bleeding gums.

Endocrine: Denies intolerance of heat or cold, changes in hair or skin texture.
Psychiatric: Patient Health Questionnaire 2 (PHQ-2) in the past 2 weeks. He denies feeling down or sad mood. He also denies loss of interest in his usual activities.

Physical Examination

General: Well-nourished, well-groomed Caucasian male appearing stated age.
Vital signs: Height 72 inches, weight 182 pounds. Body mass index (BMI) 23.4. Temperature 98.2°F, blood pressure 122/80, heart rate 76 regular, respiratory rate 14 at rest, O_2 saturation on room air 99% at rest.
Skin: Warm/dry. No jaundice, rash, or lesions.
Eyes: Sclera clear; conjunctiva, no injection, no exophthalmos.
Ears: Canals clear, no cerumen. Tympanic membranes (TMs) no erythema, bulging/retraction.
Nose: Slightly deviated septum, nares intact, moist. No sinus tenderness.
Mouth/pharynx: Membranes moist, adequate dentition, no missing or damaged teeth. Slight thin, clear postnasal drainage. Slight pharyngeal erythema. Tonsillar tissue left 1+, right 2+ nonexudative. No lesions of tongue or buccal mucosa. No halitosis.
Neck: Supple. Thyroid expected size, shape, and consistency. Enlarged anterior cervical lymph nodes, soft, tender to palpation; right side nodes larger than left. Posterior cervical, submandibular, and submental nodes nonpalpable.
Cardiac: Regular rhythm. No gallop, murmurs, or rubs.
Respiratory: Clear to auscultation bilaterally without wheezes or crackles.
Abdomen: Scaphoid, soft, bowel sounds occurring every 2 to 3 seconds in all quadrants. No organomegaly or tenderness.
Extremities: Pedal pulses present bilaterally, no edema or calf tenderness, capillary refill 1 to 2 seconds in digits.
Neurologic: Alert, oriented to person, place, time, and situation. Appears to be adequate historian. Thought coherent. No tremors noted. Cranial nerves II to XII grossly intact. Gait smooth, coordinated. Romberg negative. No pronator drift. Muscle tone 3/5 upper/lower extremities. Reflexes: Biceps: 1+ bilaterally, triceps 1+ bilaterally. Knees: 2+ bilaterally. Ankles: 1+ bilaterally. Plantar: Down bilaterally.

1. Mr. Summers complains of recurrent sore throat, hoarseness, lymphadenopathy, and fatigue over a period of 6 months. What additional information will the health care provider need to glean to guide his care? Describe potential barriers to care that may be encountered by Mr. Summers in his interactions with the health care providers and system

The "reason for seeking care" is a brief phrase or sentence in the patient's own words describing his or her reason for interacting with the health care provider.[1] By shifting away from "chief complaint" language the encounter is framed in a positive manner rather than establishing that the patient is complaining.[1] Subsequently, the history of present illness (HPI) delves further into the chief complaint and is guided methodically by the provider to encourage the patient to provide additional information regarding his illness and experience. The provider may use a mnemonic device such as OLD CARTS (onset, location/radiation, duration, character, aggravating factors, relieving factors, timing, and severity) to assist in expanding and clarifying the history. The responses need to be recorded in the patient's own words. Explore terms the patient uses to ensure an accurate portrayal of the patient and record of his symptoms. Avoid interpreting the patient's words into medical terms.

Additional concerns during the patient/provider encounter are the ability of the patient to participate fully in the interview and examination process. Evaluating the patient's hearing and communication skills and mental status early in the interview affects the success and outcome of the patient/provider interaction. Establish the patient's ability to provide his own history and direct his own care.[1]

Ensure the setting is quiet, private, well lit, and at a comfortable temperature. Avoid interruptions or distractions created by equipment, technology, or furniture. Position yourself at the same height or lower than the patient with an opportunity for eye contact to balance the power in the interaction.[1] According to Jarvis,[1] if the health care provider is standing during the interview, the stance can suggest that the provider is impatient; it also places the patient in an inferior or subservient position, impairing communication.

Providing patient-centered care requires the provider to ascertain the patient's expectation of the visit.[2] Once this information is elicited, the provider can proceed with additional questions, examination, and shared planning of care. It is important to explain to the patient that you will be taking notes or using an electronic health record during the interview. Describe the interview procedure and request permission to proceed.

Additional questions to ask Mr. Summers may include:

- How can I best help you today? (Asking this question helps establish the patient's expectations of today's visit.)
- Do think your sore throat is related to heartburn or GERD?
- How often do you experience these symptoms?
- Do you cough at night?
- In your past experiences with the sore throat and enlarged lymph nodes, have you ever had a fever?
- In the past when experiencing a sore throat, have you ever had a swab collected to test for strep throat or other testing?
- Do you feel that food gets stuck after you swallow it or do you feel like you have trouble swallowing?
- Have you had to change the way you eat or drink because of your sore throat?
- Have you ever had a health care provider use a tool or scope to look at your throat or esophagus?
- What kind of changes have you noticed in your voice?

Case Study, Continued

Further conversation with Mr. Summers indicates that he would like a different antibiotic. "Amoxicillin doesn't seem to be getting rid of whatever this is." He answers that he has not had a throat swab or other diagnostic testing related to his sore throat or enlarged lymph nodes. "They just give me Amoxicillin and tell me to come back if I'm not better. I always get better but it comes back." He has never had an esophagogas-troduodenoscopy (EGD). He feels that his GERD is well controlled with the OTC ranitidine. He denies that he has had to alter his eating habits and denies feeling that food gets stuck in his esophagus.

2. Based on Mr. Summers' history and physical examination, what differential diagnoses should be considered?

Mr. Summers' symptoms are complex because of comorbidities and duration of symptoms. With recurrent pharyngitis, the etiology could be a bacterial, fungal, or viral infection or possibly a malignancy. Atypical symptoms of GERD, including chronic laryngitis and recurrent pharyngitis, must be considered.[3] The persistent lymphadenopathy could indicate recurrence of bacterial or viral infection, malignancy, or a structural abnormality.

3. What is the Patient Health Questionnaire-2?

The provider is aware that the PHQ-2 is a screening tool used to identify depression symptoms.[4] Today's result does not indicate concerning mood symptoms.

4. What diagnostic testing should be considered?

A rapid streptococcal test along with a pharyngeal culture would assist the provider in identifying bacterial or fungal causes of pharyngitis. Testing for the Epstein–Barr virus or Epstein–Barr heterophile antibodies to identify mononucleosis would also be helpful. A complete blood count (CBC) to identify infection or malignancies of the hematopoietic system should also be considered. A thyroid-stimulating hormone (TSH) is indicated because he does have a history of hypothyroidism.

Ordering an ultrasound (US) or computed tomography scan (CT) of the soft tissues of the neck to measure the size of the lymph nodes is a consideration to identify appearance or structural conditions that would require a biopsy to rule out malignancy. The health care provider initially decides to check Mr. Summers' laboratory tests and throat culture before ordering a US, but the provider notes that the enlarged lymph node is concerning because of size, location, and recurrence. Mr. Summers will require follow-up to ensure complete resolution even if Mr. Summers' diagnostic testing reveals an infectious process.

Each encounter by a patient in the primary care setting provides an opportunity to review the chart for the patient's last laboratory studies and offer recommended screening studies appropriate for age, gender, and family history. Mr. Summers is 62 years old and has a family history of CAD and DM II. Information about his renal and hepatitis function can also assist the provider in selection of medication should antibiotic therapy be indicated.

The health care provider discusses these concerns and a tentative plan to determine the cause of the symptoms with Mr. Summers. The patient expresses understanding of the reasoning for having the tests and agrees to have fasting labs the next morning.

5. Mr. Summers' rapid strep test is negative. The Epstein–Barr heterophile antibody test is also negative. The complete blood count, complete metabolic profile, lipid profile, and thyroid-stimulating hormone are noted below. The report for the throat culture will not be received for 48 hours.

CBC:
White blood count (WBC): 10.5 (4.0–11.0 K/mm^3)
Hemoglobin (Hgb): 12.3 (11–16 grams/dL)
Hematocrit (Hct): 36.4 (35%–48%)
Mean corpuscular volume (MCV): 88 (80–100 fL)
Platelets: 200 (130–400 K/mm^3)
Neutrophils % (Auto): 72 (37.0%–80.0%)
Lymphocytes % (Auto): 24 (23.0%–45.0%)
Neutrophils # (Auto): 2 (1.9–7.5 K/mm^3)
Lymphocytes #:2 (1.2–3.4 K/mm^3)

Na	140	mEq/L	Ca	9.9	milligrams/dL	Hgb A1C	5.0	%
K	4.0	mEq/L	Phosphorus	3.2	milligrams/dL	Fasting lipid profile:	—	—
Cl	95	mEq/L	AST	21	IU/L	Total cholesterol	189	milligrams/dL

CO$_2$	22	mEq/L	**ALT**	15	IU/L	**HDL**	78	milligrams/dL
BUN	14	milligrams/dL	**Alkaline phosphatase**	45	IU/L	**LDL**	105	milligrams/dL
SCr	0.8	milligrams/dL	**Total bilirubin**	0.9	milligrams/dL	**Triglycerides**	145	milligrams/dL
Fasting glucose	88	milligrams/dL	—	—	—	**TSH**	2.0	mU/L

ALT, alanine transaminase; *AST,* aspartate transaminase; *BUN,* blood urea nitrogen; *HDL,* high-density lipoprotein; *Hgb,* hemoglobin; *LDL,* low-density lipoprotein; *SCr,* serum creatinine; *TSH,* thyroid-stimulating hormone.

6. What are important considerations for the health care provider during the conversation with Mr. Summers about the diagnostic results? How do you explain the diagnostic test results to Mr. Summers? After reviewing the diagnostics with Mr. Summers what will you suggest to him as a plan of care? What socioeconomic factors may influence the decision making for Mr. Summers? What information do we need to provide so that Mr. Summers can make an informed decision?

It is important to also explain to Mr. Summers that the throat culture results will be available in approximately 48 hours. Mr. Summers should be advised that the tests do not indicate a bacterial or viral infection and that an antibiotic is not indicated to treat his symptoms. His renal, hepatic, and thyroid function are within acceptable limits and are not concerning. His fasting blood sugar is within an acceptable range and the Hgb A1C of 5.0% does not indicate prediabetes or diabetes. However, it would be reasonable to have his fasting blood sugar repeated annually because of his family history.

His cholesterol levels are also satisfactory. The health care provider explains that by calculating his cardiovascular risk score as recommended by the American College of Cardiology (ACC)/ American Heart Association (AHA),[5] Mr. Summers has a 6.6% chance of having a stroke and/ or cardiovascular event in the next 10 years. When the result of this calculation is lower than 7.5%, the ACC/AHA guidelines do not recommend statin therapy.

During this conversation with Mr. Summers, the health care provider needs to begin to introduce information regarding the potential need for additional diagnostic testing such as imaging or referral to a specialist to further evaluate the lymph nodes, recurrent pharyngitis, and hoarseness. It is important that the health care provider describe the potential diagnostics: US or CT scan of the neck region, and laryngoscopy and EGD. Assessing the patient's knowledge of specialists to ensure the information given is understood is essential.[6] Discussing the specialists and settings in which these services are provided is also an important component of patient education and patient-centered care.[2]

Two days later the pharyngeal culture and sensitivity is received. The report reads: "Normal pharyngeal flora. No streptococcal A or B detected."

Additionally, the report does not indicate that Mr. Summers has a fungal infection. He will need the additional diagnostic testing to determine the etiology of the recurrent lymphadenopathy and sore throat. Potential concerns that he might have could include insurance coverage of services, potential out-of-pocket expenses, time off work (compensated or uncompensated), and future treatment plans. Using the SHARE approach[7] for informed and participative decision making involves these steps:

- Seek the patient's participation
- Help your patient explore and consider treatment options
- Assess your patient's values and preferences
- Reach a decision with your patient
- Evaluate your patient's decision.[7]

The SHARE process improves the patient experience and adherence to treatment plans. For the health care provider, patient satisfaction is increased and quality of care is improved.[7]

Assessment/Plan

1. **Lymphadenopathy:** A US will be ordered because this is Mr. Summer's preference and because of the expense of a CT scan.
2. **GERD:** An EGD is also recommended. However, the patient prefers to wait until the US is completed. Mr. Summers comments: "One thing at a time."

Case Study, Continued

Mr. Summers has the US of the soft tissues of his neck. The report reads: There is a slightly lobulated hypoechoic solid left neck mass. This has internal blood flow. This mass is just inferior to the angle of mandible on the left. This is concerning for malignancy or enlarged lymph node, and CT could further evaluate neck for additional masses and origin of this mass. In addition biopsy may be useful. Impression: Large solid left neck mass with malignancy not excluded.

7.   How do you explain the findings of the ultrasound? What are your recommendations at this time? What diagnoses are included in your differential diagnoses based on this finding?

Explaining diagnostic results that are unexpected or unfavorable requires a careful, methodical approach. The provider should focus the delivery in a patient-centered manner, expect emotional responses, and involve the patient in future planning.[2,8] The delivery of concerning test results requires thoughtful planning and practice by the health care provider.

Health care providers may feel uncomfortable when delivering test results or a diagnosis with a poor prognosis to the patient. The SPIKES mnemonic (Fig. 13.1) was developed by oncologists to assist in the delivery of bad or unfavorable news.[8] This methodical yet empathetic approach can foster informed consent, maintain the patient's right to direct their own care, and improve the patient-provider interaction.[8]

The first step "S" in the SPIKES mnemonic includes planning for the *setting* of the delivery of diagnostic results or adverse diagnosis. The health care provider should arrange uninterrupted time, provide a comfortable setting, and sit at the patient's level. Family members should be included if the patient requests their presence.[8]

The next step, "P," delves into ascertaining the patient's *perception* and knowledge of their health. The health care provider may explore previous experiences with similar results or diagnosis. The patient's perception of the diagnosis or test results will affect their care. The health care provider will need to delve into the patient's resources and coping mechanisms in this step.[8]

Third, the "I" indicates the need for the health care provider to be *invited* by the patient to provide additional information or guidance. Medical personnel frequently assume the patient wants or needs to know everything from the onset. This assumption can be incorrect and can cause distress for the patient if they are not prepared or able to receive extensive information. Allowing the patient to invite additional information helps provide patient comfort and allows the patient to retain information.[8]

Imparting *knowledge* is the "K" section of the SPIKES mnemonic. Similar to perception, the health care provider asks about the patient's knowledge and desire for additional information. The health care provider will need to ascertain a patient's understanding of tests, potential diagnoses, and future treatments. Identifying and providing missing details or correcting misunderstandings are also addressed in this step.[8]

The fifth step of SPIKES, "E," is *emotion*. The patient may display a variety of emotional responses that the health care provider will need to respond to in an empathetic manner. The

Setting
- Find a private location.
- Sit down, turn on the lights.
- Remove barriers to full eye contact (i.e. the slit lamp).
- Minimize interruptions.
- Appear calm and attentive.
- Acknowledge family / friends, and invite them into the conversation.

Perception
- Explore what the patient already knows.
- Find out what previous physicians have told them.
- Ask whether they know the results from previous testing.
- "What did you first think when you noticed your right eye seemed blurry?"
- "What have you been worrying about?"

Invitation
- Empower the patient: ask before you tell.
- Offer to involve significant others who are not present before proceeding.
- Find out how much detail the patient prefers.
- "What would you like to know about your diagnosis?"
- "How much detail would you like about your diagnosis and treatment?"
- "Is there anyone else you would like me to talk to?"

Knowledge
- Offer a warning shot: "I'm sorry to tell you... I wish I had better news..."
- Start chronologically: "Remember when you first noticed ...?"
- Deliver information in small pieces.
- Allow for moments of silence.
- Avoid medical terminology.
- Explain the role (or lack of role) of glasses.
- Remember that patients will not absorb many details after the initial bad news.

Empathy
- Recognize patient emotions (anger, fear, shock).
- Acknowledge / validate feelings.
- "I know this isn't what you were hoping to hear."
- "This is probably a shock to you."

Summary
- Confirm understanding, and invite questions.
- Establish a follow-up plan, emphasizing that you will work together as a team.
- Offer to speak to family members.
- Identify resources for support (low vision, support groups, etc.).
- Offer HOPE when possible: symptomatic control, minimizing pain, research.
- Give contact information.

Fig. 13.1 Modified SPIKES protocol. (From Hilkert, S. M., Cebulla, C. M., Jain, S. G., Pfeil, S. A., Benes, S. C., & Robbins, S. L. [2016]. Breaking bad news: A communication competency for ophthalmology training programs. *Survey of Ophthalmology, 61*[6], 791–798; data from Baile, W. F., Buckman, R., Lenzi, R., Glober, G., Beale, E. A., & Kudelka, A. P. [2000]. SPIKES—a six-step protocol for delivering bad news: Application to the patient with cancer. *Oncologist, 5*[4], 302–311.)

patient may express anger, disbelief, denial, or sadness. Alternatively, the patient may remain silent. Empathetic responses are based in the recognition of the emotion, identifying the connection to the information delivered, and providing the patient with the space and time to process the emotion. The health care provider should allow for silence while remaining engaged and present with the patient. The health care provider should avoid other distractions in the setting during this time focusing directly on the patient.[8]

The final step, "S" includes *strategy* and *summary*. In this step the health care provider assists the patient in forming a plan that is acceptable to the patient. Respecting the patient's perspective and allowing the patient and family time to process the information and determine their own strategy are necessary. The health care provider and staff summarize the plan and provide the patient with written information to which they can refer after they have left the office. The summary also allows the health care provider to correct misinformation or misconceptions.[8]

Use of the SPIKES mnemonic can improve the patient's experience of receiving unfavorable results. The mnemonic can also foster the patient–provider relationship for future interactions. The provider can be well prepared in advance to provide compassionate, patient-centered care.

Case Study, Continued

Mr. Summers agrees to further evaluation with a CT scan of the soft tissues of his neck. The report reads:

Dynamic images through the neck demonstrate no focal brain abnormalities. Mild maxillary mucosal thickening is seen greater on the right. Mastoid air cells are clear. The nasopharynx is within normal limits. There is some residual tonsillar tissue in the palatine tonsils with some calcification seen on the left without a dominant mass seen. There is also some lingual tonsillar tissue seen at the base of the tongue. No focal mass is seen. The epiglottis is within normal limits. The aryepiglottic folks and true vocal cords are within normal limits.

The area of palpable fullness marked with BB appears to represent an enlarged deep cervical node just below the parotid gland at the left level II. This lymph node has some low–density changes within it along its anterior aspect certainly concerning for some possible areas of necrosis. Just posterior to this is a borderline deep cervical node measuring 0.96 × 0.41 cm. The jugulodigastric node on the right is upper limits in size. No other deep cervical adenopathy is seen.

No focal thyroid masses are seen. No supraclavicular adenopathy is seen.

Apical scarring is seen.

Cervical spondylosis without acute bony changes seen.

Impression: Enlarged deep cervical node at the level II region on the left with some possible areas of necrosis along its anterior aspect. A malignant node would be the diagnosis of exclusion. The source is not definitely seen with persistent tonsillar and lingular tonsillar tissues noted, which appears fairly symmetric. A mucosal mass cannot be confirmed. No focal thyroid mass or other significant adenopathy can be identified.

8. How do you explain the findings of the CT scan to Mr. Summers and his wife when they come to the office for the CT results? What are your recommendations at this time? Has your differential diagnosis changed?

Use the SPIKES mnemonic as a method to deliver the findings of the CT scan. Provide for the patient's comfort before delivering the report results. Introduce the report with a statement that indicates the news is not favorable.[8] Provide an interpretation of the CT scan report in language consistent with the patient's health literacy.[6,8] The patient and family are informed that the report indicates a likely cancer as the cause of Mr. Summer's symptoms. Indicate that the radiology report strongly suggests that the enlarged node is a malignancy, although a biopsy is necessary for a definitive diagnosis. Inquire about their perception and understanding of the test report. Allow the patient time to request additional information. If requested, the patient and his wife should be informed that there are varied types of cancer causing his symptoms and the enlarged lymph node. The enlarged node could represent a lymphoma, squamous cell carcinoma, or metastatic cancer. Provide an empathetic response to the emotion the patient displays. Discuss the possible differential diagnoses and assist in the strategic plan for expedited referral to a surgeon for a biopsy. Summarize the findings and plan with the patient, and offer written information for future reference.

Case Study, Continued

Mr. Summers and his wife express a desire to proceed with surgical consult as long as the provider is within network for his insurance benefits. He is scheduled with the general surgeon at the local hospital for further evaluation and treatment in 2 days' time.

Mr. Summers has met with the general surgeon and had an US-guided biopsy of the lymph node. The biopsy findings suggest metastatic, poorly differentiated carcinoma. The patient was subsequently referred to oncology. The consult notes indicate the patient has been diagnosed with Stage 3 Tx N1 M0 squamous cell cancer of the throat/tonsillar tissue that is human papilloma virus positive. He has also been evaluated by otolaryngology (ENT) and gastroenterology (GI). The ENT performed a laryngoscopy with no abnormalities noted. The GI performed EGD with notable gastritis, but the biopsies were negative for malignancy. Helicobacter pylori *testing was also negative. The patient was advised to stop the ranitidine and was started on omeprazole 40 milligrams po daily. Mr. Summers will receive chemotherapy and radiation therapy under the direction of oncology.*

After the chemotherapy has been completed and surgery has been performed to remove the remaining tonsillar tissue, the patient was noted to be losing weight. Megestrol (Megace) 125 milligrams/mL 5 mL po one time a day was prescribed by oncology. Subsequently the patient developed a deep vein thrombosis (DVT) and was hospitalized because of megestrol use. The megestrol has been discontinued. You are now seeing the patient in the primary care office to manage warfarin as the patient is transitioned from enoxaparin (Lovenox) to warfarin. On discharge from the hospital Mr. Summers' international normalized ratio (INR) is 1.9. He will be seen in your office the next day. The hematology/oncology specialist directs that the warfarin therapy is to continue for 3 months because the DVT was medication related.

Mr. Summers' current medications per medication reconciliation:

Warfarin (Coumadin) 5 milligrams po daily

Enoxaparin (Lovenox) 150 milligrams/mL injected subcutaneously daily until the INR is 2 to 3 × 2 consecutive days.

Omeprazole 40 milligrams po daily

Levothyroxine 112 micrograms po daily

Miralax 17 grams in 4 ounces of fluid daily

Physical Examination

General: Mr. Summers presents to your office to check PT/INR. His wife accompanies him. He received his Lovenox injection today, which was administered by his wife.

Vital signs: Height 72 inches, weight 162 pounds. BMI 20.8. Temperature 98.0°F, blood pressure 128/78, heart rate 76 regular, respiratory rate 16 at rest, O_2 saturation on room air 99% at rest. Today his INR is 2.5, and his warfarin dose is 5 milligrams. The PHQ-2 is administered indicating that in the past 2 weeks Mr. Summers has felt down or depressed almost every day but that he has not lost interest in usual activities.

Skin: Warm/dry. No jaundice, rash, or lesions.

Eyes: Sclera clear; conjunctiva, no injection, no exophthalmos.

Ears: TMs no erythema, bulging/retraction.

Nose: Slightly deviated septum, nares intact, moist.

Mouth/pharynx: Membranes moist, adequate dentition, no missing or damaged teeth. Slight thin, clear post nasal drainage is present. Slight pharyngeal erythema is noted. Tonsillar tissue is surgically absent. No lesions of tongue or buccal mucosa are noted. No halitosis.

Neck: Supple. Thyroid expected size, shape, and consistency. Enlarged anterior cervical lymph nodes, soft, tender to palpation, right-side nodes larger than left. Posterior cervical, submandibular, and submental nodes are nonpalpable.

Cardiac: Regular rhythm, No gallop, murmurs, or rubs.

Respiratory: Clear to auscultation bilaterally without wheezes or crackles.

Extremities: Pedal pulses are present bilaterally. There is no edema or calf tenderness. Capillary refill occurs at 1 to 2 seconds in digits.

Neurologic: Alert, oriented to person, place, time, and situation. The patient appears to be an adequate historian. Thought is coherent. No tremors noted. Cranial nerves II to XII are grossly intact. Gait is smooth and coordinated.

9. Describe your expected plan of care for Mr. Summers related to deep vein thrombosis diagnosis and treatment. What patient education is needed related to warfarin (Coumadin)? What is the significance of the PHQ-2 results?

The goal INR range is 2 to 3 for DVT.[9] The primary care provider is aware that for a patient on day 5 of warfarin therapy and an INR of 2.0 to 3.0, no change in the dose is necessary. Warfarin 5 milligrams po today is ordered, and he will return to the office for another INR tomorrow. If the INR remains within the goal range, the enoxaparin (Lovenox) will be discontinued.[9]

Patient education for warfarin and enoxaparin includes discussion regarding symptoms of excessive anticoagulation that the patient should report promptly to the primary care provider or seek emergency evaluation and treatment. The patient should be instructed to check stools for bright red blood or a dark, black appearance. Urine that is darker than usual or visible blood in the urine should be reported. Nosebleeds, rashes, and bruising are also symptoms of over anticoagulation.[10]

The patient should also be instructed about dietary considerations to provide a consistent source of vitamin K that can antagonize the anticoagulant effect of warfarin. The U.S. Department of Agriculture maintains an Internet database reporting vitamin K levels (available at https://ndb.nal.usda.gov/ndb/nutrients/report?nutrient1=430&nutrient2=&nutrient3=&fg=&subset=0&offset=0&sort=c&totCount=4878&measureby=m). If the patient does not have Internet access, materials may be printed by the provider or a dietician consult may be arranged.[10]

The PHQ-2 has a positive response of depressed or down mood nearly every day, indicating the need for completion of an additional diagnostic questionnaire. The PHQ-9 is a diagnostic tool that helps identify a depression diagnosis and symptoms for targeted therapy.[11]

The results of today's PHQ-9 completed by Mr. Summers include:

1. Little interest or pleasure in doing things: 0 (not at all)
2. Feeling down, depressed or hopeless: 3 (nearly every day)
3. Trouble falling or staying asleep or sleeping too much: 0 (not at all)
4. Feeling tired or having little energy: 1 (several days)
5. Poor appetite or overeating: 3 (nearly every day)
6. Feeling bad about yourself, or that you are a failure or have let yourself or family down: 1 (several days)
7. Trouble concentrating on things, such as reading the newspaper or watching TV: 0 (not at all)
8. Moving so slowly that people could have noticed. Or the opposite, being so fidgety or restless that you have been moving around a lot more than usual: 0 (not at all)
9. Thoughts that you would be better off dead or of hurting yourself in some way: 0 (not at all)

If you checked off *any* problems, how *difficult* have these problems made it for you to do your work, take care of things at home, or get along with other people? Answer: Somewhat difficult. Total score is 8, indicating moderate depression

10.   How do you explain the PHQ-9 results to Mr. Summers? After reviewing the PHQ-9 with Mr. Summers, what will you suggest to him as a plan of care? What socioeconomic factors may influence the decision making for Mr. Summers? What information do we need to provide so that Mr. Summers can make an informed decision? How do we describe the role of therapy in the treatment of depression?

Primary care providers have an opportunity to provide early identification and treatment of depression.[12] After assessing for comorbid disease processes, suicidal ideation, and substance abuse, the primary care provider may suggest a selective serotonin reuptake inhibitor (SSRI) medication and offer collaborative treatment with a mental health professional for therapy.[12,13] Early identification and treatment are identified as highly effective in the patient achieving remission from depression symptoms within the first two steps of the STAR*D algorithm.[13]

Case Study, Continued

Mr. Summers elects to start on a medication for depression and agrees to consultation with a clinical psychologist for therapy. A consultation request is initiated. The psychologist's office will contact the patient directly to schedule for the patient's convenience. After discussing the various SSRIs including fluoxetine, paroxetine, citalopram, and sertraline, the patient chooses sertraline for treatment.

11.   The primary care provider knows that the serotonin uptake inhibitor and serotonin-norepinephrine reuptake inhibitor classes of medication have similar efficacy, so rational drug selection is based on patient preference, side effect profile, and medication expense.[14] What is the starting dose and titration for sertraline? What patient education will Mr. Summers need regarding the medication? When should we see Mr. Summers in the office again to address depression? What information should be provided about psychologists or counseling professionals?

The starting dose of sertraline is 50 milligrams po daily with an increase of 25- to 50-milligram increments weekly with a maximum of 200 milligrams po daily.[15] Older adult patients may require a lower starting dose (e.g. 25 milligrams po daily). The primary care provider can follow up in 1 week to assess for patient response to the sertraline, including adverse effects, increase in suicidal or homicidal ideation, and ability to adhere to treatment plan.[14] During this visit the provider can also verify that the patient has scheduled with a psychologist or professional to provide counseling services. Reevaluation of depression symptoms should be performed at approximately 4 weeks; patients with more severe symptoms may require a shorter visit interval.[16]

The primary care provider should be familiar with the side effect profile of the medication. For many medications in the SSRI class, the side effects include nausea, dizziness, nervousness, sexual dysfunction, hyponatremia, and weight gain.[15] Assessment for side effects includes patient interview and report, measurement of weight with each visit, and periodic laboratory monitoring.

The prescribing provider must be aware of potential life-threatening effects of psychotropic medications, including serotonin syndrome, cardiac arrhythmias, and withdrawal syndrome. Serotonin syndrome occurs when the brain has excess serotonin. A variety of causes have been established, including drug-to-drug interactions, prescribing an initial dose that is too high, or increasing the medication dose too quickly. Initial symptoms include diaphoresis, nausea, or diarrhea and they can progress to mental confusion, autonomic and musculoskeletal system problems, and death. The patient will require supportive care while the medication is withdrawn.[16]

A thorough understanding of the counseling professionals is needed to ensure appropriate referral and provide patient education so the patient knows what to expect from the professional. Psychologists are prepared at the doctoral level to provide counseling services and psychological evaluation and diagnosis using a variety of validated tools. For counseling, a variety of techniques may be used depending on the diagnosis and the patient's needs. Psychological evaluation may include intelligence, personality traits, cognition, vocational, and neuropsychological function.[17] In a few states in the United States psychologists have the authority to prescribe psychotropic medications after completing additional training.[18]

Additional professionals also provide counseling services, including social workers, licensed professional counselors, mental health counselors, nurse psychotherapists, psychiatric/mental health clinical nurse specialists, marital/family therapists, and pastoral counselors. Most of these professions are prepared with education at the master's degree level or higher.[19] Should the primary care provider determine that the patient requires prescription management beyond the knowledge and comfort of the primary care provider, the patient may be referred to a psychiatric provider. Psychiatric providers with specialized training in prescribing for mental or behavioral health include psychiatric mental health nurse practitioners (PMHNPs), psychiatric mental health clinical nurse specialists (PMHCNs),[20] or psychiatrists.[19] A psychiatrist is a physician who specializes in psychiatric conditions. Psychiatric providers may not provide counseling services in addition to medication management.[19] Some circumstances requiring psychiatric referral include the patient not responding to medication as expected, suicidal ideation, severe adverse effects of medication, or complex presentations of mental health disorders.[13]

Case Study, Continued

Mr. Summers presents to your office to check prothrombin time (PT)/INR (fifth day of warfarin therapy). He received his enoxaparin injection today administered by his wife.

Height 72 inches, weight 162 pounds. BMI 20.8. Temperature 98.0°F, blood pressure 128/78, heart rate 76 regular, respiratory rate 16 at rest, O_2 saturation on room air 99% at rest. Today his INR is 2.5 and his warfarin dose is 5 milligrams. The goal INR range is 2 to 3 for DVT.[9] The primary care provider is aware that for a patient on day 5 of warfarin therapy and an INR of 2 to 3, no change in the dose is necessary. Warfarin 5 milligrams po one time daily is ordered and the enoxaparin is discontinued.[8] Mr. Summers will come in weekly for a PT/INR while on warfarin until the health care provider deems the dose to be stable. At that time, Mr. Summers' PT/INR can be checked every 2 to 4 weeks if stable. If the warfarin dose is changed, the PT/INR testing will need to be increased. His warfarin will be continued for 3 months per the hematologist's recommendation.

Mr. Summers presents to your office to check PT/INR (12th day of warfarin therapy) and a recheck after initiating sertraline. He has had slight nausea with the sertraline but he feels that this is resolving. He denies nightmares, suicidal ideation, homicidal ideation, or changes in mood. He has an appointment with a clinical psychologist next week and expects that he will have psychological testing that day per their communication.

Height 72 inches, weight 162 pounds. BMI 20.8. Temperature 98.0°F, blood pressure 122/72, heart rate 72 regular, respiratory rate 16 at rest, O_2 saturation on room air 99% at rest. PHQ-9 results are unchanged. Today his INR is 2.8.

Review of Systems
General: Denies fatigue, fever, or chills.
Skin: Denies rashes or lesions, changes in texture in hair or skin.
HEENT: Denies headache, rhinorrhea, changes in vision. Does have some difficulty swallowing.
Neck: Denies pain, denies stiffness.

Respiratory: Denies cough, shortness of breath, or sputum production.

Cardiac: Denies chest pressure, pain, and palpitations.

Gastrointestinal: Denies nausea, vomiting, weight loss, diarrhea. + constipation.

Urinary: Denies urinary hesitancy, burning, and frequency.

Musculoskeletal: Denies muscle aches or joint pain.

Peripheral vascular: Denies swollen legs, calf pain, or cramps.

Neurovascular: Denies numbness, tingling, or burning in extremities.

Hematologic: Denies bruising or bleeding gums. Has not noted blood in stools or visible blood in urine.

Endocrine: Denies intolerance of heat or cold, changes in hair or skin texture.

Medications: Omeprazole 40 milligrams po daily; levothyroxine 112 micrograms po daily; Miralax 17 grams added to 4 ounces of juice po daily, sertraline 50 milligrams po daily, warfarin 5 milligrams po daily.

Physical Examination

General: Well-nourished, well-groomed Caucasian male appearing stated age.

Vital signs: Height 72 inches, weight 163 pounds. Temperature 98.4°F, blood pressure 128/78, heart rate 74 regular, respiratory rate 14 at rest, O_2 saturation on room air 99% at rest.

Skin: Warm/dry. No bruising, jaundice, rash, or lesions.

Eyes: Sclera clear; conjunctiva, no injection, no exophthalmos.

Ears: TMs no erythema, bulging/retraction.

Nose: Slightly deviated septum, nares intact, moist.

Mouth/pharynx: Mucous membranes are moist. Dentition is adequate without missing or damaged teeth. Slight thin, clear postnasal drainage is present. Slight pharyngeal erythema. Tonsillar tissue is surgically absent. No lesions of tongue or buccal mucosa. No halitosis.

Neck: Supple. Thyroid expected size, shape, and consistency. No lymphadenopathy noted.

Cardiac: Regular rhythm. No gallop, murmurs, or rubs.

Respiratory: Clear to auscultation bilaterally without wheezes or crackles.

Extremities: Pedal pulses present bilaterally, no edema or calf tenderness, capillary refill 1 to 2 seconds in digits.

Neurologic: Alert, oriented to person, place, time, and situation. Appears to be adequate historian. Thought is coherent. No tremors noted. Cranial nerves II to XII grossly intact. Gait smooth, coordinated.

12. Describe your plan of care for Mr. Summers today. What information should be provided or reinforced?

Today's plan would include continuing medications at the current dose. Reinforce the need for the patient to continue with the hematology/oncology specialist and to keep future appointments with the psychologist as scheduled. Advise him to continue to come into the office weekly to check PT/INR. Assess understanding of the indication and side effects of his medications. Providing patient-centered care[2] includes inquiring if he feels that he is able to manage the medications, appointments, and activities of daily living or has concerns that were not addressed today. Schedule the patient back in approximately 3 weeks to follow up on the sertraline. Provide and advise the patient of the process to contact the office or primary care provider should questions or problems arise before the next scheduled visit.

References

1. Jarvis, C. (2016). *Physical examination & health assessment* (7th ed.). St. Louis, MO: Elsevier.
2. Epstein, R., & Street, R. (2011). The values and value of patient-centered care. *Annals of Family Medicine*, *9*(2), 100–103.

3. University of Michigan Health Center. (2012). Guidelines for clinical care: Gastroesophageal Reflux Disease (GERD). Retrieved from http://ocpd.med.umich.edu/sites/default/files/guidelines/gerd.12.pdf.

4. Kroenke, K., Spitzer, R. L., & Williams, J. B. (2003). The Patient Health Questionnaire-2: Validity of a two-item depression screener. *Medical Care, 41*(11), 1284–1292. Retrieved from https://www.ncbi.nlm.nih.gov/pubmed/14583691.

5. American College of Cardiology/American Heart Association. (n.d.) ACCVD risk estimator [Internet-based tool]. Retrieved from http://tools.acc.org/ASCVD-Risk-Estimator/.

6. US Department of Health and Human Services. (n.d.). Health literacy: Fact Sheet. Retrieved from https://health.gov/communication/literacy/quickguide/factsbasic.htm.

7. Agency for Healthcare Research and Quality. (2017). The SHARE approach. Retrieved from https://www.ahrq.gov/professionals/education/curriculum-tools/shareddecisionmaking/index.html.

8. Baile, W. F., Buckman, R., Lenzi, R., Glober, G., Beale, E. A., & Kudelka, A. P. (2000). SPIKES. A protocol delivering bad news: Application to the patient with cancer. *The Oncologist, 5*(4), 302–311.

9. Cushman, M., Lim, W., & Zakai, N. A. (2014). *Clinical practice guide on antithrombotic drug dosing and management of antithrombotic drug associated bleeding complications in adults.* American Society of Hematology. Retrieved from http://www.hematology.org/Clinicians/Guidelines-Quality/Quick-Reference.aspx.

10. Woo, T. M., & Osborne, K. (2016). Drugs affecting the hematopoietic system. In T. M. Woo & M. V. Robinson (Eds.), *Pharmacotherapeutics for advanced practice nurse prescribers* (4th ed., pp. 414–446). Philadelphia: F. A. Davis.

11. Kroenke, K., Spitzer, R. L., & Williams, J. B. (2001). The PHQ-9: Validity of a brief depression severity measure. *Journal of General Internal Medicine, 16*(9), 606–613.

12. Huynh, N. N., & McIntyre, R. S. (2008). What are the implications of the STAR*D trial for primary care? A review and synthesis. *Primary Care Companion to the Journal of Clinical Psychiatry, 10*(2), 91–96.

13. Weber, M., & Estes, K. (2016). Anxiety and depression. In T. M. Woo & M. V. Robinson (Eds.), *Pharmacotherapeutics for Advanced practice nurse prescribers* (4th ed., pp. 897–912). Philadelphia: F. A. Davis.

14. Qaseem, A., Snow, V., Denberg, T., Forciea, M., & Owens, D. (2008). Using second generation antidepressants to treat depressive disorders: A clinical practice guideline from the American College of Physicians. *Annals of Internal Medicine, 149*(10), 725–733.

15. Stahl, S. (2017). *Stahl's essential psychopharmacology: Prescriber's guide* (6th ed.). New York: Cambridge University Press.

16. Stahl, S. (2013). *Stahl's Essential psychopharmacology: Neuroscientific basis and practical applications.* New York: Cambridge University Press.

17. American Psychological Association. (n.d.). What do practicing psychologists do? Retrieved from http://www.apa.org/helpcenter/about-psychologists.aspx.

18. American Psychological Association Practice Organization. (n.d.) About prescribing psychologists. Retrieved from http://www.apapracticecentral.org/advocacy/authority/prescribing-psychologists.aspx?_ga=2.63673641.769788747.1494674906-98486587.1494674226.

19. Mental Health America. (n.d.) Types of mental health professionals. Retrieved from http://www.mentalhealthamerica.net/types-mental-health-professionals.

20. American Psychiatric Nurses Association. (n.d.). Psychiatric mental health nurses. Retrieved from https://www.apna.org/i4a/pages/index.cfm?pageID=3292.

Weight Gain

Nancy S. Morris

Case Study Scenario/History of Present Illness

Just another "bout of diabetes" is what Mr. G, a 76-year-old man, says when he acknowledges that he has had diabetes off and on for the last 15 years. "It seems to come and go." He arrived from Nigeria 14 years ago after his wife died and lives with his daughter and her family here in the United States. His daughter came with him and explains that she thinks her father takes his medication as prescribed but, "it is the food that is difficult." Mr. G was diagnosed with a deep vein thrombosis (DVT) several years ago and was on warfarin and mistakenly understood that he should not eat any green vegetables. Although he is no longer on warfarin, he has still not resumed eating green vegetables because he "doesn't want another blood clot." He met with a dietician a few years ago but he does not want to limit his intake of some of his favorite foods like jollof rice, fried yams, fried plantains, and puff puff (deep fried sweet dough balls) as suggested because he does not want to "get too thin." He was visiting relatives in Nigeria for a few months and missed his last appointment with the nurse practitioner and thus has not been in the office for 7 months. Today, Mr. G's daughter is concerned because she noticed that his blood sugars have been higher since he returned from Nigeria about a month ago and that he gained weight. Review of the home glucometer reveals a 7-day fasting blood sugar (FBS) average of 177.

Past medical history: Hypertension, hyperlipidemia, type 2 diabetes mellitus, peripheral neuropathy, vitamin D deficiency, status post DVT in left leg (9 years ago), status post prostate cancer 10 years ago.

Medications: Amlodipine 10 milligrams daily, aspirin 81 milligrams daily, atorvastatin 20 milligrams daily, glipizide 5 milligrams daily, losartan 50 milligrams daily, metformin ER 1000 milligrams twice daily, sitagliptin 100 milligrams daily, and vitamin D 1000 units daily.

Allergies: Penicillin caused hives.

Habits: Nonsmoker, no alcohol use, and no recreational drug use.

Past surgical history: None.

Family history: Father died from malaria at age 48 years. Mother died from pneumonia age 49 years. He has four siblings who have died (two from car accidents, one from a wound infection, and one from infectious diarrhea). He has a younger sister with tuberculosis who continues to live in Nigeria.

Personal + social history: Moved from Nigeria 14 years ago when his wife died to live with his daughter and her family here in the United States. He has two other adult children living in the United States. He completed secondary education in Nigeria and worked in agriculture until age 60; he is now retired. He speaks English well.

Review of Systems

General: Feels well. No fatigue, malaise. No fever, no chills.

Skin: Skin on his feet dry in the winter, not a problem now. No rashes or abnormal moles.

Head, eyes, ears, nose, and throat (HEENT): Last eye examination was 8 months ago. No history of retinopathy. Wears glasses for reading and distance. Vision has been blurry off and on the last few months. Denies headache, dizziness, nasal congestion, epistaxis, rhinorrhea, sinus pain, sore throat, or problems hearing.

Neck: No swollen glands.

Respiratory: No cough, shortness of breath (SOB), or sleep apnea.

Cardiovascular: No chest pain, palpitations, or dyspnea on exertion. History of lower leg DVT.

Peripheral vascular: No swelling in his legs, no calf pain.

Gastrointestinal: Appetite very good, "always hungry," more thirsty than others, 18-pound weight gain this past year. No heartburn, nausea or vomiting, constipation, diarrhea, blood in stool, or hemorrhoids.

Urinary: Urinates frequently during the day and has nocturia ×2; no dysuria, hematuria, urgency, incontinence, or flank pain.

Genital/reproductive: Positive erectile disorder (but not a current concern). History of prostate cancer. Treated with radiation, monitored regularly with no recurrence to date.

Musculoskeletal: Bunion left great toe, wears shoes that do not cause pain. No back pain. No joint swelling, erythema, or increased warmth. No myalgia.

Psychiatric: No anxiety/depression. Sleeps well, feels refreshed in the morning.

Neurologic: Intermittent burning and tingling in his feet, primarily in the evening when sitting still. Not feeling a need for any medication for it at this time. No vertigo, weakness, tremor, or seizures. No memory loss. Gait stable. No falls in the past year.

Hematologic: No easy bruising.

Endocrine: Increased thirst, increased hunger, and increased urination. No hoarseness, no change in sock or glove size. Hypoglycemia in the past, but not for a "long time." Weight gain this past year.

Physical Examination

General: Obese black man, alert, and responding to questions with some history details provided by his daughter.

Vitals: Weight 192 pounds, height 5′5″. Body mass index (BMI) 31.9. Blood pressure (BP) sitting in chair 138/86, pulse 88 regular, respiration rate 20 unlabored. Temperature 98.4°F.

Skin: No acanthosis nigricans, no breaks in skin integrity, and no rashes or abnormal lesions.

HEENT: Thinning hair, eyes with clear conjunctiva, sclera nonicteric, pupils equal and reactive to light and accommodation, extraocular movements (EOMs) intact, funduscopic examination with no arteriovenous (AV) nicking, and no cotton wool spots. Nares clear and patent, no sinus tenderness. Mouth with moist mucous membranes. Teeth intact. Uvula midline. Ears with easily visualized pinkish gray tympanic membrane with normal bony landmarks easily visible, minimal yellow cerumen, gross hearing intact. Thyroid midline with no enlargement; no cervical adenopathy.

Cardiovascular: Normal S1, S2 with regular rate and rhythm, no murmurs, gallops, or rubs.

Lungs: Clear to auscultation.

Abdomen: Obese, bowel sounds in all four quadrants, soft, no hepatosplenomegaly.

Back: No tenderness over vertebrae or paraspinal muscles, no costovertebral angle (CVA) tenderness.

Extremities: Skin intact on both feet, minimal edema both ankles.

Neurological: Slightly widened stance with steady gait, posture slightly bent forward. Get Up and Go test normal. Romberg negative.

Laboratory results from yesterday: Serum glucose 186 milligrams/dL, hemoglobin (Hgb) A1C 10% (reflects average glucose of 240).

ASSESSMENT AND PLAN

1. Based on the history and physical examination results, what are the possible causes (differentials) for the patient's current condition?

Mr. G presents with type 2 diabetes with hyperglycemia (supported by elevated Hgb A1C of 10% and peripheral neuropathy). With reported FBSs this past week that average approximately 177 milligrams/dL, the nurse practitioner would have expected his Hgb A1C to be closer to 7.8%. It is important to think about the why behind this discrepancy. It may be that his blood glucose is higher at other times of the day, contributing to an overall higher average blood glucose of 240, which would be consistent with the Hgb A1C of 10%. He may have a previously undiagnosed Hgb variant, which can confound Hgb A1C depending on the assay method used. Hgb C and Hgb S variants are found in approximately 7% of Africans. Hgb variants may hinder interpretation of Hgb A1 because of altered red blood cell (RBC) turnover.[1] In addition to falsely elevated Hgb A1C caused by Hgb variants, a falsely low Hgb A1C can be seen in conditions that increase RBC turnover/shorten RBC life span, such as end-stage renal disease, acute and chronic blood loss, and hemolytic anemia.[2]

Another consideration is that during his recent 3-month visit to Nigeria his diet was significantly different and caused high glycemia, which has improved since his return to the United States this past month but is reflected in today's A1C. One cultural belief in Nigeria is that being overweight is a sign of wellness and financial security,[3] and efforts to lose weight are often questioned by family and community members. He gained weight while in Nigeria; it would be helpful to know more specifics about dietary intake over the last several months.

Because some medications can affect blood glucose, the nurse practitioner wants to know about any change to medications over the last few months. How consistently did he take prescribed medications? Did he run out when he was in Nigeria? It would also be important to ask specifically about any infections in the last several months because infection leads to an increase in cortisol and adrenaline with subsequent increase in the production of glucose. The nurse practitioner needs more information to interpret and make decisions about how to help him manage his diabetes.

2. What components of the history or physical examination are missing?

Given the complexity of managing diabetes, his increasing age, worsening glycemic control, and knowledge that diabetes increases the incidence of all-cause dementia,[4] it is important to assess his cognitive status. Since a Montreal Cognitive Assessment (MoCA) test[5] was done when he first came to this practice 2 years ago, it is reasonable to repeat the MoCA and compare it with baseline. Another option would be to conduct a Mini-Cog,[6] which is a screen for cognitive impairment that has little education or race bias and a short administration time. Cognitive screening is important because the results will affect decisions regarding management goals and management strategies.

Older adults with diabetes are a high-priority population for depression screening.[7] Asking the two-item Patient Health Questionnaire (PHQ)-2[8] is a reasonable approach to screening for depression.

American Diabetes Association (ADA) guidelines[9] recommend annual examinations of the feet. This should include assessment of skin integrity, vascular status (pedal pulse), loss of sensation using a 10-g monofilament, and at least one of the following: pinprick, temperature, or vibration perception using a 128-Hz tuning fork.

3. What diagnostics are necessary for the patient at this time?

Today it is important to assess his renal function (serum creatinine and estimated glomerular filtration rate [eGFR], and urinary albumin-to-creatinine ratio) because the nurse practitioner may make medication changes and will want to know current renal function. Also, liver function tests (LFTs) have not been checked within the past year. With the unexplained discrepancy between his home glucometer readings and his A1C results, the nurse practitioner may want to check for an Hgb variant with a serum Hgb electrophoresis. If he was not taking his medications consistently over the past 3 months, however, the decision may be to have him take more frequent home blood glucose readings and reassess before ordering an Hgb electrophoresis. Getting some home blood glucose readings 2 hours after eating would also help the nurse practitioner identify postprandial rises in blood glucose, which will aid decision making regarding the most appropriate drug therapy.

4. What treatments would you recommend for this patient?

Before making a treatment plan it is important to clarify glycemic treatment goals. If life expectancy is such that he would benefit from intensive treatment management and cognitive and physical function are adequate to perform such interventions, and the patient, via shared decision making, chooses to achieve more intensive glycemic target goals, it is appropriate to do so. However, if comorbidities are such that a benefit from reducing the risk of microvascular complications is less likely to be realized, less stringent glycemic control is reasonable. The goal should always be to prevent acute complications including hypoglycemia, dehydration, poor wound healing, and hyperglycemic hyperosmolar coma.[10]

Given Mr. G's overall physical function, adequate social support, lack of depression (based on the results of the PHQ-2), no significant cognitive impairment (MoCA score of 29/30), and relatively well-controlled risk factors, it is reasonable to consider an A1C goal less than 7.5% with reevaluation at any time should his health status change. With this goal it is clear something needs to be done to improve his glycemic control. It is important to obtain missing information before making any changes to his drug therapy and to sort out the discrepancy between his reported home blood glucose results and his A1C in the office today.

Lifestyle counseling is recommended at every encounter. The nurse practitioner wants to encourage 150 min/week of moderate-intensity exercise spread over 3 days/week plus flexibility and strength training two times a week.[11] In addition, it is suggested that when sedentary, he engage in some light activity such as walking, leg extensions, or overhead arm stretches every 30 minutes; specifically he should not sit for more than 90 minutes at any one time.[11] With the noted weight gain, it is important to explore his dietary intake and, if agreeable, he may benefit from medical nutrition therapy (MNT) from a dietician to discuss overall dietary intake, type and quantity of carbohydrates, and options consistent with his cultural preferences. Today it is important to clarify that he can eat and enjoy green vegetables with vitamin K, which he thought he had to avoid while taking warfarin. The message is that while on warfarin his vitamin K intake needs to be consistent week to week, but not that he needed to avoid foods high in vitamin K.

He agrees to laboratory work today to assess renal function and LFTs, which have not been checked in 12 months, and will follow up in 7 to 10 days with more frequent home blood glucose monitoring results. His daughter will review his medications and his system for taking them to be sure he is not missing any doses. In addition, he agrees to consider options for increasing his activity level and is willing to meet with a dietician.

In traditional belief systems in many African countries, diabetes is thought to be curable and symptoms that persist or recur after a "cure" are typically thought of as a recurrence of diabetes.[3] Suggesting Mr. G meet with a certified diabetes educator for culturally specific diabetes education might be helpful. Diabetes education and support are important not only when diabetes is initially diagnosed but whenever patients are ready to review or learn more about managing their health.

Case Study, Continued

One week later the patient returns to discuss laboratory results, review his glucometer results, and consider ongoing treatment plans.

His daughter found out that her father had many dietary indiscretions the 2 months he was in Nigeria and was eating a higher than usual amount of carbohydrates. Further discussion about his concern about becoming "too thin" reveals that his perception of body size is consistent with many middle-age and older Nigerians who prefer a body figure that is overweight compared with a body figure of desired weight.[12] While visiting in Nigeria, his well-intentioned relatives were trying to "fatten him up a bit." He does not perceive his body weight as a concern at this time. When asked about any plans to increase his activity level, he explains that he will begin taking a 15-minute walk in the afternoon, but he has not started this yet. He also had run short of his medications while in Nigeria and was not taking all of them every day. He picked up refills 5 weeks ago and has been taking them consistently since his return. This week his daughter purchased a weekly pill box and helped her father set up his medications to help keep track of his medication use. His MoCA was scored at 29/30. The PHQ-2 was negative. Results of laboratory work: creatinine 1.43 milligrams/dL, GFR 47 mL/min, albumin-to-creatinine ratio 25 milligrams/gram. LFTs are within normal limits (WNL). His BP is 138/84. Past week of home glucometer results with 7-day average of 200 milligrams/dL are seen in the subsequent table.

	FBS	2 Hours After Breakfast	2 Hours After Lunch	2 Hours After Dinner	Bedtime
Tuesday	185	220	230	240	232
Wednesday	162	180	244	266	220
Thursday	180	175	202	210	216
Friday	168	160	216	188	192
Saturday	178	200	210	225	202
Sunday	186	190	196	204	185
Monday	140	—	—	—	—

FBS, Fasting blood sugar.

5. What are your next steps?

According to the ADA,[13] diabetes self-management education (DSME), diabetes self-management support (DSMS), MNT, education on physical activity, guidance on routine immunizations, and psychosocial care are the foundation of diabetes management. With an A1C goal of ~7.5% (and a recent A1C of 10%), it is clear attention to lifestyle changes and adjustment to his medications are necessary. Although this past week his average blood sugar was 200 (based on his home blood glucose monitor), it is still above the goal. Given his cultural beliefs regarding body size, it may be beneficial to discuss healthy food choice goals rather than focusing on weight goals at this time. It is important to support his decision that he and his daughter, who does most of the food shopping and cooking, meet with the dietician, and this has been scheduled for the following week. His daughter suggests his plan for a daily walk is not realistic given his dislike for being outside when it is "too hot" and "too cold." Providing information about local exercise programs for older adults, like the SilverSneakers Program at the YMCA or the many offerings at senior centers, may be more realistic for him.

There are several pharmacologic options to help with glycemic management. The nurse practitioner can explain the goals recommended by the ADA of an FBS between 80 and 130, postprandial blood glucose of less than 180, and bedtime blood glucose close to 150.[13] He is not interested at this time in considering any injectable options such as a GLP-1 or insulin. Although the ADA guidelines suggest insulin as one option with an A1C of 10%, the discrepancy between last week's home glucometer readings and his reluctance to take an injection prompt the decision to try and optimize oral agents and lifestyle changes at this time. He can continue the metformin unless his GFR drops to less than 30 mL/min/1.7 m².[14] If he were to have an iodinated contrast imaging procedure, he should not take the metformin before the procedure and his GFR should be reevaluated 48 hours later to be sure it is stable before restarting the metformin. He has been taking 100 milligrams of sitagliptin daily. Sitagliptin requires dosage adjustments based on renal function. For patients with moderate renal insufficiency (GFR 30–50 mL/min/1.7 m²) the maximum dose of sitagliptin is 50 milligrams once daily; thus this change should be recommended today.

Mr. G is also taking 5 milligrams of glipizide daily. Although glipizide has a risk of hypoglycemia and is associated with weight gain, it is inexpensive and has worked well for him in the past. The nurse practitioner contemplated switching from the glipizide to an SGLT-2, but Mr. G. is not willing to try a new medicine today and is concerned about the added cost. He favors staying with the glipizide as he has been on it for a time with no problems. Given his elevated blood glucose, the nurse practitioner decides to add 2.5 milligrams of glipizide before dinner in addition to the 5 milligrams of glipizide he takes before breakfast, which Mr. G is agreeable to instead of adding a new drug. Recognizing the potential risk of hypoglycemia, the nurse practitioner reviews the signs and symptoms of hypoglycemia with Mr. G and his daughter and what to do should it occur.[13] Common symptoms of hypoglycemia (glucose less than 70 milligrams/mL) include new onset of sweating, chills, tremors, irritability, hunger, weakness, fatigue, headache, confusion, or lightheadedness. Mr. G should check his blood glucose if he experiences any of these symptoms, and if low, he should consume 15 grams of simple carbohydrates and recheck his blood glucose in 15 minutes. If his blood glucose is still low, he should eat another 15 grams of simple carbohydrates with a goal of getting his blood glucose above 90. If his next planned meal is more than 1 hour away, he should consume a small snack. Mr. G and his daughter are both able to repeat back the key aspects of hypoglycemia recognition and management, confirming their understanding of the nurse practitioner's explanation. They agree to follow up in 3 months, at which time it will be appropriate to recheck his A1C and evaluate his response to the changes agreed on today.

Case Study, Continued

Three months later Mr. G and his daughter return, having met with the dietician twice and having joined a Tai Chi class at the local Senior Center. He has been taking his medications as prescribed. Suggestions given by the dietician have led to some changes in his eating, which he is willing to continue because he has seen some improvement in his glucose levels. He has, however, experienced hypoglycemia six times (during the late afternoon and during the night) this past month. He eats carbohydrates when this occurs and subsequently finds his blood glucose elevated when next checked. His weight is 191 pounds, height 5'5", and BMI 31.9. BP is 136/86. Results of blood work he had drawn 2 days ago are creatinine 1.8 milligrams/dL GFR 44 mL/min, and A1C 8.3%. Past week of home glucometer results with 7-day average of 190 milligrams/dL are seen in the subsequent table.

	FBS	2 Hours After Breakfast	2 Hours After Lunch	2 Hours After Dinner	Bedtime
Tuesday	135	175	188, 67 at 3:30	265	210
Wednesday	140	200	—	225	182
Thursday	145	180	140, 64 at 4:00	263	200
Friday	160	176	232	—	192
Saturday	172	225	252	201	188
Sunday	148	202	210	175	190
Monday	150	180	—	—	—

FBS, Fasting blood sugar.

6. What are your priorities for this visit?

Physical activity: He has been going to Tai Chi once a week, which helps with strength and balance. He would benefit from aerobic exercise and he expresses some interest in joining a walking group at the Senior Center, which the nurse practitioner encourages him to consider. In addition to the exercise, the socialization would likely be beneficial. He has documented neuropathy, so it is essential to consider the shoes he is wearing at Tai Chi and what he will wear for walking. He confirms that he still has burning in his feet sometimes at night but it is not too bothersome. The nurse practitioner emphasizes the importance of inspecting his feet regularly. He has mild loss of protective sensation, making inspection of the bottom of his feet with a mirror or inspection by another person important.

Diet: He has made some changes to his diet and his blood glucose readings are improving, but he has not yet lost any weight. Key today is to explore his motivation toward improving his health by decreasing his weight. Enlisting the support of his daughter to further explore the cultural perspective of overweight being associated with good health is one option. Consideration of a goal of losing 10% of his body weight, which will contribute to health improvement, may be more acceptable than trying to get his BMI to less than 25 at this time. He has a follow-up scheduled with the dietician, which the nurse practitioner encourages him to attend.

Glycemia: Mr. G's home blood glucose readings are more consistent with the A1C, ruling out a previous concern about an Hgb variant. The discrepancy seen a few months ago likely reflects his dietary indiscretion and inconsistency in use of medications 2 of 3 months before drawing the A1C. He has made good progress, but the hypoglycemia is a concern and his A1C is still higher than goal. Hypoglycemia is a significant risk because it could result in a fall with subsequent injury that could significantly affect his physical function. Although he was reluctant to try a new medication before, the nurse practitioner now suggests a GLP-1, liraglutide, which may not only improve his A1C with little risk of hypoglycemia but also result in weight loss, a slight decrease in BP, and a decrease in negative cardiovascular outcomes.[15,16] Contraindications to a GLP-1 include a history of thyroid cancer or multiple endocrine neoplasia syndrome type 2 (MEN2), which he does not have. He is hesitant to consider an injection, but after seeing the demo-pen he is willing to give it a try. The nurse practitioner prescribes liraglutide 0.6 milligrams daily for 1 week followed by 1.2 milligrams daily if tolerated. When he begins the liraglutide he will stop the sitagliptin and decrease the glipizide so that he is only taking 2.5 milligrams of glipizide twice a day. The nurse practitioner shares the potential side effect of nausea and vomiting but advises that they usually do not persist and he should contact his provider with any concerns. A daily FBS and sporadic checks of his blood glucose at different times of the day over the next 3 months should be encouraged.

Cardiovascular risk: Includes hypertension (he is below goal), dyslipidemia (he is on a moderate dose statin; last lipid profile 14 months ago and is actively trying to eat a healthy diet), albuminuria (WNL 3 months ago), smoking (not applicable [N/A]), and a family history of premature heart disease (N/A), should be assessed at a minimum once a year.[17] Although it has been 14 months since his lipid profile was checked, the decision to wait another 3 months is made recognizing that he did not take the statin regularly the 3 months he was in Nigeria, and it is best to assess the response based on regular use. Continue the 81 milligrams daily of aspirin as recommended by the ADA[16] given his atherosclerotic cardiovascular disease. Mr. G is asked to return for follow-up in 3 months and to obtain laboratory work to include an A1C, lipid profile, and a basic metabolic panel (BMP) 2 days before his next appointment.

Case Study, Continued

A phone call 2 weeks later reveals that he is tolerating the liraglutide with no side effects and his FBSs are running between 130 and 150. This is still higher than goal, but the decision is made to keep him at 1.2 milligrams of liraglutide daily for now as he continues to work on lifestyle changes

Three months later Mr. G and his daughter return happy with his progress. He has been consistently following the changes to his diet recommended by the dietician. He notes that he does not seem to be as hungry as he used to be and he gets full easier so he is not eating as much. He has made some friends at the Senior Center and has continued with his weekly Tai Chi and the walking group. He has gotten more comfortable with the daily injection of the liraglutide 1.2 milligrams and continues with metformin 1000 milligrams twice a day and glipizide 2.5 milligrams twice daily. No hypoglycemia in the last few months. No change in his peripheral neuropathy. His weight is 182 pounds, BMI 30.3 (down 9 pounds over last 3 months). His BP is 134/84. Laboratory results from 2 days ago include an A1C of 7.8%. His total cholesterol is 180, triglycerides are 170, high-density lipoprotein (HDL) is 34, and his low-density lipoprotein (LDL) is 100. Sodium 139 mmol, potassium 4.5 mmol, chloride 102 mmol, carbon dioxide 28 mmol, anion gap 9, glucose 168 milligrams/dL, blood urea nitrogen (BUN) 34 milligrams/dL, creatinine 1.41 milligrams/dL, GFR 48, and calcium 9.4 milligrams/dL (notation made of the normal potassium level because he is taking an angiotensin receptor blocker [ARB]).

Past week of home glucometer results with 7-day average of 178 milligrams/dL are shown in the subsequent table.

	FBS	2 Hours After Breakfast	2 Hours After Lunch	2 Hours After Dinner	Bedtime
Tuesday	125	200	225	210	190
Wednesday	138	195	176	—	210
Thursday	136	—	198	260	200
Friday	128	187	200	220	188
Saturday	126	—	185	195	168
Sunday	134	183	228	—	156
Monday	118	—	—	—	—

FBS, Fasting blood sugar.

7. What are your priorities for this visit?

Physical activity: Continue to support his engagement in physical activity; he is doing Tai Chi once a week and the walking group twice a week. Explore the possibility of walking three times per week.

Diet: Acknowledge his success with weight loss and the improvement to his overall health. Reevaluate his carbohydrate intake and selection of high-nutrient food choices.

Glycemia: No hypoglycemia, which is good. His FBSs are close to goal most of the time, but he is still experiencing postprandial hyperglycemia. GLP-1 agonists decrease postprandial glucose through several mechanisms including delay in gastric emptying, stimulation of glucose-dependent insulin secretion, and suppression of glucagon production.[15] The decision is made to increase the dose of liraglutide to 1.6 milligrams daily, continue metformin 1000 milligrams twice daily, and to decrease the glipizide to 2.5 milligrams in the morning only.

Cardiac risk factors: His BP is well controlled. His lipid profile is acceptable. To continue with a healthy dietary intake that is low in salt, regular physical activity, and aspirin, atorvastatin, and losartan.

Eye examination: He should continue with annual dilated eye examination.[13]

Immunizations: It is October and time to recommend an influenza vaccine consistent with the Centers for Disease Control and Prevention (CDC) Advisory Committee on Immunization Practices.[18] He has already received both pneumococcal vaccines.

Follow-up: 3 months. Plan to check A1C 2 days before next appointment.

Case Study, Continued

Mr. G and his daughter return 3 months later. With the colder winter weather he has not been getting to the Senior Center as consistently and thus not exercising as much. In addition, he says on the days he joins the walking group he does not feel "as well" and specifically describes four episodes of hypoglycemia after walking. He feels better after he has something to eat. His feet have been bothering him with burning and tingling at times during the day and in the evening. His daughter reports that the entire family has benefited from changes to their diet, and they are all adjusting to lower-carbohydrate food choices. Although Mr. G. was reluctant to lose weight initially, he now understands the relationship of his weight to his blood glucose and is happy with the outcomes of the weight loss he has achieved. He saw his eye doctor last month and brought a report with him that indicates no retinopathy. Review of his glucometer shows fewer blood sugar checks. His A1C is 7%. Weight 175 pounds (down 17 pounds since return from Nigeria) and BMI is 29.1. His BP is 132/82. Past week of home glucometer results with 7-day average of 158 milligrams/dL are listed in the subsequent table.

	FBS	2 Hours After Breakfast	2 Hours After Lunch	2 Hours After Dinner	Bedtime
Tuesday	135	148	135, 62 at 3:00	210	265
Wednesday	138	162	—	185	—
Thursday	118	—	160	—	158
Friday	122	188	166	182	178
Saturday	118	150	175	—	166
Sunday	126	148	—	188	—
Monday	120	—	—	—	—

FBS, Fasting blood sugar.

8. What are the priorities for this visit?

The standard follow-up for adults with diabetes is every 3 months until glycemia is well controlled, at which time it can decrease to every 4 to 6 months. His blood glucose is at goal; however, the recurrence of hypoglycemia is a concern and it is important to monitor his weight, BP, peripheral neuropathy, cognitive status, physical functioning, and renal function on a regular basis, so it is important at this time to see him every 3 months.

Glycemia: Today it is essential that the nurse practitioner review his medications, diet, and activity level to discern factors that may be contributing to hypoglycemia. Of the three medications Mr. G is taking for diabetes the glipizide is the one most commonly associated with hypoglycemia. Given his decreased weight, change in diet, and more consistency with his activity level, a recommendation is made to stop the glipizide today. He will continue with metformin 1000 milligrams twice a day and liraglutide 1.6 milligrams daily.

Physical activity: He has decreased his activity level, which he explains is because he was not feeling so well after walking (likely related to hypoglycemia but important to think about coronary artery disease as well) and worsening symptoms of neuropathy. The nurse practitioner should encourage ongoing exercise, and hopefully stopping the glipizide will take care of feeling poorly after walking if it is related to hypoglycemia. Emphasize that he should always check his blood glucose to rule out hypoglycemia whenever he is not feeling well.

Peripheral neuropathy: He complains of intermittent tingling and a burning sensation in both feet; there is no discomfort in his calves. It is most bothersome when sitting still. Examination of his feet reveals intact skin, palpable pedal pulses, callus formation on the balls of both feet, and a bunion on his right foot. He also has loss of protective sensation supported by monofilament and vibratory testing. His pain is worse when sitting still and at night. Glucose control is one component of managing neuropathy, although it is not likely to reverse existing symptoms. He does not want to consider medication therapy. Given the importance of keeping him physically active, the nurse practitioner refers him to a physician colleague with a request that he be seen and certified for a pair of therapeutic diabetic shoes, which is considered durable medical equipment (DME) and covered by Medicare.[19] The 2015 American Association of Clinical Endocrinologists (AACE) guidelines[20] recommended that if a patient has large-fiber neuropathies, orthotics and strength, gait, and balance training may be beneficial. For small-fiber neuropathies consider the use of foot protection (padded socks), supportive shoes/orthotics, regular foot inspection, prevention of heat/cold injury, and emollient creams for dry skin.[20]

Follow-up: Mr. G is asked to come back in 3 months but to call sooner if he continues to experience hypoglycemia or if he continues to not feel well with walking. Every 3 months it is important to assess his activity level, dietary intake, medication use, home blood glucose monitoring results, hypoglycemia, cognitive status, BP, weight, and A1C.[11] Annually he should be screened for depression, diabetes distress, microvascular and macrovascular complications, and have a fasting lipid profile (FLP), LFT, spot urinary albumin-to-creatinine ratio, serum creatinine, and eGFR.[11] In addition he should have an annual funduscopic examination, thyroid palpation, a comprehensive foot examination, and routine dental care.[11] Diabetes education and support are needed on an ongoing basis. Given the complexity of diabetes management and need for ongoing guidance as the disease progresses, having a team approach is likely to best serve Mr. G and his daughter.

References

1. Rhea, J. M., Molinaro, R., & Roberts-Wilson, T. K. (2012). Impact of hemoglobin variants on HbA1c interpretation: Do we assume too much? *MLO: Medical Laboratory Observer, 44*(68), 10, 12 passim: quiz 20. http://www.mlo-online.com/impact-of-hemoglobin-variants-on-hb-a1c-interpretation-do-we-assume-too-much.php.
2. Radin, M. S. (2014). Pitfalls in hemoglobin A1c measurement: When results may be misleading. *Journal of General Internal Medicine, 29*(2), 388–394. https://www.ncbi.nlm.nih.gov/pmc/articles/PMC3912281/.
3. Chinenye, S., & Obera, A. O. (2013). Socio-cultural aspects of diabetes mellitus in Nigeria. *Journal of Social Health and Diabetes, 1*(1), 15–21. http://www.joshd.net/text.asp?2013/1/1/15/109833.
4. Kirkman, M. S., Briscoe, V. J., Clark, N., Florez, H., Haas, L. B., … Swift, C. S. (2012). Diabetes in older adults. *Diabetes Care, 35*(12), 2650–2664.
5. Nasreddine, Z., Phillips, N. A., Bedirian, V., Charbonneau, S., Whitehead, V., … Chertkow, H. (2005). The Montreal cognitive assessment MoCA: A brief screening tool for mild cognitive impairment. *Journal of the American Geriatrics Society, 53*(4), 695–699.
6. Borson, S., Scanlan, J., Brush, M., Vitaliano, P., & Dokmak, A. (2000). The mini-cog: A cognitive "vital signs" measure for dementia screening in multi-lingual elderly. *International Journal of Geriatric Psychiatry, 15*(11), 1021–1027.
7. Kimbro, L. B., Mangione, C. M., Steers, W. N., Kenrik Duru, O., McEwen, L., … Ettner, S. L. (2014). Depression and all-cause mortality in persons with diabetes mellitus: Are older adults at higher risk? Results from the Translating Research into Action of Diabetes Study. *Journal of the American Geriatrics Society, 62*(6), 1017–1022.
8. Kroenke, K., Spitzer, R. L., & Williams, J. S. (2003). The Patient Health Questionnaire-2: Validity of a two-item depression screener. *Medical Care, 41*, 1284–1294.
9. American Diabetes Association. (2016). Section 9. Microvascular complications and foot care. *Diabetes Care, 39*(Sl), S72–S80.

10. American Diabetes Association. (2016). Older adults. *Diabetes Care, 39*(S1), S81–S85.
11. Colberg, S. R., Sigal, R. J., Yardley, J. E., Riddell, M. C., Dunstan, D. W., ... Tate, D. F. (2016). Physical activity/exercise and diabetes: A position statement of the American Diabetes Association. *Diabetes Care, 39*(11), 2065–2079.
12. Okoro, E. O., & Oyejola, B. A. (2008). Body image preference among Nigerians with type 2 diabetes. *Practical Diabetes International, 25*(6), 228–231.
13. American Diabetes Association. (2016). Section 3. Foundations of care and comprehensive medical evaluation. *Diabetes Care, 39*(S1), S23–S35.
14. FDA Drug Safety Communication. FDA revises warnings regarding use of the diabetes medicine metformin in certain patients with reduced kidney function. Retrieved from www.fda.gov.
15. Eng, C., Kramer, C. K., Zinman, B., & Retnakaran, R. (2014). Glucagon-like peptide-1 receptor agonist and basal insulin combination treatment for the management of type 2 diabetes: A systematic review and meta-analysis. *Lancet, 384*(9961), 2228–2234.
16. Marso, S. P., Danies, G. H., Brown-Frandsen, K., Kristense, P., Mann, J. F. E., ... Buse, J. B. (2016). Liraglutide and cardiovascular outcomes in type 2 diabetes. *The New England Journal of Medicine, 375,* 311–322.
17. American Diabetes Association. (2016). Cardiovascular disease and risk management. *Diabetes Care, 39*(S1), S60–S71.
18. Centers for Disease Control and Prevention (CDC). (2017). Advisory Committee on Immunization Practices. http://www.cdc.gov/vaccines/schedules.
19. Centers for Medicare & Medicaid Services. Is my test, item, or service covered? Therapeutic shoes or inserts. Retrieved from https://www.medicare.gov/coverage/therapeutic-shoes-or-inserts.html.
20. Abrahamson, J. J., Barzilay, J. I., Blonde, L., Bloomgarden, Z. T., Bush, M. A., ... Umpierrez, G. (2015). AACE/ACE comprehensive diabetes management algorithm. *Endocrine Practice, 21*(4), e1–e10. https://www.aace.com/files/aace_algorithm.pdf.

Knee Pain

Terry Mahan Buttaro

Case Study Scenario

SKILLED NURSING FACILITY DAY 1

Mr. Johnson, a 77-year-old Jamaican male, was admitted to the skilled nursing facility (SNF) at 10 p.m. last evening, 6 days after a total right knee arthroplasty at the local hospital. He was a late admission because he was anemic after the surgery and required two units of packed red blood cells before hospital discharge. His orders were approved over the phone with the patient's covering physician in the nursing facility.

SKILLED NURSING FACILITY DAY 2: A.M.

The next morning, the physician, concerned about such a late-night admission, requests that one of the nurse practitioners or physician assistants on the team make a medically necessary visit and see Mr. Johnson early in the day and then update him on the patient's condition.[1]

The health care provider scheduled to see patients that day in the facility reviews Mr. Johnson's hospital discharge paperwork and his medications. The orthopedic surgeon's report recommended skilled nursing care because of Mr. Johnson's age and the fact that he lives alone. The discharge summary reveals that his blood pressure was low after surgery and both the amlodipine and hydrochlorothiazide were discontinued. Additionally, his blood sugars postoperatively were low and the patient's glipizide and linagliptin were also discontinued.

Mr. Johnson's Medication Reconciliation at Skilled Nursing Facility

Preoperative medications:
  Lisinopril 10 milligrams orally (po) each day
  Hydrochlorothiazide 25 milligrams po daily
  Metoprolol XL 50 milligrams po daily
  Amlodipine 2.5 milligrams po daily
  Pantoprazole (Protonix) 30 milligrams po daily
  Metformin 1000 milligrams po once a day
  Glipizide XL 5 milligrams po every morning.
  Linagliptin (Tradjenta) 5 milligrams po daily
  Atorvastatin 80 milligrams po daily
  Warfarin 2 milligrams po daily
  Acetaminophen 1000 milligrams po twice a day
  Ferrous sulfate 325 milligrams po daily
Postoperative discharge medications:
  Lisinopril 10 milligrams po daily
  Metoprolol XL 50 milligrams po daily
  Pantoprazole (Protonix) 30 milligrams po daily

Metformin 1000 milligrams po once a day

Atorvastatin 80 milligrams po daily

Ferrous sulfate 325 milligrams po daily with orange juice

Warfarin 2 milligrams po daily

Oxycodone and acetaminophen 5/325 milligrams 1 tablet po every 4 to 6 hours as needed (prn) for moderate pain

Oxycodone acetaminophen 5/325 milligrams 2 tablets po every 4 to 6 hours prn for severe pain. *Not to exceed 4 grams acetaminophen daily.*

Allergies: Erythromycin: elevated liver enzymes.

1. What are the essential factors the health care provider should consider when caring for patients throughout the transitions of care?

For patients of all ages, safety across the transitions of care is a paramount concern. The transition from hospital to home or another health care facility is often the most problematic. Medication changes are common, and communication among health care providers at least initially can be limited to the patient's discharge instructions. Additionally, a patient's health literacy and possible cognitive and sensory impairment (especially hearing) combined with the complexity of discharge instructions increase the possibility of adverse events. For these reasons, it is especially important for the health care provider caring for patients at the transitions of care to be attentive to:

- patient culture, language, and health literacy;
- any deficits in a patient's attention, memory, word finding, or executive functioning;
- medication safety (e.g., high-risk medications and medication complexity);
- patient–provider communication; and
- provider–provider communication.[2]

Admission Skilled Nursing Note

General: 77-year-old male transferred to an SNF late last evening from Mercy Hospital status post total right knee replacement 7 days ago.

Past medical/surgical history: Positive for anemia, gastrointestinal (GI) bleeding related to Barrett esophagus, atrial fibrillation, hypertension, hypercholesterolemia, type 2 diabetes, and osteoarthritis. Appendectomy age 11.

Personal and social history: Widower, lives alone. Four stairs into the house, bedroom on the second floor. Two sons live nearby. Former cigarette smoker, stopped 40 years ago per patient. Occasional beer.

Review of Systems

General: Bilateral knee pain all the time. Right greater than left and worse after physical therapy. Tired, but denies fever, chills.

Skin: Denies rashes or lesions.

Head, eyes, ears, nose, and throat (HEENT): Reading glasses only. Denies dizziness, weakness, visual changes, or neck pain.

Respiratory: Denies cough or shortness of breath.

Cardiac: Denies chest pressure, pain, or palpitations.

Gastrointestinal: Last bowel movement? 5 days ago (patient not quite certain). Denies heartburn, difficulty swallowing, nausea, vomiting, or abdominal pain.

Urinary: Nocturia one to two times each night. Denies burning on urination or frequency.

Musculoskeletal: Bilateral knee pain, more constant on the right (surgical knee), some occasional back pain.

Peripheral vascular: Denies swollen legs, calf pain.

Neurovascular: Denies numbness, tingling.

Hematologic: Denies rectal bleeding, black stools, easy bruising, or bleeding gums.

Endocrine: Denies low blood sugar feeling, sweating, or thirst.

Psychiatric: Denies anxiety, depression.

Physical Examination

General: Overweight, older male sitting in wheelchair in no acute distress. Requires two-person assist to transfer from wheelchair to bed for examination.

Vital signs: Height not obtained. Weight 195 pounds. Temperature 96.8°F. Blood pressure 128/62 sitting. Heart rate 80 irregular, respiratory rate 20 at rest, O_2 saturation on room air 95%.

Skin: Warm/dry. No jaundice, rash, or acute lesions.

Eyes: Sclera clear; conjunctiva, no injection.

Ears: Hearing seems diminished. Improved if he is facing speaker.

Nose: No rhinitis or sinus tenderness.

Mouth: Membranes moist, teeth some staining, no postpharyngeal erythema or exudate. No lesions of tongue or buccal mucosa.

Neck: Supple. No masses, lymphadenopathy, thyroid enlargement, or tenderness.

Cardiac: S1, S2 irregular. No gallop, murmurs, or rubs.

Respiratory: Clear to auscultation without rales, wheezes, or rhonchi.

Abdomen: Obese, appears distended. Bowel sounds +, but diminished. No organomegaly. No tenderness, rebound, or guarding. No cough or bump tenderness.[3] Rectal examination: No stool in rectal vault.

Extremities: Right knee: Vertical surgical incision with 18 staples. Positive edema and tenderness, slight erythema at incision edges, but no exudate. Range of motion, flexion, and extension are limited by edema and discomfort. Pedal pulses present and symmetric bilaterally. No calf edema or tenderness bilaterally.

Neurologic: Alert, oriented to person, place, and time. Thoughts coherent, speech fluent. Appropriately answering questions during examination. Lower extremities: Sensation intact bilaterally to pain and light touch. Position sense is intact.

ASSESSMENT/PLAN

2. What, if any, information about Mr. Johnson's postoperative status is missing in the patient history and review of systems? What are the essential components of the abdominal examination?

a. Mr. Johnson's laboratory results from the hospital (both preoperatively and postoperatively) would be helpful to monitor trends.

b. Orthostatic vital signs should be checked.

c. Patient should be asked if has had a recent fall or injury or if he has traveled recently.[4] Additional information includes learning if he is belching frequently or passing flatus. Lack of flatus (i.e., obstipation) is concerning because in combination with abdominal pain and vomiting, it can be a sign of a mechanical bowel obstruction.[3]

d. A thorough physical examination (i.e., head to toe) is necessary for all patients with abdominal pain or a suspected abdominal disorder. The patient should be draped and lying on a flat surface for the abdominal portion of the physical. The physical should be conducted in the correct order (inspection, auscultation, percussion, and palpation). The patient should be asked to cough or the stretcher or bed bumped by the examiner (eliciting pain that would suggest peritonitis).[4] A rectal and possibly testicular examination should also be performed, if indicated.[4]

e. Hospital documentation of constipation concern and/or treatment for constipation during hospitalization should be determined if not included in the discharge summary.

f. Actual measurement of operative knee flexion and extension is necessary to gauge progress during the rehabilitation period. Often, this information can be obtained together with the physical therapist.

3. What are the essential goals of care for this patient today and why?

a. A primary goal for this patient today is treatment of his constipation avoiding an ileus, if possible.

b. Obtaining hemoglobin and hematocrit values after transfusion of packed red blood cells at hospital yesterday is important to determine patient status. It is possible that the patient lost blood during surgery. However, Mr. Johnson is on anticoagulation therapy and has a history of anemia, so it is necessary to establish the current cause of his anemia if this information is not noted or clear in the discharge summary. In some instances, the patient's hospital discharge summary does not include information that might be pertinent to the patient's well-being, and the health care provider will need to communicate with the surgeon, hospitalist, or primary care provider for the answer.

c. Discuss rehabilitation plans with physical therapy. Usually, on the patient's first day in the SNF, a physical therapist will evaluate the patient and the physical therapy plan will be initiated.

4. Write the admission Assessment and Plan for Mr. Johnson.

a. Assessment/plan
  i. **Status post right total knee replacement:** Monitor wound daily. Physical therapy evaluation and treat (patient lives alone, stairs at home,? need for home safety evaluation before discharge, will discuss with physical therapy).
  ii. **Anemia:** Check with surgeon today to learn if cause of anemia was related to surgery. Repeat complete blood count (CBC)/differential and monitor.
  iii. **Constipation:** Patient has abdominal distention with minimal bowel sounds and no bowel movement for several days. He does not seem to have any discomfort and denies nausea and vomiting. Discussed situation with MD who will plan to see patient later today. Also explained concerns and projected plan of care with patient.
  iv. **Atrial fibrillation:** Adequate rate control today. Monitor prothrombin time (PT)/international normalized ratio (INR).
  v. **Type 2 diabetes mellitus:** Monitor fasting blood sugars × 3 days and prn.
  vi. **Hypertension:** Monitor; goal is 140/90, but check orthostatic vital signs for 3 days.[5]
  vii. **Family notification:** Mr. Johnson agreed to discuss patient status with his son, Larry, and the son was updated by this provider after the patient was seen today.

5. Why is the health care provider concerned about Mr. Johnson's constipation, and how should this problem be treated today?

a. Mr. Johnson's physical examination reveals abdominal distention and minimal bowel sounds. He does not have nausea, vomiting, or abdominal pain, which is fortunate, but he has not had a bowel movement in several days. It seems that Mr. Johnson's bowel dysfunction is most likely related to narcotic-induced constipation, although other causes should always be considered in the differential. Gallstone ileus is common in older adults, but Mr. Johnson does not have a known history of chronic cholecystitis and does not have the abdominal pain that is common with this type of mechanical ileus.[6] Sepsis is another possible cause that should be considered because Mr. Johnson has had recent surgery.

b. The health care provider knows that potential complications of constipation/obstipation (especially when associated with narcotics, anticholinergics, or other medications that cause constipation) include not only bowel obstruction or ileus but also ischemic colitis, megacolon, or ruptured intestine.[7,8]

c. Mr. Johnson needs to understand that if he feels nauseated, begins vomiting, or has *any* abdominal discomfort, he needs to notify the nurses immediately because he will need to be transferred to the emergency room for further evaluation.[9]

d. Treatment of Mr. Johnson's constipation should be conservative because aggressive treatment could result in ischemic colitis.[10] The opioids and other medications that cause constipation should be discontinued. Mr. Johnson should be started on scheduled acetaminophen 1000 milligrams po twice a day for his postoperative pain. His diet should be stopped, and he should take nothing by mouth (NPO) until there is evidence that his bowels are functioning. A stimulant laxative is an appropriate treatment to hopefully induce a bowel movement.[11] Other possible pharmacologic treatments include methylnaltrexone (Relistor), which is an opioid antagonist, or linaclotide (Linzess), which is a guanylate cyclase-C agonist,[11] but neither of these medications is available in the SNF. Depending on the kidneys, ureters, and bladder (KUB) x-ray results, an enema is also a possible treatment. Additional appropriate orders include NPO and intravenous (IV) fluids to maintain fluid and electrolytes while NPO.[9]

e. Necessary diagnostics include KUB to check for constipation, CBC/differential, serum electrolytes, magnesium, blood urea nitrogen (BUN), creatinine, and PT/INR.[9]

6. Why is it important to check Mr. Johnson's laboratory values and a KUB? What is the goal INR for Mr. Johnson after his surgery?

a. Both hyperglycemia and hypokalemia have been associated with ileus,[12] although high levels of magnesium have also been associated with ileus.[13] A CBC is necessary to determine whether there is an infectious process and monitor Mr. Johnson's hemoglobin and hematocrit.

b. Mr. Johnson has a history of atrial fibrillation. His goal INR is 2.5 with a range of 2 to 3. Maintaining an INR as close to 2.5 as possible is important to prevent both a stroke and GI bleeding.

7. Write a health care provider's orders for Mr. Johnson today.

Mr. Johnson's medications were approved by the physician last night when the patient was initially admitted to the nursing facility.

Postoperative discharge medications:

Lisinopril 10 milligrams po daily

Metoprolol XL 50 milligrams po daily

Pantoprazole (Protonix) 30 milligrams po daily

Metformin 1000 milligrams po once a day

Atorvastatin 80 milligrams po daily

Ferrous sulfate 325 milligrams po daily with orange juice

Warfarin 2 milligrams po daily

Oxycodone and acetaminophen 5/325 milligrams 1 tablet po every 4 to 6 hours prn for moderate pain

Oxycodone acetaminophen 5/325 milligrams 2 tablets po every 4 to 6 hours prn for severe pain. *Not to exceed 4 grams acetaminophen daily.*

Today's orders should include:

a. Admit to Skilled Nursing Pavilion.

b. NPO, sips of water only for oral medications.

c. CBC/differential, chemistry profile, serum magnesium, PT/INR, and KUB STAT.

d. IV $D_5\frac{1}{2}$ normal saline at 100 cc/hr.

e. Bisacodyl (Dulcolax) 10 milligrams po now.[11] If no bowel movement, notify health care provider.

f. Discontinue ferrous sulfate 325 milligrams po daily.

g. Notify health care provider with today's KUB and laboratory results.

h. Accu-Check every morning for next 3 days and prn if patient has symptoms of low blood sugar.

i. Notify health care provider/physician immediately if patient has *any* abdominal discomfort, nausea, or vomiting because the patient will need urgent emergency room evaluation and hospitalization.

j. Physical therapy evaluation and treatment. Encourage ambulation, if patient is able, because ambulation will help treat constipation.

k. Discontinue oxycodone and acetaminophen 5/325 milligrams 1 tablet po every 4 to 6 hours prn for moderate pain.

l. Discontinue oxycodone acetaminophen 5/325 milligrams 2 tablets po every 4 to 6 hours prn for severe pain.

m. Start acetaminophen 1000 milligrams po every 12 hours for pain. If patient is having pain that affects activities or sleep, notify health care provider.

n. Orthostatic vital signs (blood pressure and heart rate) first sitting, then standing today and tomorrow.

DIAGNOSTIC RESULTS

KUB: + stool impaction and ileus
Hematology:
WBC: 11 (4.0–11.0 (K/mm³)
RBC: 3.10 (4.20–6.10 M/mm³)
Hgb: 8.5 (13.8–17.0 grams/dL)
Hct: 30.6 (37.0%–48%)
MCV: 91.1 (80–100 fL)
MCH: 25.3 (27.0–34.0 pg)
RDW: 17.3 (11.5%–15%)
Platelet count: 153 (130–400 K/mm³)
Remainder of CBC within normal limits

Chemistry:
Sodium: 134 (136–145 mmol/L)
Potassium: 3.3 (3.4–5.1 mmol/L)
Chloride: 98 (98–107 mmol/L)
Carbon dioxide: 22 (22–32 mmol/L)
BUN: 25 (5–23 milligrams/dL)
Creatinine: 1.3 (0.4–1.0 md/dL)
Estimated GFR: 50.2 mL/min/1.73 m² (mL/min)
Random glucose: 128 H (74–118 milligrams/dL)
Magnesium: 2.0 (1.7–2.4 milligrams/dL)
INR: 2.4

BUN, Blood urea nitrogen; *GFR,* glomerular filtration rate; *Hgb,* hemoglobin; *Hct,* hematocrit; *INR,* international normalized ratio; *KUB,* kidneys, ureters, and bladder; *MCH,* mean corpuscular hemoglobin; *MCV,* mean corpuscular volume; *RBC,* red blood cell count; *RDW,* red cell distribution width; *WBC,* white blood cell count.

8. Mr. Johnson's diagnostic results are faxed to the skilled nursing facility, and the health care provider is called with the results. Discuss any abnormalities that are concerning, and describe what actions the health care provider should take at this time.

■ The KUB results indicate that Mr. Johnson has an ileus, which is an intestinal blockage, somewhere in the bowel (Fig. 15.1).

■ His CBC does not suggest an infection. He is still anemic. His anemia warrants further monitoring, but it is not serious enough to require a transfusion of packed red blood cells.

■ The chemistry profile indicates a slightly elevated serum glucose, although Mr. Johnson was not NPO when the laboratory tests were drawn. Additionally, he has mild hyponatremia, hypokalemia, and stage 3 chronic kidney disease. His serum magnesium is normal.

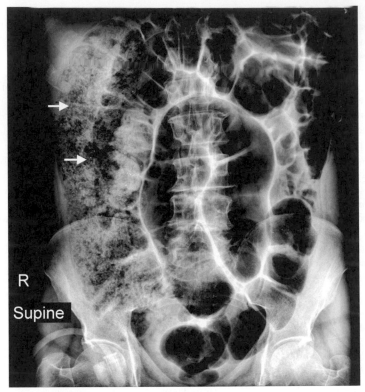

Fig. 15.1   Plain abdominal x-ray shows ileus mainly in small intestine and fecal material in colon with small dense particles *(arrows)*. R, Right. (From Davarani, S. S., & Mirfazaelian, H. [2016]. An unusual cause of abdominal pain. *Journal of Emergency Medicine, 52*[3], e73.)

Case Study, Continued

SKILLED NURSING FACILITY DAY 2: LATE AFTERNOON

The covering physician and the health care provider meet at the nursing facility to reevaluate Mr. Johnson. Mr. Johnson's IV orders were changed earlier when his serum potassium results (3.2) were reported to the health care provider. At that time, his IV fluid was changed to IV D₅ ½ normal saline with 30 mEq KCl at 100 cc/hr to increase his serum potassium to a recommended goal of 4.0 mmol/L. for patients with an ileus.⁹ The health care provider also learned from the surgeon that there was more blood loss during surgery than was expected, which is why Mr. Johnson received the two units of packed red blood cells.

History of Present Illness
   General: Mr. Johnson complains that he is hungry, but states he still did not move his bowels. He denies fever, chills, nausea, vomiting, or abdominal pain.

Physical Examination
   General: Overweight, older male lying in bed in no acute distress.
   Vital signs: Temperature 97.6°F. Blood pressure 138/62 sitting, 142/70 standing. Heart rate 78, irregular with no orthostatic changes. Respiratory rate 20 at rest, O₂ saturation on room air 94%.

Skin: Warm/dry. No rash.

Eyes: Sclera clear; conjunctiva, no injection.

Mouth: Membranes moist. No lesions of tongue or buccal mucosa.

Neck: Supple. No masses, lymphadenopathy, thyroid enlargement, or tenderness.

Cardiac: S1, S2 irregular. No gallop, murmurs, rubs.

Respiratory: Clear to auscultation without rales, wheezes, or rhonchi.

Abdomen: Obese, distended. Rare bowel sounds, barely audible. No organomegaly, tenderness, or rebound. No pain with cough.

Extremities: Right knee incision; + edema, + staples. Minimal erythema at wound edges. No exudate. Pedal pulses present. No edema or calf tenderness.

ASSESSMENT/PLAN

9. Based on Mr. Johnson's afternoon assessment by the physician and health care provider, what are possible considerations for his continued plan of care?

The options are discussed with Mr. Johnson. An enema is a possible treatment, but there is no guarantee that the enema will precipitate a bowel movement. The health care provider also expresses concern about the possibility that the patient will develop abdominal pain during the night and the need for urgent hospitalization will be delayed. Urgent/emergent hospitalization can possibly be prolonged because the covering nurse will first need to call the on-call physician, who may not know the patient, and explain the situation. Once the physician okays the hospitalization, the nurse then must call the family, ready the transfer paperwork, and then call the ambulance. It is unclear how long the skilled nursing requirements for transfer would take in the middle of the night, and for this reason it is decided to send the patient to the emergency room for further evaluation now.

Mr. Johnson is transferred to the emergency room and while there develops some abdominal discomfort. The surgical team is notified and a computed tomography (CT) of the abdomen is obtained. The CT results suggest ischemic colitis, and Mr. Johnson is taken to the operating room. The surgical findings revealed left-sided ischemic colitis, and a bowel resection and temporary colostomy were performed.[10] The ischemic colitis was likely caused by medications that cause constipation, although other causes of ischemic colitis are possible. Older adults have varied risk factors for ischemic colitis (e.g., age, comorbidities), but the causes of ischemic colitis are myriad and can include, among others, emboli, thrombosis, mechanical obstruction, vasculitis, shock, and surgical trauma.[10]

Case Study, Continued

READMISSION TO SKILLED NURSING FACILITY FOR REHABILITATION

Mr. Johnson spent the next 9 days in the hospital and was then readmitted to the SNF. During his hospitalization, the hospital sliding scale insulin protocol was ordered.

History of Present Illness

General: This is a 77-year-old widower 15 days status post right knee replacement, 9 days status post left-sided bowel resection and colostomy secondary to ischemic colitis associated with constipation.

Past medical history: + hypertension, type 2 diabetes mellitus, atrial fibrillation, hypercholesterolemia, osteoarthritis, Barrett esophagus, and GI bleed.

Review of Symptoms

Feels weak, tired, little appetite, some abdominal discomfort with movement. Denies fever, chills, headache, dizziness, difficulty swallowing, chest discomfort or pain, rapid heart rate, shortness of breath, cough, nausea, vomiting, diarrhea, urinary burning or frequency, calf pain, or other concerns.

Physical Examination

General: Alert, older male lying in bed. No acute distress.

Vital signs: Temperature 98°F. Blood pressure 134/68; heart rate 68, irregular; respiratory rate 16 at rest, O_2 saturation on room air 94%.

Skin: Warm/dry. No rash.

Eyes: Sclera clear; conjunctiva, no injection.

Mouth: Membranes slightly dry. No lesions on lips, tongue, or buccal mucosa.

Neck: Supple. No masses, lymphadenopathy, goiter, or bruits.

Cardiac: S1, S2 irregular. No gallop, murmurs, or rubs.

Respiratory: Diminished at bases, but clear to auscultation without rales, wheezes, or rhonchi.

Abdomen: Obese, soft. + colostomy bag with some stool. Bowel sounds positive throughout. No organomegaly or tenderness.

Extremities: Right knee incision, suture line well healed and approximated, staples still present. Pedal pulses present. No edema or calf tenderness.

Admitting Orders

1. Admit to skilled nursing.
2. Physical therapy evaluation and treat; status post right knee replacement and abdominal surgery.
3. CBC/differential, chemistry profile, PT/INR in 7 days.
4. Lisinopril 10 milligrams po daily.
5. Metoprolol XL 50 milligrams po daily.
6. Pantoprazole (Protonix) 30 milligrams po daily.
7. Metformin 1000 milligrams po once a day.
8. Atorvastatin 80 milligrams po daily.
9. Ferrous sulfate 325 milligrams po daily with vitamin C 500 milligrams po daily.
10. Warfarin 2 milligrams po daily.
11. Acetaminophen 1000 milligrams po twice a day.
12. Daily morning blood sugar and at 4 p.m. Discuss with health care provider if greater than 200.
13. Weekly weight. Discuss with health care provider if there is weight loss.
14. Colostomy care.
15. Physical therapy/occupational therapy evaluation and treat.
16. Encourage patient to get out of bed for all meals.
17. Call ortho for follow-up appointment for staple removal.

10.   What other orders should be considered for Mr. Johnson? Should he be started on sliding scale insulin while in the rehab unit? Should older patients in skilled nursing facilities or long-term care facilities be restricted to a diabetic diet, or should Mr. Johnson have a regular diet? Do patients on metformin require B$_{12}$ supplementation? Why or why not?

Every patient's medical regimen should be individualized, and this includes diabetes treatment in older adults. Metformin is recommended even for elderly patients as long as renal function is adequate. Other oral antidiabetes medications also can be considered, although every attempt should be made to limit polypharmacy (defined as greater than five medications a day), simplify medication complexity, and avoid hypoglycemic episodes.[14] In general, concerns about the risks of hypoglycemia negate the benefit of isolated sliding scale insulin regimens for older adults with type 2 diabetes living in these facilities.[15,16] Basal insulin is appropriate when indicated, with a fixed dose of insulin at mealtime, if necessary (e.g., 2 units regular insulin for patients with blood sugar greater than 250 milligrams/dL).[16] According to Munshi and colleagues (2016), easing dietary restrictions is also recommended because this cohort of patients does not always eat well and comorbidities (e.g., renal insufficiency) increase their risk of hypoglycemia, resultant confusion, and falls. For that reason a regular diet is usually recommended in SNFs.[16]

Mr. Johnson is taking metformin, and there is a risk of B_{12} deficiency in patients taking this medication. To avoid the neuropathy or anemia associated with long-term use of metformin, it is recommended to check serum B_{12} before initiating metformin and then monitor B_{12} levels at least once a year.[17,18] Patients with symptoms associated with B_{12} deficiency but low normal serum B_{12} levels (e.g., 200–400 pg/mL) should have methylmalonic acid and homocysteine levels checked.[18] Mr. Johnson's primary care office can be called to learn if he had recent serum B_{12} or methylmalonic acid and homocysteine levels, or the B_{12} level can be ordered and drawn with his other laboratory tests.

11.   Mr. Johnson had a partial colectomy and temporary colostomy just a week after a right knee replacement. What information is important for the health care provider to consider when caring for Mr. Johnson during this admission?

Skilled nursing rehabilitation goals include improving an older adult's function after hospitalization and preparing the patient for discharge home. This goal is not always possible. A great deal depends on the patient's prehospitalization status, but the illness (e.g., infection, surgery) or disorder causing the hospitalization, as well as the hospitalization itself, can affect the patient in multiple ways. Determining Mr. Johnson's cognitive and functional status during the readmission process is important, but other possible factors affecting discharge home should be considered. These include age, presence of depression, and even marital status.[19]

The health care provider readmitting Mr. Johnson needs to be aware that two hospitalizations in such a short period of time could certainly affect his recovery. The second hospitalization would be expected to result in further weakness and muscle loss, especially in his lower extremities. These changes would be caused by both the immobilization and a possible reduction in food intake and protein synthesis associated with his hospitalization and abdominal surgery.[20] The psychological impact and physiologic components of colostomy care are additional stressors for any patient, but in older adults who live alone stoma care can be overwhelming.

A team approach to rehabilitation is always recommended, but before Mr. Johnson is even seen by the health care provider today, a discussion about resources is necessary. Physical and occupational therapy, as well as consultation with nursing and the facility nutritionist, are important first steps. Learning the nurses' familiarity with stoma care and availability of an ostomy care consultant will also be helpful. The early benefit of an ostomy consultant cannot be understated.[21] Patients and families both have problems dealing with ostomy care (e.g., leakage, skin irritation, bag failure) and adjustment to the colostomy in general.[21] Most health care providers (including primary care physicians, nurse practitioners, physicians assistants, nurses, and medical assistants) feel equally inept and also need the support of an ostomy care specialist.[21] Ideally, the ostomy specialist is consulted immediately so that the health care provider can discuss the benefits of the consultation with the patient during the patient encounter today.

The other important consideration is being certain that the patient with a colostomy has adequate privacy. A private room is very helpful for the patient with a colostomy, and having a regular nurse each shift who is comfortable with colostomy care will help allay the patient's anxiety and help the patient feel more comfortable with colostomy care.

If an ostomy specialist is not readily available, reviewing colostomy care with the nursing staff and then including the pertinent steps of skin care should be included in the patient orders. This is important because caregivers who are comfortable and familiar with colostomy care can help allay a patient's anxiety and encourage the patient to learn how to best care for the stoma. Two online references that might help both patients and nursing staff include *Basic Ostomy Skin Care: A Guide for Patients and Healthcare Providers* available at http://www.cdss.ca.gov/agedblinddisabled/res/VPTC2/8%20Paramedical%20Services/Basic_Ostomy_Skin_Care.pdf and *Ostomy Care 2017* available at https://www.youtube.com/watch?v = gOeW3h8Xjzo.

Case Study, Continued

Feeling more comfortable after talking with the ostomy specialist and the health care team at the SNF, the health care provider goes to visit Mr. Johnson. The health care provider knows that it is first important to sit and just talk with Mr. Johnson, ask him about the events associated with his hospitalization, and ask how he is feeling now. Mr. Johnson is quiet at first, then comments: "It was a terrible experience. I never thought all this would happen. If I knew I never would have had the surgery, and I won't have surgery again just to get rid of this thing!"

Not certain what to say, the health care provider listens to Mr. Johnson and then asks him if he met with a colostomy specialist in the hospital. Learning that he did not, the health care provider communicates concern about his situation and explains the plan to have the ostomy specialist meet with him later that day. For now, the health care provider asks first if he has any questions. After answering his questions, the health care provider asks to look at the stoma and skin around it (i.e., peristomal skin) to be certain it looks healthy. As the provider does the assessment, she explains how important it is to keep the skin healthy (no irritation or rashes) and how careful skin cleansing, cautious drying with a cool hairdryer, and carefully applying stoma powder and skin sealant before applying the wafer and pouch helps protect the skin.

The health care provider finishes the assessment and explains to Mr. Johnson that the ostomy specialist will be in to see him and that he can ask the nurses to call her if he has any questions not answered today. She also tells him she will be back to double check on how things are going early next week, but also explains that the covering physician at the SNF will be in to see him later this week. Mr. Johnson is also reassured that he can ask the nurses to call the health care provider team if there are any concerns.

The health care provider writes a note and orders:

1. *regular diet*
2. *add B_{12} to next week's laboratory tests*
3. *consult ostomy specialist*
4. *ostomy care per ostomy specialist*

SECOND POSTOPERATIVE VISIT BY HEALTH CARE PROVIDER AFTER MR. JOHNSON'S ABDOMINAL SURGERY

One week later the health care provider makes scheduled rounds at the SNF. Mr. Johnson was seen by the orthopedic surgeon, and the staples were removed. The orthopedic surgeon noted that Mr. Johnson had fairly good extension of the right knee, although he was not yet at 0 degrees, which is the goal for full extension. His flexion goal is 90 degrees or more, and the physical therapist states he is making progress. Physical therapy also agrees that a home visit and home safety evaluation would be beneficial before the patient is discharged home. Having one of Mr. Johnson's sons present would also be beneficial if there are home safety concerns that the son could help with (e.g., removing scatter rugs, installing safety bars in bathroom if needed). The projected discharge date is unclear, however. The nurses state that Mr. Johnson is "managing" but remark that he does seem impatient and angry at times.

Today, Mr. Johnson denies complaints but tells the health care provider he needs to go home. The health care practitioner explains that for safety reasons Mr. Johnson needs to be able to manage the colostomy care, be able to toilet, and be able to go up and down stairs safely before discharge. He sighs and replies, "I can't afford to stay here much longer."

12. Why is Mr. Johnson concerned about the cost of his rehabilitation?

Patients with Medicare A must have a qualified (not observation) inpatient hospitalization for 3 days and require skilled nursing care to qualify for rehabilitation in a nursing home or SNF. Medicare will pay for the costs of skilled nursing care for the first 20 days, but after that the patient will need to pay $164.50 (the required copay from day 21 to day 100) each day.[22] A patient could be eligible for skilled nursing care for a total of 100 days, but the patient would be responsible for those copay costs ($164.50 × 80 days = $13,560). Some patients have Medigap and Medicare Advantage and could have additional coverage, but Mr. Johnson does not have either of these plans.

13. What are other options of care for Mr. Johnson if he continues to need skilled nursing care but cannot or will not remain in the skilled nursing facility because of costs?

Patients do have the right (unless deemed incompetent to make their own health care decisions) to leave a hospital or skilled nursing center, but it is always wise to work closely with patients and families to make the transition home as smooth as possible. The health care provider believes that Mr. Johnson has used 8 days of his 20 covered Medicare days (i.e., the first initial rehab night after his knee replacement and now he is at day 8 of his admission after his abdominal surgery). Mr. Johnson has several (i.e., 11, if the health care provider calculated correctly) days left before his paid Medicare 20 days expires. It is possible he can achieve the safety goals and continue to manage his colostomy care independently during that time. Discussing options with Mr. Johnson and his sons is one option. For example, how much support can his family realistically provide after discharge, is there a possibility that Mr. Johnson could live with one of the sons for a while if safety goals are not achieved before then, and how much community support is available (e.g., visiting nursing)?

Case Study, Continued

The health care provider asks Mr. Johnson if staying with one of his sons is an option. Mr. Johnson responds: "They don't really have the room and it would be hard with the colostomy. I need to go to my own place." The health care provider asks Mr. Johnson to be patient but adds, "Keep working with therapy and taking care of the colostomy. For today, let me ask you some questions and then I'll examine you and see what we can do to try to get you home. I cannot promise, but we can try."

Review of Symptoms. Feels stronger and has less pain in his right knee since surgery. Colostomy is working, and "I'm managing pretty OK." Denies weakness, headache, dizziness, poor appetite, difficulty swallowing, chest pain, palpitations, shortness of breath, cough, abdominal pain, heartburn, nausea, vomiting, constipation, loose stool, urinary burning or frequency, calf pain, or difficulty sleeping.

Physical Examination
   General: Alert, sitting in chair by his bed. Able to get up with walker and get into bed for examination. No acute distress.
   Vital signs: Temperature 97.6°F. Blood pressure 142/70 sitting, 136/68 standing. Heart rate 72, respiratory rate 22, O_2 saturation on room air 96%.
   Skin: Warm/dry. Area around colostomy appears intact, no erythema or obvious lesions.

Eyes: Sclera clear; conjunctiva, no icterus or injection.

Mouth: Membranes moist. No lesions on lips, tongue, or buccal mucosa.

Neck: Supple. No masses, lymphadenopathy, goiter, or bruits.

Cardiac: S1, S2, irregular. No gallop, murmurs, or rubs.

Respiratory: Breathing easily. Clear to auscultation without rales, wheezes, or rhonchi.

Abdomen: Obese, soft, + colostomy bag with a small amount soft brown stool. Bowel sounds present. No organomegaly or tenderness.

Extremities: Right knee incision, suture line well healed. Still slight edema. Pedal pulses present. No edema or calf tenderness.

13. Write the assessment and plan for the health care provider's visit today with Mr. Johnson based on the health care provider's conversation with Mr. Johnson and the patient's review of systems, physical examination, and laboratory results.

Assessment/Plan

1. **Status post right knee replacement:** Seen by ortho, staples removed, making progress with therapy.
2. **Status post abdominal surgery:** With temporary colostomy secondary to possible constipation-induced ischemic colitis.
3. **Anemia:** Improving. Continue iron and monitor.
4. **Low normal B$_{12}$:** Suspect this is related to metformin, but will check methylmalonic acid and homocysteine.
5. **Atrial fibrillation:** INR 2.8 today on warfarin 2 milligrams po daily. Would prefer his INR to be closer to 2.5 so will plan warfarin 1 milligram po today only and then 2 milligrams po daily. Repeat PT/INR 1 week.
6. **Electrolytes:** Stable.
7. **Chronic kidney disease:** Stage 3A. Monitor.
8. **Type 2 diabetes mellitus:** Fasting serum glucose report today 120. Plan Hgb A1C before discharge.
9. **Discharge plans:** He would like to go home soon for financial reasons. Discussed goals with patient (safe ambulation, stairs, and colostomy care). Will discuss home safety evaluation with physical therapy.

Patient Orders

1. Serum methylmalonic acid and homocysteine tomorrow.
2. Discontinue previous warfarin orders.

Hematology	Chemistry
WBC: 10.2 (4.0–11.0 (K/mm³)	Sodium: 141 (136–145 mmol/L)
Hgb: 10.8 (13.8–17.0 grams/dL)	Potassium: 4.0 (3.4–5.1 (mmol/L)
Hct: 32.8 (37.0%–48%)	Chloride: 101 (98–107 mmol/L)
MCV: 91.1 (80–100 fL)	Carbon dioxide: 26 (22–32 mmol/L)
MCH: 27.8 (27.0–34.0 pg)	BUN: 29 (5–23 milligrams/dL)
RDW: 19 (11.5%–15%)	Creatinine: 1.5 (0.7–1.2milligrams/dL)
Platelet count: 200 (130–400 K/mm³)	Glucose: 120 H (74–118 milligrams/dL)
	eGFR: 48.9 mL/min
	B$_{12}$: 217 (180–914 pg/mL)
	PT/INR 31.4/2.8

BUN, Blood urea nitrogen; *eGFR,* estimated glomerular filtration rate; *Hgb,* hemoglobin; *Hct,* hematocrit; *INR,* international normalized ratio; *MCH,* mean corpuscular hemoglobin; *MCV,* mean corpuscular volume; *PT,* prothrombin time; *RDW,* red cell distribution width; *WBC,* white blood cell count.

3. Today only, warfarin 1 milligram po.

4. Starting tomorrow, warfarin 2 milligrams po daily.

5. PT/INR in 1 week.

Case Study, Continued

THIRD POSTOPERATIVE VISIT BY HEALTH CARE PROVIDER AFTER MR. JOHNSON'S ABDOMINAL SURGERY.

It has been 1 week since the health care provider saw Mr. Johnson and he has only four more days (of 20) of Medicare-covered skilled care. The provider knows that he went with physical therapy yesterday for a home visit and is anxious to learn how the visit went. The nurses remark to the health care provider that he is planning to go home this week, but also comment that the visit went reasonably well. The physical therapist also feels that he did well. There is a half bath on the first floor, and the sons are renting a hospital bed for their father. Some rugs were removed, and one of his sons is putting in a handheld shower and safety bars in the upstairs bathroom. A shower chair was also ordered. Everyone's concern though, is what will happen if he needs help with his colostomy at night. With this knowledge in mind the health care provider goes to see Mr. Johnson.

Mr. Johnson is sitting in his room reading the newspaper when the health care provider knocks on the door and enters his room. He puts down his paper, smiles, and says: "The visit home went well. When can I go home?" They talk for a bit as the health care provider goes through the review of systems and then asks Mr. Johnson how the colostomy care is going. "I don't like it, but I do it because I want to go home. The specialist was here yesterday and told me the skin looks good. I haven't really had too many problems. I think I can manage no matter what."

The health care provider returns to the nursing station to review Mr. Johnson's laboratory results. His INR today is 2.3. Over the past 7 days (i.e., day one, he received 1 milligram of warfarin po, then days two through six he received 2 milligrams of warfarin po daily) for a total of 13 milligrams in 7 days.

These are the results of the methylmalonic acid and homocysteine laboratory diagnostics:

Methylmalonic acid: 305 (70–270 nmol/L)

Homocysteine: 21 (5–15 μmol/L)

When a patient has a low serum B_{12} level, it is reasonable to check both methylmalonic acid and homocysteine. When both of these laboratory results are elevated (i.e., methylmalonic acid and homocysteine), a diagnosis of B_{12} deficiency is confirmed.[23] The likely cause in this patient is metformin therapy, and the recommended treatment is vitamin B_{12} 1000 micrograms po daily.

Review of Symptoms. Occasionally takes "Tylenol" for knee pain after a hard rehab session. Colostomy is working. Not sleeping so well lately because of noises at night. Denies fever, chills, dizziness, weakness, trouble swallowing, heartburn, chest pain, shortness of breath with exertion, cough, abdominal pain, nausea, vomiting, constipation, loose stool, urinary burning or frequency, calf pain.

Physical Examination

General: Alert, pleasant male, no acute distress.

Vital signs: Weight 196 pounds. Temperature 97°F. Blood pressure 136/72 sitting, 142/76 standing. Heart rate 68, respiratory rate 20, O_2 saturation on room air 96%.

Skin: Warm/dry. No rash.

Eyes: Sclera clear; conjunctiva, no icterus or injection.

Mouth: Membranes moist. No lesions on lips, tongue, or buccal mucosa.

Neck: Supple. No masses, lymphadenopathy, or bruits.

Cardiac: S1, S2 irregular. No gallop, murmurs, or rubs.

Respiratory: Clear throughout. No rales, wheezes, or rhonchi.

Abdomen: Obese, soft, + stick on colostomy bag. No evidence of erythema or rash at bag site. Bowel sounds throughout. No tenderness. No organomegaly.

Extremities: Right knee incision, suture line well healed. Slight edema. Pedal pulses present. Sensation intact. No edema or calf tenderness.

14.   Mr. Johnson received 13 milligrams of warfarin over the past 7 days and his INR today is 2.3. What orders should the health care provider write for Mr. Johnson's warfarin dose today? Based on the health care provider's conversation with Mr. Johnson and his physical examination, is discharge home in 4 days a reasonable goal for this patient? What additional information, if any, is needed before discharge is planned?

When Mr. Johnson was taking 2 milligrams of warfarin po daily, his INR was 2.8. At that time, the health care provider decided to give Mr. Johnson 1 milligram of warfarin for 1 day, and then 2 milligrams po daily for the next 6 days. It is reasonable to continue Mr. Johnson on warfarin 1 milligram po today, then 2 milligrams po daily. It also would not be unreasonable to have Mr. Johnson take 2 milligrams of warfarin po daily. Warfarin is easily affected by diet, especially green leafy vegetables, so diet and a new medication is always a concerning variable. It is also important to keep medication regimens as simple as possible for patients to prevent misunderstandings and adverse drug reactions.

After speaking with Mr. Johnson, one of his sons, the nurses, the ostomy specialist, and the physical and occupational therapists, the health care provider decides that discharge home with visiting nurses, physical therapy, and an appointment with the primary care provider soon after discharge is reasonable. The health care provider takes the time to discuss discharge plans with Mr. Johnson, and he agrees that the health care provider can talk to Mr. Johnson's son about the discharge plans. The health care provider also calls the visiting nurses' association and Mr. Johnson's primary care provider so that everyone has a clear understanding of Mr. Johnson's health care problems and the plan of care.

15.   What orders, if any, are necessary before Mr. Johnson's discharge home?

To be certain that discharge home is appropriate, laboratory diagnostics are sometimes indicated. Normally, cholesterol levels and Hgb A1C are checked every 3 months by the primary care provider, so those laboratory tests may or may not be necessary depending on the length of stay in the nursing facility. Mr. Johnson has had a problem with anemia and electrolytes during his hospitalizations and rehabilitation stays, so it would be reasonable to recheck the CBC/differential, serum electrolytes, and renal status if not recently checked. His laboratory results were checked within the past 2 weeks and his electrolytes, renal status, Hgb and hematocrit were all improved at that time. His PT/INR has also been stable, so repeating these tests now does not seem necessary, although it is not necessarily wrong to recheck them. When patients go home though, diets often change and a follow-up PT/INR should be drawn within the first week home to be certain that the patient's PT/INR is within goal. The visiting nurses can be asked to obtain a CBC/differential, chemistry profile, and PT/INR during a home visit to Mr. Johnson and have the laboratory results sent to the primary care provider.

Today's Orders

1. Start vitamin B_{12} 1000 micrograms po daily.
2. Continue warfarin 2 milligrams po daily.

16. Write the discharge summary and discharge orders for Mr. Johnson.

Mr. Johnson is a 77-year-old widower with a past medical history of anemia, atrial fibrillation, GI bleed related to Barrett esophagus, type 2 diabetes mellitus, hypercholesterolemia, hypertension, and osteoarthritis admitted to Manor Village, which is an SNF, 19 days ago after a right total knee replacement and 7-day hospitalization at Mercy Hospital. His surgery was uneventful, but he did require two units of packed red blood cells before hospital discharge because of surgical blood loss. On day one of his rehabilitation, Mr. Johnson complained of constipation, which was likely opioid induced. He was sent to the emergency room that evening, and the abdominal CT suggested ischemic colitis. He had emergency abdominal surgery and colostomy that evening. He was hospitalized for 9 days and then returned to the SNF for rehabilitation.

During his skilled nursing stay, he did well with rehabilitation and learned to manage his colostomy independently. His anemia has improved, and his vital signs, PT/INR, serum glucose, serum electrolytes, BUN, and creatinine have been stable. He will be discharged home with visiting nurse visits. The visiting nurses will check his PT/INR, CBC/differential, and chemistry profile within 5 days of discharge home, and he has a scheduled appointment in your office within 7 days of discharge.

Discharge Orders
1. Discharge home with visiting nurses and physical therapy for continued rehabilitation and colostomy care.
2. Fax discharge summary, discharge orders, and laboratory reports to Mr. Johnson's primary care provider.
3. CBC/differential, chemistry profile, PT/INR in 5 days.
4. Lisinopril 10 milligrams po daily.
5. Metoprolol XL 50 milligrams po daily.
6. Pantoprazole (Protonix) 30 milligrams po daily.
7. Metformin 1000 milligrams po once a day.
8. Atorvastatin 80 milligrams po daily.
9. Ferrous sulfate 325 milligrams po daily with vitamin C 500 milligrams po daily.
10. Warfarin 2 milligrams po daily.
11. B_{12} 1000 micrograms po daily.
12. Acetaminophen 100 milligrams po twice daily prn.
13. Follow-up appointment with primary care provider in 7 days.
14. Follow-up appointment with orthopedics in 3 weeks.

References
1. Department of Health and Human Services. Centers for Medicare and Medicaid Services. (2013). Physician delegation of tasks in skilled nursing facilities (SNFs) and nursing facilities (NFs). Retrieved from https://www.cms.gov/Outreach-and-Education/Medicare-Learning-Network-MLN/MLNMattersArticles/downloads/SE1308.pdf.
2. Buttaro, T. M. (2016). Transitional care. In T. M. Buttaro, J. Trybulski, P. Polgar-Bailey, & J. Sandberg-Cook (Eds.), *Primary care: A collaborative practice* (5th ed.). St. Louis, MO: Elsevier.
3. Brownson, E. G., & Mandell, K. (2014). The acute abdomen. In G. M. Doherty (Ed.), *CURRENT diagnosis & treatment: surgery* (1st ed.). New York: McGraw-Hill. Retrieved from http://accessmedicine.mhmedical.com.ezproxy.simmons.edu:2048/content.aspx?bookid=1202&sectionid=71519979.
4. Donroe, J. (2017). Abdominal exam IV. Acute abdominal pain assessment. JoVE Science Education Database. *Essentials of Physical Examinations II*. Retrieved from https://www.jove.com/science-education/10120/abdominal-exam-iv-acute-abdominal-pain-assessment.
5. Armstrong, C. (2014). JNC 8 guidelines for the management of hypertension in adults. *American Family Physician, 90*(7), 503–504.

6. Tavakkoli, A., Ashley, S. W., & Zinner, M. J. (2015). Small Intestine. In F. Brunicardi, D. K. Andersen, T. R. Billiar, D. L. Dunn, J. G. Hunter, J. B. Matthews, et al. (Eds.), *Schwartz's principles of surgery* (10th ed.). New York: McGraw-Hill.

7. Betts, C. (2016). Constipation. In T. M. Buttaro, J. Trybulski, P. Polgar-Bailey, & J. Sandberg-Cook (Eds.), *Primary care: A collaborative practice* (5th ed.). St. Louis, MO: Elsevier.

8. Stern, S. C., Cifu, A. S., & Altkorn, D. (Eds.), (2014). Abdominal pain. *Symptom to Diagnosis: An Evidence-Based Guide* (3rd ed.). New York: McGraw-Hill. Retrieved from http://accessmedicine. mhmedical.com.ezproxy.simmons.edu:2048/content.aspx?bookid=1088&sectionid=61696569.

9. Ansari, P. (2017). Ileus. Retrieved from http://www.merckmanuals.com/professional/gastrointestinal-disorders/acute-abdomen-and-surgical-gastroenterology/ileus.

10. Washington, C., & Carmichael, J. C. (2012). Management of ischemic colitis. *Clinics in Colon and Rectal Surgery, 25*(4), 228–235.

11. Lee, L. A., & Shieh, E. (2016). Constipation. In S. C. McKean, J. J. Ross, D. D. Dressler, & D. B. Scheurer (Eds.), *Principles and practice of hospital medicine* (2nd ed.). New York: McGraw-Hill. Retrieved from http://accessmedicine.mhmedical.com.ezproxy.simmons.edu:2048/content.aspx?bookid=1872&sectionid=146976018.

12. Common Laboratory Tests. (2014). In R. F. LeBlond, D. D. Brown, M. Suneja, & J. F. Szot (Eds.), *DeGowin's diagnostic examination* (10th ed.). New York: McGraw-Hill. Retrieved from http://accessmedicine.mhmedical.com.ezproxy.simmons.edu:2048/content.aspx?bookid=1192&sectionid=68671769.

13. Bringhurst, F., Demay, M. B., Krane, S. M., & Kronenberg, H. M. (2014). Bone and mineral metabolism in health and disease. In D. Kasper, A. Fauci, S. Hauser, D. Longo, J. Jameson, & J. Loscalzo (Eds.), *Harrison's principles of internal medicine* (19th ed.). New York: McGraw-Hill. Retrieved from http://accessmedicine.mhmedical.com.ezproxy.simmons.edu:2048/content.aspx?bookid=1130&sectionid=79753494.

14. Sandberg-Cook, J. (2016). Aging and common geriatric syndromes. In T. M. Buttaro, J. Trybulski, P. Polgar-Bailey, & J. Sandberg-Cook (Eds.), *Primary care: A collaborative practice* (5th ed.). St. Louis, MO: Elsevier.

15. Lipska, K. J., Ross, J. S., Miao, Y., Shah, N. D., Lee, S. J., & Steinman, M. A. (2015). Potential overtreatment of diabetes mellitus in older adults with tight glycemic control. *JAMA Internal Medicine, 175*(3), 356–362.

16. Munshi, M. N., Florez, H., Huang, E. S., Kalyani, R. R., Mupanomunda, M., Pandya, N., et al. (2016). Management of Diabetes in long-term care and skilled nursing facilities: A position statement of the American Diabetes Association. *Diabetes Care, 39*(2), 308–318.

17. Chapman, L. E., Darling, A. L., & Brown, J. E. (2016). Association between metformin and vitamin B12 deficiency in patients with type 2 diabetes: A systematic review and meta-analysis. *Diabetes and Metabolism, 42*(5), 316–327.

18. Kibirige, D., & Mwebaze, R. (2013). Vitamin B12 deficiency among patients with diabetes mellitus: Is routine screening and supplementation justified? *Journal of Diabetes and Metabolic Disorders, 12*, 17.

19. Everink, I. H. J., van Haastregt, J. C. M., van Hoof, S. J. M., Sofie, J. M., Schols, J. M. G. A., & Kempen, G. I. J. M. (2016). Factors influencing home discharge after inpatient rehabilitation of older patients: A systematic review. *BMC Geriatrics*. Retrieved from https://bmcgeriatr.biomedcentral.com/articles/10.1186/s12877-016-0187-4.

20. English, K. L., & Paddon-Jones, D. (2010). Protecting muscle mass and function in older adults during bed rest. *Current Opinion in Clinical Nutrition and Metabolic Care, 13*(1), 34–39.

21. Hendren, S., Hammon, K., Glasgow, S. C., Perry, W. B., Buie, D., Steele, S. R., et al. (2015). Clinical practice guidelines for ostomy surgery. *Dis Colon and Rectum, 58*(4), 375–387.

22. Sollitto, M. (2017). How long does Medicare cover care in a skilled nursing facility? Retrieved from https://www.agingcare.com/articles/medicare-coverage-of-skilled-nursing-facility-153265.htm.

23. Hauser, S. L., & Ropper, A. H. (2014). Diseases of the Spinal Cord. In D. Kasper, A. Fauci, S. Hauser, D. Longo, J. Jameson, & J. Loscalzo (Eds.), *Harrison's principles of internal medicine* (19th ed.). New York: McGraw-Hill. Retrieved from http://accessmedicine.mhmedical.com.ezproxy.simmons.edu:2048/content.aspx?bookid=1130&sectionid=79756110.

Insomnia

Susan Sanner ▪ Terry Mahan Buttaro

Case Study Scenario/History of Present Illness

Mr. Harry Handley is a 72-year-old African American male who has been managed at your office for the past year for his essential hypertension (HTN). As a new provider replacing his previous health care provider who left the practice, you have been assigned to be his primary care provider. He presents today with a new complaint of insomnia, anxiety, forgetfulness, and shortness of breath, especially when completing light house and yard work. He is accompanied by his daughter who shares her concerns about her father's recent general irritability and forgetfulness. She mentions that the last time she visited her father at his house, she noted that his daily medications that she set up in the pill organizer were still there. When questioned, he became irritated and shared that he had often forgotten to take some of his medications but was not sure which ones because "the pills all look the same" when he looks at the pill organizer.

You determine that Mr. Handley was last seen in the office 8 months ago for his annual physical examination, which was then noted to be unremarkable. At his annual examination, he indicated that for the past 6 months he had been walking 1 hour at least three times a week with his Silver Sneaker's group and had actually lost 8 pounds over the last 3 months. His medications were reviewed at that visit and no changes were made because of the excellent control of his blood pressure (BP). Before leaving the office that day, he made his annual appointment for the same day next year.

Today, his daughter, Laurie, tells you, "My father's activity level has decreased. He has not walked with his walking group in over a month and just seems to not be interested in even completing his daily routine. He did not even plant a spring garden this year." She also shares that she is concerned about him living alone and is planning on asking Mr. Handley to come and live with her, her spouse, and his grandchildren.

When speaking with Mr. Handley, he reports that he gained at least 7 pounds over this last month and admits that part of his irritability is related to the shortness of breath that he experiences when walking, which has prevented him from keeping up with his friends in the walking group. He also reported that he was not fully aware of missing doses of his medications until his daughter discussed it with him. He attributes his insomnia and forgetfulness to his decreased activity and his shortness of breath caused by weight gain because of his curtailed activity.

Medications: Atenolol 25-milligram tablet by mouth (po) daily, Centrum Silver 1 tablet po daily, and Tamsulosin 0.4 milligrams po daily.

Allergies: No known drug allergies; no food or latex allergies; no environmental allergies.

Habits: Former smoker that quit 25 years ago; drinks a beer or a glass of red wine with dinner once or twice a month; denies illicit drug use. Walks at least three times per week with his Silver Sneaker's group up until approximately 1 month ago when he began experiencing shortness of breath.

Past medical history: Essential HTN, hyperlipidemia, and benign prostatic hypertrophy (BPH).

Past surgical history: Bilateral cataract surgery 5 years ago.

Family history: Father died at age 84 of myocardial infarction (MI), had HTN, hyperlipidemia, and congestive heart failure (CHF). Mother died at age 64 of breast cancer. Brother age 68, HTN and BPH. One child, daughter age 45, who is overweight and prediabetic, and alive and well.

Personal and social: Accountant, retired 7 years ago, and widowed 3 years ago. Has one grown daughter and two teen grandchildren. He lives alone in a house. He graduated college with a BBA degree with a concentration in accounting.

Review of Systems

General: Reports weight gain of 7 pounds over past month. Has fatigue, especially on exertion. No appetite changes, fever, chills, or injury. Sleeps on and off during the night with 3 to 4 hours of uninterrupted sleep.

Skin: Denies lesions, rashes.

Head, eyes, ears, nose, and throat (HEENT): Seasonal allergies. Tinnitus left ear, hearing loss right ear restored after cerumen impaction removed. Dental: full set of dentures that fit well with chewing and swallowing. Last eye examination 2 years ago. Denies vision changes, sinus pain, rhinitis, sore throat, dysphagia, ear pain, or pressure.

Neck: Denies pain, stiffness, and swollen glands.

Respiratory: Reports shortness of breath. Denies cough or wheezing. Props on two pillows at night for sleeping.

Cardiac: Denies chest pain or heart palpitations. Has dyspnea on exertion (DOE). Denies dizziness.

Gastrointestinal: + heartburn, denies nausea/vomiting, constipation, hemorrhoids, black tarry stools, or rectal bleeding.

Genitourinary (GU): Hesitancy, nocturia two to three times a night. Denies urgency, burning, and hematuria. Denies dribbling/incontinence, and penile discharge. Denies history of sexually transmitted infection (STI).

Peripheral vascular: Lower legs are now puffy. Denies calf pain, ulcers.

Musculoskeletal: Has intermittent right knee pain along medial joint lines and aching in knee joint. Has intermittent low back ache and muscle tightness. Denies radiation of pain, numbness, tingling, or leg weakness. Denies joint swelling, redness, instability, popping, and locking.

Neurologic: Denies headache, vertigo, forgetfulness, numbness, and tingling.

Psychiatric: Reports insomnia, irritability, and anxiety. Denies lack of interest or feeling depressed or sad.

Hematologic: Denies bruising, history of blood transfusions in past.

Endocrine: Denies heat or cold intolerance, excessive thirst or urination, or increased appetite, sweating.

Physical Examination

General: Well-groomed, attentive African American male in no apparent distress. Affect and responses appropriate.

Vital signs: Height 72 inches, weight: 248 pounds (112.49 kg). Basal metabolic index (BMI) 33.6. BP (left arm) 156/94. Pulse 84 regular, respiratory rate 20, O_2 saturation 96% on room air.

Skin: No lesions, ulcers, or rashes.

Head: Normocephalic, atraumatic.

Eyes: Without redness or discharge.

Nose, sinuses: Nares clear, mucosa pink, moist without lesions. Sinuses nontender to percussion and palpation.

Mouth: + dentures. Membranes moist without lesions or discoloration, posterior pharynx without injection or exudate.

Ears: Bilateral ears with a small amount of cerumen. Bilateral tympanic membranes (TMs) gray with cone of light at 7 o'clock.

Neck: Supple. Thyroid smooth, nonenlarged. No lymphadenopathy.

Cardiac: S1 and S2, regular rate, with +S3, no S4.

Respiratory: Respiratory rate 18 even, fine crackles noted in both lung bases, otherwise lungs clear to auscultation. No rales, wheezes, or rhonchi.

Abdomen: Soft, rounded, positive bowel sounds in all quadrants. Nondistended, nontender, without hepatosplenomegaly.

Musculoskeletal: Full range of motion of all joints with crepitus noted. Bilateral knees with active flexion. Joints are smooth without erythema or edema, nontender to palpation. Some stiffness and pain of knees noted when moving from sitting to standing.

Extremities: Skin warm, dry, uniform color. 1+ pretibial pitting edema bilaterally. Skin: Lower legs smooth with minimal hair distribution, no varicosities.

Neurologic: Alert, 1/3 word recall. Gait: Smooth, coordinated movements.

ASSESSMENT AND PLAN

1. Based on the history and physical examination results, what are the possible causes (differential diagnosis) for the patient's current condition?

- Mr. Handley presents to the office today with complaints of insomnia, anxiety, forgetfulness, and shortness of breath. He is accompanied by his daughter, who is concerned about his missed medications because of forgetfulness. His last office visit was 8 months ago in which he presented with excellent BP control and an unremarkable examination.
- The report of insomnia, anxiety, forgetfulness, and shortness of breath may be from a variety of causes; therefore the patient requires a comprehensive evaluation to determine an accurate patient profile to guide diagnosis and treatment.
- To identify potential differential diagnoses for this patient, review closely what is known currently about Mr. Handley from today's visit. Also, factor in his previous state of health on his last office visit and seek to determine what may have caused these changes in his health status:
  1. Decreased activity.
  2. DOE.
  3. Crackles in both lungs.
  4. Seven-pound weight gain over the last month, 1+ pitting pretibial edema
  5. Irritability, insomnia, and forgetfulness.
  6. BP 156/94 mm Hg; average BP readings presented by the patient via home monitoring at last visit were 130/70 to 136/78 mm Hg.
  7. Presence of S3 on cardiac examination.
  8. Increased nocturia.
  9. Obesity.

It is possible that Mr. Handley's weight gain, fluid retention, DOE, and crackles in the left lung base could be related to CHF. Although there is no single sign or symptom that is diagnostic for heart failure, clinical findings can be evaluated to confirm heart failure and to determine its cause. A diagnosis of heart failure could explain his decreased activity and elevated systolic and diastolic BP.[1]

In terms of Mr. Handley's irritability, insomnia, and forgetfulness, these also could be related to CHF. Decreased oxygenation caused by his presumptive heart failure signs and symptoms could result in mental status changes. Depression is common in aging and more prevalent in patients who have heart failure because the symptoms can affect the patient's functional status and overall quality of life, which can trigger depression.[2] Depression also may reduce a patient's ability to cope and manage heart failure, resulting in poorer health outcomes.[2] Detection of depression is complicated in patients with heart failure because of symptom overlap between heart failure and depression, including fatigue and insomnia. Therefore heart failure guidelines recommend the regular assessment of depression during the patient workup and treatment of heart failure.[2]

The patient's history indicates risk factors for diabetes including his family history and personal history of HTN and obesity.[3]

An assessment of his functional and mental status (which seems to have declined), his ability to perform activities of daily living (ADLs), and screening for depression and dementia may provide valuable information to determine his ability to manage his medical treatment effectively while living alone. A thorough review of Mr. Handley's past medical records to assess previous labs and screenings is necessary. On today's visit, a complete physical examination along with appropriate diagnostic laboratory work and other tests will be needed to fully investigate all symptoms.

2. What components of the history or physical examination are missing?

Mr. Handley is currently being treated for HTN with atenolol. His BP should be rechecked in both arms sitting. The BP in the highest arm should be documented, and Mr. Handley should also have his BP checked standing to determine whether his systolic blood pressure (SBP) decreases 10 or more points, which makes him at risk for falls. The provider will need further information from the physical examination to assess his cardiovascular function.

Mr. Handley has a family history of hyperlipidemia, HTN, and CHF. A careful review of his current medications will help determine whether he is on the appropriate antihypertensive regimen. A thorough assessment of all components of the cardiovascular system is required starting with the funduscopic examination to look for signs of hypertensive retinopathy (narrowing and straightening of terminal vessels, arteriovenous [AV] nicking, and the proliferative changes associated with diabetes.). Although Mr. Handley does not have a family history of diabetes mellitus type II (DM II), he presents with increased urinary frequency, which is a symptom of diabetes, but it is also a symptom associated with heart failure.

The cardiac examination should not only include the more precise BP examination detailed previously, but it is important that the health care provider auscultate all five cardiac landmarks and document findings. Auscultation of the heart should be performed both sitting and supine because cardiac murmurs may be identified in one but not another position. Palpation of the point of maximum impulse (PMI) is necessary because a downward and/or laterally displaced PMI can indicate left ventricular hypertrophy (LVH), which is associated with poorly controlled HTN.[4] Palpation additionally should be performed bilaterally on all peripheral arteries for symmetry and quality of pulsations. The temporal, carotid, aorta, renal, iliac, and femoral arteries should be auscultated for the presence of bruits.

The complaint of weight gain and dyspnea indicates the importance of determining whether Mr. Handley has jugular vein distention (JVD) and hepatojugular reflux. The abdominal aorta should be assessed for location of pulsation and approximate width because Mr. Handley's age and HTN history are risk factors for an abdominal aortic aneurysm.[4]

The risk for diabetes requires that the health care provider also assess for signs of neuropathy by performing the monofilament test on both of Mr. Handley's feet, checking vibratory sense on both lower extremities and the Achilles reflex bilaterally. However, it is important to note that in older adults it is sometimes necessary to spread out the physical examination over two or more visits to not exhaust the patient. His high BP and possible heart failure are the more serious concerns at today's visit.

3. What diagnostics are necessary for this patient at this time?

Mr. Handley reports DOE, and the physical examination reveals the presence of bibasilar rales (i.e., crackles) and 2+ pitting pretibial edema. His signs and symptoms indicate that he should be evaluated for CHF. The health care provider rechecks Mr. Handley's BP sitting and standing and notes there are no orthostatic changes, but his BP does increase when he stands to 162/100. Mr. Handley does not have other positive examination findings, so the health provider continues to be concerned with Mr. Handley's elevated BP and possible heart failure.

Initial tests to be evaluated include B-type natriuretic peptide level, complete blood count, liver function studies, a complete metabolic panel, and serum magnesium. Electrocardiography and chest radiography should also be performed.[5] An echocardiogram should also be ordered because it is the most practical and available diagnostic test available to assess the patient's valvular and left ventricular function.[5] Additional diagnostic testing for heart failure could include a Holter monitor if arrhythmias are suspected and a sleep study if Mr. Handley snores, has a history of daytime sleepiness, or his trouble sleeping at night has been long-standing.

Mr. Handley's history of HTN and family history of cardiovascular disease indicate the importance of ordering a lipid profile and his risk for atherosclerotic cardiovascular disease risk (ASCVD) calculated using the Pooled Cohort Equation.[6-7] A thyroid-stimulating hormone (TSH) with free T_4 should also be checked. His age, obesity, and family history of hyperlipidemia indicates that he should be screened for diabetes with a hemoglobin (Hgb) A1C.[8]

Other appropriate screenings include administering the Patient Health Questionaire-9 (PHQ-9) to identify depression and the Mini-Cog assessment to screen for any underlying cognitive impairment. Again, it is most important to set priorities, and today's visit needs to determine and, if necessary, treat Mr. Handley for HTN and heart failure.

4.   What treatments would you recommend for this patient?

Mr. Handley's SBP and diastolic blood pressure (DBP) are not at the recommended goal set by the Eighth Joint National Committee (JNC 8) of the National Heart, Lung, Blood Institute of the National Institutes of Health (NIH) evidence-based guidelines.[9] According to the American College of Cardiology (ACC) and the American Heart Association (AHA), Mr. Handley also has symptoms of stage C heart failure as evidenced by fatigue and DOE.[1] Because he presents with heart failure symptoms and an S3 gallop, a common physical examination finding in heart failure, an echocardiogram will be ordered to determine whether he has systolic (heart failure with reduced ejection fraction) or diastolic heart failure (heart failure with preserved ejection fraction). This information will guide the health care provider in choosing the best medications to treat Mr. Handley's symptoms. The health care provider does need to treat Mr. Handley's s HTN and dyspnea today; however, an electrocardiogram is necessary now to determine the presence of ischemia or other cardiac changes (Fig. 16.1).

Mr. Handley's electrocardiogram is discussed with the collaborating physician and does not reveal acute changes. The decision is made to add a troponin level to Mr. Handley's laboratory tests and treat his HTN and heart failure as an outpatient today and have him return for follow-up in the next few days. The recommended goal for Mr. Handley' s BP, based on his age, absence of DM, or chronic kidney disease (CKD) is SBP < 150 and DBP < 90.[9] If it is determined that he has been taking his current medications, and the current regimen is inadequate to manage his BP within the recommended goal. The recommendations of the JNC 8 reflect evidence indicating that African Americans with HTN benefit more from calcium channel blockers (CCBs) and diuretics than from a beta-blocker. The health care provider could consider adding amlodipine 2.5 to 5 milligrams po daily along with a diuretic. Amlodipine is a CCB, and they are recommended in African American patients, but the concern about heart failure persuades the health care provider to choose lisinopril, which is an angiotensin-converting enzyme (ACE) inhibitor to treat Mr. Handley's HTN. Hydrochlorothiazide is an effective diuretic in patients with CKD stage 3, but not in stage 4 or stage 5. Because the health care provider is not certain of Mr. Handley's current renal status, it is decided to start Mr. Handley on a loop diuretic, which is considered to be more effective in treating heart failure.[10]

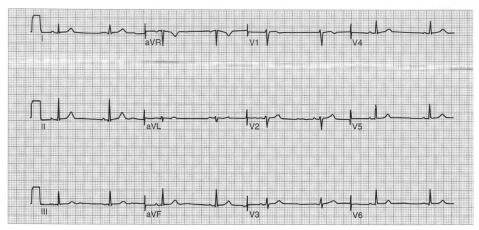

Fig. 16.1   12-lead electrocardiogram. (From Benjamin, I. J., Griggs, R. C., Wing, E. J., & Fitz, J. G. [2016]. *Andreoli and Carpenter's Cecil essentials of medicine* [9th ed.]. Philadelphia: Saunders.)

The health care provider chooses to start Mr. Handley on lisinopril 5 milligrams po daily and furosemide (Lasix) 20 milligrams po twice a day at 8 a.m. and 2 p.m. He will take his first dose of furosemide today, and he will need a repeat chemistry profile within 3 to 5 days of starting the diuretic to check for electrolyte imbalance (e.g., hyponatremia or hyperkalemia or hypokalemia).[11] An appointment is made for him to return to the office for follow-up in 5 days, but the health care provider will call Mr. Handley and his daughter if the laboratory or chest x-ray results indicate the need for Mr. Handley to be hospitalized.

The next day, the health care provider receives the results of Mr. Handley's diagnostic results, which are shown in the subsequent table. What conclusions should the health care provider make about Mr. Handley's health status?

Diagnostic Laboratory Results

Test Name	Result	Reference
Glucose	163 milligrams/dL	7–118
Hemoglobin	13.4 grams/dL	11–16
Hematocrit	40.5%	35–48
Mean corpuscular volume	89.8 fL	80.0–100.0
Mean corpuscular hemoglobin	29.7 pg	27.0–34.0
Platelet count	160 K/mm^3	130–400
Mean platelet volume	11.8 fL	9.0–11.0
Neutrophils (%)	47.4%	37.0–80.0
Lymphocytes (%)	37.9%	23.0–45.0
Monocytes (%)	8.0%	2.5–14.0
Eosinophils (%)	5.9%	0.5–4.0
Basophils (%)	0.5%	0.0–2.0
Sodium	141 mmol/L	136–145
Potassium	4.2 mmol/L	3.4–5.1
Chloride	104 mmol/L	98–107
Carbon dioxide	26 mmol/L	22–32
Anion gap	11 mmol/L	8–16
Blood urea nitrogen	19 milligrams/dL	5–23

Diagnostic Laboratory Results—cont'd

Test Name	Result	Reference
Creatinine	1.2 milligrams/dL	0.4–1.0
Estimated glomerular filtration rate	45 mL/min/1.73 m^2	—
Calcium	8.9 milligrams/dL	8.6–10.2
Magnesium	1.8 milligrams/dL	1.6–2.6
Cholesterol level	215 milligrams/dL	0–200
Triglycerides	125 milligrams/dL	0–150
HDL cholesterol	46 milligrams/dL	>65
LDL cholesterol	160 milligrams/dL	0–100
Cholesterol/HDL ratio	5	0–5
TSH	2.10 uIU/mL	0.27–4.20
Troponin T	<0.03 ng/mL	<0.3
Hgb A1C	7.2	<6.5
N-Terminal proBNP	1040 pg/mL	100–400

BNP, Brain natriuretic peptide; *HDL,* high-density lipoprotein; *Hgb,* hemoglobin; *LDL,* low-density lipoprotein; *TSH,* thyroid-stimulating hormone.

Chest X-Ray Report

Procedure: Chest x-ray: 2 views.
   History: SOB.
   Comparison: October 13, 2017.
   Findings: Cardiac silhouette enlargement. Lungs: + Kerley B lines lower posterior lung fields. Increased pulmonary vasculature. Pleura: Bilateral effusions. Bony thorax: No kyphoscoliosis.
   Impression: Cardiomegaly. Congestive heart failure.

SOB, Shortness of breath.

Mr. Handley's chest x-ray report and proBNP indicate CHF. Potential causes of his heart failure need to be determined. His white blood count is not elevated, so infection as the cause of his heart failure seems unlikely. His Hgb is normal, as is his TSH and troponin level. It is possible that HTN, diabetes, and kidney disease are contributing factors, but it is important to perform further testing to determine whether arrhythmias, coronary artery disease, or a valvular disorder is present. An echocardiogram is scheduled, but the health care provider decides that a cardiology consultation will also be helpful.

   The health care provider also notes Mr. Handley's lipid profile and suspects this is also a contributing factor in Mr. Handley's heart failure. The ACC/AHA guideline for prevention and treatment of ASCVD has classified four statin benefit categories in an effort to reduce cardiovascular events through primary and secondary prevention.[7] The recommendations indicate that treatment should be based on the individual's risk and expected benefit from statin therapy. The assessment to prescribe a statin and the intensity of the statin (based on expected percent reduction of low-density lipoprotein [LDL]) is based on the expected benefit, and specific target treatment goals are no longer recommended. High-intensity statins should reduce LDL by 50% or more, medium-intensity statins reduce LDL by 30% to 50%, and low-intensity statins reduce LDL by 30% or more.[7] According to the ACC/AHA guideline, individuals with known clinical ASCVD should be prescribed a high-intensity statin unless there is a concern for patient tolerance.[7] In

Mr. Handley's case, he is not currently taking a statin, so a high-intensity statin would seem to be appropriate. Using the ACC/AHA 10-year Cardiovascular Risk Assessment Calculator, Mr. Handley's 10-year risk of a cardiovascular event is calculated to be 49.9% (available at http://clincalc.com/cardiology/ascvd/pooledcohort.aspx).

5. Based on the health care provider's review of Mr. Handley's diagnostic testing, what are the provider's next steps in the care of Mr. Handley?

The health care provider realizes that Mr. Handley will need to be started on a high-intensity statin and aspirin 81 milligrams po daily right away. Lifestyle changes (diet and exercise) and achieving ideal weight are also highly recommended for treatment of ASCVD. The JNC 8 Dietary Approaches to Stop Hypertension (DASH) diet includes low-saturated fats (fats from animal sources) and complex carbohydrates, limiting simple carbohydrates.[9] Recommendations for exercise are for 30 minutes of sustained aerobic exercise (brisk walk or more) five or more days per week. A total of 150 minutes of weekly exercise is suggested, and there is evidence that achieving this goal over several days is superior to doing more exercise on fewer days for reducing risk and improving cardiovascular status. However, before starting an exercise regimen, Mr. Handley should have all diagnostic testing (i.e., an echocardiogram and a stress test) and cardiology consult.

Weight loss (often as little as 10% loss) can be associated with an improved BP and lipid profile.[7,12] Therefore weight loss could result in demonstrable improvement in Mr. Handley's conditions. Plant sterols and viscous fiber have shown efficacy in reducing LDL; however, their effect on cardiovascular outcomes has not been determined.[7] Including these recommendations into dietary changes are reasonable. A referral to a nutritionist can be helpful if it is determined that there are knowledge gaps and/or difficulty in applying the dietary changes into his daily routine.

Case Study, Continued

The provider decides to call Mr. Handley on the phone to see how he is doing and also asks if Mr. Handley will agree to allow the health care provider to speak to Mr. Handley's daughter. The phone call reveals that Mr. Handley feels a little less short of breath, and the provider explains that Mr. Handley did have fluid in his lungs and that his blood sugar and cholesterol levels reveal that he is at risk for a heart attack, stroke, or more problems requiring more medicines each day. Mr. Handley does not want to have the health care provider speak to his daughter about his test results, and tells the provider he is not sure about taking more medicines.

SECOND PRIMARY CARE VISIT

Mr. Handley is again accompanied by his daughter for the follow-up visit. His daughter states his breathing is better and Mr. Handley agrees, telling the health care provider that he is sleeping better and does not feel so short of breath, "but I am always in the bathroom though, and my knee and back still hurt. What are you going to do about that?" His daughter rolls her eyes and tries to cajole her father a bit.

Medications:
  Atenolol 25-milligram tablet po daily
  Centrum Silver 1 tablet po daily
  Tamsulosin 0.4 milligrams po daily
  Furosemide 20 milligrams po twice a day
  Lisinopril 5 milligrams po daily
Allergies: No known drug allergies; no food, latex, or environmental allergies.

Review of Systems

General: Sleeping better, breathing better, but "I am always going to the bathroom." Denies falls, dizziness, or weakness.

Skin: Denies itching, rash.

HEENT: Denies vision changes, ear pain or sinus pain, rhinitis, or sore throat.

Neck: Denies pain, stiffness.

Respiratory: Not as short of breath. Denies cough or wheezing.

Cardiac: Denies chest pain, palpitations, DOE, and weakness.

Gastrointestinal: Occasional heartburn, not every day; "depends on what I eat." Denies nausea/vomiting/constipation, or rectal bleeding.

Genitourinary (GU): Still some hesitancy. Up once a night. Denies urgency, burning, hematuria, or dribbling/incontinence.

Peripheral vascular: Denies calf pain, swelling.

Musculoskeletal: Still has right knee pain, which is worse "going to the bathroom all the time." Back pain is the same but "maybe a little worse getting up and down so much." Denies radiation, numbness, tingling, or leg weakness.

Neurologic: Denies headache.

Psychiatric: Denies anxiety, depression.

Physical Examination

General: Well-groomed male in no apparent distress.

Vital signs: Height 72 inches, weight 244 pounds (110.9 kg), 4-pound weight loss. Body mass index (BMI) is 33.1. BP (left arm) 148/84, (right arm) 144/80, standing BP 142/88. Heart rate 78 regular, respiratory rate 18, O_2 saturation on 96% room air.

Skin: Dry, no rash.

Head: Normocephalic; atraumatic.

Eyes: Sclera clear, no icterus.

Nose: No rhinitis or sinus tenderness.

Mouth: + dentures. Membranes moist. No lesions on tongue or buccal mucosa.

Ears: Bilateral tympanic membranes (TMs) gray with cone of light at 7 o'clock.

Neck: Supple. Thyroid smooth, nonenlarged. No lymphadenopathy, no bruits.

Cardiac: S1 and S2, regular rate. No S3, no S4.

Respiratory: Diminished at bases, but no rales, wheezes, or rhonchi.

Abdomen: Soft, + bowel sounds in all quadrants. No organomegaly or tenderness.

Musculoskeletal: + crepitus bilateral knees with flexion, no erythema or edema. + stiffness and pain when moving of and on examination table.

Extremities: Skin warm, dry, less pretibial pitting edema bilaterally.

Neurologic: Alert, conversant. No tremors.

Mr. Handley's labs today are listed in the subsequent table.

Sodium	144 mmol/L	136–145
Potassium	4.0 mmol/L	3.4–5.1
Chloride	105 mmol/L	98–107
Carbon dioxide	28 mmol/L	22–32
Anion gap	11 mmol/L	8–16
Blood urea nitrogen	22 milligrams/dL	5–23
Creatinine	1.2 milligrams/dL	0.4–1.0
eGFR	45 mL/min/1.73 m^2	—
N-Terminal proBNP	690 pg/mL	100–400

BNP, Brain natriuretic peptide; *eGFR*, estimated glomerular filtration rate.

6. Based on today's examination and diagnostic results, what are appropriate interventions for Mr. Handley's health care problems today?

- Mr. Handley's pain.
- Heart failure is improved, N-terminal proBNP is improved.
- HTN is improved.
- Stage 3A CKD.
- DM II.
- Hyperlipidemia.
- Probable coronary artery disease: cardiology and echocardiogram recommended.
- ? Mental status changes versus depression.

Case Study, Continued

Chagrined because the health care provider did not address Mr. Handley's pain at the last visit, the provider decides to address this issue first and apologizes to Mr. Handley that he did not talk about his pain or offer a treatment at the last visit.

The provider first asks if Mr. Handley has tried anything for the knee and back pain. When he answers "nothing," the provider then assesses his level of discomfort to determine its impact on his activity level. The provider recommends first trying acetaminophen extra strength (i.e., one 500-milligram tablet once or twice a day if needed) to see if that helps ease the discomfort. The provider also explains that ibuprofen or Motrin (nonsteroidal antiinflammatory drugs [NSAIDs]) are contraindicated in patients with HTN and heart failure because the BP rises when these meds are taken in older adults and can actually cause fluid in the lungs. The provider also explains that even losing a pound or two (as Mr. Handley just did) can help with knee pain, so weight loss strategies like the DASH diet could be tried and might be beneficial. If the knee pain does not get better, knee x-rays can tell if there is evidence of joint narrowing, and treatment with injectable artificial synovial fluid replacement might be an option. A referral to orthopedics based on the level of joint degeneration seen on x-ray is a reasonable plan. If the x-rays are normal, a referral to physical therapy is another possible treatment for strengthening exercises for joint support and to reverse any possible deconditioning.

The provider then explains that with the new medicines Mr. Handley's BP is better controlled and the fluid in his lungs is decreasing. He asks Mr. Handley if he remembers the name of the two new medicines that were started at the last visit. Mr. Handley has trouble with the pronunciation of his medicines, but he does remember all four of his previously prescribed medications. The health care provider explains that these medicines, plus the cholesterol medicine (atorvastatin), a baby aspirin, and metformin for diabetes, all should be continued, but it will be helpful for Mr. Handley to eat a banana or Medjool date each day or another medication (a potassium pill) might be necessary.

The CKD is explained as partly related to age, but also to the high BP, high cholesterol, and diabetes. These all can be controlled, the provider explains, with medicines and diet, and hopefully, if the knee feels better and heart continues to improve, more exercise will also help. Metformin 500 milligrams po each day with a meal is recommended to help the diabetes, and atorvastatin 40 milligrams orally each day is recommended to decrease Mr. Handley's cholesterol level. A plain uncoated baby aspirin is also recommended, but the health care provider asks Mr. Handley to call if he has any increase in heartburn, explaining that occasional heartburn is okay and possibly caused by aspirin or certain foods, but frequent heartburn (more than twice a week) would be a concern.

The provider then tells Mr. Handley that he knows this is a great deal of information and he will write all this down. He also asks Mr. Handley and his daughter if he has any questions. Mr.

Handley responds he is not so happy about "all these pills." The health care provider then asks: "Do you think it will be hard to remember all we talked about today? Are you worried about your memory at all?" Quick to respond, Mr. Handley replies: "My memory is fine. I was tired before but I feel better." His daughter chimes in that she thinks he is a bit better.

Knowing this has been a long visit, the provider asks Mr. Handley if he can just ask him a few more questions, and then administers the PHQ-2 (available at http://www.cqaimh.org/pdf/tool_phq2.pdf). Mr. Handley's score is 2, and the provider suggests he will ask him these questions again at the next visit to see if what they discussed today will help in any way. The provider also completes a Mini-Cog with the patient, which shows a normal clock and word recall of 2/3. During check out from his office visit today, the patient is given a print out of his current medications and plans for follow-up appointments and lab work.

Discharge Instructions

Medications:
    Atenolol 25-milligram tablet po daily
    Centrum Silver 1 tablet po daily
    Tamsulosin 0.4 milligrams po daily
    Furosemide 20 milligrams po twice a day
    Lisinopril 5 milligrams po daily
    Metformin 500 milligrams po daily with food
    Atorvastatin 40 milligrams po daily
    Baby aspirin 81 milligrams one po daily
    Acetaminophen 500 milligrams, 1 tablet twice a day if needed for pain
Cardiology consult: Two weeks.
Echocardiogram: As scheduled.
Follow-up blood tests: In 6 weeks, chemistry profile.
Follow-up appointment: Six weeks or earlier if any problems or questions. Please have laboratory tests before next visit.

_____

po, by mouth.

THIRD PRIMARY CARE VISIT

The patient returns six weeks later. Prior to the visit, the provider reviews the cardiology consult note as well as the echocardiogram and SPECT test results.

Cardiology Consult Note. This 72-year-old male is seen today in the office after a recent episode of heart failure treated by his primary care provider. Patient is now stable and denies shortness of breath and chest discomfort.

- *Problem 1, coronary artery disease: Recommend aggressive secondary prevention. Change atenolol to metoprolol succinate 25 milligrams po daily.*
- *Problem 2, heart failure:*
  - *Weight 240 pounds. BP stable at 136/80 today. Lungs are clear. Edema has resolved. Recommend continuing same medications. Monitor serum electrolytes, blood urea nitrogen (BUN), creatinine, and glomerular filtration rate (GFR).*
  - *Recommend patient monitor salt intake.*
  - *Recommend cardiac rehabilitation.*
  - *Holter monitor negative for arrhythmias.*
- *Problem 3, HTN: Continue lisinopril 5 milligrams po daily.*

- ***Problem 4, hypercholesterolemia:*** *Continue atorvastatin 40 milligrams po daily. Increase to 80 milligrams po daily if inadequate response to current dose.*
- ***Problem 5, DM II:*** *Increase metformin to 1000 milligrams po twice a day. Continue aspirin 81 milligrams po daily. Check urine microalbumin.*
- ***Problem 6, stage 3A CKD:*** *Monitor fluid status, serum electrolytes, BUN, creatinine, and estimated GFR (eGFR). Patient has had one episode of volume overload and risk will increase if renal function deteriorates.*

Thank you for the referral. I will plan to see the patient in follow-up in 3 months.

Dr. Hartmaker
Cardiology Associates
Third Primary Care Visit

Myocardial Gated SPECT

Indication/reason for study: Hypertension, hyperlipidemia, diabetes, and heart failure.

Findings:

Tomographic images show a distal inferolateral defect.

SPECT images show slightly abnormal left ventricular cavity size and systolic function with a calculated LVEF of 55% and with wall motion abnormalities.

Small positive area of distal left circumflex territory myocardial ischemia. No evidence for myocardial infarction. Patient should be treated aggressively for secondary prevention of coronary disease.

Impression:

Abnormal nuclear stress test.

Echocardiogram

LV wall thickness: Mild left ventricular hypertrophy
LV systolic function: Estimated LVEF 50% with slight wall motion abnormality
LV diastolic function: Impaired relaxation with normal left atrial pressure
RV function: Normal
PASP: 20 plus RA pressure, therefore about 30 mm Hg
IVC: Normal, suggestive of normal right atrial pressure

Valves:

Aortic valve: Mildly thickened; trileaflet. Normal opening
No aortic insufficiency or aortic stenosis by Doppler
Mitral valve: Normal. Trace mitral regurgitation
No mitral stenosis
Pulmonic valve: Normal. Trace pulmonic insufficiency
No pulmonic stenosis
Tricuspid valve: Normal. Trace tricuspid regurgitation
No tricuspid stenosis
Pericardium: No effusion

Impression:

Images were obtained in sinus bradycardia with a rate of 55 beats per minute and without any ectopy.

Normal left and right ventricular systolic function with an LVEF of 55% and with wall motion abnormality.

Left ventricular hypertrophy and mild left atrial enlargement suggest hypertensive heart disease.

No significant valve disease.

LV, left ventricle; *LVEF,* left ventricular ejection fraction; *PASP,* systolic pulmonary artery pressure; *RA,* right atrial; *RV,* right ventricle; *SPECT,* single-photon emission computed tomography.

7. What are the priorities for Mr. Handley's visit today?

The main priority for today's visit is to be certain Mr. Handley continues to improve and check his laboratory tests. Mr. Handley and his daughter arrive and are in good spirits. Mr. Handley has been able to start walking again with his friends and tells the health care provider he is feeling much better. His daughter agrees and states that "he is his old self, he is helping me more than I help him, that's for sure!"

Medications:
    Metoprolol tartrate 25-milligram tablet po daily
    Centrum Silver 1 tablet po daily
    Tamsulosin 0.4 milligrams po daily
    Furosemide 20 milligrams po twice a day
    Lisinopril 5 milligrams po daily
    Atorvastatin 40 milligrams po daily
    Metformin 500 milligrams po daily
    Aspirin 81 milligrams po daily
Allergies: No known drug allergies; no food, latex, or environmental allergies.

Review of Systems
    General: Sleeping better, breathing fine. Denies falls, dizziness, or weakness.
    Skin: Denies itching, rash.
    HEENT: Denies vision or hearing change, sinus pain, rhinitis, or sore throat.
    Neck: Denies pain, stiffness.
    Respiratory: Denies shortness of breath, cough, or wheezing.
    Cardiac: Denies chest pain or pressure, DOE, or weakness.
    Gastrointestinal: Denies recent heartburn, nausea/vomiting/constipation, or rectal bleeding.
    GU: Denies urgency, burning, hematuria, or dribbling/incontinence.
    Peripheral vascular: Denies calf pain, swelling.
    Musculoskeletal: Right knee pain is better. Back pain only if he stands too long.
    Neurologic: Denies headache, dizziness.
    Psychiatric: Denies anxiety, depression.

Physical Examination
    General: Well-groomed male in no apparent distress.
    Vital signs: Height 72 inches, weight: 235 pounds (110.9 kg). BMI 31.9. BP (left arm) 138/80, (right arm) 136/84, standing 138/80. Heart rate 72 regular, respiratory rate 18, O_2 saturation 96% on room air.
    Skin: Dry, no rash.
    Head: Facies symmetric.
    Eyes: Sclera clear, no icterus.
    Nose: No rhinitis or sinus tenderness.
    Mouth: + dentures. Membranes moist. No lesions on tongue or buccal mucosa.
    Ears: Bilateral TMs gray with cone of light at 7 o'clock.
    Neck: Supple. Thyroid smooth, nonenlarged. No lymphadenopathy, no bruits.
    Cardiac: S1 and S2, regular rate. No S3, no S4 or murmur.
    Respiratory: Clear. No rales, wheezes, or rhonchi.
    Abdomen: Soft, + bowel sounds in all quadrants. No organomegaly or tenderness.
    Musculoskeletal: Seems more mobile. Still some crepitus of bilateral knees with flexion, no erythema or edema.
    Extremities: Pedal pulses present bilaterally. Skin warm, dry, no edema, no lesions on either foot. Sensation with monofilament intact bilaterally. Vibration intact bilaterally.[12]
    Neurologic: Alert and oriented. No tremors.
    Laboratory tests: Mr. Handley's labs today are listed in the subsequent table.

Sodium	140 mmol/L	136–145
Potassium	3.8 mmol/L	3.4–5.1
Chloride	102 mmol/L	98–107
Carbon dioxide	28 mmol/l	22–32
BUN	20 milligrams/dL	5–23
Creatinine	1.1 milligrams/dL	0.4–1.0
Magnesium	1.8	1.6–2.6
AST/ALT	All WNL	—
N-Terminal proBNP	585 pg/mL	100–400

ALT, alanine transaminase; *AST,* aspartate transaminase; *BNP,* brain natriuretic peptide; *BUN,* blood urea nitrogen; *WNL,* within normal limits.

Mr. Handley looks well and feels well. He is losing weight and his laboratory results are stable, and there are no concerning cognitive deficits.

Assessment/Plan

- **HTN:** Patient has already changed from atenolol to metoprolol after seeing the cardiologist a month ago. Continue same meds. Recheck Chem 8 in 3 months with follow-up.
- **Heart failure:** Stable. Encourage daily weights and record them. Call if weight gain greater than 3 pounds in 3 days.
- **Hyperlipidemia:** Improving. Continue atorvastatin 40 milligrams po daily. No concerning liver function test (LFT) changes. Recheck lipid profile 3 months.
- **Hyperglycemia:** Increase metformin to 1000 milligrams po daily with plan to increase if renal status stable and no complaints of diarrhea. Continue aspirin 81 milligrams po daily. Will need Hgb A1C next visit with B_{12} level because metformin affects B_{12} absorption. Urine for microalbumin next visit. Referral given for ophthalmology appointment for dilated eye examination to check for diabetic retinopathy.
- **Stage 3 CKD:** Check renal status every 3 months.

Case Study, Continued

At this visit the health care provider also praises Mr. Handley for adhering to his medication regimen, monitoring his diet, and walking again. Mr. Handley praises his daughter. They have been going grocery shopping together to choose ingredients for heart-healthy recipes, and that has helped too.

References

1. American College of Cardiology Foundation/American Heart Association (ACCF/AHA). (2014). ACCF and AHA release guidelines on the management of heart failure. *American Family Physician, 90*(3), 186–189.
2. Eisele, M., Rakebrandt, A., Boczor, S., Kazek, A., Pohontsch, N., Okolo-Kulak, M., et al. (2017). Factors associated with general practitioners' awareness of depression in primary care patients with heart failure: Baseline results from the observational RECODE-HF study. *BMC Family Practice, 18,* 71.
3. ADA. (2016). American Diabetes Association Standards of Medical Care in Diabetes-2016. Retrieved from http://care.diabetesjournals.org/content/suppl/2015/12/21/39.Supplement_1.DC2/2016-Standards-of-Care.pdf.
4. Bickley, L., & Szilagyi, P. G. (2016). *Bates' guide to physical assessment and history* (12th ed.). Philadelphia, PA: Lippincott Williams & Wilkins.
5. Lamber, M. (2012). NICE updates guidelines on management of chronic heart failure. *American Family Physician, 85*(8), 832–883.
6. ASCVD Risk Estimator. Published 2014. Retrieved from http://tools.acc.org/ASCVD-Risk-Estimator/.

7. Stone, N. J., Robinson, J. G., Lichtenstein, A. H., et al. (2014). 2013 ACC/AHA guideline on the treatment of blood cholesterol to reduce atherosclerotic cardiovascular risk in adults: A report of the American College of Cardiology/American Heart Association Task Force on Practice Guidelines. *Journal of the American College of Cardiology, 63*(25 Pt. B), 2889–2934.

8. Mora, S. (2016). Nonfasting for routine lipid testing: From evidence to action. *JAMA Internal Medicine, 176*(7), 1005–1006. Retrieved from http://jamanetwork.com/journals/jamainternalmedicine/article-abstract/2518766.

9. James, P., Oparil, S., Carter, B., et al. (2014). 2014 evidence-based guideline for the management of high blood pressure in adults: Reports from the panel members appointed to the eighth joint national committee (JNC 8). *JAMA: The Journal of the American Medical Association, 311*(5), 507–520.

10. Casu, G., & Merella, P. (2015). Diuretic therapy heart failure—Current approaches. *European Cardiology Review, 10*(1), 42–47. Retrieved from https://www.ecrjournal.com/articles/diuretic-therapy-heart-failure-current-approaches.

11. Yancy, C., Jessup, M., Bozkurt, B., Butler, J., Casey, D., Colvin, M., et al. (2016). ACC/AHA/HFSA Focused update on new pharmacological therapy for heart failure: An update of the 2013 ACCF/AHA guideline for the management of heart failure. *Journal of the American College of Cardiology, 68*(13), 1476–1488.

12. Mullins, A. (2016). Diabetes foot exams among changes in 2016 PQRS. Family Practice Management. Retrieved from http://www.aafp.org/journals/fpm/blogs/gettingpaid/entry/diabetes_foot_exams_among_changes.html.

Fainting

Laura J. Thiem

Case Study Scenario/History of Illness

This is a 63-year-old Hispanic female, widowed. Grown children: Son 44, daughter 43, and son 40. Daughter lives with patient to share expenses.

    Grace Vieira is a 63-year-old, widowed Hispanic female who presents to the primary care office complaining of "dizziness." "I'm just sitting there, I get dizzy, and then I wake up on the floor." She denies fever, headache, shortness of breath, or other recent illnesses. Symptoms have been occurring for 2 months and occur every 2 to 3 days; "I think they are getting more frequent." She denies any other symptoms except dizziness before she "passes out." She also describes trying to sit still to prevent passing out with no improvement of symptoms, but she denies passing out more frequently with activity. During several episodes her daughter checked her blood sugars, which were "usually over 120," her blood pressure (BP), which was "around 130/80," and her pulse, which was "around 70."

Medications:
Losartan (Cozaar) 50 milligrams po daily, paroxetine (Paxil) 30 milligrams po daily, Levemir 30 units subcutaneously (SQ) every night. Regular insulin per sliding scale before meals and at bedtime: Blood sugar 0 to 150, no additional insulin; 151 to 200, 2 (two) units; 201 to 250, 4 (four) units; 251 to 300, 6 (six) units; 301 to 350, 8 (eight) units; 351 to 400, 10 (ten) units; 401 and over, 12 (twelve) units and call provider.

Allergies: Lisinopril (angioedema) and penicillin (rash).

Intolerances: Metformin (diarrhea and severe abdominal cramping).

Habits: Physical exercise includes gardening and lawn work at home. Denies alcohol, tobacco, or recreational drug use.

Past medical history: Type 2 DM, hypertension, anxiety, and obesity.

Past surgical history: Total hysterectomy for fibroid tumors.

Personal history: Widowed for 4 years. Was in a monogamous relationship with husband 45 years. Works as a Licensed Practical Nurse. She has a high school education and vocational practical nursing program. Started courses for associate's degree in nursing for Registered Nurse but did not complete a degree.

Family history: Grandparents deceased of "old age. We did not talk about illnesses then. I think they were all in their 80s." Mother deceased at age 82 after stroke, hypertension. Father deceased at age 70. "I think he had a heart attack. He was mowing and just dropped." Sibling: Brother 66 with "heart problems. He had a stent." Children: Son, 44, alive and well, substance use in past. "He's clean and sober now." Daughter, 43, has noninsulin-dependent diabetes mellitus (type 2 DM) and hypertension. Son, 40, with substance use, has been in rehab several times, relapses frequently. "He stresses me out. I'm always expecting a phone call that he's in jail or worse."

Review of Systems

    General: Admits fatigue. Denies fever or chills.

    Skin: Denies rashes or lesions, changes in texture in hair or skin.

    Head, eyes, ears, nose, and throat (HEENT): Denies headache, rhinorrhea, or changes in vision.

Neck: Denies pain or stiffness.
Respiratory: Denies cough, shortness of breath, or sputum production.
Cardiac: Denies chest pressure, pain, or palpitations.
Gastrointestinal: Denies nausea, vomiting, weight loss, diarrhea, or constipation.
Urinary: Denies urinary hesitancy, burning, or frequency.
Musculoskeletal: Denies muscle aches or joint pain.
Peripheral vascular: Denies swollen legs, calf pain, or cramps.
Neurologic: Denies numbness, tingling, or burning in extremities. Denies headache. Sleep is okay. "My family says I snore."
Hematologic: Denies bruising, bleeding gums.
Endocrine: Denies intolerance of heat or cold, changes in hair or skin texture.
Psychiatric: Patient Health Questionnaire 2 (PHQ-2) in the past 2 weeks. She denies down or sad mood. Denies loss of interest in usual activities. Generalized Anxiety Disorder 7-item (GAD-7) scale results include:
In the past 2 weeks:
1. How often have you felt nervous, anxious, or on edge? *Most days.* **2**
2. Not being able to control or stop worrying? *Most days.* **2**
3. Worrying too much about different things? *Most days.* **2**
4. Trouble relaxing? *Most days.* **2**
5. Being so restless is it hard to sit still? *Not at all.* **0**
6. Feeling afraid something awful might happen? *Several days.* **1**
   Total Score = **9** (total score 6 months ago = 4)
7. If you checked off any problems, how difficult have these problems made it for you to do your work, take care of things at home, or get along with other people? *Somewhat difficult.*

Epworth Sleepiness Scale:
- Sitting and reading: *Slight chance of dozing.* **1**
- Watching TV: *Slight chance of dozing.* **1**
- Sitting inactive in a public place (theater or meeting): *No chance of dozing.* **0**
- As a passenger in a car for an hour without a break: *Slight chance of dozing.* **1**
- Lying down to rest in the afternoon when circumstances permit: *Good chance of dozing.* **2**
- Sitting and talking to someone: *No chance of dozing.* **0**
- Sitting quietly after a lunch without alcohol: *Slight chance of dozing.* **1**
- In a car, while stopped for a few minutes in traffic: *No chance of dozing.* **0**
Total Epworth Sleepiness Score: **6**

Physical Examination
General: Well-nourished, well-groomed Hispanic female appearing stated age.
Vital signs: Height: 62 inches. Weight 182 pounds. Body mass index (BMI) 33.8. Temperature 98.2°F. BP 132/80. Heart rate 76 and regular, respiratory rate 14 at rest, O_2 saturation on room air 99% at rest.
Skin: Warm/dry. No jaundice, rash, or lesions.
Eyes: Sclera clear. Conjunctiva, no injection. No exophthalmos or nystagmus.
Ears: Hearing intact. Tympanic membranes (TMs): No erythema, bulging/retraction.
Nose: Nares intact, moist, no lesions.
Mouth/pharynx: Membranes moist, adequate dentition, missing lower molars, no damaged teeth. Slight thin, clear post nasal drainage. No pharyngeal erythema. Tonsils minimal. No lesions of tongue or buccal mucosa. No halitosis.
Neck: Supple. Thyroid expected size, shape, and consistency. Anterior cervical, posterior cervical, submandibular, and submental nodes nonpalpable.

Cardiac: S1, S2, regular rhythm. No gallop, murmurs, or rubs.

Respiratory: Clear to auscultation bilaterally. No rales, wheezes, or rhonchi.

Abdomen: Soft, bowel sounds occurring every 2 to 3 seconds in all quadrants. No organomegaly or tenderness.

Extremities: Pedal pulses present bilaterally, no edema or calf tenderness, capillary refill 1 to 2 seconds in digits. Monofilament testing performed with sensation intact bilateral feet/toes.

Neurologic: Alert, oriented to person, place, time, and situation. Appears to be an adequate historian. Thoughts coherent. No tremors noted. Cranial nerves: II to XII, grossly intact. Gait smooth, coordinated. Romberg negative. No pronator drift. Muscle tone 3/5 upper/lower extremities. Reflexes: Biceps: 1+ bilaterally. Triceps: 1+ bilaterally. Knees: 2+ bilaterally. Ankles: 1+ bilaterally. Plantar: Down bilaterally.

1. Mrs. Vieira complains of dizziness and syncope with increasing frequency over a period of 2 months. What additional information will the health care provider need to obtain to guide her care? Describe potential barriers to care that may be encountered by Mrs. Vieira in her interactions with the health care providers and system?

The history of present illness (HPI) expands on the reason for her visit. The provider inquires methodically to encourage the patient to provide additional details about her illness, symptoms and experience. Use of a mnemonic such as OLD CARTS (onset, location/radiation, duration, character, aggravating factors, reliving factors, timing, and severity) helps the patient and provider in reviewing various details and clarifying the history. Record the patient's responses in her own words without interpreting into medical language. Seek explanation for unfamiliar terms to ensure an accurate portrayal of the patient and documentation of her symptoms.[1]

On entering the room evaluate the patient's hearing and communication skills, as well as mental status, early in the interview to address any impairment that would affect the patient/provider interaction. Establish the patient's reliability as a historian and ability to direct her own care.[2] Ascertain the patient's health literacy. Health literacy includes evaluation of basic literacy skills, health topics, and patient understanding of these topics. Assessment of the patient's health literacy offers the health care provider the opportunity to alter the interaction to meet the literacy needs of the patient. Meeting patients at their level of understanding is more likely to result in the patient retaining and using the information provided in the visit.[3]

Inquire about the patient's comfort in the setting. Arrange to decrease interruptions or distractions. Elicit the patient's expectation of the visit. Determining the patient's expectation assists the provider in adjusting the agenda to address the patient's expectation as a provision of patient-centered care.[4] Patient-centered care incorporates the patient's expectations and the provider's process of differential diagnosis. The provider can proceed with additional questions, examination, and shared planning of care.

Be aware of barriers created by equipment, technology, or furniture. Inform the patient if you will be taking notes or using an electronic health record during the interview. Explain the interview procedure and request permission to proceed. Provide a quiet, private, well-lighted setting that is a comfortable temperature. To balance the perceived power in the interview the provider should be seated at the same height or lower than the patient with opportunity for eye contact. If the provider is standing or sitting higher than the patient, the patient may feel inferior or subservient impairing communication. If the provider remains standing during the interview, the patient may suspect that the provider is rushed or impatient.[2]

Additional questions to ask Mrs. Vieira may include:

- How can I best help you today? Establishes expectation.
- What concerns you most about these episodes?
- How are these episodes limiting you in your life?

- Have you had any recent medication changes by other providers (increase or decrease of dosages, different medications)?
- Are you under specialty care?
- Has anyone in your family ever described similar symptoms?
- Can you describe what happens when you are dizzy? Do you feel like the room is spinning? Do you feel like you are spinning? Do you feel like you are going to pass out?
- Do you experience any changes in your vision during the episodes of dizziness?

Case Study, Continued

Further conversation with Mrs. Vieira indicates that she is concerned that these symptoms are serious and may indicate a problem with her heart. Today's expectations include blood work and referral to cardiology. She is embarrassed by the episodes. She is afraid to drive or go to public places because she does not know when she will pass out. No one in her family has ever had similar episodes. She has not had any recent medication changes. She has not been seen by any specialists except for a screening colonoscopy at age 50. She denies spinning sensations. She describes the feeling as light-headed. She denies symptoms with position changes or when she is in bed. She denies changes in vision during episodes.

2. Based on Mrs. Vieira's history and physical examination, what differential diagnoses should be considered?

Mrs. Vieira's symptoms, medications, and comorbidities require a thorough evaluation of the dizzy complaint. The differential diagnoses can include syncope related to hypotension, hypoglycemia, hyponatremia, anemia, thyroid disease, cardiac arrhythmia, heart disease, or adverse effects of medications. Vertigo differentials include benign paroxysmal positional vertigo, Meniere's disease, vestibular neuronitis, labyrinthitis, acoustic neuroma, perilymph fistula, cholesteatoma, acute illness, medications, or psychogenic disorders.[1] Additional disease processes to be considered include cerebellar or brainstem dysfunction, syphilis, seizure disorder, migraine activity, and multiple sclerosis.[1]

3. What additional physical examination should be performed?

Additional information can be obtained by performing orthostatic BPs, visual acuity examination, and Dix–Hallpike maneuvers.[1] These examination techniques assist the provider in isolating causes of the dizzy complaint. Positive findings can direct the provider in appropriate diagnostic testing and referral.

Findings for the additional physical examination:
- Orthostatic BP readings: Supine: 148/80, sitting 146/80, and standing 144/78.
- Visual acuity: 20/40 in both eyes with glasses.
- Dix–Hallpike negative.

4. What is the Patient Health Questionnaire-2?

The PHQ-2 is a two-question screening tool used to identify symptoms of depression. A positive score on the PHQ-2 indicates a need for additional depression screening.[5] Today's result does not indicate a depressed mood.

5. What is the Generalized Anxiety Disorder-7?

The GAD-7 is a screening tool used to identify symptoms of anxiety. With a score of 0 to 7, anxiety is unlikely, but a score of 8 and above indicates anxiety.[6]

6. What is the Epworth Sleepiness Scale?

The Epworth Sleepiness Scale is a self-reporting scale to measure daytime drowsiness, which is an indicator for obstructive sleep apnea.[7] The interpretation is as follows:

0 to 7: It is unlikely that you are abnormally sleepy.

8 to 9: You have an average amount of daytime sleepiness.

10 to 15: You may be excessively sleepy depending on the situation. You may want to consider seeking medical attention.

16 to 24: You are excessively sleepy and should consider seeking medical attention.[7]

Over 15% of the US population is affected by sleep-disordered breathing.[4] As a result, health problems including injury, hypertension, and impaired cognition occur. Sleep apnea is also connected to metabolic syndrome, cardiovascular disease, and mortality.[8] Polysomnography is recommended for a score of 16 or higher.[8]

7. What diagnostic testing should be considered?

With the history and physical findings as noted previously, additional testing is indicated. A complete blood count (CBC), basic metabolic panel (BMP), thyroid-stimulating hormone (TSH), hemoglobin (Hgb) A1C, and lipid panel can assist the provider in evaluation of anemia, hyponatremia, hypoglycemia, and thyroid disease and the status of glycemic control. Consider a urine drug screen to rule out substance use. An electrocardiogram (ECG) can assist the provider in determining the presence of arrhythmia or other heart conditions. A computed tomography scan (CT) or magnetic resonance image (MRI) of the brain assists the provider in ruling out brain lesions.[1] A polysomnography can identify causes of snoring.

Case Study, Continued

Mrs. Vieira agrees to laboratory testing and an ECG in the office. The results of the random (nonfasting for patient's convenience) CBC, BMP, lipid profile, Hgb A1C, RPR, urine drug screen, and TSH include:

CBC:

> White blood cells (WBCs): 10.5 (4.0–11.0 K/mm^3)
>
> Hgb: 12.3 (11–16 grams/dL)
>
> Hematocrit (Hct): 36.4 (35%–48%)
>
> Mean corpuscular volume (MCV): 88 (80–100 fL)
>
> Platelet count: 200 (130–400 K/mm^3)
>
> Neutrophils % (Auto): 72 (37.0%–80.0%)
>
> Lymphocytes % (Auto): 24 (23.0%–45.0%)
>
> Neutrophils # (Auto): 2 (1.9–7.5 K/mm^3)
>
> Lymphocytes #: 2 (1.2–3.4 K/mm^3)

Urine drug screen is negative. Syphilis rapid plasma reagin (RPR) test is negative. ECG shows normal sinus rhythm, left ventricular hypertrophy, and no acute findings (Fig. 17.1).

Basic Metabolic Panel

Na	140	mEq/L
K	4.0	mEq/L
Cl	95	mEq/L
CO$_2$	22	mEq/L
BUN	14	milligrams/dL
Serum creatinine	0.8	milligrams/dL
Random glucose	144	milligrams/dL
Hgb A1C	7.6	%

BUN, Blood urea nitrogen; *Hgb,* hemoglobin.

Random Lipid Profile

Total cholesterol	200	milligrams/dL
HDL	78	milligrams/dL
LDL	105	milligrams/dL
Triglycerides	200	milligrams/dL
TSH	2.0	mU/L

HDL, High-density lipoprotein; *LDL,* low-density lipoprotein; *TSH,* thyroid-stimulating hormone.

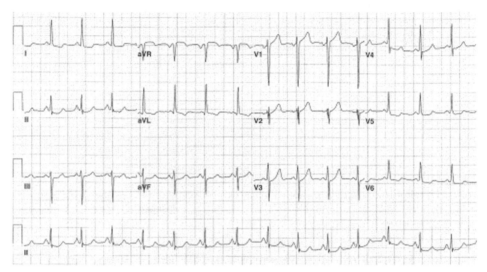

Fig. 17.1 Left ventricular hypertrophy. (From Demangone, D. [2006]. ECG manifestations: Noncoronary heart disease. *Emergency Medicine Clinics North America, 24*[1], 113–131.)

8. What diagnoses can be deleted from the previous differential diagnoses? Are there diagnoses to be added?

Based on the additional testing in the office anemia, hyponatremia, thyroid disorders, syphilis, and substance use can be ruled out. Hypoglycemia, seizure disorder, narcolepsy, adrenal disorders, orthostatic hypotension, and cardiac arrhythmia remain in the differential as the patient is asymptomatic during the visit.

9. How do you explain the diagnostic test results to Mrs. Vieira? After reviewing the diagnostics with Mrs. Vieira, what will you suggest to her as a plan of care? What socioeconomic factors may influence the decision making for Mrs. Vieira? What information do we need to provide so that Mrs. Vieira can make an informed decision?

Mrs. Vieira should be advised that the tests do not reveal a cause for her symptoms. All values for blood counts, kidney, and thyroid function are within acceptable limits at this time. Cholesterol levels will need to be repeated fasting in the future to determine whether intervention is indicated. The blood glucose and Hgb A1C indicate adjustments are needed in glycemic control. Urine drug screen is negative. Inquire about GAD-7 findings and offer medication adjustment or counseling if patient agrees. Begin the conversation of additional imaging or referral to further evaluate left ventricular hypertrophy and for testing beyond the capacity of the primary care office. Assess the patient's knowledge of specialists to ensure the information given is appropriate.[3] Discuss the specialists and settings who provide the indicated services.

Mrs. Vieira will need additional diagnostic testing to determine the etiology of the syncope. Potential concerns that she may have could include time off work (compensated or uncompensated), if the providers and testing centers are covered under her insurance plan, potential out-of-pocket expenses, and future treatment plans. The SHARE approach to enhance the patient's informed and participative decision making involves these steps:

- Seek the patient's participation
- Help your patient explore and consider treatment options
- Assess your patient's values and preferences
- Reach a decision with your patient
- Evaluate your patient's decision[9]

The SHARE process improves the patient's experience and adherence to treatment plans. For the health care provider, patient satisfaction is increased and quality of care is improved.[9]

ASSESSMENT/PLAN

1. **Syncope:** Per the patient's expectations and her symptoms, cardiology consultation will be arranged. CT of the brain will be ordered. If these tests are inconclusive, consider electro-encephalography (EEG), MRI of the brain, and/or neurology consultation.
2. **Type 2 DM:** Future appointment to discuss management.
3. **Hypertension:** Future appointment to discuss management.
4. **Hyperlipidemia:** Future appointment for fasting lipid profile and to discuss management.
5. **Anxiety:** Medication change or increase offered and declined at this time. Counseling referral offered and declined at this time.

PATIENT EDUCATION/HEALTH PROMOTION

1. Lifestyle changes discussed during visit include reduction of intake of animal products including meats, cheese, and eggs and increasing physical activity as possible with current symptoms.
2. The patient is instructed to summon emergency medical services for new or worsening symptoms.
3. The patient is advised not to drive until etiology of syncope is determined.
4. The patient is advised to take paroxetine daily and to call if increasing symptoms of anxiety, thoughts of hurting herself, or someone else occur. Do not stop or increase medication without talking with your health care provider.
5. The hospital/imaging center will call you to schedule the CT of the brain. Please call us if you have not received a call within a week.
6. The cardiologist's office will call you to schedule the consultation. Please call us if you have not received a call within a week.

Case Study, Continued

Mrs. Vieira has a CT of the brain. The report reads that there is a no midline shift of mass effect. No extraaxial fluid collection or intraparenchymal hemorrhage. Gray–white matter differentiation is preserved. Ventricles and sulci are normal for patient age. The impression is no acute intracranial abnormality is noted.

10.   What diagnoses are now excluded in your differential diagnoses based on this finding? How do you explain the findings of the computed tomography test to Mrs. Vieira? What are your recommendations at this time?

The diagnoses of mass effect or stroke can be eliminated from the differential diagnosis. Mrs. Vieira should be informed that the CT does not indicate findings of mass or stroke. Advise her that she will need to follow through with the cardiology consultation as planned.

Case Study, Continued

Two weeks later Mrs. Vieira and her daughter present to your office to discuss the CT findings and to follow up on diabetes and lipid management. She reports that she is having an average of two to three syncopal episodes per day. The cardiology appointment is scheduled for next week.

  Medications: Losartan 50 milligrams daily, Paxil 30 milligrams daily, and Levemir 30 units every night. Regular insulin per sliding scale before meals and at bedtime: Blood sugar 0 to 150, no additional insulin; 151 to 200, 2 (two) units; 201 to 250, 4 (four) units; 251 to 300, 6 (six) units; 301 to 350, 8 (eight) units; 351 to 400, 10 (ten) units, and 401 and over, 12 (twelve) units and call provider.

They bring home glucose readings for the past week that are charted in the following table.

Day	BP	Before Breakfast/Insulin	Noon/Insulin	Before Supper/Insulin	Bedtime/Insulin
Thursday	150/80	144/0 units	152/2	—	240/4
Friday	148/72	180/2 units	160/2	—	236/4
Saturday	162/78	188/2 units	150/0	288/6 (family dinner)	224/4
Sunday	152/74	202/4 units (family dinner Saturday)	164/2	—	188/2
Monday	130/78	144/0	150/2	—	150/0
Tuesday	132/80	152/2	164/2	—	302/8 (potluck at work)
Wednesday	144/78	200/2	200/4 (candy at work)	—	188/2

BP, Blood pressure.

Review of Systems
  General: Admits fatigue. Denies fever or chills.
  Skin: Denies rashes or lesions, changes in texture in hair or skin.
  HEENT: Denies headache, rhinorrhea, or changes in vision.
  Neck: Denies pain, denies stiffness.
  Respiratory: Denies cough, shortness of breath, or sputum production.
  Cardiac: Denies chest pressure, pain, or palpitations.
  Gastrointestinal: Denies nausea, vomiting, weight loss, diarrhea, or constipation.
  Urinary: Denies urinary hesitancy, burning, or frequency.
  Musculoskeletal: Denies muscle aches or joint pain.
  Peripheral vascular: Denies swollen legs, calf pain, or cramps.
  Neurologic: Denies numbness, tingling, or burning in extremities. Denies headache. Sleep is unchanged.
  Hematologic: Denies bruising, bleeding gums.
  Endocrine: Denies intolerance of heat or cold, changes in hair or skin texture.

Physical Examination
  General: Well-nourished, well-groomed Hispanic female appearing stated age.

Vital signs: Height: 62 inches, weight 180 pounds. BMI 32.9. Temperature 98.8°F. BP 134/84. Heart rate 80 regular, respiratory rate 14 at rest, O_2 saturation on room air 98% at rest.

Skin: Warm/dry. No jaundice, rash, or lesions.

Eyes: Sclera clear. Conjunctiva, no injection. No exophthalmos or nystagmus.

Ears: TMs: No erythema, bulging/retraction. Hearing intact.

Nose: Nares intact, moist, no lesions.

Neck: Supple. Thyroid expected size, shape, and consistency. Anterior cervical, posterior cervical, submandibular, and submental nodes nonpalpable.

Cardiac: Regular rhythm. No gallop, murmurs, or rubs.

Respiratory: Clear to auscultation bilaterally.

Extremities: Pedal pulses present bilaterally, no edema or calf tenderness, capillary refill 1 to 2 seconds in digits.

Neurologic: Alert, oriented to person, place, time, and situation. Appears to be adequate historian. Thought coherent. No tremors noted. Cranial nerves: II to XII grossly intact. Gait smooth, coordinated.

Psychiatric: PHQ-2 in the past 2 weeks. She denies down or sad mood. Denies loss of interest in usual activities. GAD-7 scale results include:

In the past 2 weeks:

1. How often have you felt nervous, anxious or on edge? *Most days.* **2**
2. Not being able to control or stop worrying? *Most days.* **2**
3. Worrying too much about different things? *Most days.* **2**
4. Trouble relaxing? *Most days.* **1**
5. Being so restless is it hard to sit still? *Not at all.* **0**
6. Feeling afraid something awful might happen? *Several days.* **1**
   Total Score = **8** (last score **9**, score 6 months ago = **4**)
7. If you checked off any problems, how difficult have these problems made it for you to do your work, take care of things at home, or get along with other people? *Somewhat difficult.*

11. Describe your expected plan of care for Mrs. Vieira related to type 2 diabetes mellitus, hyperlipidemia, anxiety, and syncope treatment.

Assessment/Plan

Type 2 DM: Inquire about barriers that prevent Mrs. Vieira from testing her blood glucose and administering sliding scale insulin four times a day. The American Diabetes Association (ADA[10]) and the American Association of Clinical Endocrinologists (AACE[11]) offer different algorithms for management of type 2 DM. Explore various options for improving glycemic control with the patient. Consider increasing the basal insulin, adding bolus doses, or adding an insulin sensitizer such as metformin.[10,11] Both algorithms stress lifestyle changes including dietary changes and exercise as ongoing treatment strategies in addition to pharmacotherapeutic measures. Consider endocrinology consult. Patient declines changes at this time. She will try to check her blood sugar and administer sliding scale insulin four times a day. Glycemic control is also based on age. For patients under 65, the target Hgb A1C goal is 7 or below. In patients at risk for hypoglycemia or who have limited life expectancy or multiple comorbidities, a Hgb A1C goal of 8 may be appropriate.[12]

Hypertension: The AACE[11] recommends BP control to a mean of 131/70. Patient declines medication changes today.

Hyperlipidemia: Mrs. Vieira's risk of arteriosclerotic cardiovascular disease risk is 10.1% as calculated using the risk calculator from the American College of Cardiology and American Heart Association.[13] Because of the risk of heart attack or stroke for a score over 5% along with known history of type 2 DM with a Hgb A1C over 7.5, Mrs. Vieira is a candidate for high-intensity statin therapy.[13] Patient declines medication today. Patient will discuss with cardiology. Patient states that she will try to eliminate cheese and reduce other animal products from her diet.

Anxiety: Today's GAD-7 indicates a lower score than 2 weeks ago. The primary care provider should continue to monitor for a side effect profile of the medication, paroxetine. For many medications in the selective serotonin reuptake inhibitor (SSRI) class, side effects include nausea, dizziness, nervousness, sexual dysfunction, hyponatremia, and weight gain.[14] The prescriber should monitor for potential life-threatening effects of psychotropic medications including serotonin syndrome, cardiac arrhythmias, and withdrawal syndrome.[14] Patient declines medication adjustment today. Patient declines counseling consultation at this time.

Syncope: Encourage patient to keep cardiology appointment. Consider neurology consult. Return to clinic in 2 to 4 weeks to review home blood glucose log.

PATIENT EDUCATION/HEALTH PROMOTION

1. Lifestyle changes discussed during visit include reduction of intake of animal products including meats, cheese, and eggs and increasing physical activity as possible with current symptoms.
2. The patient is instructed to summon emergency medical services for new or worsening symptoms.
3. The patient is advised not to drive until etiology of syncope is determined.
4. The patient is advised to take paroxetine daily. Call if increasing symptoms of anxiety or thoughts of hurting herself or someone else occur. Do not stop or increase medication without talking with your health care provider.

Case Study, Continued

Mrs. Vieira has seen the cardiologist. The cardiologist has forwarded the following reports and communication:

Carotid Doppler impression is mild bilateral atherosclerotic plaquing without a hemodynamically significant stenosis.

Echocardiogram conclusions:

1. *Left ventricle: Systolic function was normal. Wall motion was normal. Normal diastolic function.*
2. *Aortic valve: Structurally normal valve. Trileaflet. There was no stenosis. No regurgitation.*
3. *Mitral valve: Structurally normal valve. No regurgitation.*
4. *Pericardium, extracardiac. There was no pericardial effusion.*

Cardiology note: Syncope and dizziness with an episode here with documented normal pulse and BP actually being on the high side. These findings rule out cardiac cause for her symptomology. Her other testing included carotid duplex and echocardiogram, which are unremarkable. No further cardiology workup is indicated. We have noted atherosclerotic cardiovascular disease (ASCVD) risk score of 10.1% and recommended high-dose statin therapy. Patient agrees to this plan. Atorvastatin 80-milligram tablets, #30 with one (1) refill is sent by electronic prescribing to the patient's preferred pharmacy. Patient is to follow with primary care provider in approximately 1 month for repeat lipid profile and hepatic enzymes. In light of elevated BP readings noted in patient's home monitoring log and our findings in the clinic, an additional medication will be added. Hydrochlorothiazide 25-milligram tablet #30 with one (1) refill is sent to the pharmacy. Patient is instructed to continue home monitoring and to follow up with primary care provider for laboratory tests and medication adjustments. We will see patient back on an as-needed basis for additional symptoms or concerns.

12. Based on this communication from cardiology, what diagnoses are excluded from the differential diagnoses? What is your plan for Mrs. Vieira?

The diagnoses excluded from the cardiology evaluation include hypotension, heart disease, and arrhythmia. Medication side effect of paroxetine is also ruled out with normal ECG and echocardiogram. The next steps in Mrs. Vieira's plan include elimination of the remaining differential diagnoses: benign paroxysmal positional vertigo, Meniere's disease, vestibular neuronitis, labyrinthitis, acoustic neuroma, perilymph fistula, cholesteatoma, psychogenic disorders, cerebellar or brainstem dysfunction, seizure disorder, migraine activity, and multiple sclerosis. After discussing the cardiologist's findings with Mrs. Vieira, she elects for neurology consult.

Case Study, Continued

Mrs. Vieira has been seen by Neurology, which conveys the following test results and communication.

MRI brain:

> *Findings: Ventricles, sulci, and basilar cisterns appear normal. No evidence for recent ischemic infarct, hemorrhage, mass effect or abnormal enhancement. No abnormal extraaxial fluid collections. There are appropriate vascular flow voids identified.*
>
> *Impression: Normal MRI head examination.*

EEG: Unremarkable.

Ambulatory EEG: "Episodes are nonepileptic in nature."

Magnetic resonance angiography (MRA): Denied by insurance carrier.

Neurology note: Syncopal episodes are not neurogenic in nature because testing has ruled out neurologic events. We discussed increased level of stress as contributing to these episodes. Offered referral to therapist, but she has declined.

Mrs. Vieira and her daughter present to your office to discuss the cardiology and neurology consults and follow up on diabetes and lipid management. Mrs. Vieira states that she has been very careful about her diet, checking her BP and blood sugars, and taking her sliding scale insulin. "It looks like my numbers are coming down. When do we check the hemoglobin A1C again?" Syncopal episodes continue at the rate of one to "several times of day." They express their concerns: "No one so far has found anything for me passing out. What d1o we do now?"

> **Medications:** Atorvastatin 80 milligrams daily, losartan 50 milligrams daily, Paxil 30 milligrams daily, and Levemir 30 units every night. Regular insulin per sliding scale before meals and at bedtime: Blood sugar 0 to 150, no additional insulin; 151 to 200, 2 (two) units; 201 to 250, 4 (four) units; 251 to 300, 6 (six) units; 301 to 350, 8 (eight) units; 351 to 400, 10 (ten) units; 401 and over, 12 (twelve) units and call provider.

They bring home glucose readings for the past week. The home chart reads as follows:

Day	BP	Before Breakfast/Insulin	Noon/Insulin	Before Supper/Insulin	Bedtime/Insulin
Thursday	148/80	148/0 units	152/2	188/2	200/4
Friday	148/72	180/2 units	108/0	178/2	188/2
Saturday	146/78	188/2 units	150/0	168/2	178/2
Sunday	150/74	158/2 units	164/2	168/2	192/2
Monday	150/78	144/0	150/2	102/0	158/2
Tuesday	146/80	148/0	158/2	188/2	168/2
Wednesday	148/78	172/2	178/2	—	156/2

BP, Blood pressure.

Review of Systems

General: Admits fatigue. Denies fever or chills.

Skin: Denies rashes or lesions, changes in texture in hair or skin.

HEENT: Denies headache, rhinorrhea, or changes in vision.

Neck: Denies pain, denies stiffness.

Respiratory: Denies cough, shortness of breath, or sputum production.

Cardiac: Denies chest pressure, pain, or palpitations.

Gastrointestinal: Denies nausea, vomiting, weight loss, diarrhea, or constipation.

Urinary: Denies urinary hesitancy, burning, or frequency.

Musculoskeletal: Denies muscle aches or joint pain.

Peripheral vascular: Denies swollen legs, calf pain, or cramps.

Neurologic: Denies numbness, tingling, or burning in extremities. Denies headache. Sleep is unchanged.

Hematologic: Denies bruising, bleeding gums.

Endocrine: Denies intolerance of heat or cold, changes in hair or skin texture.

Physical Examination

General: Well-nourished, well-groomed Hispanic female appearing stated age.

Vital signs: Height 62 inches. Weight 180 pounds. BMI 32.9. Temperature 97.8°F. BP 140/80. Heart rate 78 regular, respiratory rate 14 at rest, O_2 saturation on room air 97% at rest.

Skin: Warm/dry. No jaundice, rash, or lesions.

Eyes: Sclera clear. Conjunctiva, no injection. No exophthalmos or nystagmus.

Ears: Hearing intact.

Cardiac: Regular rhythm. No gallop, murmurs, or rubs.

Respiratory: Clear to auscultation bilaterally.

Neurologic: Alert, oriented to person, place, time, and situation. Thought coherent. No tremors noted. Cranial nerves II to XII grossly intact. Gait smooth, coordinated.

Psychiatric: PHQ-2 in the past 2 weeks. She denies down or sad mood. Denies loss of interest in usual activities. GAD-7 scale results include:

In the past 2 weeks:

1. How often have you felt nervous, anxious, or on edge? *Most days.* **2**
2. Not being able to control or stop worrying? *Most days.* **2**
3. Worrying too much about different things? *Most days.* **2**
4. Trouble relaxing? *Most days.* **1**
5. Being so restless is it hard to sit still? *Not at all.* **0**
6. Feeling afraid something awful might happen? *Several days.* **1**
   Total Score = **8** (last score **8**, score 7 months ago = **4**)
7. If you checked off any problems, how difficult have these problems made it for you to do your work, take care of things at home, or get along with other people? *Somewhat difficult.*

13. Describe your expected plan of care for Mrs. Vieira related to type 2 diabetes mellitus, hyperlipidemia, hypertension, anxiety, and syncope treatment. What information should be provided or reinforced?

Assessment/Plan

Type 2 DM: Recognize the effort Mrs. Vieira has made in home glucose monitoring and reinforce her current plan. Consider increasing basal insulin.[10,11] Patient declines changes at this time. Next Hgb A1C will be in 3 to 4 months. Mrs. Vieira is willing to consult with endocrinology to rule out adrenal disorders that could contribute to syncope.

Hypertension: The mean of Mrs. Vieira's home BP readings is 148/77. Although this is an improvement, further adjustment may be needed per the ADA,[10] AACE,[11] and Eighth Joint National Commission (JNC 8) guidelines.[15] Patient declines medication changes today.

Hyperlipidemia: Continue the atorvastatin as prescribed by cardiology. Continue lifestyle measures. Return to the clinic in 2 weeks for laboratory studies such as lipid profile and hepatic enzymes.

Anxiety. Today's GAD-7 indicates the same score as 2 weeks ago. The primary care provider should continue to monitor for the side effects profile of paroxetine. Patient declines medication adjustment today. Patient declines counseling consultation at this time.

Syncope: Schedule with endocrinology and inner ear specialty otolaryngologist.

Return to clinic in 2 to 4 weeks to review home blood glucose, BP log, and laboratory tests to follow the start of the new medication, atorvastatin.

PATIENT EDUCATION/HEALTH PROMOTION

1. Lifestyle changes discussed during visit include reduction of intake of animal products including meats, cheese, and eggs and increasing physical activity as possible with current symptoms.
2. The patient is instructed to summon emergency medical services for new or worsening symptoms.
3. The patient is advised not to drive until etiology of syncope is determined.
4. The patient is advised to take paroxetine daily. Call if increasing symptoms of anxiety and thoughts of hurting herself or someone else occur. Do not stop or increase medication without talking with your health care provider.
5. Signs and symptoms of low BP are discussed. Return to clinic if any occur.
6. Signs and symptoms of low blood sugar are discussed. Discussed appropriate foods to improve blood sugar.[8] Summon emergency services if blood sugar remains low.
7. Signs and symptoms of high blood sugar are discussed. Notify office or summon emergency medical services if any occur.
8. Adverse effects of atorvastatin discussed. Return to clinic if experiencing muscle aches or weakness or if having abdominal pain or jaundice.

Case Study, Continued

Mrs. Vieira has seen the inner ear specialist and the endocrinologist. Subsequently she was referred to an electrophysiologist and pulmonologist. The reports and communication are as follows:

Inner ear specialty: No inner ear disorder is noted. Normal oculomotor testing. She had an episode of syncope sitting up from the Dix–Hallpike maneuver, although the Dix–Hallpike was normal. Her positional testing results were also normal. Caloric testing was performed indicating a peripheral vestibular weakness in the left ear. These results must be interpreted with the perspective that she had just had a syncopal episode. Although the patient is having recurrent syncope with disequilibrium, there are no peripheral vestibular disorders that cause syncopal episodes. Therefore it is my opinion that her symptoms are more likely to have a central nervous system (CNS), cardiovascular, or vasomotor etiology. I will see her back on an as-needed basis.

Endocrinology: Primary care office notes, consultation notes, and laboratory studies are reviewed. Orthostatics are positive. Systolic BP dropped by 20 points. She lost consciousness during deep breaths for lung examination, but regained consciousness within 30 seconds. No seizure movements, no incontinence occurred. Thyroid function tests are normal, 24-hour urine metanephrines negative, plasma metanephrines negative, and catecholamines negative. No adjustment is made in her medications at this time. She is to return in 3 months. Encouraged to follow current plan of diabetes management closely. Patient states that she did not have a 24-hour event monitor during cardiology workup. I am going to refer her to an electrophysiologist for further evaluation and treatment as indicated.

Electrophysiology: No evidence that episodes are cardiovascular in nature. Even monitor is negative, although several syncopal episodes are noted in the diary. I suspect sleep apnea may have a role in her syncopal episodes based on the extensive workup she has been provided. I am requesting a consult from pulmonology and will schedule polysomnography.

Pulmonology: Chest film shows the heart size and pulmonary vascularity are within the upper range of normal. The lungs are clear with no acute chest process. There are no effusions. Impression is posteroanterior and lateral chest reveal no acute process.

Epworth Sleepiness Scale Score: 6

Polysomnography: Total recording time 7 hours 57 minutes. Awakenings 14. Sleep-onset latency 34.5 minutes. SaO_2 awake average is 97%, and lowest SaO_2 is 84%.

SaO_2 Table

Desaturations Statistics		Saturation Levels	
Desaturation (%)	Number of Events	Saturation Levels	Minutes
≥2	288	Time below 95%	1:22
≥3	287	Time below 90%	0:11
≥4	239	Time below 89%	0:07
≥5	195	Time below 85%	0:00:36

Respiratory Events: Rapid Eye Movement/Nonrapid Eye Movement

Parameter	REM	NREM	Sleep
Apneas	0	74	74
Hypopneas	1	223	224
Apneas + hypopneas	2	297	298
Duration in apnea	0	19	19
Duration in hypopnea (minutes)	0.4	82.7	83.1
Duration in apnea + hypopnea (minutes)	0.4	101.7	102.1
AHI per hour	1.4	50.8	45.4
Respiratory Arousal Index	0	5.3	4.7
AHI per hour at CPAP 0	—	—	120.4

AHI, Apnea/Hypopnea Index; *CPAP*, continuous positive airway pressure; *NREM*, Nonrapid eye movement; *REM*, rapid eye movement.

Pulmonology interpretation of polysomnography: Epworth Sleepiness Scale 6/24. Sleep architecture: Stage 1 sleep 11.1%, stage 2 sleep 75.5%, stage 3 sleep 2.7%, and rapid eye movement (REM) stage sleep 10.8%. Heart rate: 49 to 87 beats/min, average 60. No arrhythmias noted in study. Limb movements: 231 total movements in study with an average of 7.3 limb movements per hour. The arousal index was 9 events per hour. Snoring: There was loud continuous snoring throughout the study. Oxygen saturation: Average oxygen was 97% with a low of 84%. 294 total respiratory disturbances: 220 hypopneas, 48 obstructive apneas, 20 mixed apneas, and 25 central apneas. The longest duration of apnea was 31 seconds. The overall Apnea/Hypopnea Index (AHI) was 120 events per hour. The AHI of 120 events per hour is consistent with severe obstructive sleep apnea. The patient underwent a continuous positive airway pressure (CPAP) titration portion of their study with a titration range of 5 to 11 cm of water pressure. The ideal pressure was 10 cm of water pressure. On this pressure the patient slept 40 minutes. There was REM sleep seen, and the residual AHI was 3 events per hour. The patient used a large mask during their study and tolerated this well.

Recommendations

1. CPAP at 10 cm of water pressure with large mask and using a ramp feature and heated humidity.
2. Download CPAP data in 4 to 6 weeks for compliance and efficacy.
3. Avoid CNS depressant medications because this can alter the degree of sleep disordered breathing.
4. Because of a BMI of 32.9, weight loss to a normal BMI would be indicated as a part of adjunctive treatment.
5. If the patient continues to complain of excessive daytime sleepiness, she should be cautioned about driving and operating hazardous machinery.

Pulmonology (two weeks after polysomnography): Improvement and resolution of symptoms with initiation of CPAP. Epworth Sleepiness Scale = 6.

Case Study, Continued

Mrs. Vieira and her daughter present to your office to discuss the inner ear/otolaryngology, endocrinology, and pulmonology consults and follow-up on diabetes and lipid management. They note that syncopal episodes have resolved with the use of CPAP. "I feel so much better! I will never go without it." Mrs. Vieira continues to work on glycemic control with dietary measures, glucose monitoring, and sliding scale insulin. Additionally, she continues to monitor her BP at home.

    Medications: Atorvastatin 80 milligrams daily, losartan 50 milligrams daily, Paxil 30 milligrams daily, and Levemir 30 units every night. Regular insulin per sliding scale before meals and at bedtime: Blood sugar 0 to 150, no additional insulin; 151 to 200, 2 (two) units; 201 to 250, 4 (four) units; 251 to 300, 6 (six) units; 301 to 350, 8 (eight) units; 351 to 400 10, (ten) units; and 401 and over, 12 (twelve) units and call provider.

They bring home glucose readings for the past week. The home chart reads as follows:

Day	BP	Before Breakfast/ Insulin	Noon/Insulin	Before Supper/ Insulin	Bedtime/Insulin
Thursday	138/80	138/0 units	152/2	168/2	188/2
Friday	138/72	150/2 units	108/0	158/2	168/2
Saturday	136/78	168/2 units	130/0	158/2	158/2
Sunday	130/74	138/0	134/0	148/0	172/2
Monday	130/78	134/0	130/0	128/0	138/0
Tuesday	136/80	138/0	138/0	168/2	148/0
Wednesday	138/78	152/2	158/2	134/0	136/0

BP, Blood pressure.

Review of Systems

    General: Denies fatigue. Denies fever or chills.
    Skin: Denies rashes or lesions, changes in texture in hair or skin.
    HEENT: Denies headache, rhinorrhea, or changes in vision.
    Neck: Denies pain, denies stiffness.
    Respiratory: Denies cough, shortness of breath, or sputum production.
    Cardiac: Denies chest pressure, pain, or palpitations.
    Gastrointestinal: Denies nausea, vomiting, weight loss, diarrhea, or constipation.
    Urinary: Denies urinary hesitancy, burning, or frequency.
    Musculoskeletal: Denies muscle aches or joint pain.
    Peripheral vascular: Denies swollen legs, calf pain, or cramps.

Neurologic: Denies numbness, tingling, or burning in extremities. Denies headache. Sleep is improved. "I didn't know I had a problem until I started with CPAP."
Hematologic: Denies bruising, bleeding gums.
Endocrine: Denies intolerance of heat or cold, changes in hair or skin texture.

Physical Examination
General: Well-nourished, well-groomed Hispanic female appearing stated age.
Vital signs: Height 62 inches. Weight 178 pounds. BMI 32.6. Temperature 98.2°F. BP 130/78. Heart rate 76 regular, respiratory rate 14 at rest, O_2 saturation on room air 97% at rest.
Skin: Warm/dry. No jaundice, rash, or lesions.
Eyes: Sclera clear. Conjunctiva, no injection. No exophthalmos or nystagmus.
Ears: Hearing intact.
Cardiac: Regular rhythm. No gallop, murmurs, or rubs.
Respiratory: Clear to auscultation bilaterally.
Neurologic: Alert, oriented to person, place, time, and situation. Thought coherent. No tremors noted. Cranial nerves II to XII grossly intact. Gait smooth, coordinated.
Psychiatric: PHQ-2 in the past 2 weeks. She denies down or sad mood. Denies loss of interest in usual activities. GAD-7 scale results include:
In the past 2 weeks:
1. How often have you felt nervous, anxious or on edge? *Several days.* **1**
2. Not being able to control or stop worrying? *Several days.* **1**
3. Worrying too much about different things? *Several days.* **1**
4. Trouble relaxing? *Several days.* **1**
5. Being so restless is it hard to sit still? *Not at all.* **0**
6. Feeling afraid something awful might happen? *Not at all.* **0**
   Total Score = **4** (last score **8**, score 8 months ago = **4**)
7. If you checked off any problems, how difficult have these problems made it for you to do your work, take care of things at home, or get along with other people? *Not very difficult.*

Fasting Lipid Profile and Liver Function Tests

Total cholesterol	188	milligrams/dL
HDL	78	milligrams/dL
LDL	90	milligrams/dL
Triglycerides	150	milligrams/dL
AST	21	IU/L
ALT	15	IU/L
Alkaline phosphatase	45	IU/L
Total bilirubin	0.9	milligrams/dL

ALT, Alanine transaminase; *AST,* aspartate transaminase; *HDL,* high-density lipoprotein; *LDL,* low-density lipoprotein.

14. Describe your expected plan of care for Mrs. Vieira related to type 2 diabetes mellitus, hyperlipidemia, hypertension, anxiety, syncope, and obstructive sleep apnea treatment. What information should be provided or reinforced?

Assessment/Plan
Type 2 DM: Recognize the effort Mrs. Vieira has made in home glucose monitoring and reinforce her current plan. Consider increasing basal insulin.[10,11] Patient declines changes at this time. Next Hgb A1C will be in 3 months.

Hypertension: The mean of Mrs. Vieira's home BP readings is 148/77. Although this is an improvement, further adjustment may be needed per the ADA,[10] AACE,[11] and JNC 8 guidelines.[15] Patient declines medication changes today.

Hyperlipidemia. Continue the atorvastatin as prescribed by cardiology. Continue lifestyle measures. The lipid profile indicates improvement; the hepatic profile remains within normal limits.

Anxiety: Today's GAD-7 is a 4 from a previous 8. The primary care provider continues to monitor for side effects profile of the medication, paroxetine. Patient declines medication adjustment today.

Syncope: Continue with CPAP.

Obstructive sleep apnea: Continue with CPAP. Follow with pulmonology as previously scheduled.

PATIENT EDUCATION/HEALTH PROMOTION

1. Lifestyle changes discussed during visit include reduction of intake of animal products including meats, cheese, and eggs and increasing physical activity as possible with current symptoms.
2. The patient is instructed to summon emergency medical services for new or worsening symptoms.
3. The patient is advised to take paroxetine daily. Call if increasing symptoms of anxiety or thoughts of hurting herself or someone else occur. Do not stop or increase medication without talking with your health care provider.
4. Signs and symptoms of low BP are discussed. Return to clinic if any occur.
5. Signs and symptoms of low blood sugar are discussed. Discussed appropriate foods to improve blood sugar.[9] Summon emergency services if blood sugar remains low.
6. Signs and symptoms of high blood sugar are discussed. Notify office or summon emergency medical services if any occur.
7. Adverse effects of atorvastatin discussed. Return to clinic if experiencing muscle aches or weakness or if having abdominal pain or jaundice.

Return to clinic in 3 months to review home blood glucose, BP log and laboratory tests to follow medications and glycemic control.

References

1. Dains, J. E., Baumann, L. C., & Scheibel, P. (2016). *Advanced health assessment and clinical diagnosis in primary care.* St. Louis, MO: Elsevier.
2. Jarvis, C. (2016). *Physical examination & health assessment* (7th ed.). St. Louis, MO: Elsevier.
3. US Department of Health and Human Services, Office of Disease Prevention and Health Promotion. (n.d.). Health literacy: Fact Sheet. Retrieved from https://health.gov/communication/literacy/quickguide/factsbasic.htm.
4. Epstein, R., & Street, R. (2011). The values and value of patient-centered care. *Annals of Family Medicine, 9*(2), 100–103.
5. Kroenke, K., Spitzer, R. L., & Williams, J. B. (2003). The Patient Health Questionnaire-2: Validity of a two-item depression screener. *Medical Care, 41*(11), 1284–1292. Retrieved from https://www.ncbi.nlm.nih.gov/pubmed/14583691.
6. Spitzer, R. L., Kroenke, K., Williams, J. B., & Lowe, B. (2006). A brief measure for assessing generalized anxiety disorder: the GAD-7. *Archives of Internal Medicine, 166*(10), 1092–1097.
7. Johns, M. W. (1991). A new method for measuring daytime sleepiness: The Epworth Sleepiness Scale. *Sleep, 14*(6), 540–545.
8. Colten, H. R., & Alteveogt, B. M. (Eds.), (2006). *Institute of medicine. Sleep disorders and sleep deprivation: an unmet public health problem.* Washington, DC: National Academies Press.

9. Agency for Healthcare Research and Quality. (2017). The SHARE approach [Website]. Retrieved from https://www.ahrq.gov/professionals/education/curriculum-tools/shareddecisionmaking/index.html.
10. American Diabetes Association. (2017). Pharmacologic approaches to glycemic treatment. *Diabetes Care, 40*(Suppl. 1), S64–S74. Retrieved from https://doi.org/10.2337/dc17-S011.
11. American Association Clinical Endocrinologists. (2017). *Consensus statement by the American Association of Clinical Endocrinologists and American College of Endocrinology on the comprehensive Type 2 Diabetes Management Algorithm – 2017 Executive Summary.* Jacksonville, FL: Author. Retrieved from https://www.aace.com/sites/all/files/diabetes-algorithm-executive-summary.pdf.
12. American Diabetes Association. (2013). Standards of medical care in diabetes—2013. *Diabetes Care, 36*(Suppl. 1), S11–S66.
13. American College of Cardiology/American Heart Association. (2014). ASCVD risk estimator [Web-based tool]. Retrieved from http://tools.acc.org/ascvd-risk-estimator/.
14. Stahl, S. (2013). *Stahl's essential pharmacology: Neuroscientific basis and practical applications.* New York: Cambridge University Press.
15. James, P. A., Oparil, S., Carter, B. L., Cushman, W. C., Dennison-Himmelfarb, C., Handler, J., et al. (2014). 2014 evidence-based guideline for the management of high blood pressure in adults: Report from the panel members appointed to the Eighth Joint National Committee (JNC-8). *JAMA: The Journal of the American Medical Association, 311*(5), 507–520.

Pain/Burning Sensation on Back

Randy M. Gordon

Case Study Scenario/History of Present Illness

Mary Miller, a 70-year-old Caucasian female, presents to the office complaining of waking up with a painful, burning sensation on her left back 2 days ago. She reports working in her garden 3 days earlier. Mrs. Miller denies any known insect stings or bites and does not recall exposure to any chemicals or irritating plants, although she reports having had poison ivy multiple times before without having seen it in her garden. She rates her discomfort as 6 out of 10 and states that her skin in extremely tender to touch. Any pressure applied to the skin results in stabbing pain. She has a history of atopic dermatitis (AD) and occasionally experiences flare-ups, such as when she changes laundry soap. She reports having worn a newly purchased top on the day she was gardening. She denies having washed the top before wearing it. Today she describes a new area of discomfort under her left arm and along her left flank. She is unable to see her back easily, so she cannot describe what her skin looks like. She reports having taken over-the-counter acetaminophen for discomfort last evening without much improvement. For weeks she has been busily preparing and looking forward to a trip to Florida to visit her week-old grandson.

Medications: Lisinopril 10 milligrams daily, multiple herbal supplements, and hydrocortisone 1% cream prn.

Allergies: No known medication, food, or environmental allergies.

Immunizations: Reports having received childhood vaccinations. Received flu shot this year. Received Zostavax 10 years ago.

Habits: Denies smoking or illegal substance use. Drinks 1 to 2 glasses of wine with dinner 2 to 3 times a week.

Past medical history: Obesity, hypertension, AD, chronic lymphocytic leukemia (CLL) stage I diagnosed in 2003 (follows regularly with hematologist/oncologist but is not being treated currently).

Childhood illnesses: Does not recall details, possible varicella age 5.

Past surgical history/hospitalization: Denies surgical history or hospitalization.

Family history: Father died age 90 from congestive heart failure. Mother died age 72 from breast cancer. Grandparents died of "natural causes." No siblings.

Personal and social history: Retired business owner. Married but separated and living alone. She has three sons; two have hypertension but are otherwise healthy.

Review of Systems

General: Reports feeling "tired." Denies fever, chills, weakness, or unexplained weight changes.

Skin: Occasional skin rashes.

Head, eyes, ears, nose, and throat (HEENT): Denies headache, dizziness, vision or hearing difficulties, sinus pain, nasal congestion, or sore throat.

Neck: Denies neck pain or lumps.

Respiratory: Denies shortness of breath or cough.

Cardiac: Denies chest pain or palpitation.

Gastrointestinal: Denies difficulty swallowing, heartburn, nausea, vomiting, or diarrhea.

Urinary: Denies urinary burning, frequency, or flank pain.
Musculoskeletal: Denies back pain, leg pain, or joint pain.
Peripheral vascular: Denies swollen legs or calf pain.
Neurovascular: Denies fainting, numbness, or tingling.
Hematologic: Denies easy bruising, bleeding gums, or history of anemia.
Endocrine: Denies temperature intolerance, sweating, or thirst.
Psychiatric: Denies changes in mood or depression.

Physical Examination
  General: Obese female sitting on examination table in a patient gown. No acute distress.
    Height 5 feet 2 inches. Weight 170 pounds.
  Vital signs: Temperature 98.5°F (orally). Blood pressure 126/78. Heart rate 80 regular, respiratory
    rate 18 at rest, O_2 saturation on room air 99%.
  Skin: Unilateral erythematous, macular-papular eruption involving the lower left back and
    flank. No streaking. Warm and tender to light palpation. Slight swelling is noted in rash
    area, but no punctate to suggest insect bite/sting. No other skin abnormalities noted to
    body.
  Eyes: Sclera white. Conjunctiva pink without injection.
  Ears: Tympanic membranes (TMs): No erythema, bulging/retraction.
  Nose: No rhinitis or sinus tenderness.
  Mouth: Membranes moist, good dentition, no postpharyngeal cobblestoning or erythema.
    No lesions of tongue or buccal mucosa.
  Neck: Supple. Without masses, lymphadenopathy, thyroid enlargement, or tenderness.
  Cardiac: Rapid regular S1, S2. No S3, S4, murmurs, or rubs.
  Respiratory: Clear to auscultation in all lobes.
  Abdomen: Rounded, soft, bowel sounds positive. No tenderness or organomegaly.
  Extremities: Nontender, shotty lymph nodes bilateral axilla. Pedal pulses present bilaterally.
    No edema or calf tenderness.
  Psychiatric: Alert and oriented × 4. Appropriate affect.

Assessment/Plan

1. Based on the history and physical examination, what are the possible etiologies (differential diagnoses) of Mrs. Miller's presenting complaint?

Based on the history and physical examination, several etiologies warrant exploration. Mrs. Miller reports working in her garden and a history of acute allergic contact dermatitis (ACD) secondary to poison ivy. ACD is characterized by pruritic papules and vesicles on an erythematous base. Individuals with ACD typically develop the condition within a few days of exposure in areas that were exposed directly to the allergen. In this case the patient was unaware of direct exposure, which lessens, although it does not exclude, the diagnosis as a potential differential.

AD, also known as eczema, may predispose a patient's skin to irritation by numerous exogenous triggers. Mrs. Miller reports wearing a new top before she washed it. Although the manufacturer's chemicals in an unwashed article of clothing may be an aggravating trigger for skin irritation, the provider would expect to find widespread dermatitis involving any skin surface area that was in contact with the irritant. The focused distribution of the skin rash only along the patient's left scapula and left flank makes this etiology doubtful. Skin irritation consistent with AD is pruritic and not generally described as burning or painful, as in this case.

Many patients confuse an insect bite with a sting and may use the terms interchangeably. A bite is usually from mouth parts and occurs when an insect is agitated to defend itself or when an insect seeks to feed. Bites from mosquitoes, fleas, and mites are more likely to cause itching than pain. In a local reaction, the patient may complain of discomfort, itching, moderate or severe pain, erythema, tenderness, warmth, and edema of tissues surrounding the site. In a severe local reaction, complaints include generalized erythema, urticaria, and pruritic edema. In this case Mrs. Miller denied having seen any insects. Physical examination did not identify any punctate to suggest an insect sting or bite, making this etiology less likely.

The provider should consider a more likely etiology that is not contingent on acute external exposure to the environment. Herpes zoster is caused by the varicella zoster virus (VZV), which causes an acute skin rash in adults, especially immunocompromised patients.[1] The age-related increased incidence of herpes zoster and its complications is thought to be a result of the decline in cell-mediated immunity. During the preeruptive phase, one early symptom of herpes zoster is paresthesia, which occurs as a result of infection, inflammation, and compression along the dermatomal distribution of the spinal cord.[2] This sensory phenomenon may appear along one or more skin dermatomes and lasts 1 to 10 days (average 48 hours). The thoracic dermatomes, specifically T5 and T6, and the cervical dermatomes are the most commonly affected in all age groups (45% and 23%, respectively). Along the thoracic dermatomes, the pain may simulate cardiac pain, appendicitis or other intraabdominal disease, or sciatica. Other associated symptoms include malaise, myalgia, headache, photophobia, and, uncommonly, fever.[1]

2. What skin rash characteristics are associated with herpes zoster during the preeruptive phase?

The preeruptive phase may precede a skin eruption by 72 hours. This phase begins with patchy erythema, which evolves into papular lesions. Skin changes may be indistinguishable from other exanthems or skin rashes. Vesicles are not noted during the preeruptive phase, which can make diagnosis difficult if based on cutaneous manifestation.[3]

3. What are the diagnostic criteria for herpes zoster?

In most patients, confirming the diagnosis via laboratory testing usually has no utility because most tests are time-consuming, lack specificity, or are unavailable outside of research facilities. In select patient populations, however, the presentation of herpes zoster may vary. Pain may be absent or the rash may be atypical with limited area of dermatomal involvement or failure of vesicles to appear (zoster sine herpete); therefore selective testing may be necessary to increase diagnostic accuracy. This is particularly true in VZV-vaccinated patients. If the diagnosis is questionable, the provider may order a Tzanck test, which is a rapid way to determine the presence of the varicella virus and can be performed in the office. This test does not distinguish between the herpes simplex virus and VZV. The direct fluorescent antibody (DFA) test is another rapid test that can be performed in the office. A viral culture may also be ordered. DFA and molecular assays are the most commonly used tests for reactivation. Culture is less sensitive than DFA. Polymerase chain reaction (PCR) analysis, which detects the DNA sequence of the virus, along with an antibody titer are diagnostic tests preferred over culture because of greater sensitivity.[1] Molecular assay is rapid for detection with clinical relevance to be determined. Molecular assays with different formats are the main tools for the differentiation between wild-type and vaccine strains. Serology is mostly useful for the determination of immunity status. Serology tests and cultures may not be available in all practice settings and results may take several days to weeks to acquire.[2]

4. In this case, what precipitating factors may have contributed to a herpes zoster episode?

After initial varicella infection, usually as a child, the virus remains dormant in the dorsal nerve root. How the virus remains in the body or subsequently reactivates is not well understood.

Reactivation is thought to be influenced by a multitude of factors, such as the patient's age, trauma, surgery, and chronic comorbid diseases like rheumatoid arthritis and inflammatory bowel disease.[1] Age is the most significant risk factor, presumably related to a loss of components of VZV-specific cell-mediated immunity response because of aging (i.e., immune senescence) possibly combined with waning immunity that might occur over time after the initial varicella infection.[4] Once reactivated, the virus travels from the nerve body to the endings in the skin producing vesicles. Patients with a compromised immune system are at higher risk for herpes zoster. Mrs. Miller has CLL, which is a monoclonal disorder characterized by a progressive accumulation of functionally incompetent lymphocytes.[5] This condition also places Mrs. Miller at increased risk of developing disseminated herpes zoster. Although rare, disseminated herpes zoster is defined as 20 (or more) lesions appearing outside either the primarily affected dermatome or dermatomes directly adjacent to it. Along with the skin, other organs, such as the liver or brain, may also be affected (causing hepatitis or encephalitis, respectively), which makes the condition potentially lethal.[6] Anecdotal references to psychological or physiologic stress as a causative factor remain unproven by research. Mrs. Miller has been preparing to travel for a planned visit with her son and newborn grandson. The physical and psychological stress of a significant life event, even an event that is happily anticipated, may be a contributing factor for a herpes zoster episode. Persons with severe physical limitations and older women are thought to be a higher risk.[1]

5.   What management interventions are necessary for this patient at this time?

It is important for the provider to have a high index of suspicion for herpes zoster, particularly in the preeruptive phase. Although the course of the herpes zoster episode is self-limiting, effective therapies can reduce the extent and duration of symptoms, and possibly the risk of chronic sequelae. The Centers for Disease Control and Prevention (CDC) offers guidelines for therapy.[4] The goals of therapy for herpes zoster are to shorten the clinical course, provide analgesia, prevent complications, and decrease the incidence of postherpetic neuralgia (PHN). Therapeutic choices generally depend on the host's immune state and on timing regarding the presentation of zoster. Conservative therapies include nonsteroidal antiinflammatory drugs (NSAIDS), wet dressings with 5% aluminum acetate (Burow solution) applied for 30 to 60 minutes four to six times daily, and lotions (such as calamine). Treatment is of greatest benefit in immunocompromised patients and persons older than 50 years of age. Mrs. Miller meets these criteria and therefore warrants treatment.

Mrs. Miller presented to the office approximately 48 to 72 hours after the onset of symptoms. Ideally, antiviral agents should be initiated within 72 hours of symptom onset to have the most beneficial effect, decrease the length of time for new vesicle formation, minimize the number of days to attain complete crusting, and reduce the days of acute discomfort.[1,4] Several studies found antiviral therapy to be beneficial even when started beyond the traditional 72-hour therapeutic window, which supports initiating antiviral therapy for herpes zoster regardless of the time of presentation. Acyclovir and its derivatives (valacyclovir, famciclovir, and penciclovir) are safe and effective in treating active disease and preventing PHN.[4] Their mechanism of action involves preventing VZV replication through inhibition of viral DNA polymerase. Some studies suggested that valacyclovir and famciclovir may be superior to acyclovir in resolving pain and accelerating cutaneous healing.[4] However, the development of acyclovir-resistant viral strains suggests a need for newer agents. The duration of antiviral treatment in studies has ranged from 7 to 21 days. For immunocompetent patients, a 7- to 10-day course of acyclovir or a 7-day course of famciclovir is appropriate, with longer courses for immunocompromised patients.[1,4,6] The provider prescribes famciclovir 500 milligrams by mouth every 8 hours for a 7-day course.

Although debated by the research, orally administered corticosteroid may provide modest benefits in reducing the acute pain of herpes zoster and the incidence of PHN. Prednisone used in conjunction with acyclovir has been shown to reduce the pain associated with herpes zoster.

The likely mechanism involves decreasing the degree of neuritis caused by active infection and, possibly, decreasing residual damage to affected nerves. The provider prescribes the suggested dosing schedule of 30 milligrams orally twice daily on days 1 through 7, then 15 milligrams twice daily on days 8 through 14, and then 7.5 milligrams twice daily on days 15 through 21.[4,6]

The pain associated with herpes zoster ranges from mild to excruciating. Patients with mild to moderate pain may respond to over-the-counter analgesics. Patients with more severe pain may require the addition of a narcotic medication. A regular dosing schedule results in better pain control. Topical lidocaine (Xylocaine) applied to intact skin and nerve blocks have been reported to be effective in reducing pain. Referral to a pain specialist, or even hospitalization and administration of epidural analgesics, should be considered for incapacitating pain. Application of topical creams or lotions and drying agents during the preeruptive and eruptive phases may not be tolerated well by patients with acute pain and should be recommended accordingly. No evidence indicates that topical antiviral therapy or corticosteroids without systemic antiviral therapy have a role in treatment of zoster.

Patients with uncomplicated zoster should be advised to keep the rash clean and dry, to avoid topical antibiotics, and, if possible, to keep the rash covered. They should alert their provider if the rash worsens or they have a fever, which could indicate bacterial superinfection.

6. What do you recommend regarding travel and exposure to others during this time?

During the preeruptive and eruptive phases, Mrs. Miller should be counseled to avoid direct skin contact with immunocompromised persons, pregnant women, and individuals with no history of chickenpox infection (including infants). Physical activity should be encouraged as tolerated. If contact with other persons is unavoidable, the lesions should be covered with a nonadherent, absorbent dressing to decrease the potential inadvertent spread of the virus. Dressings with exudate must be discarded appropriately and clothing laundered daily.

7. When is it appropriate to follow up with Mrs. Miller?

In this case the presenting physical skin findings are questionable for the diagnosis. It is essential to request that the patient follow up in 24 to 48 hours so that the provider may reevaluate the patient's skin and monitor the rash for evolution. It is important to note that the evolution of the skin eruption may not be halted by having received the herpes zoster vaccination, especially if the vaccination was received 5 or more years earlier.

Case Study, Continued

The provider orders a viral culture to determine if the patient's rash is caused by VZV. Ideally, a culture should be collected from a newly formed vesicle with a minimal amount of exudate or crust. Adequate collection of specimens from maculopapular lesions in vaccinated persons can be challenging. However, a recent study comparing a variety of specimens from the same patients vaccinated with one dose suggests that maculopapular lesions collected with proper technique can be highly reliable specimen types for detecting VZV.[7] In the absence of vesicles, the culture is collected from a maculopapular lesion on the patient's left back using the following procedure guidelines[8]:

     Specimen collection materials: A sterile cotton swab and polyester or rayon on a plastic shaft are recommended.

     Collection/transport container: Universal Transport Medium (UTM), store at room temperature and use before expiration date (written on the UTM collection device).

     Collection of a clinical sample:

         1. Select a lesion or lesions that are fluid filled to be sampled. In the absence of fluid-filled lesions, pick the crusts of lesions that appear partially crusted over, put them into the UTM, and follow on from step 4.

2. If the site is ulcerated or infected, remove the crust and discard, remove the pus with a sterile swab, and follow on from step 4 with a fresh sterile swab.
3. Clean area with sterile water or saline, if required. Do not use alcohol or other skin disinfectants to clean the area.
4. Using a sterile needle or disposable scalpel, and gently de-roof the vesicle.
5. Use the sterile swab to collect the fluid and swab the base of the lesion to collect cellular material in which the virus is present. (If multiple distinct sites [e.g., face, chest, etc.] are being sampled, use separate swabs for each site, and put each swab into a separately labeled UTM container.)
6. Place the swab(s) into the UTM and screw the cap on tightly to prevent leakage of the transport medium. (It may be necessary to cut the top of the swab so that the cap will screw down completely.)
7. Label the swab container(s) with the patient's full first and last name and the site of the lesion.
8. Complete a laboratory requisition with the required patient information.
9. Keep samples refrigerated (35–48°F) after sample collection and transport at ambient temperature.

Primary Care Office Visit: Day 3

Mrs. Miller returns to the primary care office. She reports feeling more tired than during the previous visit and suspects that she may be running a fever. Her discomfort level is 2 out of 10 and she is sleeping better at night. Mrs. Miller also reports that the skin rash is larger and involves her lower back on the left and has begun to blister and ooze a clear fluid (Fig. 18.1). She continues to take the antiviral medication as directed. Although she does not feel like traveling, she wants to know if she should keep her plans to go to Florida to visit her son and new grandson.

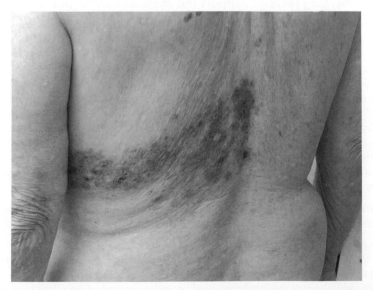

Fig. 18.1   Varicella zoster. (From Li, A. W, Yin, E. S., Stahl, M., Kim, T. K., Panse, G., Zeidan, A. M., & Leventhal, J. S. [2017]. The skin as a window to the blood: Cutaneous manifestations of myeloid malignancies. *Blood Reviews, 31*[6], 370–388.)

Focused Review of Systems

　General: Reports feeling "more tired" with fever. Denies chills, weakness, or unexplained weight changes.

　Skin: Expanding painful rash as reported previously.

　Mouth: Denies oral lesions or sore throat.

　Neck: Denies neck pain or lumps.

　Respiratory: Denies shortness of breath or cough.

　Cardiac: Denies chest pain or palpitation.

Focused Physical Examination

　General: Obese female sitting on examination table in a patient gown holding gown away from body to prevent touching her left side.

　Vital signs: Temperature 101.2°F (orally). Blood pressure 118/66. Heart rate 102 regular, respiratory rate 20 at rest, and O_2 saturation on room air 97%.

　Skin: Unilateral erythematous, vesicular lesions in groups and clusters involving the left lower back above the buttock extending around under left arm and left abdomen. Lesions do not cross the midline of the body. Weeping and exudate noted to lesions on back. No streaking. Warm and tender to light palpation.

　Mouth: Membranes moist, good dentition, no posterior pharyngeal cobblestoning or erythema. No lesions of tongue or buccal mucosa.

　Neck: Supple without masses, lymphadenopathy, thyroid enlargement, or tenderness.

　Cardiac: Rapid regular S1, S2. No S3, S4, murmurs, or rubs.

　Respiratory: Clear to auscultation all lobes.

　Abdomen: Rounded, soft, bowel sounds positive. No tenderness or organomegaly.

　Extremities: Nontender, shotty lymph nodes bilateral axilla. Pedal pulses present bilaterally. No edema or calf tenderness.

　Psychiatric: Alert, appropriate affect.

　Laboratory results: The viral culture is positive for VZV.

8. What emerging findings support the diagnosis of herpes zoster?

Since her initial visit, Mrs. Miller's rash continues to evolve and now includes vesiculation indicative of the eruption phase. In its classical manifestation, the signs and symptoms of zoster are usually distinctive enough to make an accurate clinical diagnosis once the rash has appeared. The low-grade fever and malaise coupled with the unilateral dermatomal distribution of clustered vesicles should help exclude other differential diagnoses. The hallmark or classic physical examination findings associated with herpes zoster occur during the acute eruptive phase, which is marked by the following:

- Grouped herpetiform vesicles developing on the erythematous base (the classic finding).
- Cutaneous findings typically appear unilaterally, stopping abruptly at the midline of the limit of sensory coverage of the involved dermatome.
- Vesicular involution occurs and the vesicles initially are clear but eventually cloud, rupture, crust, and involute and resolve over 10 to 15 days.[1,3]

9. How do you advise Mrs. Miller regarding continued care and her travel plans to visit her newborn grandson?

Mrs. Miller must be advised to complete her antiviral medication and corticosteroid regimens. Although the rash will likely continue to evolve, the provider reassures her that the medication is working to slow viral replication. Mrs. Miller should also be instructed to practice good hygiene, wound care, and continue her analgesic medication as directed. Zoster lesions contain high concentrations of VZV that can be spread, presumably by the airborne route, and cause primary varicella in exposed susceptible persons. Localized zoster is only contagious after the rash erupts and until the lesions crust. Regarding travel and intimate contact with others, the CDC recommends that persons with localized zoster avoid contact with susceptible persons at high risk for severe varicella in household and occupational settings until lesions are crusted.[4] Therefore Mrs. Miller should be counseled to delay travel until her lesions are well crusted.

Primary Care Office Visit: Day 14

Mrs. Miller is being seen today for a planned follow-up visit. She reports that her skin eruption on her flank was almost healed but is now getting worse again. She developed a red, pus-filled bump on her midflank. She also reports increased warmth and tenderness with a red line around the bump. She denies fever or chills. She denies having squeezed or manipulated the bump since she discovered it yesterday.

Focused Physical Examination
Skin: Examination of the left midflank reveals an erythematous, subcutaneous, nonfluctuant abscess measuring 2.6×2.8 cm. Moderate induration and warm to touch. No streaking. Light palpation results in spontaneous rupture with purulent, yellow pus. No odor.

10. What is the most appropriate next course of action?

The next best intervention is to collect a specimen from the draining abscess for culture and sensitivity (C&S). A microbiological culture is used to determine the type of organism (if any), its abundance in the sample being tested, or both. It is one of the primary diagnostic methods of microbiology and used as a tool to determine the cause of infectious disease by letting the agent multiply in a predetermined medium. Anticipating the potential need for antibiotics, a complete blood count (CBC) to assess for infection and a comprehensive metabolic panel (CMP)-14 to determine liver and kidney function and electrolyte and acid/base balance are ordered.

Day 17

The CBC, CMP-14, and microbiology report from the wound culture are available (Tables 18.1–18.3).

11. How do you interpret the culture and sensitivity report and what medication do you prescribe for Mrs. Miller?

A C&S report contains the name of the organism, source of the specimen, antimicrobials used to treat that organism, the sensitivity to each agent (e.g., S = sensitive, I = intermediate, R = resistant), and if the organism is a suspected extended spectrum β-lactamase (ESBL) producer. If there is a suspected ESBL organism, the clinician should seek confirmation before giving an antimicrobial because it may actually be resistant in vivo if it is true. If the organism is proven not to be an ESBL producer, then the antimicrobial agent may be used.[9] The report will specify if the organism has inducible β-lactamase (IB) properties, indicated as (S) for susceptible next to the antimicrobial (for example, ceftriaxone) but will also have IB listed after the (S). Some laboratories may list IB next to the minimum inhibitory concentration (MIC) value of the organism.[9] Although the provider may initially choose this antimicrobial because it appears sensitive, it will rapidly become resistant because of the β-lactamase properties of the organism (as will other β-lactams).[9] Unlike the potential ESBL-producing organism, any antimicrobial listed with IB should be avoided, including other β-lactams. There was no growth on day 1, day 2 shows a gram-negative rod identified, and day 3 shows that an additional organism (a gram-positive cocci) was isolated. The final report identified light growth of *Proteus mirabilis* and a multidrug-resistant organism (in this case methicillin-resistant *Staphylococcus aureus* [MRSA]).

TABLE 18.1 Microbiology Culture and Sensitivity Report

Site: Left back.
Preliminary 1: Day 1, no growth.
Preliminary 2: Day 2, gram-negative rods isolate. ID and MIC to follow.
Preliminary 3: Day 3, gram-positive cocci isolated. ID and MIC to follow.
Organism 1: *Proteus mirabilis.*
Organism 2: *MRSA.*
Final results: Very light growth of *P. mirabilis* and *MRSA.*

| | Organism 1 | | Organism 2 | |
| | *P. mirabilis* | | MSRA | |
Antibiotics	*MIC*	*Interpretation*	*MIC*	*Interpretation*
Amoxicillin/clavulanic acid	≤8/4	S	—	—
Amp/Sub	≤8/4	S	≤8/4	R
Ampicillin	≤2	S	—	—
Cefazolin	≤8	S	—	—
Cefepime	≤8	S	—	—
Ceftriaxone	≤8	S	>32	R
Cefuroxime	≤4	S	—	—
Ciprofloxacin	≤1	S	>2	R
Clindamycin	—	—	>4	R
Daptomycin	—	—	≤0.5	S
Erythromycin	—	—	>4	R
Gentamicin	2	S	≤4	S
Imipenem	≤4	S	—	—
Levofloxacin	≤2	S	>4	R
Linezolid	—	—	≤1	S
Oxacillin	—	—	>2	R
Piperacillin/tazobactam	≤16	S	—	—
Rifampin	—	—	≤1	S
Tetracycline	>8	R	≤4	S
Trimethoprim/ sulfamethoxazole	≤2/38	S	≤0.5/9.5	S
Vancomycin	—	—	1	S

MIC, Minimum inhibitory concentration; *MRSA,* methicillin-resistant *Staphylococcus aureus; POS,* positive; *R,* resistant; *S,* susceptible interpretation; μg/mL (milligrams/L).

Retrieved from https://health.wyo.gov/publichealth/infectious-disease-epidemiology-unit/healthcare-associated-infections/infection-prevention-orientation-manual/antibiotic-stewardship/

It is important for the provider to understand the MIC value adjacent to the sensitivity interpretation (S, I, or R). The MIC is the minimum concentration at which an antimicrobial inhibits visible growth of the organism.[9] The report does not provide information regarding whether the organism is actually killed. Susceptibility in vitro does not uniformly predict clinical success in vivo. If the organism is resistant, this will often, but not always, correlate with treatment failure. The only true measure of bacterial response to an antibiotic is the clinical response of the patient. A report of "susceptible" indicates that the isolate is likely to be inhibited by the usually achievable concentration of an antimicrobial agent when the recommended dosage is used. For this reason, MICs of different agents for a particular organism are not directly comparable. A common misconception when interpreting the C&S report is to assume that the choice antibiotic is the one with the lowest MIC number.[9] In reality, the MIC interpretations are specific to both the organism and the antimicrobial agent. Interpretation of quantitative susceptibility tests is based on the relationship of the MIC to the achievable concentration of antibiotic in body fluids

TABLE 18.2 **Complete Blood Count With Differential/Platelet**

Test	Result	Flag	Units	References Interval
WBC	5.7	—	×10E3/μL	4.0–10.5
RBC	5.27	—	×10E3/μL	4.10–5.60
Hemoglobin	15.4	—	grams/dL	12.5–17.0
Hematocrit	44.1	—	%	36.0–50.0
MCV	84	—	fL	80–98
MCH	29.2	—	pg	27.0–34.0
MCHC	34.9	—	grams/dL	32.0–36.0
RDW	13.7	—	%	11.7–15.0
Platelets	268	—	×10E3/μL	140–415
Neutrophils	47	—	%	40–74
Lymphocytes	46	—	%	14–46
Monocytes	6	—	%	4–13
Eosinophils	1	—	%	0–7
Basophils	0	—	%	0–3
Neutrophils (absolute)	2.6	—	×10E3/μL	1.8–7.8
Lymphocytes (absolute)	2.6	—	×10E3/μL	0.7–4.5
Monocytes (absolute)	0.4	—	×10E3/μL	0.1–1.0
Eosinophils (absolute)	0.1	—	×10E3/μL	0.0–0.4
Basophils (absolute)	0.0	—	×10E3/μL	0.0–0.2
Immature granulocytes	0	—	%	0–1
Immature granulocytes (absolute)	0.0	—	×10E3/μL	0.0–0.1

MCH, Mean corpuscular hemoglobin; *MCHC,* mean corpuscular hemoglobin concentration; *MCV,* mean corpuscular volume; *RBC,* red blood cell; *RDW,* red cell distribution width; *WBC,* white blood cell.

TABLE 18.3 **Comprehensive Metabolic Panel-14**

Test	Result	Flag	Units	References Interval
Glucose, serum	84	—	milligrams/dL	65–99
BUN	16	—	milligrams/dL	5–26
Creatinine, serum	1.06	—	milligrams/dL	0.76–1.27
eGFR	>59	—	mL/min/1.73	>59
BUN/creatinine ratio	15	—	—	8–27
Sodium, serum	141	—	mmol/L	135–145
Potassium, serum	4.4	—	mmol/L	3.5–5.2
Chloride, serum	101	—	mmol/L	97–108
Carbon dioxide, total	23	—	mmol/L	20–32
Calcium, serum	9.9	—	milligrams/dL	8.7–10.2
Protein, total, serum	7.6	—	grams/dL	6.0–8.5
Albumin, serum	4.9	—	grams/dL	3.5–5.5
Globulin, total	2.7	—	grams/dL	1.5–4.5
A/G ratio	1.8	—	—	1.1–2.5
Bilirubin, total	1.8	High	milligrams/dL	0.0–1.2
Alkaline phosphatase, serum	65	—	IU/L	25–150
AST (SGOT)	30	—	IU/L	0–40
ALT (SGPT)	32	—	IU/L	0–55

A/G, Albumin/globulin ratio; *ALT,* alanine transaminase; *AST,* aspartate transaminase; *BUN,* blood urea nitrogen; *eGFR,* estimated glomerular filtration rate; *SGOT,* serum glutamic oxaloacetic transaminase; *SGPT,* serum glutamic pyruvate transaminase.

with the dosage given for a given organism. It should not be assumed that the antimicrobial with the lowest MIC is always the best one to choose.[9]

Based on the C&S report, the provider should select a 7- to 10-day course of trimethoprim/sulfamethoxazole (TMP/SMX) as the best antimicrobial agent in this case. Sulfonamides can cause severe skin and blood problems in elderly patients and should generally be used with caution and for the shortest time possible. Review of her CBC and CMP reveals no concern for renal impairment. The provider prescribes TMP/SMX 160 to 800 milligrams (1 double-strength tablet) orally every 12 hours for 7 days.

Telephone Follow-up Call: Day 23

You speak with Mrs. Miller via telephone to check her status and assess her response to treatment. She reports that her lesions are almost healed and the majority are well crusted. Her fever has resolved, and her pain has diminished to a 3 out of 10. She is on day 6 of a 7-day course of TMP/SMX. You advise Mrs. Miller to complete her regimen and report any concerns or side effects.

Primary Care Office Visit: 6 Months

Mrs. Miller presents to the office for a scheduled follow-up appointment. She reports that although her skin lesions have been healed for at least 4 to 5 months, she continues to have pain and tenderness on her left flank. Occasionally she experiences an additional burning sensation in the area of the rash; however, the pain is constant. She took her pain medication as directed, with some improvement. She wants to know what treatment options are available and if she should receive the herpes zoster vaccination again.

12.   What is the most likely etiology for Mrs. Miller's complaint?

PHN is the most common complication of herpes zoster. Several studies have indicated that the risk for PHN among persons with zoster increases with age, particularly for persons 50 years of age or older. The risk for experiencing at least 2 months of pain from PHN increased 27.4-fold among patients over the age of 50 compared with younger patients.[4] People with compromised or suppressed immune systems are more likely to have complications from herpes zoster. In this case Mrs. Miller has CLL; therefore she is more likely to have symptoms that last longer.

13.   How can you determine the degree or severity of Mrs. Miller's pain?

Pain associated with PHN occurs in three broad categories: spontaneous pain that is ongoing (e.g., continuous burning pain), paroxysmal shooting or electric shock-like pains, and evoked sensations that are pathologic amplifications of responses to light touch and other innocuous stimuli (mechanical allodynia) or to noxious stimuli (mechanical hyperalgesia). Treatment selection should be guided by pain characteristics per individual patient. The Zoster Brief Pain Inventory (ZBPI) is a validated and convenient tool for the purpose of determining patient's PHN pain and to guide treatment decisions.[10]

14.   What treatment options may improve her symptoms?

Numerous treatments are available to manage the pain associated with PHN. Treatment is based on symptom control. Unfortunately, PHN pain may persist for years or for life, and medication is often required over prolonged periods. It is important to monitor the effect of interventions on pain intensity and to modify or discontinue treatments that do not result in appreciable pain relief or that have adverse effects in excess of the benefit.

Topical therapy alone is reasonable to consider as first-line treatment for mild pain. It is sometimes used in combination with systemic drugs when pain is moderate or severe, although data are lacking from randomized trials comparing combination topical and systemic therapy with either therapy alone. Patches containing 5% lidocaine are approved for the treatment of PHN in Europe and the United States. Capsaicin 0.075% cream may be helpful. However, its use is limited because it must be applied four times daily for a number of consecutive days and it causes a short-term burning or stinging sensation and erythema when applied. Patients must be instructed to apply to intact skin only and wash hands carefully to avoid inadvertent contact with sensitive mucous membranes and the eyes.[11]

Acetaminophen and NSAIDs are generally considered to be ineffective for neuropathic pain. In addition, long-term NSAID use is not recommended in older adults because of the increased risk of renal dysfunction. There is evidence to support the use of tricyclic antidepressants; however, this recommendation is off-label. The Food and Drug Administration (FDA) has approved antiepileptic drugs gabapentin and pregabalin for the treatment of PHN.[11] Although some clinical trial data have suggested that opioids (morphine and oxycodone) are effective in PHN, a more recent Cochrane review concluded that there was not enough convincing, unbiased evidence of a benefit of oxycodone in treating the disorder. PHN patients are often elderly and have other diseases for which they are taking medication. Narcotics should not be used for long-term management unless absolutely necessary. Providers must exercise particular caution when prescribing medications for these patients. Therefore collaboration with pain management specialists is recommended with regard to treatment regimens. As a best practice strategy, providers should seek the most current treatment guidelines for practice.[11]

15. Is she an appropriate candidate for repeat vaccination with Zostavax?

Certain studies suggest a recurrence herpes zoster rate that is comparable to the rate of initial episodes.[4] Research suggests that the vaccine's effectiveness declined with time and after 8 years no longer works to prevent disease. Other studies found that initial vaccination is more efficacious in persons aged 60 to 69 years, which suggests that persons who received vaccination earlier or later than these years may benefit from repeat vaccination. Although the safety and efficacy of zoster vaccine have not been assessed in persons with a history of zoster, different safety concerns are not expected in this group. More research is warranted, and recent study results support further investigation of zoster vaccination administration in early versus later age and of booster doses for elderly individuals at an appropriate interval after initial immunization against herpes zoster.[12] Shingrix, the new adjuvanted zoster vaccine, is now available and recommended for patients who have had a previous vaccination with the zoster vaccine (Zostavax).

References

1. Blair, G. (2017). Herpes zoster (shingles). In T. M. Buttaro, J. Trybulski, P. Polgar-Bailey, & J. Sandberg-Cook (Eds.), *Primary care: A collaborative practice* (5th ed., pp. 284–286). St. Louis, MO: Elsevier.
2. Dunphy, L. M., Winland-Brown, J., Porter, B., & Thomas, D. (2015). *Primary care: Art and science of advanced practice nursing*. Philadelphia, PA: FA Davis.
3. Wolff, K., Johnson, R. A., & Saaverdra, A. P. (2013). *Fitzpatrick's color atlas and synopsis of clinical dermatology* (7th ed.). New York, NY: McGraw-Hill.
4. Harpaz, R., Ortega-Sanchez, I., & Seward, J. (2008). Prevention of herpes zoster: Recommendations of the advisory committee on immunization practices (ACIP). *Morbidity and Mortality Weekly Report, 77*, 1–16. Retrieved from https://www.cdc.gov/mmwr/PDF/rr/rr5705.pdf.
5. Mir, M. A. (2016). Chronic lymphocytic leukemia. Retrieved from http://emedicine.medscape.com/article/199313-overview.

6. Giridhar, K. V., Shanafelt, T., Tosh, P. K., Parikh, S. A., & Call, T. G. (2016). Disseminated herpes zoster in chronic lymphocytic leukemia (CLL) patients treated with B-cell receptor pathway inhibitors. *Leukemia & Lymphoma*, 1–4.

7 National Center for Immunization and Respiratory Diseases (NCIRD). (2016). Interpretation of laboratory tests for VZV. Retrieved from http://www.cdc.gov/chickenpox/hcp/lab-tests.html#interpretation.

8. Alberta Health Services. (2013). Sample type and collection guidelines for herpes simplex virus (HSV) and varicella zoster virus (VZV) testing. Retrieved from http://www.provlab.ab.ca/Insert_Sample_type_Collection_HSV_VZV_June_2015.pdf.

9. Burk, K. (2014). The bacterial culture and sensitivity report. Retrieved from https://health.wyo.gov/wp-content/uploads/2016/02/22-16294_WYIPOM_Section_12_Antimicrobial_Stewardship_FINAL.pdf.

10. Coplan, P., Schmader, K., Nikas, A., Chan, I., Choo, P., … Oxman, M. (2004). Development of a measure of the burden of pain due to herpes zoster and postherpetic neuralgia for prevention trials: Adaptation of the brief pain inventory. *The Journal of Pain*, 5(6), 344–356.

11. Johnson, R. W., & Rice, A. S. (2014). Postherpetic neuralgia. *The New England Journal of Medicine*, *371*(16), 1526–1533.

12. Levin, M. J., Schmader, K. E., Pang, L., Williams-Diaz, A., Zerbe, G., Canniff, J., et al. (2016). Cellular and humoral responses to a second dose of herpes zoster vaccine administered 10 years after the first dose among older adults. *The Journal of Infectious Diseases*, *213*(1), 14–22.

Practice Case Studies in Multimorbidity Management

Basic Case Studies

Heartburn

Karen L. Dick

Instructions

After reviewing the case study, please jot down your notes or preliminary answers in the spaces provided. When you are ready to submit your answers for grading and reflective expert feedback for evaluation, go to http://www.evolve.elsevier.com/DickAndButtaro/ to complete this case.

Case Study Scenario/History of Present Illness

A 71-year-old man comes to the clinic today as an add-on urgent visit. He reports having two separate episodes this past week of heartburn. The first episode occurred 3 days ago when he was carrying a bag of dog food into the house from his car, and the second one occurred while he was sitting at his computer after dinner last night. On both instances there were no other associated symptoms: he denies shortness of breath, diaphoresis, or radiation to other areas. He is not sure how long the first episode lasted because he continued to put away groceries, and after about 20 minutes the heartburn subsided, although he found himself belching on and off for the next hour before dinner. The episode last evening occurred after dinner, and subsided only after he chewed four calcium carbonate tablets he found in his medicine cabinet. He recalls in the past that he had used Maalox a few years back when he experienced similar symptoms during a trip to Mexico.

    Medications: Ocuvite 1 tablet daily, losartan 50 milligrams 1 daily, Norvasc (amlodipine) 5 milligrams daily, tamsulosin 0.4 milligrams per day, fluticasone 50 micrograms/act 1 spray both nostrils, twice daily, as needed.

    Allergies: Keflex: rash. Lisinopril: cough.

    Habits: Never smoked, occasional cigar, 1 to 2 glasses wine with dinner every night.

    Past medical history: Macular degeneration, benign prostatic hypertrophy (BPH), hypertension (HTN), and allergic rhinitis.

    Past surgical history: Right knee anterior cruciate ligament (ACL) tear in college.

    Family history: Father died age 80 of chronic obstructive pulmonary disease (COPD). Mother died age 84 of HTN, depression, and osteoarthritis.

    Personal and social history: Defense attorney, single, never married. Lives alone, has a girlfriend.

Review of Systems

    General: Feels well today, no fever/chills/weakness.

    Skin: Denies rashes or lesions.

    Head, eyes, ears, nose, and throat (HEENT): Constant runny nose, occasional sinus pain, occasional sore throat, no headache.

    Respiratory: Denies cough, wheeze, hemoptysis, or shortness of breath.

    Cardiac: Denies previous episodes of chest discomfort before this past week, no palpitations, no weakness, no syncopal episodes.

    Gastrointestinal: Denies nausea/vomiting.

    Urinary: Denies dysuria, hematuria. Has nocturia × 2.

    Musculoskeletal: Daily right knee pain, wears a knee band.

    Neurologic: Denies headache, dizziness.

Physical Examination

   General: Well appearing, in no acute distress, pleasant.

   Vital signs: Height: 72 inches (182.8 cm). Weight: 220 pounds (99.7 kg). Blood pressure (BP): 178/80 left arm, and 176/78. Heart rate 70, O_2 saturation 99%.

   Skin: No lesions.

   Neck: Supple, no lymphadenopathy, thyroid nonpalpable.

   Respiratory: Clear to auscultation. No rales, wheezes, or rhonchi.

   Cardiac: Regular rate, S1, S2; no S3, S4. No murmurs, rubs, or gallops.

   Abdomen: Soft, bowel sounds +, nondistended, nontender to palpation.

   Extremities: Trace pedal edema, pedal pulses 2+ bilaterally, right knee with flexion to 100 degrees.

ASSESSMENT AND PLAN

1. Based on the history and physical examination results, what are the possible causes (differential diagnosis) for the patient's current condition?

Differentials

2. What components of the history or physical examination are missing?

History

Physical Examination

3. What diagnostics are necessary for this patient at this time?

Case Study, Continued

The patient provides more information on further questioning. He has had no surgeries since his ACL repair in college, and he has tried to stay active. There is no family history of clotting disorders or coronary heart disease or hyperlipidemia. He has been under a lot of stress recently at work because of an impending trial date, and reports that he has been eating more processed foods, getting little sleep, and has been "living on coffee." He knows that he has gained some weight but he does not know how much. He also reports that he had injured his "bad" knee a few months ago while playing tennis, and has been taking Aleve (naproxen) twice a day for about 2 months, admitting that on really bad days he takes it three times a day. He said when the injury on the tennis court happened, his friends took him to a local urgent care center where he had films of the knee done and was told that it was negutive for fracture or other acute issues. He has had no change in his bowel pattern and he denies melena. He denies a sore throat or difficulty swallowing. Additional findings on examination include no tenderness or pain on palpation to the chest wall, there is no JVD or carotid bruits, and peripheral pulses are 2+. The ECG shows normal sinus rhythm, rate 68, PR interval 0.16 seconds, QT interval 0.22 seconds, no ST elevation or depression, and normal R wave progression. This ECG was compared with a prior one done in the office 2 years ago and shows no changes.

4. What additional diagnostics would you order based on the additional history provided?[1]

5. What treatments would you recommend for this patient?[2,3]

6. What are your next steps?

Second Office Visit

The patient returns in a week and reports that he has not had the stress test yet, and he is unable to schedule it because of his court schedule. He has had no further episodes of heartburn. He has been taking the omeprazole once a day since he was last seen. He first noted some loose stool during the first few days, but his bowel pattern is back to baseline. The CBC results showed no anemia, and the stool for OB was negative. He has been trying to substitute decaffeinated coffee but says he still has to have a large cup in the morning. He knows he should lose weight, but his knee pain is preventing him from playing tennis. His BP today is still elevated at 164/80 left arm and 160/78 right arm. There are no orthostatic changes. Additional physical examination findings today include:

Skin: No lesions or rash.

Neck: No JVD.

Respiratory: Clear to auscultation. No rales, wheezes, rhonchus.

Cardiac: Regular rate, S1, S2; no S3, S4. No murmurs, rubs, or gallops.

Abdomen: Soft, nondistended, nontender to palpation.

Extremities: Right knee with a small anterior effusion, no warmth, redness, and no crepitus. There is some tenderness over the medial joint line and limited flexion.

7. **What additional history would be helpful here?**[4]

Case Study, Continued

The patient admits to still taking daily Aleve (naproxen) for his knee pain, saying, "It's the only thing that helps." The link between elevated BP and chronic use of an NSAID is reviewed with the patient who had the idea that it could affect his blood pressure readings. The provider discusses with the patient the possibility of having to add a third medication to his regime to lower his blood pressure. In addition, the provider talks to the patient about needing to find ways to lower his stress level, which can also be contributing to elevated readings. A discussion of his dietary habits also takes place. The patient reports he knows he overeats because of stress that is primarily caused by his job, and he is particularly fond of eating several handfuls of mixed nuts after dinner when he does his preparation work for court. He reports that the way he has combated stress previously was to play tennis, but because his knee pain has been bothering him, he has stopped and he admits to having gained 15 pounds over the last 6 months. The patient agrees to switch to acetaminophen for the knee pain. He describes the pain as only occurring with movement. He has no pain at rest. He does not notice if the pain is worse at different times of the day. He does note that he has some trouble going from sitting to standing if he has been sitting for long periods of time. He originally used ice when the injury first occurred, but now uses a heating pad every once in a while when he has time. He tells the provider that his girlfriend has always tried to get him to go to yoga classes with her as a way to relax. He jokes that maybe he will try some yoga breathing and see if that helps. He does not want to have to take another BP medication and wants to try cutting out the Aleve and mixed nuts first. He is scheduled to return in 2 weeks for a repeat BP check.

8. What are the priorities for the next visit?

Third Office Visit

The patient returns in 2 weeks, reporting that he has stopped taking Aleve, and he has switched to extra-strength acetaminophen but that it does not really seem to work as well. He has been trying to be mindful in terms of watching his intake of salt and high-calorie foods. He has had no further episodes of heartburn and reports taking omeprazole daily. He says that he has been thinking about stress reduction and what he believes will help him the most is if he can get back to playing tennis. He has also been thinking about his weight and believes if he can get back on track with exercise he could be better about his food choices, but admits that he does not really know how to begin. His BP readings today are 150/76 left arm, 148/70 right arm. No orthostasis.

9. What other options might be considered for the patient's knee pain?

10. What referrals would be appropriate here?

Case Study, Continued

The patient agrees to make an appointment with an orthopedic surgeon who is the son of one of his colleagues. He is also given information about a nutritionist who works with the practice, and he says he will make an appointment once his current court case is over within the next few weeks. He continues to be adamant that he does not want to take another BP medication and vows to work on his stress level, as he hopes that will help. He was encouraged by the decrease in his readings by coming off the Aleve and cutting back his sodium intake. An appointment is made for 1 month later.

Fourth Office Visit

The patient returns 1 month later, having seen the orthopedic surgeon, and tells the provider that he has had a magnetic resonance imaging (MRI) scan and was told he had a right knee meniscus tear. The surgeon has recommended arthroscopy but recommends that the patient see his primary care provider to arrange a stress test before the surgery to rule out any cardiac disease. His BP readings today are 168/78 in the left arm and 166/78 in the right arm. His weight is up 2 pounds to 222 pounds. The provider discusses concern regarding the continued elevation in BP. The patient reluctantly agrees to a change in his medications but does not want to take a diuretic because he fears that it will add to his nocturia. A decision to increase amlodipine to 10 milligrams daily is made. The patient is scheduled to return to the clinic in 2 weeks. The provider speaks to the patient again about needing to schedule a stress test. The patient admits that he does not think he can walk on the treadmill for the test, saying he was too embarrassed to mention it because he had always considered himself to be athletic. The provider explains that a stress test with nuclear imaging can be done and the patient does not have to walk on a treadmill for the test. A myocardial perfusion imaging scan (MPI) is ordered.

The patient misses his 2-week appointment because he was called out of town, but he returns in 4 weeks. In the interim, the provider has received the results of the stress test, which reveal the following. There is normal distribution of the radiopharmaceutical throughout the left ventricle on both the stress and resting imaging. Wall motion of the left ventricle appeared normal. The computer calculated left ventricular end diastolic volume was 84 ml, and the computer calculated left ventricle ejection fraction was 60%. Impression was normal myocardial perfusion scan.

11. **What are the priorities for this visit?**

Fifth Office Visit

The patient reports that he has been taking Ultram (tramadol) given to him by the orthopedic surgeon for his knee pain, but he does not like the way it clouds his thinking, so he has been taking it only at night. He continues to take acetaminophen twice a day. The date for the knee arthroscopy and meniscus repair has been set for next week. He has been taking the increased dose of Norvasc as ordered. He has been watching what he eats: he had seen the nutritionist who reviewed low-carbohydrate, low-fat food options. He is quite happy with himself having lost 7 pounds over the last month. He also continues to take omeprazole and has not had any heartburn symptoms. The provider reviews the results of the stress test and today's BP readings. The patient is looking forward to getting his knee "taken care of" so he can resume playing tennis and walking the dog. He hopes that it will help him continue to lose weight. His physical examination reveals the following:

    General: Well appearing, in no acute distress, pleasant.

    Vital signs: Height: 72 inches (182.8 cm). Weight: 215 pounds (97.5 kg). BP: 140/80 left arm and 142/78 in the right arm. Heart rate 70, O_2 saturation 99%.

    Respiratory: Clear to auscultation.

    Cardiac: Regular rate, S1, S2; no S3, S4. No murmurs, rubs, or gallops.

    Abdomen: Soft, non-distended, nontender to palpation.

    Extremities: Trace pedal edema, pedal pulses 2+ bilaterally.

12. **What ongoing issues will be the focus of future visits?**

Sixth Visit 2 Months Later, 4 Weeks Postoperative

The patient returns for check of his BP, knee pain, and reflux symptoms. He reports that the meniscus repair surgery went well but that the surgeon told him there was scarring from the previous ACL reconstruction surgery that was contributing to the knee pain. He had to take time off from work and spent many days at home, and went back to previous habits of drinking caffeinated coffee, not paying attention to what he was eating, and had resumed taking Aleve because it was the only thing that really helped his knee pain. He says the pain is much improved, and he is moving better, but he still relies on the Aleve at night when the knee discomfort seems to be worse. He knows he has gained weight, and he is discouraged and feels like he is going backward. Says he is still having PT and has progressed to a cane.

Medications: Taking: Ocuvite 1 tablet daily, losartan 50 milligrams per day, Norvasc (amlodipine) 10 milligrams per day, tamsulosin 0.4 milligrams per day, extra-strength acetaminophen 500 milligrams 2 tablets 1 to 2 times a day "when I think of it," and Aleve 200 milligrams 2 tablets at bedtime.

Not taking: Fluticasone 50 micrograms/act 1 spray both nostrils twice a day as needed, tramadol (he does not know the dose), and omeprazole.

Review of Systems
General: Feels "down" today, denies fever/chills/weakness.
Skin: Denies rashes or lesions.
HEENT: Chronic rhinitis, worse lately.
Respiratory: Denies cough, wheeze, hemoptysis, or shortness of breath.
Cardiac: No chest pain, palpitations, or shortness of breath.
Gastrointestinal: No nausea/vomiting, has had increased belching with heartburn twice this past week.
Urinary: No dysuria, hematuria.
Musculoskeletal: Has right knee pain with movement, which has been improving since surgery but gets worse by the end of the day. Not sleeping well unless he takes pain medication. Reports knee is stiff in the morning, and it takes a while to get moving.
Neurologic: Slight frontal headache, has had two episodes over the last 2 weeks, no dizziness.

Physical Examination
General: Well appearing, in no acute distress, pleasant.
Vital signs: Height: 72 inches (182.8 cm). Weight: 230 pounds (104 kg). BP: 188/80 left arm, and 186/78 right arm. Heart rate 76, O_2 saturation 98%.
Skin: No lesions.
Neck: Supple, no lymphadenopathy, thyroid nonpalpable.
Respiratory: Clear to auscultation. No rales, wheezes, or rhonchi.
Cardiac: Regular rate, S1, S2; no S3, S4. No murmurs, rubs, or gallops.
Abdomen: Soft, bowel sounds +, nondistended, nontender to palpation.
Extremities: Trace pedal edema, pedal pulses 2+ bilaterally, right knee with three scabbed over incisions.

13.   What are the patient's current problems identified at this visit?

14.   How would you address each problem?

Case Study, Continued

The patient returns 1 week later for a BP check. He reports that he had a long discussion with his girlfriend, and he feels better. "I know what I have to do." He says he has switched back to the acetaminophen for pain relief at night, and has been really trying to watch his salt intake and make better food choices. The PT who has been working with him has indicated that he is getting ready to discharge him and that he has made good progress and that his level of knee discomfort at night will continue to lessen.

   Medications: Taking: Ocuvite 1 tablet daily, losartan 100 milligrams daily, Norvasc 10 milligrams daily, tamsulosin 0.4 milligrams daily, extra-strength acetaminophen 500 milligrams 2 tablets 1 to 2 times a day.

Physical Examination

   General: Well appearing, in no acute distress, pleasant.
   Vital signs: Height: 72 inches (182.8 cm). Weight: 227 pounds (103 kg). BP: 156/80 left arm, and 158/78 right arm. Heart rate 76, O_2 saturation 98%.
   Skin: No lesions, rash.
   Respiratory: Clear to auscultation.
   Cardiac: Regular rate, S1, S2; no S3, S4. No murmurs, rubs, or gallops.

15.   Would you make any changes to the patient's blood pressure regimen today? Why or why not?[5]

ONLINE ANSWER SUBMISSION

When you are ready to submit your answers for grading and reflective expert feedback for evaluation, go to http://www.evolve.elsevier.com/DickAndButtaro/ to complete this case.

References

1. ACC/AHA. (2002). Guideline update for exercise testing: Summary article. *Circulation, 106*, 1883–1892.
2. Katz, P., Gerson, L., & Vela, M. (2013). Guidelines for the diagnosis and management of gastroesophageal reflux disease. *The American Journal of Gastroenterology, 108*(3), 308–328.
3. Sostres, C., Gargallo, C., Arroyo, M., & Lanas, A. (2010). Adverse effects of non-steroidal anti-inflammatory drugs on upper GI tract. *Clinical Gastroenterology, 24*(2), 121–132.
4. Johnson, A., Nguyen, T., & Day, R. (1994). Do nonsteroidal anti-inflammatory drugs affect blood pressure? A meta-analysis. *Annals of Internal Medicine, 121*(4), 289–300.
5. James, P. A., Oparil, S., Carter, B. L., et al. (2014). 2014 evidence-based guideline for the management of high blood pressure in adults: report from the panel members appointed to the eighth Joint National Committee (JNC 8). *JAMA: The Journal of the American Medical Association*, doi:10.1001/jama.2013.284427. [published online 18 December 2013].

Back Pain

Nicole Eckerson

Instructions

After reviewing the case study, please jot down your notes or preliminary answers in the spaces provided. When you are ready to submit your answers for grading and reflective expert feedback for evaluation, go to http://www.evolve.elsevier.com/DickAndButtaro/ to complete this case.

Case Study Scenario/History of Present Illness

B.R., a 73-year-old white male, comes into the internal medicine office for a regular check-up for his blood pressure (BP), chronic kidney disease (CKD), and elevated cholesterol. During the course of the visit, the patient mentions that he has had chronic back pain for many years and had seen a pain management doctor in the past for epidural steroid injections. He notes that these were very helpful for his pain, but the pain management doctor has moved and he has not seen a new pain management provider since. He has not taken any medication for the back pain, although he does state that Tylenol and ibuprofen have not helped in the past and he denies any trauma precipitating this chronic pain and denies any acute exacerbation of the pain. He also notes that the back pain is no worse than usual, and he is not having any numbness or tingling and no bowel or bladder incontinence. He denies any consistent aerobic exercise but states he is consistently working in the garden and doing yardwork. He currently rates the pain at approximately 5 to 6/10 and states it does not usually hinder him from most activities of daily living, although sometimes it makes gardening difficult. He takes extra-strength Tylenol on occasion but says that "it doesn't really help." He would like to try epidural steroid injections again.

Medications: Atorvastatin 40 milligrams po daily, vitamin B$_{12}$ 1000 micrograms po daily, paroxetine 40 milligrams po daily, and extra-strength acetaminophen 500 milligrams po 2 tablets daily.

Allergies: No known drug allergies (NKDA).

Social history: Patient is unmarried, although he does have a long-term girlfriend. He is retired. He smokes cigarettes, approximately 1 pack a day and has a pack-year history of about 50 years. Denies any illicit drug use.

Family history: Sister: hyperlipidemia. Mother: died at age 88 of colon cancer. Father: died of old age at 99.

Past medical history: Anxiety, dysthymia, hyperlipidemia, heart murmur related to mild aortic stenosis diagnosed at age 68. Chronic back pain, prediabetes, carpal tunnel syndrome, and Lyme disease. Paroxysmal supraventricular tachycardia diagnosed at age 62 not requiring any ablation or cardioversion, but patient stopped taking a beta-blocker after 3 years. CKD stage 3.

Past surgical history: Carpal tunnel release left hand at age 69. Arthroscopic patellofemoral and medial compartment chondroplasties right knee at age 69. Cervical spine surgery at age 63. Tonsillectomy/adenoidectomy as a child. Right inguinal hernia repair at age 58.

Review of Systems

Constitutional: He reports no fever, no night sweats, no significant weight gain, no significant weight loss, and no exercise intolerance. No fatigue.

Head, eyes, ears, nose and throat (HEENT): He reports runny nose and frequent sneezing.

Respiratory: He reports no cough, no wheezing, no shortness of breath, and no coughing up blood.

Cardiac: Patient reports known heart murmur, but reports no chest pain, no arm pain on exertion, no shortness of breath when walking, no shortness of breath when lying down, and no palpitations.

Abdomen: He reports no abdominal pain. No constipation, diarrhea, or change in bowels.

Musculoskeletal: He reports back pain (neck and lower back). He reports numbness (in hands only, denies any numbness or tingling in lower extremities).

Neurologic: No dizziness and no headaches.

Psychological: Positive for anxiety. Denies suicidal ideation (SI) or homicidal ideation (HI).

Physical Examination

General appearance: Healthy-appearing, well-nourished, and well-developed older adult male. Ambulation: ambulating normally.

Vital signs: BP 144/82 left arm, recheck 152/70 left arm. Heart rate (HR) 86, respiratory rate (RR) 16, O_2 saturation 98% on room air (RA). Temperature 98.5°F. Body mass index (BMI) 28.6.

Psychiatric: Appropriate insight and good judgment. Mental status: normal mood and affect and active and alert.

Head: Normocephalic and atraumatic.

Lungs: Breath sounds normal, good air movement. No wheezes, rales, crackles, or rhonchi.

Cardiovascular: Normal S1 and S2, regular rate and rhythm (RRR). Grade II systolic murmur best auscultated at right upper sternal border. No rubs or gallops.

Musculoskeletal: No rashes or scarring noted. Normal movement of all extremities. Positive tenderness in posterior neck.

Back: Thoracolumbar appearance: no abnormalities. Full range of motion back flexion, extension, and lateral extension. Negative straight leg raise. Positive paravertebral tenderness.

Extremities: No cyanosis, edema, varicosities, or palpable cords.

Neurologic: Normal gait and station. Normal sensation lower extremities.

Back: Thoracolumbar appearance: no abnormalities, negative straight leg raise. Positive paravertebral tenderness, no rashes or scarring noted.

1. Based on this patient's history and physical examination findings, what are B.R.'s current problems?

2.   What elements are missing from this patient's history, review of systems, and physical examination?

3.   When considering B.R.'s current complaint of back pain, what should the health care provider include in the differential diagnosis? What red flag diagnoses are possible?

Case Study, Continued

Further discussion with B.R. reveals that he had been on some kind of medication for his kidneys in the past, although he "can't remember what it was called" and stopped taking it because he did not feel any different on the medication and he did not want to pay for a medication that "was not doing anything." He has seen a nephrologist in the past who started him on this medication, but he has not seen the nephrologist in a long time.

He also states that the back pain began around 6 years ago at age 66 and it is consistent throughout the day and worse after doing activity and feels a little better after resting. His last epidural injection was approximately 18 months ago, and he had a CT done about 3 months before the injection. He cannot remember what kind of surgery he had on his neck.

His last A1C was done 2 months ago and he remembers it was 6.1%. His last dilated eye examination was 3 months ago, and the patient reports that "everything was fine."

He reports starting to take vitamin B_{12} about 2 months ago because his girlfriend told him he should.

He was treated for Lyme disease 3 years ago with 3 weeks of antibiotics, and he denies any further problems since then.

He occasionally has a beer (maybe two to three times a month) and denies any falls or history of falling. He denies any headache, swelling in legs, or vision changes.

4. What diagnostics should the health care provider order at this time? Why are these necessary?

Case Study, Continued

UA and urine for microalbumin done in office reveal no abnormalities and microalbumin is normal.

The abdominal examination is negative for any CVA or urinary bladder tenderness. An abdominal aortic pulse is very faintly palpable and there are no pulsatile masses. There are no abdominal bruits.

DTRs of lower extremities are 2+, and sensation and muscular strength are intact.

5. Are there any diagnoses that can be excluded based on this information?[1]

6. What is the working diagnosis at this time?

7. What further instructions and treatment plan should be discussed with B.R.?[2]

8. What are the provider's next steps?[3,4]

Case Study, Continued

The patient is adamant that he does not want a medication to help him quit smoking at this time, but he promises he will try to cut back. The patient does have his laboratory work done as scheduled the next day.

- *CBC shows no anemia and platelets are in normal range, differential unremarkable.*
- *Lipid panel shows total cholesterol 182; high-density lipoprotein (HDL) 50; triglycerides 158; and low-density lipoprotein (LDL) 100, which is an improvement from previous fasting lipid panel.*
- *CMP reveals blood urea nitrogen (BUN) 25, creatinine 1.55, and glomerular filtration rate (GFR) 44, indicating Stage 3B moderate kidney disease. All other values are within the normal range.*
- *Vitamin B$_{12}$ is 653.*
- *These results are given to the patient on the telephone and he is encouraged to follow up with his nephrologist. The patient gives verbal consent for these laboratory results to be faxed to his nephrologist.*

The patient returns as scheduled in 2 weeks for BP recheck. He has started physical therapy and states that he has not really seen much relief for his back pain, and states the scheduled Tylenol is not helping his back pain. He still denies any numbness or tingling in his lower extremities or bowel or bladder incontinence. He states that he is not taking any pain medication other than acetaminophen for his back pain. He does state that he has been avoiding salt but has not increased his physical activity at all. He also notes that he has been checking his BP every other day using his neighbor's cuff and it has been ranging in 140s/70s. He has also tried to cut back on his cigarette usage but is still smoking about three-quarters of a pack per day.

His BP is still elevated, 144/82 on left arm, recheck left arm 142/84, and HR 82.

His abdominal US is negative for any aneurysm.

Review of Systems

Constitutional: No fever, no night sweats, no significant weight gain, no significant weight loss, and no exercise intolerance. No fatigue.

Respiratory: No cough, no wheezing, no shortness of breath, and no coughing up blood.

Cardiac: No chest pain, no shortness of breath when walking.

Musculoskeletal: Back pain is intermittent, dull, without radiation, continues to be hard standing for long periods.

Neurologic: No dizziness and no headaches.

Physical Examination

General: Alert, comfortable, pleasant.

Lungs: No wheezes, rales/crackles, or rhonchi. Breath sounds normal, good air movement.

Cardiovascular: Normal S1 and S2, no rubs or gallops. RRR and grade II systolic murmur best auscultated at right upper sternal border.

Extremities: No cyanosis, edema, varicosities, or palpable cord.

Neurologic: Normal gait and station, normal sensation. 2+ DTRs lower extremities.

Back: No obvious abnormalities, no tenderness. Straight leg raise negative.

9. **What further steps should be considered for B.R.'s back pain?**

10.   What interventions are indicated for B.R.'s hypertension and chronic kidney disease?

11.   What further information could aid B.R. in his smoking cessation plan?

Case Study, Continued

Three weeks later, the patient returns for an urgent sick visit with acute onset of back pain. He denies any trauma or injury, stating that "he woke up this morning like this." While walking into the examination room, he is in obvious discomfort.

BP 178/80

HR 88

RR 20

O_2 saturation 97% on RA

Temperature 98.2

He explains that he has been continuing to do physical therapy with some relief but has not gone this week. He also states that he has not seen pain management yet, although he does have an appointment scheduled. He tried taking Tylenol for his back pain this morning with no relief, and states his pain is about 8/10. He still denies any numbness or tingling in his lower extremities and denies any bowel or bladder incontinence. He is asking for "something really strong" to take the pain away. He does report that he has been taking his lisinopril daily but forgot to take it this morning because he was so preoccupied with his back pain.

Physical Examination
  Vital signs: BP 178/80, HR 88, RR 20.
  O$_2$ saturation: 97% on RA.
  Temperature: 98.2.
  General appearance: Older male with moderate distress, having trouble sitting on chair, prefers to stand during the visit.
  Lungs: Clear to auscultation.
  Cardiovascular: Normal S1 and S2, no rubs or gallops. Grade II systolic murmur best auscultated at right sternal border.
  Neurologic: Gait is stiff, normal sensation. 2+DTRs lower extremities.
  Back: Decreased lateral flexion, rotation, and extension, diffuse paravertebral tenderness. Straight leg raise and contralateral straight leg raise are negative.

12.   What diagnostics or referrals are appropriate at this visit?

13.   What, if any, medications should be offered to B.R. for pain relief at this time?[5]

14.   What are the concerns associated with prescribing opioids for older adults?[8]

15.   What should be done about the patient's blood pressure at this time?

Case Study, Continued

The patient is given a prescription for tramadol 50 milligrams po one to two times daily for pain. Dispense #14 and no refills. The statewide drug prescription monitoring database is checked before writing the prescription, and the patient is educated on possible side effects and fall risk. He is also instructed to keep appointment with pain management.

He has a lumbar MRI done and results shows grade 1 anterolisthesis of L5 on S1 associated with L5 pars defects. No significant central narrowing at this level; however, there is foraminal narrowing with mild mass effect on exiting L5 nerve roots. Mild central and lateral recess narrowing and foraminal narrowing with lateral disk/osteophytes abutting exiting nerve roots at L3–L4 and L4–L5.

16. Based on these results, what are the next steps in managing B.R.'s pain?

Case Study, Continued

B.R. returns for a follow-up visit after seeing the neurosurgeon and pain management. He received a corticosteroid injection in his lower back at his pain management appointment, which has given him good pain relief. He reports that the neurosurgeon states he is not a good candidate for surgery because it likely would not really help his symptoms.

His BP at this visit is now 136/72, and he reports daily adherence taking his lisinopril 10 milligrams by mouth each day. He still is eating a low-salt diet but has not really started doing any sort of exercise, although he is now feeling well enough to start gardening again.

His BMP results reveal his potassium level is 4.3 and his kidney function shows BUN 23, creatinine 1.3, and GFR 47, which is a mild improvement from the previous chemistry profile.

He has not stopped smoking, although he is down to a half pack of cigarettes daily. He still is refusing to take any kind of medication therapy to help him quit smoking.

He also states he has started to get an annoying dry cough that is nonproductive. This cough has been going on for about 3 weeks. He denies any fevers, chills, or sick contacts. He explains that he does not feel ill at all, but the cough is annoying to him and others.

Review of Systems

Constitutional: No fever, no night sweats, no significant weight gain, no significant weight loss, and no exercise intolerance. No fatigue.

Vital signs: BP 136/72, HR 83, RR 16, O_2 saturation 98% on RA, temperature: 98.1°F.

Respiratory: Dry, nonproductive cough. No real pattern to it, not worse at night. No wheezing, no shortness of breath.

Cardiac: No chest pain, no shortness of breath when walking.

Musculoskeletal: Back pain is intermittent, dull, without radiation, continues to be hard standing for long periods.

Neurologic: No dizziness and no headaches.

Physical Examination

General appearance: Well appearing, conversant, comfortable.

Lungs: Clear to auscultation. No rales, wheezes, or rhonchi.

Cardiovascular: Normal S1 and S2, no rubs or gallops. Grade II systolic murmur best auscultated at right upper sternal border.

Musculoskeletal: Normal movement of all extremities. Extremities: no cyanosis, edema, varicosities, or palpable cord.

Neurologic: Normal gait and station, normal sensation. 2+/4+ DTRs in the lower extremition

Back: No obvious abnormalities, no tenderness to lower back, straight leg raise negative, full range of motion extension, flexion, lateral extension, and rotation.

17.   What diagnoses are included in the differential based on B.R.'s review of systems and physical examination today?

18.   What further review of system, physical examination, and diagnostics should be done to rule out or rule in diagnoses?

Case Study, Continued

On further examination, patient denies any nasal congestion, sore throat, or rhinorrhea. He also denies any heartburn, change in taste, or difficulty swallowing. He states his last chest x-ray was many years ago and there is no record of it in the chart. ENT examination reveals patent nares, no obstruction or deviated septum, no nasal discharge, no posterior pharyngeal erythema or cobblestoning, and no sinus tenderness. Abdominal examination is positive for normal bowel sounds in all four quadrants, no tenderness or masses palpated. In-office spirometry is normal with first second of forced expiration (FEV$_1$)/forced vital capacity (FVC) ratio 91%, FVC 3.57 L, and FEV$_1$ 3.26 L.

19. Are there any diagnoses that can be ruled excluded based on B.R.'s examination today?[9]

20. What are the next steps?

Case Study, Continued

Lisinopril 10 milligrams daily is changed to losartan 25 milligrams daily. A chest x-ray is done. The patient returns in 2 weeks to go over results. He reports that his cough is nearly completely resolved and his BP is still well controlled at 136/70, HR 82. He also brings his home electronic BP cuff to be checked for accuracy and it is found to have nearly identical readings to in-office manual BP. He states that he is now down to half a pack of cigarettes daily and is still refusing any medication for smoking cessation.

His chest x-ray is negative for any acute disease and there are no suspicious nodules or infiltrates noted.

21. What is the definitive diagnosis for B.R.'s cough?

22. What are some ongoing issues for B.R. that will need continued attention at future visits?[10]

ONLINE ANSWER SUBMISSION

When you are ready to submit your answers for grading and reflective expert feedback for evaluation, go to http://www.evolve.elsevier.com/DickAndButtaro/ to complete this case.

References

1. Strand, V., & Singh, J. A. (2017). Evaluation and management of the patient with suspected inflammatory spine disease. *Mayo Clinic Proceedings, 92*(4), 555–564.
2. Patel, N. D., Broderick, D. F., Burns, J., Deshmukh, T. K., Fries, I. B., Harvey, H. B., et al. (2015.) ACR appropriateness criteria low back pain. *American College of Radiology*. Retrieved 6/28/17 from https://acsearch.acr.org/docs/69483/Narrative/.
3. LeFevre, M. L., on behalf of the U.S. Preventive Services Task Force. (2014). Screening for abdominal aortic aneurysm: U.S. Preventive Services Task Force Recommendation Statement. *Annals of Internal Medicine, 161*(4), 281–290.
4. Caboral-Stevens, M. F., & Rosario-Sim, M. (2014). Review of the Joint National Committee's recommendations in the management of hypertension. *The Journal for Nurse Practitioners, 10*(5), 552–559.
5. American Geriatrics Society 2015 Beers Criteria Update Expert Panel. (2015). American Geriatrics Society 2015 Updated Beers Criteria for potentially inappropriate medication use in older adults. *Journal of the American Geriatrics Society, 63*(11), 2227–2246.
6. McManus, M. S., & Wynter-Minott, S. (2017). Guidelines for chronic kidney disease: Defining, staging, and managing in primary care. *The Journal for Nurse Practitioners, 13*(6), 400–410.
7. Halloran, L. (2014). Managing chronic pain: Useful tools and approaches. *The Journal for Nurse Practitioners, 9*(3), 184–185.
8. Gladkowski, C. A., Medley, C. L., Nelson, H. M., Tallie Price, A., & Harvey, M. (2014). Opioids versus physical therapy for management of chronic back pain. *The Journal for Nurse Practitioners, 10*(8), 552–559.
9. Gahbauer, M., & Keane, P. (2009). Chronic cough: Stepwise application in primary care practice of the ACCP guidelines for diagnosis and management of cough. *Journal of the American Academy of Nurse Practitioners, 21*(8), 409–416.
10. Aberle, D. R., Adams, A. M., Berg, C. D., Black, W. C., Clapp, J. D., Fagerstrom, R. M., et al. (2011). Reduced lung-cancer mortality with low-dose computed tomographic screening. *The New England Journal of Medicine, 365*(5), 395–409.

Worsening Shortness of Breath With Activity

Tracy Murray

Instructions

After reviewing the case study, please jot down your notes or preliminary answers in the spaces provided. When you are ready to submit your answers for grading and reflective expert feedback for evaluation, go to http://www.evolve.elsevier.com/DickAndButtaro/ to complete this case.

Case Study Scenario/History of Present Illness

This patient is being seen as a new patient to your practice. He and his wife recently moved to this location to be closer to his daughter and grandchildren. This is a visit to establish care, and you have no prior medical records available at this time. He is accompanied by his wife. Mr. G. is a 72-year-old Caucasian male here to establish care. While you are obtaining his medical history, his wife jumps in and says he does not have the same energy he had a few months ago and becomes "easily winded." Mr. G. shrugs it off as nothing and says he thinks he is just out of shape. He does admit though that he cannot sustain the level of activity that he once did without getting short of breath. It has gotten worse over the last 3 months. The feeling resolves after several minutes of resting. The patient states there is no associated chest pain, wheezing, cough, nausea, or diaphoresis.

The couple lives in a newly built single-story ranch home. His usual walk from the bedroom to the kitchen (about 100 feet) does not bother him, but walking up the slightly inclined driveway does. He used to walk regularly on his treadmill for 2 miles per day without any complaints; however, he admits that over the last year the distance has gradually decreased. He has not walked on the treadmill for at least 3 months but attributes that to "being too busy" with the recent move. He is tired most of the day.

Medications: Metformin 1000 milligrams po twice daily, lisinopril 10 milligrams po once daily, amlodipine 10 milligrams po daily, omeprazole 20 milligrams po once daily, tamsulosin 0.4 milligrams po at bedtime, atorvastatin 20 milligrams po at bedtime, vitamin D_3 2000 IU once po daily, Centrum silver once po daily, and ibuprofen 600 milligrams po twice a day as needed for pain.

Allergies: Keflex (rash).

Past medical history: Type 2 diabetes mellitus (DM), gastroesophageal reflux disease (GERD), hyperlipidemia, hypertension (HTN), benign prostatic hypertrophy (BPH), and osteoarthritis (OA) in bilateral knees.

Past surgical history: Right total knee replacement 5 years ago. Tonsillectomy as a child.

Habits: Former smoker of 1 pack per day (PPD) × 25 years; he quit 30 years ago. Drinks an occasional beer while watching Sunday night football. No illicit drugs.

Social and personal history: Married × 50 years, retired mechanical engineer. Two daughters, both healthy.

Family history: Father died age 51 from colon cancer, mother died age 70 from congestive heart failure (CHF). He is not sure how his grandparents died. No siblings.

Review of Systems

General: + fatigue and + weight gain (10 pounds in 6 months). Denies fever, chills, or diaphoresis.

Head, ears, eyes, nose, and throat (HEENT): Denies headaches, nasal congestion, rhinorrhea, otalgia, sore throat, or dysphagia.

Neck: Denies neck pain or swelling in lymph nodes.

Respiratory: + shortness of breath (SOB) with moderate exertion, which resolves with rest. Denies recent respiratory infection, cough, or wheezing. Former smoker. Denies hemoptysis. Had "exercise-induced" asthma as a child.

Cardiac: Denies chest pain, palpitations, orthopnea, paroxysmal nocturnal dyspnea (PND), leg pain, or claudication. He does complain of bilateral lower leg swelling when he is on his feet for most of the day or eats a high-sodium meal.

Gastrointestinal: Denies nausea, vomiting, diarrhea, or dysphagia. + heartburn (controlled with omeprazole), + mild constipation.

Urinary: Denies dysuria or incontinence. + nocturnal frequency (controlled with tamsulosin).

Musculoskeletal: Denies back pain or leg pain. + bilateral knee pain (left greater than right) because of OA.

Neurologic: Denies dizziness, syncope, weakness, or numbness and tingling.

Endocrine: + DM type II. Monitors blood sugars once daily and reports readings range from 90 to 120 before breakfast. Denies heat or cold intolerance. Reports fatigue "all the time."

Skin: Denies rashes or lesions, but complains of dry skin.

Psychiatric: Denies history of depression or anxiety. Denies trouble falling or staying asleep, but does not feel well rested. Wife reports that he does snore most nights. Takes one to two short naps (1–2 hours) per day.

Physical Examination

General: Elderly well-developed, obese white male in no apparent distress. Well-groomed and appropriately dressed.

Vital signs: Height 6'2". Weight 250 pounds. Body mass index (BMI) 32.1. Temperature 97.0°F. Blood pressure 160/95 in right arm and 165/98 in left arm, heart rate 70 regular, respiratory rate 16 at rest, O_2 saturation 96% on room air.

HEENT: Normocephalic, pupils equal, round, and reactive to light. No conjunctival erythema or drainage. Sclera white. Tympanic membranes (TMs) without erythema, bulging, or retraction. No rhinitis or nasal turbinate swelling. No tenderness over frontal or maxillary sinuses. Posterior pharynx without injection. Surgically absent tonsils. Mucosal membranes moist without lesions, teeth in good repair.

Neck: Supple. No masses, lymphadenopathy, thyroid enlargement, or tenderness. No jugular venous distension (JVD).

Cardiac: Regular rhythm without murmurs, gallops, or rubs. Normal S1 and S2. No S3 or S4. Pedal and posterior tibial pulses strong bilaterally. No calf swelling or tenderness. Bilateral peripheral edema in lower legs, 2+ nonpitting.

Respiratory: Anterior and posterior lungs clear to auscultation, no wheezes or crackles. Normal respiratory excursion with equal symmetry. No dullness or hyperresonance to percussion. No evidence of cyanosis or clubbing in fingernails.

Abdomen: Obese. Positive active bowel sounds. Soft, nontender. No ascites or hepatojugular reflux. No organomegaly.

Musculoskeletal: No kyphoscoliosis. No joint swelling. Moderate crepitus left knee with range of motion (ROM).

Skin: Warm and dry. No rashes or acute lesions. Vertical surgical scar over right knee.

Neurologic: Alert and oriented. Cranial nerves (CNs) II to XII intact. Strength full and sensation intact to bilateral upper and lower extremities. Deep tendon reflexes (DTRs) 2+ and symmetric throughout.

Psychiatric: Mood and demeanor appropriate.

ASSESSMENT AND PLAN

1. Based on the history and physical examination results, what are the possible causes (differential diagnoses) of Mr. G.'s dyspnea?[1]

2. What are other noncardiopulmonary causes that could be considered?[1]

3. What are Mr. G.'s risk factors for cardiopulmonary diseases?

4. What workup should be considered initially for the chief complaint of dyspnea on exertion?[1]

5. When the cause of dyspnea is not apparent, what initial laboratory and diagnostic studies could be ordered and why?[2]

Case Study, Continued

Mr. G. is sent to the *local outpatient diagnostic facility for testing, and a follow-up appointment is scheduled the following day to review the results. Because of his diabetic history, the health care provider also ordered a Hemoglobin A1C to determine his glucose control because his previous records are unavailable.*

Results of Initial Testing

COMPLETE BLOOD COUNT WITH DIFFERENTIAL

Component	Result	Standard Range
WBC	6.0	4.5–13.0 K/mm^3
RBC	**3.29**	4.10–5.30 m/mm^3
HGB	**11.0**	12.0–16.0 grams/dL
Hematocrit	**35**	36.0%–49.0%
MCV	**75.0**	78.0–102.0 fL
MCHC	**29.3**	31.0–37.0 grams/dL
RDW	13.4	9.0%–15.0%
Platelets	179	130–400 K/mm^3
Neutrophils	32	30.0%–70.0%
Lymphs	45	21.0%–51.0%
Monocytes	9.2	0%–14.0%
EOS	2.0	0.0%–7.0%
Basophils	0.5	0.0%–2.0%
Abs Neutrophils	2.0	1.8–8.0 K/mm^3
Lymphs (absolute)	3.8	1.2–5.2 K/mm^3
Monocyte absolute	0.4	0.2–1.1 K/mm^3
Abs eosinophils	0.1	0.0–0.6 K/mm^3
Abs basophils	0.0	0.0–0.3 K/mm^3

Abs, Absolute; *EOS,* eosinophils; *HGB,* hemoglobin; *MCHC,* mean corpuscular hemoglobin concentration; *MCV,* mean corpuscular volume; *RBC,* red blood cell; *RDW,* red cell distribution width; *WBC,* white blood cell.

Comprehensive Metabolic Panel

Component	Results	Reference Range
Glucose	83	65–99 milligrams/dL
BUN	12	6–24 milligrams/dL
Creatinine	0.7	0.57–1.00 mf/dL
eGFR non-African American	>90	>59 mL/min/1.73
BUN/creatinine ratio	17	9–23
Sodium	142	134–144 mmol/L
Potassium	4.3	3.5–5.3 mmol/L
Chloride	102	96–106 mmol/L
Carbon dioxide	29	18–29 mmol/L
Calcium	9.5	8.7–10.2 mmol/L
Total protein	6.8	6.0–8.5 grams/dL
Albumin	4.6	3.5–5.5 grams/dL
Globulin, total	2.2	1.5–4.5 grams/dL
Albumin/globulin ratio	2.1	1.2–2.2
Bilirubin, total	0.3	0.0–1.2 milligrams/dL
Alkaline phosphatase	102	39–117 IU/L
AST	19	0–40 IU/L
ALT	12	0–32 IU/L

ALT, Alanine transaminase; *AST,* aspartate transaminase; *BUN,* blood urea nitrogen; *eGFR,* estimated glomerular filtration rate.

Thyroid-Stimulating Hormone With Reflex to Free T$_4$

Component	Result	Reference Range
TSH	7 4	0.45–4.50 uIU/mL
Free T4	4.5	4.5–12.5 u/dL

TSH, Thyroid-stimulating hormone.

Chest X-Ray

No acute infiltrates or consolidations are seen. Cardiac and mediastinal silhouettes are normal. No hilar enlargement is evident. Osseous thorax is intact.

12-Lead Electrocardiogram

Normal sinus rhythm with heart rate of 85.

Hemoglobin A1C

Component	Result	Reference Range
Hgb A1C	6.0%	<5.7%, normal 5.8%–6.4%, prediabetic >6.5%, diabetic
Urine microalbumin ratio	<30	<30 micrograms/milligrams creatinine

Hgb, Hemoglobin.

When Mr. G. returns to your office the following day, these vital signs are obtained. Height 6'2", weight: 250 pounds, BMI 32, temperature 97.1°F, blood pressure (BP) 168/96 in right arm and 165/97 in left arm, heart rate 90 and regular, respiratory rate 16 breaths per minute at rest and 26 breaths per minute postwalking of 10 feet in office, and O$_2$ sat 96% and 90% on room air, respectively. He reports that nothing has changed since his visit yesterday except swelling in his legs. He reports that he took his grandkids to the county fair last evening and he ate "a lot of fair food." They only stayed an hour because he was too tired to "keep up with the kids." A focused cardiopulmonary examination reveals 1+ pretibial edema bilaterally but is otherwise negative.

6. Based on the previous information, provide a current problem list for Mr. G.'s most concerning issues.

7.   Knowing that a chest x-ray and electrocardiogram are sometimes inadequate in distinguishing between heart and lung disease as the cause for chronic dyspnea, what additional tests should the practitioner consider?[2]

Case Study, Continued

The need for further testing is discussed with Mr. G. because the initial results do not rule out the possibility of a cardiac or pulmonary source for his symptoms. The provider advises him that he will have a BNP, PFT, echocardiogram, and pharmacologic cardiac stress test with myocardial perfusion scan performed. Any abnormal findings will be discussed with him to determine any additional steps for his plan.

8.   Identify the areas of additional concern (physical examination, review of systems, laboratory results) and explain how each might contribute to Mr. G.'s overall complaints. Identify any further testing that is necessary based on the abnormal results.[3]

Mr. G. is sent out of the office today with a laboratory requisition for BNP, CBC w/diff, ferritin, stool for hemoccult × 3 (with directions), TSH, FT$_4$, anti–TPO (antithyroid peroxidase antibodies), and lipid panel. He is instructed to monitor his BP daily and bring his readings to his next visit. He is also given written instructions to observe a low-sodium diet and instructed to wear support hose and elevate his lower extremities with the occurrence of edema. The echocardiogram, PFTs, and cardiac stress test are to be arranged by office staff for later this week and a follow-up appointment is scheduled on next Monday. The following Monday, Mr. G. returns to review all of his test results. His vital signs, focused physical examination, and results are in the subsequent tables.

CBC With Differential

Component	Result	Standard Range
WBC	5.9	4.5–13.0 K/mm^3
RBC	**3.10**	4.10–5.30 m/mm^3
Hemoglobin	**10.9**	12.0–16.0 grams/dL
Hematocrit	**33**	36.0%–49.0%
MCV	**73**	78.0–102.0 fL
MCHC	**28.2**	31.0–37.0 grams/dL
RDW	11.4	9.0%–15.0%
Platelets	202	130–400 K/mm^3
Neutrophils	35	30.0%–70.0%
Lymphs	47	21.0%–51.0%
Monocytes %	9.0	0%–14.0%
EOS	2.0	0.0%–7.0%
Basophils	0.6	0.0%–2.0%
Abs neutrophils	2.1	1.8–8.0 K/mm^3
Lymphs (absolute)	3.9	1.2–5.2 K/mm^3
Monocyte (absolute)	0.6	0.2–1.1 K/mm^3
Abs eosinophils	0.0	0.0–0.6 K/mm^3
Abs basophils	0.0	0.0–0.3 K/mm^3

Abs, Absolute; *EOS*, eosinophils; *MCHC*, mean corpuscular hemoglobin concentration; *MCV*, mean corpuscular volume; *RBC*, red blood cell; *RDW*, red cell distribution width; *WBC*, white blood cell.

Serum Ferritin

Component	Result	Standard Range
Serum ferritin	**18**	24–336 ng/dL

Brain Natriuretic Peptide

Component	Result	Standard Range
BNP	50	<125 pg/mL

Thyroid Studies

Component	Result	Standard Range
TSH	**10.0**	0.45–4.50 uIU/Ml
FT$_4$	**1.2**	4.5–12.5µ/dL
Anti-TPO antibodies	Negative	Negative

FT$_4$, Free thyroxine; *TPO*, thyroid peroxidase; *TSH*, thyroid-stimulating hormone.

Lipid Panel

Component	Result	Standard Range
Total cholesterol	220	>200, higher risk 170–199, borderline <170, desirable
LDL	110	>130, higher risk 110–129, borderline <100, desirable
HDL	25	31–76 milligrams/dL
TG	179	38–152 milligrams/dL

HDL, High-density lipoprotein; *LDL,* low-density lipoprotein; *TG,* total glucose.

Hemoccult × 3

Component	Result	Standard Range
Hemoccult card 1	+	–
Hemoccult card 2	+	–
Hemoccult card 3	+	–

Echocardiogram

1. Left ventricle: The cavity size was normal. Wall thickness was normal. Systolic function was normal. The estimated ejection fraction was 55%. Wall motion was normal; there were no regional wall motion abnormalities. Left ventricular diastolic function parameters were normal.
2. Mitral valve: The annulus was mildly calcified. The leaflets were normal thickened.
3. Right ventricle: The cavity size was normal. Systolic function was normal.
4. Pulmonic valve: There was trivial regurgitation.
5. Pulmonary arteries: Systolic pressure was normal.
6. Bubble study revealed no intracardiac shunt.

Pulmonary Function Tests

The FVC, FEV_1, and FEV_1/FVC ratio are all within normal limits. There is minimal bronchodilator response. Lung volumes and diffusion capacity are normal. SaO_2 on room air is 97%. Flow volume loop is normal.

Impression: Normal pulmonary function test with no evidence of obstructive nor restrictive ventilator defect.

FEV_1, forced expiratory volume in 1 second; *FVC,* forced vital capacity.

Lexiscan Stress With Myocardial Perfusion

The patient was pharmacologically stressed with a 0.4 milligram Lexiscan injection. At 10–15 seconds, 10.2 mCi of technetium 99m-labeled sestamibi was given intravenously. SPECT images of the myocardium were obtained at least 30 minutes postinjection. Resting SPECT images with gating were acquired at least 30 minutes after the injection of 30.0 mCi of technetium 99m-labeled sestamibi.

Findings: The overall quality of the study was good. Left ventricular cavity size was normal on stress and rest studies. Images obtained poststress demonstrate homogenous tracer distribution throughout the myocardium. The rest images are unchanged. The gated images demonstrate uniform wall motion and myocardial thickening. The ejection fraction is 65%.

SPECT, Single-photon emission computed tomography.

Home Blood Pressure Log × 1 Week

Day (Morning)	Systolic	Diastolic	Pulse
Tuesday	159	70	80
Wednesday	169	86	72
Thursday	174	90	69
Friday	166	85	74
Saturday	171	88	83
Sunday	153	79	81
Monday	170	86	70

Focused Review of Systems

General: + continued fatigue. No additional weight gain since last visit.

Neck: Denies neck pain or swelling in lymph nodes.

Respiratory: + SOB with moderate exertion, which resolves with rest.

Cardiac: Denies chest pain, palpitations, orthopnea, PND, leg pain, or claudication. Intermittent lower extremity edema is still present, but he describes it as less noticeable. He is watching a low-sodium diet but does not wear the support hose because they are too hot.

Gastrointestinal: + mild to moderate constipation.

Endocrine: + DM type II. Blood sugars continue to average 90 to 120 before breakfast. Fatigue continues.

Focused Physical Examination

General: Elderly well-developed, obese white male in no apparent distress. Well groomed and appropriately dressed.

Vital signs: Height 6'2", weight 251 pounds, BMI 32.1. Temperature: 97.0°F. Blood pressure 150/89 in right arm and 152/90 in left arm. At this visit, no orthostatic changes. Heart rate 78 regular, respiratory rate 16 at rest, O_2 saturation 97% on room air.

Neck: Supple. No masses, lymphadenopathy, thyroid enlargement, or tenderness. No JVD.

Cardiac: Regular rhythm without murmurs, gallops, or rubs. Normal S1 and S2. No S3 or S4. Pedal and posterior tibial pulses strong bilaterally. No calf swelling or tenderness. Bilateral peripheral edema in lower legs, 1+ nonpitting.

Respiratory: Anterior and posterior lungs clear to auscultation, no wheezes or crackles. Normal respiratory excursion with equal symmetry. No dullness or hyperresonance to percussion. No evidence of cyanosis or clubbing in fingernails.

Abdomen: Obese, soft, nontender. Positive active bowel sounds. No ascites or hepatojugular reflux. No organomegaly.

9. After carefully considering these test findings, identify Mr. G.'s current problem list.[4,5]

10.   What is the likely etiology of Mr. G.'s dyspnea?

11.   What changes and/or new recommendations would you make to Mr. G.'s plan?

Nurse Visit

Mr. G. returns for a nurse visit in 2 weeks and brings a log of his latest BP readings as shown in the subsequent table.

Home Blood Pressure Log × 2 Weeks

Day (morning)	Systolic	Diastolic	Pulse
Tuesday	159	86	00
Wednesday	155	87	72
Thursday	164	90	69
Friday	150	82	74
Saturday	147	74	83
Sunday	146	72	81
Monday	140	70	70
Tuesday	142	72	74
Wednesday	139	70	76
Thursday	136	68	70
Friday	132	71	69
Saturday	134	74	72
Sunday	136	70	77
Monday	135	65	75

Case Study, Continued

Height: 6'2", weight: 246 pounds, BMI 31.6. Temperature 97.2°F. BP 130/78 in right arm and 132/76 in left arm, heart rate 72 regular without orthostatic changes, respiratory rate 16 at rest, and O$_2$ saturation 97% on room air. He has an appointment in 2 days for the EGD/colonoscopy and next week for a sleep study. He is already scheduled for a follow-up with you in 2 weeks. Before he leaves, the office nurse is given a new prescription for Mr. G.'s BP medication (no changes) and a laboratory requisition to have a CBC, TSH/FT$_4$, and CMP before his next visit.

When Mr. G. returns to the office for his next follow-up visit, the following information is reported. Height 6'2", weight: 242 pounds, BMI 31.1. Temperature 97.1°F. BP 128/66 in right arm and 130/67 in left arm, heart rate 70 and regular without orthostatic changes, respiratory rate 16 breaths per minute at rest and 20 breaths per minute postwalking of 10 feet in office, and O$_2$ saturation 97% and 94% on room air, respectively. Additionally, the subsequent reports were obtained.

Sleep Study Results

Description:

The total recording time was 424.0 minutes. The total sleep time was 373.0 minutes. There was a total of 44.0 minutes of wakefulness after sleep onset for a slightly reduced sleep efficiency of 88.0%. The latency to sleep onset was short at 7.0 minutes. The R sleep onset latency was prolonged at 203.0 minutes. Sleep parameters, as a percentage of the total sleep time, demonstrated that 3.5% of sleep was in N1 sleep, 79.2% in N2, 4.6% in N3, and 12.7% in R sleep. There was a total of 320 arousals for an arousal index of 51.5 arousals per hour of sleep, which was elevated. Respiratory monitoring demonstrated a frequent mild to moderate degree of snoring in all positions. There were a total of 434 apneas and hypopneas for an AHI of 69.8 apneas and hypopneas per hour of sleep. The REM-related AHI was 66.9/h of REM sleep compared with an NREM AHI of 70.2/h. The average duration of the respiratory events was 35.7 seconds with a maximum duration of 112.0 seconds. The respiratory events occurred in all positions. The respiratory events were associated with peripheral oxygen desaturations on the average to 78%, declining to the high 60s during REM sleep. The lowest oxygen desaturation associated with a respiratory event was 57%. Additionally, the baseline oxygen saturation during wakefulness was 90%, during NREM sleep averaged 88%, and during REM sleep averaged 85%. The total duration of oxygen <90% was 223.1 minutes and <80% was 46.0 min.

Cardiac monitoring: Did not demonstrate transient cardiac decelerations associated with the apneas. There were no significant cardiac rhythm irregularities.

Sleep Study Results—cont'd

Periodic limb movement monitoring: Did not demonstrate periodic limb movements.

Impression:

This routine overnight polysomnogram demonstrated the presence of significant obstructive sleep apnea with an overall AHI of 69.8 apneas and hypopneas per hour of sleep. The respiratory events were associated with peripheral oxygen desaturations on the average to 78%, declining to the high 60s during REM sleep. The lowest oxygen desaturation associated with a respiratory event was 57%. There was a slightly reduced sleep efficiency, elevated arousal index, increased awakenings, and failure to progress into the deeper stages of sleep. These findings would appear to be caused by the obstructive sleep apnea.

Recommendations:

1. A CPAP titration would be recommended because of the severity of the sleep apnea.
2. Additionally, would recommend weight loss in a patient with a BMI of 31.6.

AHI, Apnea hypopnea index; *BMI,* body mass index: *CPAP,* continuous positive airway pressure; *NREM,* nonrapid eye movement; *REM,* rapid eye movement.

Esophagogastroduodenoscopy Findings

Impression: Moderate erosive gastritis. Biopsy is negative for *Helicobacter pylori*.
Recommendations:
No NSAIDs.
Increase omeprazole to 40 milligrams daily.
OK to start $FeSO_4$ as ordered by PCP.

NSAID, Nonsteroidal antiinflammatory drug; *PCP,* primary care physician.

Colonoscopy Findings

Impression: An 8-mm sessile serrated adenoma without dysplasia was found in the ascending colon. A single-piece polypectomy was performed using a cold snare. The polyp was completely removed. A 15-mm slow bleeding sessile serrated adenoma without dysplasia was found in the ascending colon. A piecemeal polypectomy was performed using a cold snare. The polyp was completely removed.
Recommendations:
Recall colonoscopy in 3 years
High-fiber diet

Complete Blood Count With Differential

Component	Result	Standard Range
WBC	5.9	4.5–13.0 K/mm³
RBC	**3.75**	4.10–5.30 m/mm³
Hemoglobin	**11.3**	12.0–16.0 grams/dL
Hematocrit	**35**	36.0%–49.0%
MCV	**75**	78.0–102.0 fL
MCHC	31.0	31.0–37.0 grams/dL
RDW	11.4	9.0%–15.0%
Platelets	202	130–400 K/mm³
Neutrophils	35	30.0%–70.0%
Lymphs	47	21.0%–51.0%

Continued

Complete Blood Count With Differential—cont'd

Component	Result	Standard Range
Monocytes %	9.0	0%–14.0%
EOS	2.0	0.0%–7.0%
Basophils	0.6	0.0%–2.0%
Abs neutrophils	2.1	1.8–8.0 K/mm^3
Lymphs (absolute)	3.9	1.2–5.2 K/mm^3
Monocyte (absolute)	0.6	0.2–1.1 K/mm^3
Abs eosinophils	0.0	0.0–0.6 K/mm^3
Abs basophils	0.0	0.0–0.3 K/mm^3

Abs, Absolute; *EOS,* eosinophils; *MCHC,* mean corpuscular hemoglobin concentration; *MCV,* mean corpuscular volume; *RBC,* red blood cell; *RDW,* red cell distribution width; *WBC,* white blood cell.

Comprehensive Metabolic Panel

Component	Results	Reference Range
Glucose	76	65–99 milligrams/dL
BUN	14	6–24 milligrams/dL
Creatinine	0.7	0.57–1.00 mf/dL
eGFR non-African American	>90	>59 mL/min/1.73
BUN/creatinine ratio	16	9–23
Sodium	140	134–144 mmol/L
Potassium	4.0	3.5–5.3 mmol/L
Chloride	104	96–106 mmol/L
Carbon dioxide	26	18–29 mmol/L
Calcium	9.6	8.7–10.2 mmol/L
Total protein	6.8	6.0–8.5 grams/dL
Albumin	4.6	3.5–5.5 grams/dL
Globulin, total	2.2	1.5–4.5 grams/dL
Albumin/globulin ratio	2.1	1.2–2.2
Bilirubin, total	0.3	0.0–1.2 milligrams/dL
Alkaline phosphatase	110	39–117 IU/L
AST	24	0–40 IU/L
ALT	18	0–32 IU/L

ALT, Alanine transaminase; *AST,* aspartate transaminase; *BUN,* blood urea nitrogen; *eGFR,* estimated glomerular filtration rate.

Thyroid-Stimulating Hormone With Reflex to Free T$_4$

Component	Result	Reference Range
TSH	**4.9**	0.45–4.50 uIU/mL
Free T$_4$	**4.4**	4.5–12.5 µ/dL

TSH, Thyroid-stimulating hormone.

Mr. G. reports having less fatigue and more motivation and energy overall but still has some dyspnea with physical activity. He reports that his edema has resolved and his daily BP recordings are ranging from 130 to 140/70 to 80. He joined Weight Watchers last week and is committed to losing weight and has set a goal weight to reach 225 pounds within 6 months. He also joined the YMCA and plans to participate in their Silver Sneaker program at least 3 days per week. A focused cardiopulmonary examination shows that the lower extremity edema has resolved. The remainder of the examination was also normal.

The provider reviews the results of his recent sleep study and colonoscopy. The patient reports he started with the continuous positive airway pressure (CPAP) at night. He also states that he started on ferrous sulfate after his colonoscopy and noted that his omeprazole was increased to 40 milligrams daily by his gastroenterologist.

12. What is your assessment and plan for Mr. G. today?

At his 6-week follow-up visit, he reports a significant improvement in his dyspnea since starting an aerobic conditioning program. His fatigue has resolved. He is more motivated and he reports no edema in his legs. Mr. G.'s BP has remained at goal (<140/90), and he is tolerating his medications without adverse effects. His weight today is 240 pounds. BP is 131/68, pulse 68, respiratory rate 16, O_2 saturation 98% on room air. Laboratory results are seen in subsequent tables.

Comprehensive Metabolic Panel

Component	Results	Reference Range
Glucose	70	65–99 milligrams/dL
BUN	12	6–24 milligrams/dL
Creatinine	0.6	0.57–1.00 milligrams/dL
eGFR non-African American	>90	>59 mL/min/1.73
BUN/creatinine ratio	14	9–23
Sodium	139	134–144 mmol/L
Potassium	4.1	3.5–5.3 mmol/L
Chloride	104	96–106 mmol/L
Carbon dioxide	28	18–29 mmol/L
Calcium	9.5	8.7–10.2 mmol/L
Total protein	6.9	6.0–8.5 grams/dL
Albumin	4.2	3.5–5.5 grams/dL
Globulin, total	2.1	1.5–4.5 grams/dL
Albumin/globulin ratio	2.0	1.2–2.2
Bilirubin, total	0.3	0.0–1.2 milligrams/dL
Alkaline phosphatase	108	39–117 IU/L
AST	22	0–40 IU/L
ALT	14	0–32 IU/L

ALT, Alanine transaminase; *AST,* aspartate transaminase; *BUN,* blood urea nitrogen; *eGFR,* estimated glomerular filtration rate.

Thyroid-Stimulating Hormone With Reflex to Free T$_4$

Component	Result	Reference Range
TSH	2.8	0.45–4.50 uIU/mL
Free T$_4$	8.3	4.5–12.5 µ/dL

TSH, Thyroid-stimulating hormone.

Hemoglobin A1C

Component	Result	Reference Range
Hgb A1C	5.8%	<5.7%, normal 5.8–6.4%, prediabetic >6.5%, diabetic

Lipid Panel

Component	Result	Standard Range
Total cholesterol	196	>200, higher risk 170–199, borderline <170, desirable
LDL	95	>130, higher risk 110–129, borderline <100, desirable
HDL	30	31–76 milligrams/dL
TG	147	38–152 milligrams/dL

HDL, High-density lipoprotein; *Hgb,* hemoglobin; *LDL,* low-density lipoprotein; *TG,* total glucose.

Complete Blood Count With Differential

Component	Result	Standard Range
WBC	6.2	4.5–13.0 K/mm^3
RBC	**4.0**	4.10–5.30 m/mm^3
Hemoglobin	**11.8**	12.0–16.0 grams/dL
Hematocrit	36	36.0%–49.0%
MCV	80	78.0–102.0 fL
MCHC	33	31.0–37.0 grams/dL
RDW	11.4	9.0%–15.0%
Platelets	198	130–400 K/mm^3
Neutrophils	30	30.0%–70.0%
Lymphs	47	21.0%–51.0%
Monocytes %	9.0	0%–14.0%
EOS	2.0	0.0%–7.0%
Basophils	0.6	0.0%–2.0%
Abs neutrophils	2.1	1.8–8.0 K/mm^3
Lymphs (absolute)	3.9	1.2–5.2 K/mm^3
Monocyte (absolute)	0.6	0.2–1.1 K/mm^3
Abs eosinophils	0.0	0.0–0.6 K/mm^3
Abs basophils	0.0	0.0–0.3 K/mm^3

Abs, Absolute; *EOS,* eosinophils; *MCHC,* mean corpuscular hemoglobin concentration; *MCV,* mean corpuscular volume; *RBC,* red blood cell; *RDW,* red cell distribution width; *WBC,* white blood cell.

Serum Ferritin

Component	Result	Standard Range
Serum ferritin	38	24–336 ng/dL

The provider reviews his laboratory results and explains that his parameters are desirable now.

His prescriptions are renewed today (no changes) and he continues to be encouraged with his efforts to lose weight and increase activity. He is to return in 3 months for a routine check-up with labs done before appointment (CBC, CMP, and TSH/FT$_4$).

ONLINE ANSWER SUBMISSION

When you are ready to submit your answers for grading and reflective expert feedback for evaluation, go to http://www.evolve.elsevier.com/DickAndButtaro/ to complete this case.

References

1. Parshall, M. B., Schwartzstein, R. M., Adams, L., Banzett, R. B., Manning, H. L., Bourbeau, J., et al.; on behalf of the ATS Committee on Dyspnea. (2012). An official American Thoracic Society statement: Update on the mechanisms, assessment, and management of dyspnea. *American Journal of Respiratory and Critical Care Medicine, 185*(4), 435–452.
2. Wahls, S. (2012). Causes and evaluation of chronic dyspnea. *American Family Physician, 86*(2), 173–182.
3. Short, M., & Domagalski, J. (2013). Iron deficiency anemia: Evaluation and management. *American Family Physician, 87*(2), 98–104.
4. Stone, N. J., Robinson, J., Lichtenstein, A. H., Bairey Merz, C. N., Lloyd-Jones, D. M., Blum, C. B., et al. (2013). ACC/AHA Guideline on the treatment of blood cholesterol to reduce atherosclerotic cardiovascular risk in adults. *Journal of the American College of Cardiology*, doi:10.1016/j.jacc.2013.11.002.
5. James, P., Oparil, S., Carter, B., et al. (2014). Evidence-based guideline for the management of high blood pressure in adults. Report from the panel members appointed to the Eight Joint National Committee (JNC8). *Journal of the American Medical Association, 311*(5), 507–520.

Hallucinations

Jemecia C. Braxton-Barrett ■ Dawn Carpenter

Instructions

After reviewing the case study, please jot down your notes or preliminary answers in the spaces provided. When you are ready to submit your answers for grading and reflective expert feedback for evaluation, go to http://www.evolve.elsevier.com/DickAndButtaro/ to complete this case.

Home-Based Primary Care Initial Visit

VA Home-Based Primary Care (HBPC) is a unique home care program that provides comprehensive, interdisciplinary, primary care in the homes of veterans with complex medical, social, and behavioral conditions. In contrast to other home care systems that target patients with short-term remediable needs and provide episodic, time-limited skilled services, HBPC targets patients with complex, chronic, progressively disabling diseases and provides comprehensive, long-term home care.[1]

HBPC is designed to serve the chronically ill through the months and years before death, providing primary care, palliative care, rehabilitation, disease management, and coordination of care services. The heath care team consists of physicians, nurse practitioners, physician assistants, nurses, social workers, nutritionists, and physical and occupational therapists

Case Study Scenario/History of Present Illness

Mrs. Williams is an 81-year-old African American married female veteran with dementia who lives at home with her husband. The HBPC provider received a call from Mr. Williams regarding his wife's complaints of seeing things over the past 3 to 4 days. The husband reports his wife is more confused and is now seeing family members in their home and in a car out in front of their home. He reports the patient is not acting like herself and that his wife says that the family members she sees come and go throughout the day. Mr. Williams reports his wife denies complaints of fever, chills, chest pain, nausea, vomiting, or diarrhea. The HBPC provider made a home visit to assess Mrs. Williams' condition.

1. What are differential diagnoses for an acute change in mental status?

It is important to start with a list of differential diagnoses to guide questions during the history and physical examination. The provider is concerned about the husband's reports of his wife's increased confusion and visual hallucinations. In older adults, symptoms can be vague and often do not help determine the severity of an illness or suggest the cause.

2. What questions can help the health care provider elicit a clearer understanding of this patient's complaints?

Formulating a diagnosis starts with the history of present illness (HPI). Patients should be asked questions in the OLDCAARTS (onset, location/radiation, duration, character, aggravating factors, associated symptoms, relieving factors, timing, and severity) format using their own words. OLDCAARTS is an easy mnemonic to remember when used by the provider during history taking. It is used to help define the nature of the problem and with formulating differentials diagnosis. Most importantly, OLDCAARTS can clarify what patients mean by their answers. Questions, to consider asking the patient and her husband include:

Case Study, Continued

The following history was reviewed in Mrs. Williams' chart by the health care provider, and additional history was obtained from the patient's husband.

Past medical history: Hypertension, hypercholesterolemia, glaucoma, cerebrovascular accident (CVA), TIAs, type 2 diabetes, carotid artery stenosis, vascular dementia, constipation, insomnia, and arthritis.

Past surgical/hospitalization history: Abdominal aortic aneurysm 1999 (hospitalized), carotid endarterectomy 2004 (hospitalized), CVA 2010.

Allergies: Simvastatin, fluvastatin, rosuvastatin: muscle pain. Hydrochlorothiazide: rash. Lorazepam: delirium.

Medications:
Lisinopril 20-milligram tablet po daily.
Carvedilol 6.25-milligram tablet, take one-half tablet by mouth twice a day.
Clopidogrel bisulfate 75-milligram tablet, take one tablet by mouth every day.
Acetaminophen 325-milligram tablet, take two tablets by mouth twice a day as needed for pain.
Amlodipine 5-milligram tablet po daily.
Aspirin 81 milligrams, chew 1 tablet po daily.

Atorvastatin calcium 80-milligram tablet, take one-half tablet by mouth at bedtime.

Trazodone 50-milligram one tablet po at bedtime.

Bisacodyl 5-milligram enteric-coated tablet, take one tablet by mouth every other day.

Brimonidine tartrate 0.2% ophthalmic solution, instill 1 drop in each eye twice a day.

Dorzolamide 22.3/timolol, 6.8 milligrams/mL ophthalmic solution, instill 1 drop in each eye twice a day.

Latanoprost 0.005% ophthalmic solution, instill 1 drop in each eye at bedtime.

Precision Xtra (glucose) test strip use 1 strip as directed to check blood sugar (limited to 50 strips/90 days).

Multivitamin, take 1 capsule by mouth every day.

Vitamin D 2000 units by mouth daily.

Melatonin 5 milligrams by mouth every day at bedtime for sleep.

3. Is there anything in Mrs. Williams' history thus far that puts her at risk of delirium?[2]

Immunizations: She received all of her immunizations as a child and as part of her military enlistment. She has received her yearly influenza vaccination this year and had Pneumovax 5 years ago.

Social history: Mrs. Williams is married and lives with her husband of 40 years. She has one son who lives locally. She is a past smoker; she had previously reported smoking more than a pack of cigarettes per day over a period of 20 years. However, she stopped smoking 8 years ago, and she currently does not smoke. No illegal drug use. Her husband reports that she currently drinks two or less mixed alcoholic drinks a day.

Military history: Branch of service: Mrs. Williams was a member of the Army; she was not a prisoner of war. She served during World War II as a cook. No environmental exposures.

Family history: Father died age 72 from dementia. Mother died age 76 from congestive heart failure (CHF) and myocardial infarction. Sister died age 68 from myocardial infarction. Maternal grandfather died of black lung disease. Maternal grandmother died of a stroke.

Review of Systems

General: Reports "I feel fine I just can't see that well anymore." "I can't explain the visions but they're there." "I don't feel sick; I can't hear that well anymore." "I lost my hearing in the military." Denies fevers, chills, weakness, nausea, vomiting, diarrhea, or chest pain.

Skin: She reports her skin is very thin with red blotches from accidentally hitting herself. Also describes multiple hard areas on face, arms, and hands that she is having evaluated by dermatology for skin cancer.

Head, ears, eyes, nose, and throat (HEENT): Denies headache, dizziness, sinus pain, or sore throat. Wears hearing aids.

Neck: Denies neck pain or masses.

Respiratory: Reports some instances of shortness of breath when walking without her walker. Has a chronic cough every morning.

Cardiac: Denies chest pain or palpitations.

Gastrointestinal: Reports occasional constipation. Denies difficulty swallowing, heartburn, nausea, vomiting, or diarrhea.

Urinary: Husband reports she is going to the bathroom more often and there is a strong odor to her urine. She complains of burning and pain when she urinates. Has a history of previous UTIs. She had just finished an antibiotic a month ago, but her husband does not recall its name.

Musculoskeletal: Reports joint pain and joint stiffness in the mornings. Denies back pain or leg pain.

Peripheral vascular: Denies swelling in the legs or calf area.

Neurovascular: Has had several TIAs in the past and has a history of stroke. Denies numbness or tingling.

Hematologic: Reports a history of anemia, has easy bruising and bleeding.

Endocrine: Denies sweating, excessive thirst. Has not been checking blood sugars.

Psychiatric: Husband reports previous episodes of depression and visual hallucinations.

Physical Examination

Vital signs: Temperature: 100.8°F (orally). Heart rate 112 regular, respiratory rate 24, blood pressure (BP) 98/56 (baseline BP 138/72), and O_2 saturation on room air (RA) 94%. Pain 0. Height 66 inches (167.6 cm). Weight 157 pounds. Body mass index (BMI) 25.3.

General: Elderly African American female, sleepy but arousable in her own bed.

Skin: Thin skin with multiple hard nodules and several areas of bruising on her hands, arms, and legs.

Eyes: Unable to see any letters on the Snellen chart. On examination she is unable to detect fingers entering the field during field-of-gaze testing. She has positive discomfort with palpation of both eyes. Tonometer reading 21 mm Hg.

Ears: Tympanic membranes (TMs) with no erythema, no bulging, has hearing aids bilaterally, small amount of cerumen noted.

Nose: Turbinates intact, no erythema, no edema, no drainage noted. No rhinorrhea, no sinus tenderness.

Mouth: Membranes are moist, her upper and lower dentures are in place. Oral mucosa is moist. No erythema, no lesions on tongue and oral mucosa.

Neck: Supple, no masses, no lymphadenopathy, no thyroid enlargement, or tenderness.

Cardiac: Tachycardic S1, S2, no heaves, no S3, S4, or murmurs noted.

Respiratory: Clear but diminished in all fields. No crackles or wheezes.

Abdomen: Round, soft, positive bowel sounds in all quadrants. No masses palpated, no tenderness noted, no organomegaly noted. Slight bladder distention noted with palpation. Positive for urinary leakage during examination.

Back: No costovertebral angle tenderness.

Extremities: Pedal pulses palpable bilaterally. No edema.

Neurologic: Oriented to person only. Speech is clear. Tongue is midline. No fasciculations or tremors. Cranial nerves: II to XII no focal deficits. Muscle tone 3/5 upper/lower extremities. Reflexes: biceps 1+ bilaterally, triceps 1+ bilaterally. Knees 2+ bilaterally. Ankles 1+ bilaterally. Plantar: Down bilaterally.

During the home visit, the health care provider does a urine dipstick on Mrs. Williams, which shows +blood, +nitrites, +leukocyte esterase, and negative ketones.

4. Based on the history and physical examination, what are the most likely differential diagnoses for Mrs. Williams' presenting complaints?

5. What is the pathophysiology of a urinary tract infection and acute pyelonephritis?[3]

6.   What are systemic signs of infection?[4]

7.   Is there any reason to send Mrs. Williams to the emergency department versus medical treatment in her home?

Case Study, Continued

Mr. Williams transports his wife to the emergency department (ED). Her vital signs in triage are temperature 102.5°F, heart rate 118, respiratory rate 28, BP 96/42 right arm and 94/44 left arm, and O₂ saturation 90% on RA.

8.   What diagnostic testing is indicated at this time for Mrs. Williams? What specific information should the health care provider look for with each ordered diagnostic?[5]

9.   Please write an initial set of orders for the emergency department staff.

The following are the results of the laboratory diagnostics in the ED.

Urinalysis Clean Catch

Color: Yellow
Clarity: Hazy
Specific gravity: 1.012 (1.010–1.030)
pH: 7 (5–7)
Protein: Negative
Glucose: Negative
Ketone: Negative
Bilirubin: Negative
Blood: Negative
Nitrites: Positive, high
Urobilinogen: 2.0
Leukocyte esterase: Large, high
WBC: 104 (0–5/high-power field [hpf])
UA: Red blood cells (RBC) 5, high (0–2/hpf)
Squamous epithelial cells: 1
Bacteria: Present, high
WBC clump: Few, high

Complete Blood Count With Differential

WBC: 6.2 (5.0–10.0 × 10^3)
RBC: 4.87 (4.5–5.0 × 10^6)
Hemoglobin:13.7 (12.0–16.0 grams/dL)
Hematocrit: 42.5 (36%–48%)
Mean corpuscular hemoglobin (MCH): 28.1 (28–34)
Mean corpuscular hemoglobin concentrate (MCHC): 32.2 (32–36)
Platelets: 266 (140–400)

Differential

Neutrophils: 59.3 (37.0%–85%)
Bands: 7 (0%–3%)
Lymphocytes: 29.1 (10.0%–50.0%)
Monocytes: 8.8 (0.0%–12.0%)
Eosinophil: 3.5 (0.0%–7.0%)
Basophil: 0.3 (0.0%–3.0%)

Basic Metabolic Panel

Sodium: 137 (136–145 mmol/L)
Potassium: 4.0 (3.5–5.1 mmol/L)
Chloride: 103 (98–107 mmol/L)
Total CO_2: 29.0 (24–28)
BUN: 30 (baseline 10) (7–18 milligrams/dL)
Creatinine: 1.4, (baseline 0.8) (0.6–1.3 milligrams/dL)
Glucose: 121 (70–99 milligrams/dL)
Blood cultures: Two sets drawn
Lactate: 1.8 mmol/L. >2 mmol/L suggests hypoperfusion

Chest X-Ray

Clinical history: Fever, hypoxia, change in MS, UTI.

Comparison: None.

Technique: One anteroposterior (AP) view of the chest findings: No focal airspace consolidation, infiltrate, or pneumothorax. Hemidiaphragms are noted to be flattened. The cardiac silhouette size is prominent. Pulmonary vasculature and mediastinal structures are within normal limits (WNL). Degenerative changes in bony structures most notably in the right shoulder. Left shoulder prosthesis present.

Impression:

1. No infiltrate.
2. Flattened diaphragm consistent with chronic obstructive pulmonary disease (COPD).
3. Mild cardiomegaly.

Computed Tomography of the Head Without Contrast

History: Acute change in MS, history of dementia.

Technique: Transaxial images were obtained through the head without administration of IV contrast.

Findings: There are no prior studies for comparison. The ventricles and cisterns are enlarged consistent with history of dementia. There are no focal intracranial lesions, acute bleeding, including subdural hematoma, subarachnoid hemorrhage or epidural hematoma. There is a hypodense area representing prior ischemic stroke. There is no edema, midline shift, or extra axial fluid collections. Evaluation of an acute infarction on CT is limited. MRI is more sensitive for evaluating acute infarction.

Impression:

1. No acute intracranial abnormality.
2. Negative for bleeding, edema, or midline shift.
3. Central and cortical atrophy consistent with patient's age and dementia.
4. Previous stroke noted.

In the ED, the health care provider reviewed the patient's old records for information regarding her baseline cognitive functioning. The following assessment information was available from 2 months ago.

Assessment Measure Used

Montreal Cognitive Assessment (MoCA) 22/30, Clinical interview

MS Examination:

Appearance: WNL.

Behavior (psychomotor activity): Calm, responsive.

Attitude: Cooperative.

Level of consciousness: Alert.

Orientation: Oriented × 1.

Speech and language: Rate normal. Volume normal. Articulation normal.

Affect: Appropriate to thought content.

Mood: Euthymic.

Thought process: Directed, at times a little avoidant: for instance, when asked to remember several objects she says, "I am not good at that."

Disturbance: N.

Auditory hallucinations: N.

Olfactory: N.

Memory: "I remember things that are important to me." Short-term impaired, remote intact.

Estimated intelligence: Average.

Insight: Fair.

Cognitive functioning: Mrs. Williams completed high school and had some trade school education. She worked as a cook for many years after leaving the Army. At her initial intake, Mrs. Williams was administered the St. Louis University Mental Status (SLUMS) Examination, on which she scored 20/30. This score would place her in the range indicative of dementia. At that time, it was determined that given her visual and auditory difficulties, her functioning was estimated to be in the range of major neurocognitive disorder, which seems to be a better fit for her level of cognitive functioning. Repeat testing was recommended after the UTI, for which she is receiving treatment, resolves.

Psychological history: Mrs. Williams' records state she does not have a history of substance use or trauma and she denies symptoms or history. She does appear from records to have a past history of depression. It had been previously recommended that she should start on sertraline 25 milligrams po daily, but it is not clear that has been done.

Substance use history: None.

Tentative Diagnostic and Statistical Manual of Mental Disorders (DSM)-V diagnosis: Major neurocognitive disorder; Dementia.

10. After reading and interpreting the previous data, what should the health care provider decide is Mrs. Williams' definitive diagnosis?

11. Outline a treatment plan for Mrs. Williams' diagnosis.[3]

12. Please identify Mrs. Williams' other active problems.

13. What interventions are needed to treat active problems?

14. What are options for Mrs. Williams' disposition?

Case Study, Continued

*Based on her dehydration, UTI, relative hypotension, and risk for sepsis/septic shock, the emergency room (ER) physician has decided to place Mrs. Williams in observation overnight. In any presentation of an elderly patient with a UTI and MS changes, sepsis and septic shock must be ruled out. Signs and symptoms of SIRS include temperature >38° C or <36° C (>100.4° F or <96.8° F), heart rate >90, respiratory rate >20 or PaCO₂ <.32, and WBC >12,000 or <4000. These criteria are overly sensitive and not specific. Historically, they were considered mandatory for the diagnosis of sepsis, but they are now considered to be the **alerting symptoms**. All acutely ill patients should undergo screening for the potential diagnosis of sepsis.[4]*

15. What are the definitions of sepsis and septic shock?[5]

16. Why is it important for primary care providers to understand and recognize the signs of sepsis?[5]

Summary of Emergency Department Visit

Mrs. Williams has been seen and treated by the ER physician and managed overnight in the holding unit by the nurse practitioner. Diagnoses include recurrent UTI complicated by dehydration and delirium. She received ceftriaxone 1 gram × 2 doses and 2 L of IV fluid for hydration. Her BP responded very well after the fluid bolus. Repeat laboratory tests this morning show resolution of her dehydrated state with the BUN and creatinine returning to baseline.

She is alert and per family, at her baseline MS. She is no longer delirious or seeing people who are not there (i.e., hallucinations). Cultures have grown E. coli and sensitivities are pending. Her serum creatinine has come back down to .9. She will be converted to nitrofurantoin (Macrobid) 100 milligrams po twice daily × three more days for a total treatment of 5 days.[3] She should follow up with the HBPC primary provider in 2 to 3 days. In the meantime, the primary nurse on the HBPC team will coordinate a follow-up assessment visit in the home.

17. After seeing Mrs. Williams and reviewing the nursing note and diagnostic results, what are the essential management plans for Mrs. Williams on the day after she was discharged from the emergency department?

Home Visit Post Discharge Day 1

Mrs. Williams returns home after her ER visit and observational stay and the HBPC nurse practitioner arrives to evaluate Mrs. Williams. She finds Mrs. Williams sitting on her couch fully dressed and reports that she feels much better. She is talkative during this visit: she denies chest pain, nausea, vomiting, or diarrhea. Mrs. Williams reports that she is eating better and is using her walker to get around the house. She denies visual hallucinations. Mr. Williams confirms that she is doing much better since she has returned home. She denies complaints of burning or odor with her urine.

Physical Examination
    General: Smiling, calm, neatly dressed, sitting in chair, no acute distress.
    Vital signs: Temperature 98.4°F. Heart rate 68, BP left arm 110/68 with no orthostatic changes, respiratory rate 18, O_2 saturation 93% on RA. Weight is 158 pounds.

Cardiac: Regular rate, S1, S2, no heaves, no lifts, no murmurs noted.

Respiratory: Clear, diminished to auscultation in all fields.

Abdomen: Round, soft, positive bowel sounds in all quadrants, no masses palpated, no tenderness noted, no organomegaly noted. No flank pain elicited on examination.

Neurologic: She is alert, conversant, oriented to name and place only.

18.   What is the appropriate assessment and plan for Mrs. Williams now?

Day 4 Acute Unscheduled Home Visit

Mrs. Williams is seen again by the HBPC provider in her home for an unscheduled visit because her husband called reporting she was getting up more often through the night and last night she had a fall trying to get to the bathroom. She reports having increasing back pain but denies any visual hallucinations. She and her husband report that she finished all of her antibiotics.

Review of Symptoms

General: "I don't feel sick. I don't think I have any fevers." Denies chills but reports feeling weak. Denies chest pain.

HEENT: Denies headache, dizziness, vision or sinus pain, denies nasal congestion or sore throat.

Neck: Denies neck pain or swallowing problems.

Respiratory: Reports some instances of shortness of breath when walking without her walker, no cough or wheeze.

Cardiac: Denies chest pain or palpitations.

Peripheral vascular: Denies swelling in the legs or pain in the legs.

Genitourinary (GU): + urinary frequency with increased lower back pain, urine looks "funny."

Physical Examination

General: Older, African American female, dressed in her nightgown, sitting on the side of the bed, pale, looks uncomfortable.

Vital signs: Temperature 99°F. Heart rate 86, BP 130/70, respiratory rate 18. Weight 157 pounds. Pain 3/10.

Mouth: Membranes and tongue moist, upper and lower dentures in place, no erythema, no lesion.

Cardiac: Regular rate and rhythm C1, S2. No gallop, murmurs, or rubs.

Respiratory: Clear to auscultation. No crackles or rhonchi

Abdomen: Round, with positive bowel sounds, soft, no masses, + suprapubic tenderness, positive costovertebral angle tenderness.

Extremities: Palpable distal pedis/posterior tibial pulses, no edema.

19. Given Mrs. Williams' history, what are the most likely differential diagnoses that should be considered today?

20. How can acute uncomplicated pyelonephritis in women be treated?[6]

21. If symptoms of pyelonephritis do not improve within 3 days, or resolve but then recur, what is an appropriate plan?[6]

Case Study, Continued

Mrs. Williams completes her 7-day course of ciprofloxacin and has no further complaints. She is evaluated by urology and a recommendation is made for her to begin suppression treatment with methenamine hippurate (UREX) 1 gram po twice daily for UTI suppression.

22. How should the provider monitor efficacy of this treatment?[7]

ONLINE ANSWER SUBMISSION

When you are ready to submit your answers for grading and reflective expert feedback for evaluation, go to http://www.evolve.elsevier.com/DickAndButtaro/ to complete this case.

References

1. Edes, T., Kinosian, B., Vuckovic, N. H., Nichols, L., Becker, M., & Hossain, M. (2014). Better access, quality, and cost for clinically complex veterans with home-based primary care. *Journal of the American Geriatrics Society, 62,* 1954–1961.
2. Fick, D. M., Agostini, J. V., & Inouye, S. K. (2002). Delirium superimposed on dementia: A systematic review. *Journal of the American Geriatrics Society, 50,* 1723–1732.
3. Gupta, K., & Trautner, B. (2015). Urinary tract infections, pyelonephritis, and prostatitis. In D. Kasper, S. Hauser, J. Jameson, A. Fauci, D. Longo, & J. Loscalzo (Eds.), *Harrison's principles of internal medicine* (19th ed., pp. 861–868). New York: McGraw-Hill.
4. Mumford, R. S. (2015). Severe sepsis and septic shock. In D. Kasper, S. Hauser, J. Jameson, A. Fauci, D. Longo, & J. Loscalzo (Eds.), *Harrison's principles of internal medicine* (19th ed., pp. 1751–1759). New York: McGraw-Hill.
5. Rhodes, A., Evans, L. E., Alhazzani, W., Levy, M., Antonelli, M., Kumar, A., et al. (2016). Surviving sepsis campaign: International guideline for management of sepsis and septic shock. *Critical Care Medicine, 45,* 486–552.
6. Gupta, K., Hoonton, T. M., Naber, K. G., Wullt, B., Colgan, R., Miller, L. G., et al. (2011). Treatment of acute uncomplicated cystitis and pyelonephritis in women: A 2010 update by the Infectious Diseases Society of America and the European Society for Microbiology and Infectious Diseases. *Clinical Infectious Diseases, 52,* e103–e120. doi:10.1093/cid/ciq257.
7. Lo, T., Hammer, K., Zegarra, M., & Cho, W. (2014). Methenamine: A forgotten drug for preventing recurrent urinary tract infection in a multidrug resistance era. *Expert Review of Anti-Infective Therapy, 12*(5), 549–554.

Rhinitis

Jill Beavers-Kirby

Instructions

After reviewing the case study, please jot down your notes or preliminary answers in the spaces provided. When you are ready to submit your answers for grading and reflective expert feedback for evaluation, go to http://www.evolve.elsevier.com/DickAndButtaro/ to complete this case.

Case Study Scenario/History of Present Illness

A 68-year-old white female (Mrs. Meeker) presents to her primary care provider (PCP) for complaints of fatigue and runny nose. She denies fever, chills, myalgias, sore throat, or cough.

Medications: Acetaminophen 500 milligrams every 6 hours prn for arthritis pain, Fosamax 70 milligrams weekly, hydrochlorothiazide 25 milligrams daily, citalopram 20 milligrams daily, atorvastatin 40 milligrams at bedtime, lisinopril 20 milligrams daily, low-dose aspirin 81 milligrams daily, calcium citrate with vitamin D 500/400 milligrams twice daily, and multivitamin daily.

Allergies: Penicillin causes a rash.

Past medical history: Arthritis, hypertension, osteoporosis, depression, and hypercholesterolemia.

Past surgical history: Reduction mammoplasty 8 years ago, appendectomy 35 years ago, total abdominal hysterectomy 20 years ago because of abnormal uterine bleeding, cataract removed left eye 1 year ago, and retropubic suspension surgery 3 years ago.

Family history: Father passed away from lung cancer at age 79; mother passed away from heart attack at age 81. One older brother who is alive but has hypertension and coronary heart disease, one sister who is younger that has bipolar disorder and hypertension.

Personal and social history: Patient is married to "Randy" for the past 45 years. They have two grown boys, one is 30 years old and is married with no children; the other boy is 24 years old and not married and has no children.

Reproductive health: Gravida 2, para 2, both vaginal deliveries without complications. Birth weights were 8 pounds, menarche age 12, surgical menopause age 48.

Health maintenance/prevention: Colonoscopy 8 years ago, and screening mammogram 5 years ago. Immunizations are up to date (Pneumovax age 65, Prevnar-13 age 67, Tdap age 67, received annual influenza vaccine).

Review of Systems

General: Complains of fatigue. She states she "becomes tired more easily" and that she "can't get her housework done." Denies overt fever, but she mentions that at times she does "feel warm, but I thought it was just me"; no history or recent weight change or dietary changes. No complaints of night sweats or chills.

Head, ears, eyes, nose, and throat (HEENT): States she does have a "runny nose," but she does not pay attention to the color of the nasal drainage. Denies sinus pain, otalgia, sore throat, or headache.

Respiratory: Denies cough, wheeze, or hemoptysis.

Cardiovascular: Denies chest discomfort or pressure. No complaints of palpitations, paroxysmal nocturnal dyspnea, or lower extremity claudication.

Gastrointestinal: Denies nausea, vomiting.

Urinary: Denies dysuria, hematuria. Does have stress incontinence and infrequent nocturia.

Physical Examination

Vital signs: Blood pressure (BP) 132/78 mm Hg sitting, right arm. Heart rate 72. Temperature 98.4°F orally. Respiratory rate 18, SpO$_2$ 98% on room air. Height 65 inches. Weight 165 pounds. Body mass index (BMI) 27.5.

General: Alert and oriented, pleasant-appearing female. Appears stated age and appears in no apparent distress.

Skin: Warm and dry. No rashes or lesions noted. Well-healed scar on lower abdomen, no atypical moles noted.

Head: Atraumatic, normocephalic. No parasites noted.

Eyes: Pupils equal, round, and react to light (PERRL). Extraocular movements (EOMs) intact.

Ears: External ears are symmetric, no deformities noted.

Nose/throat: Mucosa pink and moist. Septum midline. Turbinates have no drainage noted. Poor dentition and missing a few teeth in both upper and lower jaws, does not wear dentures. Tongue appears pink. Posterior pharynx without erythema or exudates.

Neck: Neck is supple, no masses. Trachea midline. No thyroid nodules, masses, tenderness, or enlargement.

Respiratory: Lungs are clear to auscultation bilaterally; no wheezes or rhonchi noted. Chest is symmetric. Good respiratory effort with no use of accessory muscles.

Cardiac: Regular rate and rhythm. S1 and S2 audible. No S3 or S4 noted.

Neurologic: Cranial nerves (CNs) II to XII intact. Deep tendon reflexes (DTRs) 2+ throughout, gait steady and coordination normal. Oriented to person, place, and time. Memory intact. Sensory and motor levels normal, negative Babinski. No focal neurologic deficits.

1. Based on the information, what is the diagnosis?

Visit 2

Mrs. Meeker returns 4 weeks later. She tells her provider that her symptoms have not improved. She also bought a digital thermometer and has been checking her temperature daily. She reports that most days her temperature is "normal," but there have been three times since her last visit when her oral temperature was 99.0°F. She is still fatigued, and she is worried that she is not getting her work done around the house. She is afraid that this is upsetting her husband because they have been arguing more. He even slept on the sofa one evening.

Other than ongoing symptoms and an occasional low-grade fever, her review of systems is unchanged.

Vital signs: BP 102/72 mm Hg sitting, right arm. Heart rate 74. Temperature 98.6°F orally. Respiratory rate 18. SpO$_2$ 98% on room air. Height 65 inches. Weight 161 pounds. BMI 26.8.

General: Alert and oriented, pleasant-appearing female. Looks fatigued but in no apparent distress.

Skin: Warm and dry. No rashes or lesions noted. Well-healed scar on lower abdomen, no atypical moles noted.

Head: Atraumatic, normocephalic.

Eyes: PERRL. EOMs intact.

Ears: External ears are symmetric, no deformities noted.

Nose/throat: Mucosa pink and moist. Septum midline. Turbinates have no drainage noted. Poor dentition and missing a few teeth in both upper and lower jaws, does not wear dentures. Tongue appears pink. Posterior pharynx without erythema or exudates.

Neck: Neck is supple, no masses. Trachea midline. No thyroid nodules, masses, + palpable lymph node left submandibular area that measures approximately 4 × 3 cm. The lymph node is firm, nonmoveable, and slightly tender.

Respiratory: Lungs are clear to auscultation bilaterally. No wheezes or rhonchi noted.

Cardiac: Regular rate and rhythm. S1 and S2 audible. No S3 or S4 noted.

Neurologic: CNs II to XII intact. DTRs 2+ throughout. Gait steady and coordination normal. Oriented to person, place, and time. Memory intact. Sensory and motor levels normal, negative Babinski. No focal neurologic deficits.

2. Based on the ongoing symptoms and new physical examination findings, what is the next step?

3. Based on the laboratory values, what is the next step?

Case Study, Continued

The provider reviews the differential and these are the values: differential from CBC was neutrophils $7.1 \times 10^3/\mu L$, lymphocytes $7500 \times 10^3/\mu L$, monocytes $0.7 \times 10^3/\mu L$, eosinophils $0.47 \times 10^3/\mu L$, and basophils $0.10 \times 10^3/\mu L$.

The patient's previous CBC with differential was 6 months ago. The values at that time were white blood cells $9.6 \times 103/\mu L$, red blood cells $4.8 \times 106/\mu L$, hemoglobin 15.8 grams/dL, mean corpuscular volume 90 fL, mean corpuscular hemoglobin 30 pg, and platelets $190 \times 10^3/\mu L$. The differential was neutrophils $6.1 \times 10^3/\mu L$, lymphocytes $3700 \times 10^3/\mu L$, monocytes $0.4 \times 10^3/\mu L$, eosinophils $0.50 \times 10^3/\mu L$, and basophils $0.10 \times 10^3/\mu L$.

The provider notices that the patient's lymphocytes are double what they previously were 6 months ago. A normal lymphocyte range is 1000 to $3900 \times 10^3/\mu L$.

4. What components of the history, review of systems, or physical examination are missing?

Case Study, Continued

The patient denies any tobacco use but she notes that when she "worked as bartender, everyone in there smoked a lot." She does not use any illicit drugs and only has "a drink during the holidays." She previously worked as a bartender during which she was exposed to secondhand smoke. She is able to perform 100% of her ADLs independently. She has never had any transfusions. She lives in a one-story ranch-style condo with her husband and yes, she feels safe. They walk in their neighborhood every evening.

Review of Systems

Skin: Any changes in moles, any changes in nails (e.g., clubbing, spooning, or ridges)?

Eyes: Any injury, double vision, visual acuity, sudden loss of vision, tearing (unilateral and bilateral), blind spots, pain, blurred vision, vision at night, photophobia, haloes, "floaters" or "spots"?

Ears: Any pain, discharge, injury, hearing acuity, tinnitus, vertigo, balance, or wax removal?

Nose: Any nosebleeds, obstruction, discharge, changes in sense of smell, sneezing, or postnasal drainage?

Mouth/throat: Any dental difficulties, recent dental procedure, lesions, gingival hyperplasia and bleeding? Any problems with dry mouth, voice change or hoarseness, difficulty swallowing, neck stiffness or pain, masses in thyroid, or lymphadenopathy?

Respiratory: Any shortness of breath or dyspnea? What is the date of last chest x-ray?

Cardiovascular: Any syncope or near syncope?

Gastrointestinal: Any changes in appetite, dysphagia, indigestion, abdominal pain, heartburn, constipation, diarrhea, or abnormal stool (e.g., clay colored, tarry, bloody, greasy, foul smelling), flatulence, hemorrhoids, or changes in bowel habits?

Breast: Any lumps, masses, change in appearance, dimpling or retraction of any of the breast area?

Musculoskeletal: Any pain or swelling, or decreased range of motion?

Neurologic: Any dizziness, lightheadedness, convulsions, changes in mentation, difficulties with memory or speech, or disturbances in muscular coordination (ataxia, tremor)?

Mental: What is the predominant mood? Any anxiety, depression, or difficulty concentrating?

Endocrine: Any polydipsia, polyuria, polyphagia, or intolerance to heat or cold?

Case Study, Continued

She denies any changes to the skin. Denies vision changes or excessive tearing. No difficulty hearing; denies tinnitus, vertigo, or excessive wax. She does have an "occasional nosebleed that is from the dry air." No complaints of sneezing or postnasal drip. No problems with her dentures or gums. No neck stiffness or pain. She has never felt around for any swollen or tender lymph nodes. She has no difficulty swallowing or hoarseness.

She denies shortness of breath or dyspnea. She states that she has never had a chest x-ray. No complaints of syncope or near syncope. Her appetite is "normal" and she does not have any problems with dysphagia, indigestion, abdominal pain, heartburn, constipation, diarrhea, or abnormal stool or changes in bowel habits.

She has no complaints of lumps, masses, change in appearance, dimpling, or retraction in her breast area. In the musculoskeletal system, she denies pain or swelling of any joints. She has no complaints of decreased range of motion.

She notes that she has a headache about three times a year, and she thinks it is usually caused by stress. She does not have any problems with dizziness, lightheadedness, convulsions, changes in mentation, difficulties with memory or speech, or disturbances in muscular coordination. She states she is usually a "glass-half-full type of person" and denies problems with anxiety, depression, or difficulty concentrating. She denies polydipsia, polyuria, polyphagia, or intolerance to heat or cold.

Physical Examination

HEENT: Examine tympanic membrane.

Abdominal: Inspect for asymmetry or distention. Assess for color, scars, rashes, or lesions. Auscultation of all quadrants, auscultation for bruits, and percussion of all quadrants and solid organs. Palpation of abdominal area and organs.

Musculoskeletal: Inspection of range of motion and inspect joints for swelling, deformity, and muscle tone.

Lymphatic: All major lymph node chains should be examined for additional lymphadenopathy.

Neurologic: Inspect CN V and VIII and hearing.

Case Study, Continued

CNs V and VIII are normal. Tympanic membrane is pearly gray with normal cone of light. Abdomen is symmetric without distention; she has two well-healed scars on her abdomen. There are no rashes or lesions, and there are no bruits. Light and deep palpation yields no tenderness. Upper and lower extremity joints show normal range of motion without deformities or edema. Muscle tone is normal. No adenopathy or tenderness in the cervical, axillary, or inguinal lymph nodes.

5. Based on the history and physical examination results, what is the patient's condition?

6. What is your next step in the treatment plan?

7.   Why are the laboratory results not consistent with mononucleosis?[1]

8.   Why are the laboratory results not consistent with non-Hodgkin lymphoma?

9.   Based on the history and physical examination results, what are the possible causes (differential diagnoses) for the patient's current condition?[2,5]

10.   What are the diagnostics that are associated with each differential?[3,6-8]

Case Study, Continued

The patient returns 3 months later to primary care. The provider has received the report of the immuno-phenotyping, which was done on the node biopsy. It was positive for CD19, CD20, CD23, and CD5. A bone marrow biopsy was done and showed 32% of the cells stained positive for chronic lymphocytic leukemia (CLL). Based on RAI clinical stage 0 (with lymphocytosis only in her blood and marrow), she has a median survival rate of >10 years. Her oncologist has determined to take a "watchful waiting" approach.[9]

11.   What is "watchful waiting?"[10]

12.   What complications does the primary care provider need to monitor for in this patient with chronic lymphocytic leukemia?[11]

13. What physical examination areas should be routinely assessed on Mrs. Meeker and why?[11]

14. What labs should be routinely monitored in Mrs. Meeker and why?

15. What are the risk factors for chronic lymphocytic leukemia?[2]

16. What are potential complications of chronic lymphocytic leukemia?[2, 4, 12, 13, 14]

CLL may cause complications that include:

17.   How do you determine whether a patient with chronic lymphocytic leukemia needs treatment?[1]

18.   What treatment would be recommended for this patient?[14]

19. How often should patients be reassessed for changes or progression of their chronic lymphocytic leukemia?

20. What signs indicate that the patient would need treatment for chronic lymphocytic leukemia?[9]

References

1. Dillman, R. O., Garg, S., Rao, D. S., & Jones, R. (2011). *Chronic lymphocytic leukemia*. First Consult: Elsevier.
2. Haynes, A., Arnold, K. R., Aguirre-Oskins, C., & Chandra, S. (2015). Evaluation of neck masses in adults. *American Family Physician, 91*(10), 698–706.
3. Laboratory diagnosis of CMV infection for persons ≥ 12 months of age. Retrieved from https://www.cdc.gov/cmv/clinical/lab-tests.html.
4. Obel, N., Høier-Madsen, M., & Kangro, H. (1996). Serological and clinical findings in patients with serological evidence of reactivated Epstein-Barr virus infection. *APMIS: Acta Pathologica, Microbiologica, et Immunologica Scandinavica, 104*, 424.
5. Montoya, J. G. (2002). Laboratory diagnosis of *Toxoplasma gondii* infection and toxoplasmosis. *The Journal of Infectious Diseases, 185*(Suppl. 1), S73.
6. 2003). Salivary gland anatomy and physiology. In Som, P. M., & Curtain, H. D. (Eds.), *Head and neck imaging*. St. Louis, MO: Mosby.
7. Branson, B. M., & Stekler, J. D. (2012). Detection of acute HIV infection: We can't close the window. *Journal of Infectious Disease, 205*, 521–524.
8. Lewinsohn, D. M., Leonard, M. K., LoBue, P. A., Cohn, D. L., Daley, C. L., Desmond, E., et al. (2017). Official American Thoracic Society/Infectious Diseases Society of America/Centers for Disease Control and Prevention clinical practice guidelines: Diagnosis of tuberculosis in adults and children. *Clinical Infectious Diseases, 64*(2), e1–e33. doi:10.1093/cid/ciw694.
9. National Comprehensive Cancer Network. Chronic lymphocytic leukemia/small lymphocytic lymphoma. Version 1.2018 – August 21, 2017. Retrieved from http://www.nccn.org.
10. Kasper, D., Fauci, A., Hauser, S., Longo, D., Jameson, J., & Loscalzo, J. (Eds.). (2014). *Harrison's principles of internal medicine* (19th ed.). Retrieved from http://accessmedicine.mhmedical.com/content.aspx?bookid=1130&sectionid=79720864.
11. Rai, K. R., & Stilgenbauer, S. (2016). Overview of the complications of chronic lymphocytic leukemia. In *UpToDate*, T. W. Post (Ed.), *Uptodate*. Waltham, MA.
12. Chronic lymphocytic leukemia. Retrieved from https://www.mayoclinic.org/diseases-conditions/chronic-lymphocytic-leukemia/symptoms-causes/syc-20352428.
13. Eichorst, B., Robak, T., Montserrat, E., Ghia, P., Hillmen, P., Hallek, M., et al. (2015). Chronic lymphocytic leukemia: ESMO clinical practice guidelines for diagnosis, treatment and follow-up. *Annals of Oncology, 26*(Suppl. 5), 78–84. doi: https://doi.org/10.1093/annonc/mdv303.
14. How is chronic lymphocytic leukemia staged? Retrieved from https://www.cancer.org/cancer/chronic-lymphocytic-leukemia/detection-diagnosis-staging/staging.html.

Shortness of Breath

Michaela Jones

Instructions

After reviewing the case study, please jot down your notes or preliminary answers in the spaces provided. When you are ready to submit your answers for grading and reflective expert feedback for evaluation, go to http://www.evolve.elsevier.com/DickAndButtaro/ to complete this case.

Case Study Scenario/History of Present Illness

A 64-year-old male with a past medical history of hyperlipidemia and hypertension (HTN) presents to primary care for an urgent visit complaining of trouble breathing. He relates having a long-standing history of a nonproductive cough that he attributes to his smoking history. The patient describes a continuous smoking history of 32 pack-years, but states he quit when he was 62. He developed shortness of breath and wheezing about 10 years ago. He thinks he saw a doctor once who gave him an "inhaler," but he did not follow up about the breathing. He has been given medications for his high blood pressure in the past, but he is no longer taking them. He reports that he "does not like doctors." His shortness of breath has been getting worse throughout the years, and he developed a cough described as productive of a mild amount of thick white sputum.

Today, the patient's reason for presentation is because he had an episode of severe nonproductive coughing accompanied by shortness of breath and dizziness 2 weeks ago while walking home from a friend's apartment. The patient described that he had to sit at a nearby bench to catch his breath and reports the symptoms resolved after 1 to 2 minutes, but he still continues to get shortness of breath two to three times a week. He denies any wheezing or chest tightness; otherwise he states he feels "well."

Medications: None.

Allergies: No known drug, food, or environmental allergies.

Habits: Former everyday smoker, 32 pack-year history, stopped 3 years ago. Drinks two beers a week. Denies illicit drug use.

Past medical history: Hyperlipidemia, HTN.

Past surgical history: Flexor tendon surgery on fifth right digit.

Hospitalizations: None.

Trauma: None.

Family history: Father died age 81 of "natural causes." Mother died age 76 from breast cancer, but had a history of HTN and depression. He has one daughter, age 20, alive and well. He does not know anything about his grandparents' medical histories.

Social history: Patient is a married Caucasian male. Lives with wife in a one-bedroom apartment in New York. They have one daughter who is married and lives out of state. Patient is a retired firefighter.

Review of Systems

General health: Reports feeling "OK-well."

Skin: Denies rashes or lesions.

Head, ears, eyes, nose, and throat (HEENT): Denies dizziness aside from recent episode. Denies headaches or loss of consciousness. Denies change in vision, redness, discharge, history of eye infections or glaucoma, or cataracts. Denies ear pain, ringing in the ears, or difficulty hearing. Denies chronic nasal congestion, clear nasal discharge, postnasal drip, and chronic sinus pressure. Denies frequent nosebleeds. Denies throat irritation or voice hoarseness.

Neck: Denies swollen lymph nodes or glands. Denies thyroid disease.

Respiratory: Denies chest tightness. Denies hemoptysis. Sleeps in a bed with two pillows.

Cardiovascular: Denies chest pressure, pain, palpitations, or irregular heartbeat.

Gastrointestinal: Produces two well-formed bowel movements a day. Denies nausea, vomiting, abdominal pain, diarrhea, or constipation. Denies blood in stool. Tolerates food well.

Genitourinary: Denies dysuria, hematuria, or incontinence.

Musculoskeletal: Denies joint pain, stiffness, swelling, limitation of motion. History of gout or arthritis.

Extremities: Denies cyanosis or edema, numbness or tingling.

Neurologic: Denies loss of coordination, disorientation, or loss of memory.

Hematology: Denies bleeding or easy bruising.

Psychiatric: Denies decreased mood, little interest in doing things, suicidal ideation, or hallucinations.

Physical Examination

General appearance: 64-year-old Caucasian male who does not appear in acute distress. Well groomed with good hygiene.

Vital signs: Weight 164 pounds. Height 66 inches. Body mass index (BMI) 26.48. Heart rate 88, respiratory rate 20, and blood pressure 148/86 mm Hg sitting and 146/86 standing. Temperature 98.1°F. O_2 saturation 97%.

Skin: Uniformly pink in color, warm, dry, intact with good turgor. Light gray course hair. Nail beds pink with prompt capillary refill on fingers.

Eyes: Conjunctivae clear. Pupils equal, round, and reactive to light.

Mouth: Membranes moist, teeth fair repair, no lesions of tongue or buccal mucosa.

Neck: Neck supple, no lymphadenopathy. No thyromegaly. No carotid bruits. No jugular venous distention.

Chest/lungs: Nonlabored effort. Respiratory rate regular with symmetric chest expansion. Tactile fremitus equal bilaterally. No adventitious sounds bilaterally. No wheezes, rhonchi, or rales.

Cardiac: S1/S2 present, regular rate and rhythm. No S3, S4, murmurs, rubs, or gallop.

Abdomen: Abdomen symmetric, soft, nondistended. Normoactive bowel sounds in all four quadrants. Tympany predominates in all quadrants. No tenderness, masses, or palpable organomegaly present.

Neurological: Alert. Gait smooth, steady, and coordinated. Sensation is intact to pain and light touch. Cranial nerves II to XII intact. No motor or sensory deficits. Reflexes 4/4 bilaterally in upper and lower extremities and 4/4 muscle strengths in upper and lower extremities bilaterally. No cerebellar findings. No fasciculations or tremors.

Extremities: Warm and well-perfused upper and lower extremities. No edema or calf tenderness.

Psychiatric: Appearance, behavior, and speech appropriate. Alert and oriented to person, place, and time. Appropriate affect.

ASSESSMENT AND PLAN

1. Does this patient need to go to the emergency room? Why or why not?

2. Based on the history and physical examination results, what are the differential diagnoses that the health care provider should consider and why?[1]

3. What additional questions could or should the health care provider ask the patient?

4. What additional physical examination components are necessary to aid in the differential diagnoses and need for specific diagnostics?[2]

5. What diagnostics should the health care provider order and perform at this visit?[3, 4]

Case Study, Continued

The patient explains that he was a firefighter for around 25 years, wore a half-face respirator most of the time but would often take it off when talking to others, and admits he sometimes forgot to change the cartridges. He does not recall any specific exposures other than smoke, but he is not sure really. He reports he can walk four blocks and up two flights of stairs before feeling short of breath. He notices that hot weather also causes his dyspnea.

He drinks 1 small cup of coffee a day, and he reports he does not exercise. He does not restrict his diet and eats a lot of fast food. He reports he might have lost less than 5 lb in the past year, but he never weighed himself. He tolerates activities of daily living without feeling short of breath. Denies any history of clotting conditions or recent periods of immobilization. Denies recent infections, heartburn, or reflux. No family history of cancer to his knowledge.

The electrocardiogram (ECG) shows normal sinus rhythm, rate 88, PR interval 0.14 seconds, QT interval 0.20 seconds, no ST elevation or depression, and normal R wave progression.

Spirometry today shows forced vital capacity (FVC) 3.12 L (58%), forced expiratory volume in 1 second (FEV$_1$) 2.15 L (51%), and FEV$_1$/FVC 0.689. Interpretation is moderate obstruction. Postbronchodilator spirometry remained stable with <12% improvement.

6.   What is the working diagnosis for this patient? What are the criteria for this diagnosis?[5]

7.   What additional testing is now necessary? Discuss the reason for each diagnostic ordered.[6-14]

8.   What are the Global Initiative for Chronic Obstructive Lung Disease guidelines for treatment?[5]

9.   What potential pharmacologic treatment(s) should be initiated for this patient's chronic obstructive pulmonary disease?[5]

10.   What other concerns should the health care provider address for this patient's other comorbid conditions?[15]

11.   What patient education should be provided to this patient?[16-18]

12. When should the health care provider ask the patient to return to be seen in follow-up?

Second Primary Care Visit

The patient returns to the practice in 5 weeks. He has not yet completed his cardiac evaluation, stating he had an appointment but canceled it because he had a scheduling conflict and never rescheduled. His complete metabolic panel showed borderline elevated alanine transaminase (ALT)/aspartate transaminase (AST) and markedly elevated total cholesterol and low-density lipoprotein (LDL); otherwise there were no significant abnormalities.

He completed his full pulmonary evaluation, which showed moderate obstruction with stable FVC and FEV1 without significant bronchodilator response (4%), lung volumes without restriction, but elevated total lung capacity (TLV) suggestive of hyperinflation. No gas transfer defect. Moderately decreased maximal voluntary ventilation (MVV) and elevated FeNO of 66 ppb. His chest CT showed minimal air trapping; otherwise, there were no consolidation or active pulmonary disease.

His 6-minute walk test was negative. He did not schedule an appointment with palliative care.

Overall, he states he feels well and reports his shortness of breath has mildly improved. He does use his albuterol inhaler about two times a week and denies nocturnal symptoms. States his cough is mildly improved and he denies recent lower respiratory infections or COPD exacerbations requiring any emergency room or urgent care visits. He is trying to increase his exercise by walking 3 days a week.

He denies additional complaints. He has not changed his diet and reports he is "too busy" to eat healthy.

His blood pressure today is elevated at 154/88 sitting and 152/84 while standing. Spirometry is stable. His physical examination today reveals no concerning changes.

Patient's Laboratory Results

Component Results

Component	Value	References Range/Units	Status
White blood cell	3.4	3.4–10.8 × 10E^3/μL	Final
Red blood cell	4.89	4.14–5.80 × 10E^6/μL	Final
Hgb	14.6	12.6–17.7 grams/dL	Final
Hematocrit	43.6	37.5%–51.0%	Final

Continued

Component Results—cont'd

Component	Value	References Range/Units	Status
Mean corpuscular volume	89	79–97 fL	Final
Mean corpuscular Hgb	29.3	26.6–33.0 pg	Final
Mean corpuscular Hgb concentrate	33.5	31.5–35.7 grams/dL	Final
Red distributed width	13.3	12.3%–15.4%	Final
Platelet	221	150–379 × 10E³/µL	Final
Neutrophil %	48	%	Final
Lymphocyte %	40	%	Final
Monocyte %	10	%	Final
Eosinophil	2	%	Final
Basophil %	0	%	Final
Neutrophil #	1.6	1.4–7.0 × 10E³/µL	Final
Lymphocyte #	1.3	0.7–3.1 × 10E³/µL	Final
Monocyte #	0.3	0.1–0.9 × 10E³/µL	Final
Eosinophil #	0.1	0.0–0.4 × 10E³/µL	Final
Basophil #	0.0	0.0–0.2 × 10E³/µL	Final
Immature granulocytes %	0	%	Final
Immature granulocytes #	0.0	0.0–0.1 ×10E³/µL	Final
Glucose	97	65–99 milligrams/dL	Final
Urea nitrogen	21	6–24 milligrams/dL	Final
Creatinine	1.15	0.76–1.27 milligrams/dL	Final
eGFR non-African American	73	>59 mL/min/1.73	Final
eGFR African American	85	>59 mL/min/1.73	Final
BUN/creatinine	18	9–20	Final
Sodium	140	134–144 mmol/L	Final
Potassium-serum	3.7	3.5–5.2 mmol/L	Final
Chloride	101	96–106 mmol/L	Final
Carbon dioxide, total	21	18–29 mmol/L	Final
Calcium	10.0	8.7–10.2 milligrams/dL	Final
Protein total	7.3	6.0–8.5 grams/dL	Final
Albumin	4.8	3.5–5.5 grams/dL	Final
Globulin	2.5	1.5–4.5 grams/dL	Final
A/G ratio	1.9	1.2–2.2	Final
Bilirubin total	0.7	0.0–1.2 milligrams/dL	Final
Alkaline phosphatase	57	39–117 IU/L	Final
AST (SGOT)	62 (H)	0–40 IU/L	Final
ALT (SGPT)	64 (H)	0–44 IU/L	Final
Cholesterol	278 (H)	100–199 milligrams/dL	Final
Triglycerides	112 (H)	0–149 milligrams/dL	Final
HDL cholesterol	44	>39 milligrams/dL	Final
VLDL cholesterol CAL	37	5–40 milligrams/dL	Final
LDL cholesterol	194 (H)	0–99 milligrams/dL	Final
Urine specific gravity	1.015	1.005–1.030	Final
Urine pH	5.0	5.0–7.5	Final
Urine color	Yellow	Yellow	Final
Urine appearance	Clear	Clear	Final
Urine leukocyte Esterase	Negative	Negative	Final
Urine protein	Negative	Negative/trace	Final
Urine glucose	Negative	Negative	Final
Urine ketone	Negative	Negative	Final
Occult blood urine	Negative	Negative	Final
Urine bilirubin	Negative	Negative	Final
Urobilinogen	0.2	0.2–1.0 EU/dL	Final
Urine nitrite	Negative	Negative	Final
Hgb A1C	5.5	4.0–5.6%	Final

A/G, Albumin/globulin ratio; *ALT,* alanine transaminase; *AST,* aspartate transaminase; *BUN,* blood urea nitrogen; *eGFR,* estimated glomerular filtration rate; *H,* high; *HDL,* high-density lipoprotein; *Hgb,* hemoglobin; *LDL,* low-density lipoprotein; *SGOT,* serum glutamic oxaloacetic transaminase; *SGPT,* serum glutamic pyruvic transaminase; *VLDL,* very-low-density lipoprotein.

13.   Based on today's follow-up, what should the health care provider's treatment plan include?[15, 19, 20]

14.   When should the patient next be seen in follow-up and why?

Case Study, Continued

The patient presented to the laboratory as scheduled for a repeat comprehensive metabolic panel and liver panel. His chemistry profile is within normal limits. His hepatitis panel is negative. His AST is 62, and his ALT is 66.

15.   When should the patient follow up now and what are the priorities for the next visit?

Primary Care Visit 3

The patient returns in 6 months for follow-up. He reports he did not follow up because he thought he was better. He now presents with "slightly worsening" shortness of breath. He states he can only walk three blocks before he needs to stop and catch his breath. He believes he had a lower respiratory infection 1 month ago but did not follow up for a medical assessment. His cough and wheeze are stable.

Per records that were faxed over to the practice, the patient went for his cardiac evaluation soon after his last visit. His stress test was normal, echocardiogram showed mild mitral valve regurgitation, but it was essentially within normal limits. His brain natriuretic peptide (BNP) was also within normal limits. His liver tests revealed an elevated C-reactive protein (CRP), which is a marker of inflammation, but laboratory tests for autoimmune hepatitis; viral hepatitis A, B, and C; primary biliary cholangitis; hemochromatosis; and α_1-antitrypsin were negative.

He continues to exercise three times a week. He reports he tries to eat less fast food now; otherwise he keeps the same diet. Today he feels well.

Today's review of symptoms is negative except for his mentioned respiratory complaints.

Physical Examination

General appearance: 64-year-old Caucasian male who does not appear in acute distress. Well groomed with good hygiene.

Vital signs: Weight 158 pounds. Height 66 inches. BMI 26.3. Heart rate 86, respiratory rate 20. Blood pressure 139/86 mm Hg. Temperature 98.4°F.

Skin: Uniformly pink in color, warm, dry, intact with good turgor. Light gray course hair. Nail beds pink with prompt capillary refill on fingers.

Eyes: Conjunctivae clear. Pupils equal, round, and reactive to light.

Mouth: Membranes moist, no lesions.

Neck: Supple, no lymphadenopathy. No thyromegaly. No carotid bruits. No jugular venous distention.

Chest/lungs: Decreased breath sounds in upper lobes bilaterally. Nonlabored effort. Regular rate and rhythm. Symmetric chest expansion, tactile fremitus equal bilaterally. No wheezes, rhonchi, or rales.

Cardiac: S1/S2 present. Regular rate and rhythm. No S3, S4, murmurs, rubs, or gallop.

Abdomen: Abdomen symmetric, soft, nondistended. Normoactive bowel sounds in all four quadrants. No masses, tenderness, or organomegaly.

Extremities: Range of motion (ROM) full. No edema. No calf tenderness.

Spirometry today: FVC 3.00 L (57%), FEV_1 1.82 L (48%), and FEV_1/FVC 0.61. Interpretation is moderate-severe obstruction.

16. What questions should the health care provider ask the patient based on today's physical examination findings?[21]

Case Study, Continued

On questioning, the patient is taking his Spiriva 1 puff every morning. Albuterol as needed, around four times a week. He demonstrates correct use.

17. Based on the patient's history and the health care provider's physical findings, has the patient's chronic obstructive pulmonary disease status changed?[5]

18. What diagnostic tests should the health care provider order today?

19. What treatments are important for the health care provider to prescribe for this patient today?[22]

Case Study, Continued

Patient is instructed to stop tiotropium bromide and to start a new inhaler vilanterol/umeclidinium (Anoro Ellipta), 1 inhalation daily at this time. Proper use of inhaler is discussed.

20. What nonpharmacologic treatments might you consider for this patient?[23]

21. What referrals could the health care provider also consider and why?

22. What are important recommendations for a patient with suspected fatty liver disease?[24]

23.   When should the patient follow up for chronic obstructive pulmonary disease management?

Primary Care Visit 4

The patient returns in 6 weeks. The patient reports he felt some improvement with his breathing after starting umeclidinium/vilanterol (Anoro Ellipta) 62.5 micrograms/25 micrograms/actuation 1 puff daily. He also started pulmonary rehabilitation recently but states he was really reluctant to continue pulmonary rehabilitation because he feels well now. However, he decided to keep going to pulmonary rehabilitation, because his wife and daughter really want him to continue. He is using his albuterol inhaler three times a week in addition to before exercise. He is trying to exercise more, walking 4 days a week. He reports he has reduced the amount of fast food he eats and has tried to cut back his salt intake. He has an appointment scheduled to see palliative care for next month. His lipids drawn at last visit indicate a reduction in total cholesterol and LDL to within normal range, and he feels well without muscle aches or pains. He denies any recent COPD exacerbations requiring steroids, antibiotics, or emergency room or urgent care visits.

Physical Examination
General appearance: Well-groomed older male with good hygiene. No acute distress.
Vital signs: Weight: 158 pounds. Height 66 inches. BMI 26.3. Heart rate: 88, respiratory rate 20. Blood pressure 140/84 mm Hg. Temperature 98.3°F.
Skin: Warm, dry. No lesions or rash. Light gray course hair. Nail beds pink with prompt capillary refill.
Eyes: Conjunctivae clear. Pupils equal, round, and reactive to light.
Mouth: Posterior pharynx, no erythema, or exudate. No lesions tongue or buccal mucosa.
Neck: Neck supple, no lymphadenopathy. No thyromegaly. No carotid bruits. No jugular venous distention.
Chest/lungs: Decreased breath sounds in upper lobes bilaterally. Nonlabored effort. Regular rate and rhythm. Symmetric chest expansion, tactile fremitus equal bilaterally. No wheezes, rhonchi, or rales.
Cardiac: S1/S2 present. Regular rate and rhythm. No murmurs, rubs, or gallop.
Abdomen: Abdomen symmetric, soft, no distention. Bowel sounds positive in all four quadrants. No masses, no organomegaly.
Extremities: No edema or calf tenderness.
Spirometry today: FVC 3.05 L (57%), FEV_1 1.87 L (49%), and FEV_1/FVC 0.62. Interpretation is moderate-severe obstruction.

24.   What should the health care provider consider for the plan of care today?

Case Study, Continued

Telephone encounter: The health care provider calls and speaks with the patient 1 month into pulmonary rehabilitation. Patient reports he feels the same but that he feels good. He reports his breathing feels less labored and that he feels more energized. He did see palliative care and, although he does not require anything from them now, he was able to ask questions and address some of his concerns for the future if his physical status begins to decline. He has a cardiologist appointment in a few months for routine follow-up. Denies any recent acute respiratory episode or lower respiratory infection.

25.   The health care provider decides that the patient is stable and can be seen in 3 months for follow-up and have his routine annual at that time. What should the health care provider address at that visit?

ONLINE ANSWER SUBMISSION

When you are ready to submit your answers for grading and reflective expert feedback for evaluation, go to http://www.evolve.elsevier.com/DickAndButtaro/ to complete this case.

References

1. Berliner, D., Schneider, N., Welte, T., & Bauersachs, J. (2016). The differential diagnosis of dyspnea. *Deutsches Ärzteblatt International, 113*(49), 834–845.
2. Benich, J., & Carek, P. (2011). Evaluation of the patient with chronic cough. *American Family Physician, 84*(8), 887–892.
3. Bailey, K. (2012). The importance of the assessment of pulmonary function in COPD. *The Medical Clinics of North America, 96*(4), 745–752.
4. Dewar, M., Whit, R., & Curry, J. (2017). Chronic obstructive pulmonary disease: Diagnostic considerations. *Aafp.org*. Retrieved from http://www.aafp.org/afp/2006/0215/p669.html.
5. GOLD 2017 Global Strategy for the Diagnosis, Management and Prevention of COPD – Global Initiative for Chronic Obstructive Lung Disease – GOLD. (2017). Global Initiative for Chronic Obstructive Lung Disease – GOLD. Retrieved from http://goldcopd.org/gold-2017-global-strategy-diagnosis-management-prevention-copd/.
6. Zhang, X., Simpson, J., Powell, H., Yang, I., Upham, J., Reynolds, P., et al. (2014). Full blood count parameters for the detection of asthma inflammatory phenotypes. *Clinical and Experimental Allergy: Journal of the British Society for Allergy and Clinical Immunology, 44*(9), 1137–1145.
7. George-Gay, B., & Parker, K. (2003). Understanding the complete blood count with differential. *Journal of Perianesthesia Nursing, 18*(2), 96–117.
8. Köhnlein, T., & Welte, T. (2008). Alpha-1 antitrypsin deficiency: Pathogenesis, clinical presentation, diagnosis, and treatment. *The American Journal of Medicine, 121*(1), 3–9.
9. USPSTF A and B Recommendations – US Preventive Services Task Force. (2017). *Uspreventiveservicestaskforce.org*. Retrieved from https://www.uspreventiveservicestaskforce.org/Page/Name/uspstf-a-and-b-recommendations/.
10. Bell, M., Fotheringham, I., Punekar, Y., Riley, J., Cockle, S., & Singh, S. (2015). Systematic review of the association between laboratory- and field-based exercise tests and lung function in patients with chronic obstructive pulmonary disease. *Chronic Obstructive Pulmonary Diseases (Miami, Fla.), 2*(4), 321–342. http://journal.copdfoundation.org/#sthash.NtJo2ItZ.dpuf.
11. Mets, O., de Jong, P., van Ginneken, B., Gietema, H., & Lammers, J. (2011). Quantitative computed tomography in COPD: Possibilities and limitations. *Lung, 190*(2), 133–145.
12. Nackaerts, K. (2012). CT screening for lung cancer. *Lung Cancer (Amsterdam, Netherlands), 77*, S11.
13. Takigawa, N., Tada, A., Soda, R., Date, H., Yamashita, H., Endo, S., et al. (2006). Distance and oxygen desaturation in 6-min walk test predict prognosis in COPD patients. *Respiratory Medicine: COPD Update, 2*(3), 107.
14. Zoorob, R., & Campbell, J. (2017). Acute dyspnea in the office. *Aafp.org*. Retrieved from http://www.aafp.org/afp/2003/1101/p1803.html.
15. Armstrong, C. (2017). JNC8 Guidelines for the Management of Hypertension in Adults. *Aafp.org*. Retrieved from http://www.aafp.org/afp/2014/1001/p503.html.
16. Barnes, P. (2007). Chronic obstructive pulmonary disease: A growing but neglected global epidemic. *PLoS Medicine, 4*(5), e112.
17. Hanson, C., Rutten, E., Wouters, E., & Rennard, S. (2014). Influence of diet and obesity on COPD development and outcomes. *International Journal of Chronic Obstructive Pulmonary Disease, 723*.
18. Seamark, D., Seamark, C., & Halpin, D. (2017). Palliative care in chronic obstructive pulmonary disease: A review for clinicians. *NCBI*. Retrieved from https://www.ncbi.nlm.nih.gov/pmc/articles/PMC1861418/.
19. Lambert, M. (2017). ACC/AHA Release Updated guideline on the treatment of blood cholesterol to reduce ASCVD risk. *Aafp.org*. Retrieved from http://www.aafp.org/afp/2014/0815/p260.html.
20. Oh, R., & Hustead, T. (2017). Causes and evaluation of mildly elevated liver transaminase levels. *Aafp.org*. Retrieved from http://www.aafp.org/afp/2011/1101/p1003.html.
21. Pothirat, C., Chaiwong, W., Phetsuk, N., Pisalthanapuna, S., Chetsadaphan, N., & Choomuang, W. (2015). Evaluating inhaler use technique in COPD patients. *International Journal of Chronic Obstructive Pulmonary Disease, 1291*.
22. Hassan, K. (2014). Nonalcoholic fatty liver disease: A comprehensive review of a growing epidemic. *World Journal of Gastroenterology, 20*(34), 12082.

23. Corhay, J., Nguyen, D., Van Cauwenberge, H., & Louis, R. (2013). Pulmonary rehabilitation and COPD: Providing patients a good environment for optimizing therapy. *International Journal of Chronic Obstructive Pulmonary Disease, 27.*

24. Molloy, J. W., Calcagno, C. J., Williams, C. D., Jones, F. J., Torres, D. M., & Harrison, S. A. (2012). Association of coffee and caffeine consumption with fatty liver disease, nonalcoholic steatohepatitis, and degree of hepatic fibrosis. *Hepatology (Baltimore, Md.), 55*(2), 429–436.

Worsening Memory

Laura Struble

Instructions

After reviewing the case study, please jot down your notes or preliminary answers in the spaces provided. When you are ready to submit your answers for grading and reflective expert feedback for evaluation, go to http://www.evolve.elsevier.com/DickAndButtaro/ to complete this case.

Case Study Scenario/History of Present Illness

Mrs. Tucker is an 80-year-old widowed woman who lives independently in an apartment above a restaurant that she owned with her husband. She comes today, with her son David, as a new patient to the primary care clinic. Mrs. Tucker reports that she is not feeling like herself. She feels tired and does not feel like completing tasks. "I'm just getting old. My back and knees hurt more, I am forgetful, and I still miss my husband terribly."

The health care provider asks the patient whether it would be ok if you asked her son some questions about her health, and she agrees.

Mr. Tucker died suddenly 9 months ago of a heart attack. Her son David and his family moved from out of state to take over the family restaurant business. Before her husband died, David described his mother as high energy, always smiling, and a great baker who used to make a lot of the desserts for the restaurant. He states she never had any trouble keeping the financial records and felt her memory was ok. David thought things were getting back to normal after his father died, but Mrs. Tucker has "not been herself" since he moved back into town. He reports that Mrs. Tucker has a poor appetite, low energy, and sleeps a lot. She will eat some meals at the restaurant, but David noticed that she often does not cook for herself in her apartment. Mrs. Tucker told David she forgets to eat because she had a big meal at the restaurant. David reports that his mom is a very good cook, but when he encouraged her to bake her famous chocolate cake for a family celebration recently, the cake tasted terrible. David described it as flat, heavy, and very salty. He states he is worried about his mom because she used to be so social all of her life and is now more withdrawn. David also reports that Mrs. Tucker has 1 year of business school and was very sharp with numbers and figures. She used to run the cash register and kept the books for the restaurant. He noticed the financial records recently where not kept up as accurately, and when he looked at the bookkeeping records, he noticed that his father seemed to have taken over the bookkeeping for the restaurant before he died.

1. What possible risk factors may be contributing to Mrs. Tucker's fatigue and sadness?[1,2]

Check all that apply. State why or why not:
- A. History of depression
- B. Chronic medical conditions
- C. Being divorced or widowed
- D. Alcohol or substance abuse
- E. Pain

F. Stressful life events
G. Poor functional status
H. Bereavement
I. Cognitive Impairment

Answer:

Risk Factor	Identified From Mrs. Tucker's History
History of depression	
Chronic medical illness	
Being single	
Alcohol or substance abuse	
Pain	
Stressful life events	
Poor functional status	
Bereavement	
Cognitive impairment	

Case Study, Continued

Depression in older adults is often underdiagnosed because the patient focuses on various somatic complaints or cognitive symptoms and not psychological distress.[3] Given the risk factors and the son's concerns, the health care provider decides to assess Mrs. Tucker for depression by performing the Patient Health Questionnaire (PHQ)-2.[4]

Mrs. Tucker is asked the following questions.

How often over the last 2 weeks have you been bothered by the following problems?

1. *Little interest or pleasure in doing things*

2. *Feeling down, depressed, or hopeless*

The score for each question is as follows: not at all = 0; several days = 1 point; more than half the days = 2 points; and nearly every day = 3 points.

Mrs. Tucker responds she has had little interest in doing things for several days "because I am tired." She denies feeling down, depressed, or hopeless. She scores a 1 of 6 on the PHQ-2 (2 or greater is considered positive for depression). Because Mrs. Tucker scored a 1, it is not necessary to continue with the PHQ-9.[5]

Health History, Continued

Medications: Amlodipine dose is unknown, but the patient states she takes it daily. She reports she used to take other medications such as calcium and a multivitamin but decided not to take them anymore.

Allergies: No known drug allergies (NKDA).

Past medical history: Hypertension (HTN), coronary artery disease (CAD), and osteoarthritis. Patient gave vague answers to specific questions about her medical condition.

Past surgical history: Reports she does not think she had any surgeries.

Family history: Father died age 75 of a heart attack. Mother died age 85 of "old age." Sister died age 76 of chronic obstructive pulmonary disease (COPD).

Substance use history: Drinks beer or wine on social occasions. Never smoked tobacco. Denies illicit drug use.

Personal and social history: Twelfth grade education plus 1 year of business school at a community college. Met her husband on a blind date and was married for 59 years. Owned a small restaurant with her husband. She has two children: David, age 56, who runs the restaurant and is married with two kids; and Sally, 58, married and living out of state.

Review of Systems

General: Feels tired and fatigued.

Skin: Dry itchy skin, thinning hair, no rashes, no lumps, no changes in size or color of moles.

Head, ears, eyes, nose, and throat (HEENT): States slight hoarseness, but patient could not describe further. Denies headache, dizziness, or history of head injury. No vision or hearing changes. No sinus trouble or sore throat.

Respiratory: Denies shortness of breath, cough, or wheezing.

Cardiovascular: Denies chest pain but used to have "heart trouble" with heaviness in the chest. No chest discomfort for a long time. It was estimated that the heaviness stopped 5 years ago. HTN diagnosed 10 years ago. No palpitations, dyspnea, or orthopnea.

Gastrointestinal: Appetite is poor: "Not as hungry as I used to be." Constipation started approximately 6 months ago, but patient could not explain further, and reports weight is about the same. Denies heartburn, nausea, or vomiting.

Urinary: Has nocturia two to three times a night. Denies dysuria, hematuria, frequent urinary tract infections, or incontinence.

Musculoskeletal: Pain, stiffness, and muscle aches in knees and lower back. Denies history of trauma or falls.

Neurologic: Reports memory is not as good as it used to be. Denies paralysis, numbness, tremors, or seizures.

2. What assessment scale would be the most helpful in evaluating Mrs. Tucker during *today*'s visit? What are the components of this scale and how will they aid in determining Mrs. Tucker's status?

A. Instrumental Activities of Daily Living Scale[6]

B. Geriatric Depression Scale[7]

C. CAGE Substance Abuse Screening Tool[8]

D. Hendrick II Fall Risk Assessment Tool[9]

Answer:

Components of Assessment Scale	Mrs. Tucker Responses

Physical Examination

General: Alert, pleasant older female in no acute distress. She appears older than her stated age, is casually dressed, and has a stain on her shirt. She has a slight malodor.

Vital signs: Blood pressure (BP) in left arm 162/98 sitting. Heart rate 60, respirations 16, O_2 saturation on room air 96%.

Skin: Dry and coarse, no rashes, lesions, swelling, or bruising.

HEENT: Normocephalic, no nasal discharge. Auditory canals normal. No jugular vein distention (JVD) or carotid bruits, no lymphadenopathy.

Respiratory: Clear to auscultation bilaterally. No crackles or wheezing.

Cardiac: +S1/S2 and S4, regular rate and rhythm. Grade 1 murmur. No rubs or gallops.

Abdomen: Normoactive bowel sounds × 4 quadrants, soft and nontender to palpation, no organomegaly.

Extremities: Pedal pulses 1+ bilaterally, no edema, cyanosis, or skin lesions.

Musculoskeletal: Osteoarthritis findings with mild crepitus in both knees, but they are not warm or tender.

Neurologic: Cranial nerves II to XII intact, movements slightly slow but not bradykinetic, no tremors or tics noted. Muscle strength 3+ in upper and lower extremities, no pronator drift. Deep tendon reflexes are 1+ and symmetric at the triceps, biceps, and brachioradialis, 1+ and symmetric at the knees and absent at the ankles. Decreased vibratory sensation at the knees and ankles. Able to rise independently from the chair using the arm rests, is steady on her feet, walks slowly with an erect posture, narrow-based gait, and good arm swing.

3. Before performing any further tests or examinations, the health care provider needs to prioritize the list of differentials. What are the two most likely differential diagnoses related to fatigue and forgetfulness?

Differentials
   A. Acute coronary syndrome
   B. Unwitnessed head trauma
   C. Dementia
   D. Major depressive disorder
   E. Transient ischemic attack
   F. Metabolic disorder

Answer:[10-12]

4. The health care provider suspects that the patient may have possible dementia. Which specific screening test should be performed next?

   A. Mini-Mental Status Examination (MMSE)[13]
   B. Mini-Cog[14]
   C. Rapid Cognitive Screen[15]
   D. Montreal Cognitive Assessment (MoCA)[16]

Answer:[14-18]

Case Study, Continued

Mrs. Tucker agrees to complete the MoCA tool. She received an 18/30 points. Mrs. Tucker missed points in the following cognitive domains:

Attention and concentration: Missed 1 point
Executive functions: Missed 1 point
Memory: Missed 5 points
Language: Missed 0 points
Visuoconstructional skills: Missed 1 points
Conceptual thinking: Missed 0 points
Calculations: Missed 2 points
Orientation: Missed 2 points

5. What diagnostics should the health care provider consider necessary at this time and why?[19]

6.   What laboratory tests are the most important to help exclude reversible causes of dementia?[20,21]

7.   Given her history of coronary artery disease and hypertension, what other diagnostics should the health care provider order?

8.   The patient and her son are asked to return for follow-up after the test results. Is there anything important they can do before the next appointment in 2 weeks?[22]

9.   What components of the history should be asked and clarified at the next clinic visit?

10.   What other components of the physical examination would be important to include at the patient's next clinic visit that were missed during this encounter?

Test Results

   Comprehensive metabolic panel and CBC with differential were all within normal limits
   TSH 18 (range 0.35–4.94 mIU/L)
   Folate 18 (normal range 2–20 ng/mL)
   B_{12} 523 (normal range 100–700 pg/mL)
   Low-density lipoprotein (LDL) cholesterol 130 (borderline high range 130–159 milligrams/
      dL)
   Total cholesterol 198 (desirable range less than 200 milligrams/dL)
   High-density lipoprotein (HDL) cholesterol 62 (less than average risk 60 or higher)
   Triglycerides 152 (borderline high range 150–199)
   ECG: Showed mild left ventricular hypertrophy

First Return Visit

Patient reports she takes amlodipine but has run out and does not remember the dose. Her son states he is not aware of what medications the patient was on because his mom is a private person. Mrs. Tucker bought her medications at the local pharmacy, which is within walking distance of the restaurant. She admits she used to take "some kind of thyroid medicine" but did not feel it helped anything so did not refill, stating: "My husband always took care of all my medications." The patient did not remember to take her BP or record the results, and when her son tried to do it, she told him her BP was "fine."

Her son is very surprised by this. He stated, "My dad and mom did everything together, but I did not know she was having trouble handling things like her medications."

The patient tried to answer the provider's questions that were asked to clarify the history from the initial visit. David provided collateral information as well.

Patient reports that her other doctor retired and left the state so she does not have any previous medical records. She states it has been "a couple of years since I saw a dentist." Patient endorses feeling tired all the time and then is so stiff and painful when she gets up from napping that she takes Tylenol, unknown strength. Patient admits she is not taking as good of care of the apartment and is just too tired to work in the restaurant downstairs. Patient became angry when asked if she was bathing ok. "Of course I am!!! What kind of question is that?" Patient states she has not gained or lost weight but admits she has not been eating much. When asked specifically about her complaint of hoarseness, patient stated her throat does not hurt, she does not have difficulty swallowing, but her throat feels "full." Patient states she had an uncle that "was not quite right in the head but in those days it was all my mother would say." Son reminded her that her mother had dementia later in life.

While in clinic the patient is asked to call the pharmacy to find out her medications and dosages. The following information is obtained:

- *Amlodipine 5 milligrams a day (last refilled 6 months ago with no refills)*
- *Levothyroxine 50 micrograms a day (last refilled 9 months ago with no refills)*

Physical Examination

Vital signs: Highest BP sitting at rest for 5 minutes was in the left arm, 166/98. Orthostatic BP supine after resting 5 minutes in left arm was 168/96 with a pulse of 62. BP standing after 2 minutes was 158/88 with a pulse 66. Height 5'2". Weight 115 pounds. Body mass index (BMI) is 21.

Mouth: Mucous membranes moist with no mucosal lesions. Teeth/gums: Several missing teeth but no obvious caries or periodontal disease. No gingival inflammation or significant.

Pharynx: Mucosa noninflamed, no tonsillar hypertrophy or exudate.

Neck: Supple, without lesions, bruits, or adenopathy. Nontender goiter is palpable.

11. What are the diagnoses for Mrs. Tucker?

12. What treatments should the health care provider recommend for Mrs. Tucker today?

Case Study, Continued

Mrs. Tucker's son agreed to take and record her BP once a day, pick up the prescriptions, and set up her medications in a pill box.

Second Return Visit 2 Months Later

David reports that the patient's BP has been in 122 to 140/78 to 80 range. He noted the patient had not taken levothyroxine for 2 days. Her son reports that one day he noticed that the patient left the water running in the bathroom sink and the following day there was a burned pot in the sink and the kitchen smelled like smoke. He also had brought some groceries over but noted there was a lot of old food in the refrigerator that needed to be thrown out.

Mrs. Tucker reports that she feels much better. She states she is less tired and has been going downstairs and greeting all of the customers. Her son agrees and noticed a marked improvement in her energy level and thought she was finally adjusting to living without her husband, but he noted "strange things." He states these are drastic changes and his mom never had trouble like this before. When asked to elaborate, her son reports that his mother is repeating the same question right after she asked it, and once she called him at 1 a.m. asking why he was not at the restaurant yet. His mother does not seem to follow the storyline in a movie and no longer reads novels. She also does not know how to work the TV controls.

TSH level is now 6 (range 0.35–4.94 mIU/L)

The provider decides to repeat the MoCA because her thyroid function is improving.

The patient receives a score of 19/30 points. Based on the MoCA, the patient continues to have difficulty with:

Amnesia: Could not recall the five words after being distracted.

Agnosia: Said "hippo" when shown a picture of a rhinoceros.

Aphasia: Could not state 11 words that begin with the letter F in 1 minute.

Executive dysfunction: Abnormal clock draw test.

It is noted the patient has some apraxia because she had trouble turning on the TV, and her son reports she often cannot button her shirt. When Mrs. Tucker is asked what would she do if there was a fire in apartment, she replied, "I would call the fire department." She was then asked what number she would dial. She seemed to think a moment and then stated, "I would look it up in the phone book." She denied any visual or auditory hallucinations and tells the health care provider she feels safe in her apartment and no one is trying to steal from or harm her.

13.   Which of the following diagnostic tests, if any, should the health care provider now order to determine the cause of Mrs. Tucker's mental status changes?

   A. Possible noncontrast computed tomography (CT) or magnetic resonance scanning (MRI)

   B. Positron emission tomography (PET) scan

   C. Cerebrospinal fluid (CSF) and blood-based biomarkers

   D. HIV laboratory test

Answer:[23]

Case Study, Continued

The provider confers with a neurologist and orders an MRI.

   MRI findings: There is diffuse supratentorial greater than age-appropriate cerebral volume loss. There is no hydrocephalus. Nonspecific patchy T2 signal prolongation in periventricular white matter, right corona radiata, and right subcortical insular regions is also demonstrated. No intra- or extraaxial enhancing mass is seen. No areas of impeded diffusion are seen to suggest acute or subacute brain infarction. There is no intra- or extraaxial hemorrhagic collection.

   Impression:

   1. MRI brain demonstrates diffuse greater than age-appropriate parenchymal brain volume retraction in the supratentorial region.

   2. Nonspecific T2 signal changes are noted in the periventricular white matter, right corona radiata, and right subcortical insular white matter.

14.   Based on the patient's clinical presentation and MRI report, which of the following is the most likely diagnosis for Mrs. Tucker?

   A. Normal age-related changes

   B. Alzheimer's disease

   C. Vascular dementia

   D. Lewy body dementia

   E. Normal pressure hydrocephalus

Answer:

15.   What treatments should the health care provider recommend for Mrs. Tucker?[24]

16.   What nonpharmacologic interventions would be important for the health care provider to discuss with Mrs. Tucker's family?

17.   What resources would be appropriate to discuss with Mrs. Tucker's family?

18.   What ongoing issues will be the focus of future visits?

ONLINE ANSWER SUBMISSION

When you are ready to submit your answers for grading and reflective expert feedback for evaluation, go to http://www.evolve.elsevier.com/DickAndButtaro/ to complete this case.

References

1. Aziz, R., & Steffens, D. C. (2013). What are the causes of late-life depression? *The Psychiatric Clinics of North America*, *36*(4), 497–516.
2. Birrer, R. B., & Vemuri, S. P. (2004). Depression in later life: A diagnostic and therapeutic challenge. *American Family Physician*, *69*(10), 2375–2382.
3. Espinoza, R., & Kaufman, A. H. (2014). Diagnosis and treatment of late-life depression. *Psychiatric Times*, *31*(10), 18.
4. Spitzer, R. L., Kroenke, K., & Williams, J. B. (1999). Validation and utility of a self-report version of the prime-MD: The PHQ primary care study. Primary Care Evaluation of Mental Disorders. Patient Health Questionnaire. *JAMA: The Journal of the American Medical Association*, *282*(18), 1737–1744.

5. Arroll, B., Goodyear-Smith, F., Crengle, S., Gunn, J., Kerse, N., et al. (2010). Validation of PHQ-2 and PHQ-9 to Screen for major depression in the primary care population. *Annals of Family Medicine, 8*(4), 348–353.

6. Lawton, M. P., & Brody, E. M. (1969). Assessment of older people: Self-maintaining and instrumental activities of daily living. *The Gerontologist, 9,* 179–186.

7. Brink, T. L., Yesavage, J. A., Lum, O., et al. (1982). Screening tests for geriatric depression. *Clinical Gerontologist, 1,* 37–43.

8. Buchsbaum, D. G., Buchanan, R. G., Welch, J., Cantor, R. M., & Schnoll, S. H. (1992). Screening for drinking disorders in the elderly using the CAGE Questionnaire. *Journal of the American Geriatrics Society, 40,* 662–665.

9. Hendrich, A. L., Bender, P. S., & Nyhuis, A. (2003). Validation of the Hendrich II Fall Risk Model: A large concurrent case/control study of hospitalized patients. *Applied Nursing Research, 16*(1), 9–21.

10. Østergaard, S. D., Mukherjee, S., Sharp, S. J., Proitsi, P., Lotta, L. A., et al. (2015). Associations between potentially modifiable risk factors and Alzheimer disease: A Mendelian Randomization Study. *PLoS Medicine, 12*(6), e1001841.

11. Schlanger, L. E., Bailey, J. L., & Sands, J. M. (2010). Electrolytes in the aging. *Advances in Chronic Kidney Disease, 17*(4), 308–319.

12. Carnaris, G. J., Manowitz, N. R., Mayor, G., & Ridgway, E. C. (2000). The Colorado thyroid disease prevalence study. *Archives of Internal Medicine, 160,* 526–534.

13. Folstein, M. F., Folstein, S. E., & McHugh, P. R. (1975). Mini-mental state." A practical method for grading the cognitive state of patients for the clinician. *Journal of Psychiatric Research, 12*(3), 189–198.

14. Fage, B. A., Chan, C. C. H., Gill, S. S., Noel-Storr, A. H., Herrmann, N., et al. (2015). Mini-Cog for the diagnosis of Alzheimer's disease dementia and other dementias within a community setting. *Cochrane Database of Systematic Reviews,* (2), Art. No. CD010860.

15. Malmstrom, T. K., Voss, V. B., Cruz-Oliver, D. M., Cummings-Vaughn, L. A., Tumosa, N., et al. (2015). The Rapid Cognitive Screen (RCS): A point-of-care screening for dementia and mild cognitive impairment. *The Journal of Nutrition, Health & Aging, 19*(7), 741–744.

16. Nasreddine, Z. S., Phillips, N. A., Bedirian, V., Charbonneau, S., Whitehead, V., et al. (2005). The Montreal Cognitive Assessment, MoCA: A brief screening tool for mild cognitive impairment. *Journal of the American Geriatrics Society, 53*(4), 695–699.

17. Mitchell, A. J., & Malladi, S. (2010). Screening and case finding tools for the detection of dementia. Part I: Evidence-based meta-analysis of multidomain tests. *The American Journal of Geriatric Psychiatry, 18*(9), 759–782.

18. Trzepacz, P. T., Hochstetler, H., Wang, S., Walker, B., Saykin, A. J., et al. (2015). Relationship between the Montreal Cognitive Assessment and Mini-Mental State Examination for assessment of mild cognitive impairment in older adults. *BMC Geriatrics, 15,* 107.

19. Small, G. W., Rabins, P. V., Barry, P. P., Buckholtz, N. S., DeKosky, S. T., Ferris, S. H., et al. (1999). Diagnosis and treatment of Alzheimer disease and related disorders consensus statement of the American Association for Geriatric Psychiatry, the Alzheimer's Association, and the American Geriatrics Society. *JAMA: The Journal of the American Medical Association, C278*(16), 1363–1371.

20. Knopman, D. S., DeKosky, S. T., Cummings, J. L., et al. (2001). Practice parameter: Diagnosis of dementia (an evidence-based review). Report of the Quality Standards Subcommittee of the American Academy of Neurology. *Neurology, 56*(9), 1143–1153.

21. Mount, D. B. (2014). Fluid and Electrolyte Disturbances. In D. Kasper, A. Fauci, S. Hauser, D. Longo, J. Jameson, & J. Loscalzo (Eds.), *Harrison's Principles of Internal Medicine* (19th ed.). New York: McGraw-Hill. Retrieved from http://accessmedicine.mhmedical.com.ezproxy.simmons.edu:2048/content.aspx?bookid=1130&sectionid=79726591.

22. American Red Cross. (2017). Monitoring your blood pressure at home. http://www.heart.org/HEARTORG/Conditions/HighBloodPressure/KnowYourNumbers/Monitoring-Your-Blood-Pressure-at-Home_UCM_301874_Article.jsp#.WSG6Vje1vDC. (Obtained 18 May 2017).

23. Peterson, R. C., Stevenson, J. C., Ganguli, M., et al. (2001). Practice parameters: Early detection of dementia: Mild cognitive impairment (an evidence based review). Report of the Quality Standards Subcommittee of the American Academy of Neurology. *Neurology, 56*(9), 1133–1142.

24. American Psychiatric Association. (2007). *Practice guideline for the treatment of patients with Alzheimer's disease and other dementias* (2nd ed.). Arlington,: American Psychiatric Association.

Swelling

Marjorie Crabtree ▪ Susan Feeney

Instructions

After reviewing the case study, please jot down your notes or preliminary answers in the spaces provided. When you are ready to submit your answers for grading and reflective expert feedback for evaluation, go to http://www.evolve.elsevier.com/DickAndButtaro/ to complete this case.

Case Study Scenario/History of Present Illness

Marian Wilson, a 71-year-old Caucasian female, presents to the clinic for a routine follow-up visit for her hypertension (HTN) and diabetes mellitus (DM). She is an established patient of the practice; however, she is new to you because her primary care provider (PCP) has moved out of state. Mrs. Wilson states she feels well. She checks her blood pressure (BP) two to three times a month on her home BP machine and it averages 130/80 at home. Mrs. Wilson also checks her blood sugars three to four times a week, and she reports they are "in goal" and are as follows: fasting glucose from 110 to 130, postprandial 130 to 150, and bedtime 150 to 160. She tries to limit "sugar" in her diet, but states she eats an orange daily for potassium to help her with her "water pill."

During her visit, Mrs. Wilson shares that she has had right lower leg achiness and "puffiness" for the past month. She denies similar achiness, puffiness, or swelling on her left lower leg. She has also noted some dry skin over this area that can be itchy at times. She applies moisturizer to the area daily, after her shower; however, this does not seem to help with the swelling or itchiness. She says she often wakes up scratching the area at night. Mrs. Wilson states she wants to keep active and has been going to the gym three times week for the past year and participates in a cardiovascular fitness class for ages 65 and over, once a week.

Medications: Hydrochlorothiazide (HCTZ) 12.5 milligrams po daily, amlodipine 10 milligrams po daily, metformin 750 milligrams po twice daily with food, calcium 1000 milligrams po daily, vitamin D 1000 units po daily, and ASA 81 milligrams po daily.

Allergies: None.

Past medical history: HTN × 10 years, diabetes type II × 3 years.

Family history: Father: Diabetes, cerebrovascular accident (CVA) age 82, died at age 83. Mother: Depression, fibromyalgia, varicosities, currently resides in an assisted living facility at age 92. Brother age 68, HTN, and dyslipidemia. Sister age 65, rheumatoid arthritis, varicosities, and HTN.

Social history: Married for 40 years to her husband, Stanley. Retired elementary school teacher, volunteers at local soup kitchen twice a week. Remote history cigarette smoking × 10 years (1 pack per day), quit at age 35.

Review of Systems

General: Denies fever, chills, or pain.

Heart: Denies palpitations, chest pain.

Respiratory: Denies shortness of breath, cough.

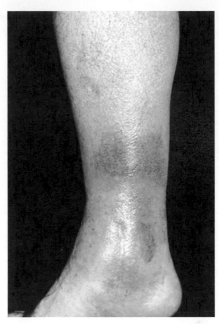

Fig. 8.1 Chronic venous insufficiency manifesting as marked erythema and edema, which is often called stasis dermatitis. (From Fitzpatrick, J. E., & Morelli, J. G. [2016]. *Dermatology secrets plus [5th ed.]*. Philadelphia: Saunders.)

Gastrointestinal (GI): Denies pain, bloating, gastroesophageal reflux disease (GERD), constipation, or diarrhea.

Genitourinary (GU): Denies dysuria, frequency.

Gynecologic (GYN): Menopause age 55, denies vaginal bleeding.

Skin: Has had eczema intermittently in the past (hands and behind knees). Basal cell cancer removed from upper back 18 months ago.

Peripheral vascular: Occasional bilateral ankle swelling, darkening of skin on the both ankles over the past few years. Denies previous clotting disorders or deep vein thrombophlebitis.

Physical Examination

General: 71-year-old well-developed female, in no distress, appears stated age.

Vital signs: BP 138/84 left arm and 134/82 right arm. Heart rate (HR) 80, respiratory rate 18. Height 5 feet 5 inches. Weight 182 pounds. Body mass index (BMI) 30.3.

Cardiac: 80 regular rate, S1, S2, no S3, S4. No murmurs, rubs, or gallops.

Respiratory: Clear, no rales, rhonchi, or wheezes.

Abdomen: Soft, bowel sounds present throughout. Nontender, nondistended, and no bruits.

Extremities: 1+ edema bilaterally lower legs and ankles. Bronze discoloration bilateral medial malleoli, and no induration, warmth, or blanching noted. Right lower leg with scattered erythematous patches (Fig. 8.1). Left medial ankle, mild bronze discoloration, and no warmth, induration, exudate, or blanching.

1.   Based on Mrs. William's history and physical examination results, what are the possible causes (differential diagnosis) for the patient's current conditions?[1-3]

2.   What components of the history or physical examination are missing?[2,4-6]

PATIENT RESPONSE

Additional History and Review of Systems. *Mrs. Wilson tells you that, along with ASA, calcium, and vitamin D, she rarely takes over-the-counter medications. She takes one to two ibuprofen less than once a month for rare headache or muscle ache after exercise. She does not believe she has ever been on an ACEI or an ARB. She has been on amlodipine for over 5 years and was increased from 5 milligrams to 10 milligrams daily 3 years ago. She was started on HCTZ at that time as well. She reports that she was offered a statin by her previous PCP, but she refused because her husband had muscle aches on this medication and she was not interested.*

Mrs. Wilson drinks socially, one to two glasses (3–4 ounces per glass) of red wine once or twice a month. She denies ever using illicit drugs. Diet recall reveals fresh fruits and vegetables at her meals, but she does snack on salty chips and nuts throughout the day and likes canned soups for lunch. Otherwise, she does not eat a lot of prepared foods and makes her food from "scratch" most of the time. Patient states that she has been using an antibacterial soap for daily showers. She showers at the gym after her class. She wears gym socks under her sneakers.

She does have varicose veins in her feet and ankles. She does get ankle edema with prolonged standing. She has an achy and heaviness feeling in both lower legs, right worse than left. However, she denies specific pain, redness, or warmth noted at any time in either calf. She denies any pain in her ankles but does state the area on her right ankle is tender and bothersome at times. Mrs. Wilson states that her leg symptoms are better when she sits for a while, especially if she puts her feet up and when she awakens in the morning, but the discomfort worsens as the day progresses and if she stands for long periods.

Physical Examination. *Her pedal and dorsalis pedis pulses are 2+ bilaterally. She has nontender, nonerythematous protruding varicosities of bilateral lower legs, ankles, and feet. She does not have any evidence of scarring (atrophie blanche) on either leg (upper or lower). Her diabetic monofilament examination and vibratory sensation are within normal limits. Her bilateral foot examination reveals that skin is smooth and dry without cracking. She has no signs of DVT or JVD. Her breathing is nonlabored.*

3. Based on the history and physical examination findings, what are the likely diagnoses for Mrs. Wilson at this time? How does the health care provider support the diagnoses?[2,7,8]

4. **What diagnostics are necessary for this patient at this time?**[7,8]

5. **What treatments would you recommend at this time for Mrs. Williams?**[1,2,4-10]

6.   What information should the health care provider discuss with Mrs. Williams about stasis dermatitis?[1,2,7]

7.   What do health care providers need to know about ordering compression stockings?[1,2,7,8,11]

8. What do you as Mrs. Williams' health care provider need to teach your patient about compression stockings?[7]

9. What are the priorities for Mrs. William's next visit?[4-6]

Case Study, Continued

Stasis dermatitis: *The patient returns 3 weeks later. She states that the right leg area was much better with compression stockings and prescription corticoid steroid ointment. She states, however, that the area has worsened over the past week. She complains that the "itchiness" returned in the area and that there is a clear drainage from a small open area on her right ankle. She has been* applying over-the-counter antibiotic ointment to the area for the past 4 to 5 days to "prevent infection." She tells you that she stopped the steroid ointment about 1 week ago because her itching improved significantly. She has been using the compression stockings during the day, but does not like to wear them to her gym class because she feels self-conscious. She wears gym socks during exercise class and then applies her stockings after she showers.

Diabetes mellitus: Patient reports the following home blood sugars: fasting average <105 and 2-hour postprandial average are in the 140 range. She has continued her metformin as prescribed.

HTN: Her home BP average is 130/80. She stopped the amlodipine and started lisinopril 10 milligrams daily 2 weeks ago. Denies cough or any new symptoms. She has continued HCTZ 12.5 milligrams daily.

BMI 30: She has had family visiting recently and was not able to make changes to her diet.

Mrs. Wilson had her fasting laboratory tests drawn 2 weeks ago. They are as follows: CBC/differential is within normal limits; CMP is within normal limits; fasting glucose is 112; TSH is 3.2; A1C is 6.6; and lipids are total cholesterol 202, triglycerides 172, low-density lipoprotein (LDL) 167, and high-density lipoprotein (HDL) 42.

Physical Examination

General: Patient is alert, cooperative, and relaxed.

Vital signs: BP 130/82 right arm and 128/80 left arm. Temperature 98.6°F, HR 88, respiratory rate 18. Height 5 feet 5 inches. Weight 182 pounds. BMI 30.3.

Cardiac: 72 regular rate, S1, S2, no S3, S4. No murmurs, rubs, or gallops.

Lungs: Clear to auscultation. No rales, wheezes, or rhonchi.

Extremities: Right medial malleolus 4 cm hyperpigmented, scaling patch with a 0.5-cm open area with clear drainage. Increased pain with flexion of the ankle. Trace edema bilaterally. Bilateral feet: Normal monofilament and vibratory sensation.

10.   Based on Mrs. William's history and physical examination results, what are the possible causes (differential diagnosis) for the patient's current condition?[1,2,10]

11.   What components of today's history or physical examination are missing?

Patient Response. *Patient states she washes with antibacterial soap daily in the shower. She states she does not like petrolatum jelly because it is too oily. She had been applying the steroid ointment once daily before she stopped using it. She is not using any devices to assist with applying stockings.*

She started applying the antibiotic ointment 5 days ago and has noticed an increase in the itchiness since then. About 2 days ago she noted the discharge and tenderness from the area.

Physical Examination
- General appearance: Observe gait, favoring of affected side.
- Right ankle: Any warmth, erythema, or odor noted? What is the depth of the open area: Excoriation (minimal loss of epidermis), erosion (loss of epidermis), or ulceration (loss of epidermis and dermis)?
- What is your assessment of the patient's varicosities today? Any worsening?
- Does she have any edema? Where is it? Is it pitting? Has it worsened?
- How are her peripheral pulses? Any changes from last assessment? Any signs/symptoms consistent with PAD?
- Does patient have any lymphadenopathy or lymphangitis?
- Examine bilateral lower extremities/feet and skin. Neurologic examination (sensory, motor).

Additional Physical Examination Findings. *There is no lymphadenopathy in either lower extremity. Trace edema bilaterally. The open area has no induration, but the area is 2 mm deep, exposing the dermis. Her lymph glands are within normal limits, and there is no lymphangitis. Peripheral pulses are +2 bilaterally, and extremities are warm to touch with normal capillary refill (<2 seconds).*

12. Based on patient's history and physical examination results, what diagnoses should you consider?

13. What diagnostics should be considered?

14. What treatments would you recommend?[4-7,9,10,12-14]

15. What referrals would be appropriate here?[2,7,16]

16.   What other options might be considered for the patient's concerns?

17.   What ongoing issues will be the focus of future visits?[9,10,15]

Case Study Continued

Mrs. Williams returns 4 days later complaining of increased pain and drainage from her right lower leg over the past 3 days. She has been busy and had difficulty scheduling an appointment with the wound clinic, but she did schedule her first appointment next week. She states she stopped the over-the-counter antibiotic ointment and antibacterial soap and resumed the steroid ointment. She has been using the topical cream on her ulcer as prescribed but has not been using a bandage over the ulcer because the bandage makes it difficult to put her compression stockings on. She has been wearing her compression stockings and elevating her leg as much as possible. She was going to the gym as usual but did not go the past 2 days because she has not felt well. She feels fatigued but denies chills, fever, or lack of energy. Her home blood sugars for the past week have increased, and now her fasting blood sugars are in the 130 range and those 2 hours after a meal are in the 160 range. Her home BPs have also been slightly higher, in the 140/90 range. She has not started statin. The culture and sensitivity (C&S) results are back and are positive for methicillin-resistant Staphylococcus aureus (MRSA).

General: BP 134/82 left arm. Temperature 99.9°F. HR 92, respiratory rate 18. Height 5 feet 5 inches. Weight 184 pounds. BMI 30.3.

Cardiac: 92 regular rhythm and rate, S1, S2. No S3, S4. No murmurs, rubs, or gallops.

Lungs: Clear to auscultation without rales, wheezes, or rhonchi.

Lymph: Right inguinal nodes 1 cm, tender, and moveable.

Extremities: Right medial ankle with erythematous, hyperpigmented area surrounding a 2-cm open (superficial) draining area with mucopurulent discharge. The area is tender to palpation with mild, nonpitting edema and increased pain with range of motion (ROM) of ankle. Left ankle examination unchanged from previous examination.

18. Based on Mrs. Williams' history and physical examination results today, what are the priority differential diagnoses (i.e., red flags) for her current condition?

19. What, if any, components of her history and/or physical examination are missing?

Patient Response. *Mrs. Williams states the area becomes more red in the evening, and the area is always tender regardless of time of day. Occasionally she notices a sharp pain in her right calf and just above her right ankle, which is sometimes a 4 to 5 out of 10, but the pain subsides quickly. She has noticed a small amount of purulent drainage from the wound. Her right leg is a little achy (2–3 out of 10) sometimes, but she is able to walk and bear weight without a problem.*

Physical Examination

  Lymph: No lymphadenopathy in the popliteal and inguinal nodes, bilaterally.

  Extremities: Right lower medial ankle ulceration 3 mm wide × 3 to 4 mm deep exposing the dermis, which is an increase in depth and width since 4 days ago. The surrounding area is without induration, fluctuance, or pustule noted. Right and left calf circumference measurements are equal, and calves are not erythematous, warm, or tender to palpation. Pulses pedal and postpopliteal 2+ bilaterally. Sensation within normal limits bilaterally.

20. Based on Mrs. Williams' complaints and the physical examination findings, what is your assessment?

21.   What diagnostics are necessary for this patient at this time?

22.   What additional diagnostics would you order based on the additional history provided previously?[8]

23. **What treatments would you recommend?**[3,5,15-17]

24. **What are further considerations necessary in the care of Mrs. Williams?**

25.   **What additional history would be helpful?**

26.   **What referrals would be appropriate here?**

27. What are the priorities for Mrs. Williams' next visit?

Case Study Continued

Patient returns 2 days later. States she is feeling better. She is having less leg pain. The area continues to be moist, but with clear drainage. Her ankle is less swollen. She has been taking her TMP-SMX DS twice daily. Her wound care clinic appointment date is tomorrow. She has not returned to the gym, but walks daily in her neighborhood. Her home blood sugars continue to be elevated; fasting range is 140 and 2 hours after a meal they are 180. Her home BP average is 130/85. She states she increased metformin to 1000 milligrams po twice daily and started simvastatin. She denies cough, diarrhea, or GI upset and denies muscle ache.

CBC showed normal hemogram: White blood cells (WBCs) were 8000 (elevation) and neutrophils 70% (slight elevation) with 1% bands (normal). Basic metabolic panel (BMP) was normal except for random blood glucose at 136.

The Doppler study report is back. It is positive for insufficiency, venous reflux, and negative for DVT. There is no occlusion noted. The greater saphenous vein (GSV) caliber is 8 mm (normal is <4 mm in diameter).

Physical Examination

General: BP 138/78. Temperature 98.6°F. HR 76, respiratory rate 18. Height 5 feet 8 inches. Weight 185 pounds.

Heart: 76 regular rhythm and rate, S1, S2, no S3, S4. No murmurs, rubs, or gallops.

Lungs: Clear to auscultation.

Abdomen: Soft, bowel sounds positive, nontender.

Lymph: No lymphadenopathy in inguinal and popliteal bilaterally.

Extremities: Right medial ankle erythema, hyperpigmented area with 2-cm ulcer, moist area with clear discharge, tender to palpation. There is 1-cm surrounding erythema, mild nonpitting edema, and no pain with ROM of ankle.

28.   What do you need to know about interpreting Doppler study reports?[11]

29.   What do you need to teach the patient about venous insufficiency and the potential for skin ulcers?[2,7,11]

30. What further suggestions should be discussed with Mrs. Williams at today's visit?[11,18]

Case Study Continued

Patient returns 1 week later. She states she now has no pain in the ankle and that she is wearing an Unna boot. She explains that they did a study to measure her arteries before they applied the boot, and that the test results were normal. The plan is that she will continue to go to the wound care clinic weekly. She has been taking metformin 1000 milligrams twice po daily and her home blood sugars are now within normal range. She also has been taking the lisinopril, metformin, and simvastatin as prescribed. Her home BPs are now in the 130/78 range. She is eating about 1500 calories per day. She has made an appointment to see a nutritionist.

General: BP 138/78. Temperature 98.6°F. HR 76, respiratory rate 18. Height 5 feet 8 inches. Weight 182 pounds.

Heart: 76 regular rate and rhythm, S1, S2, no S3, S4. No murmurs, rubs, or gallops.

Lungs: Clear to auscultation all fields.

Abdomen: Soft, bowel sounds present throughout, nontender.

Lymph: No lymphadenopathy in the inguinal and popliteal bilaterally.

Extremities: The Unna boot is removed for the examination. Right medial ankle: Toes are warm, the ulcer has pink granulation tissue on edges and is now 1 cm in size. Surrounding erythema has resolved, and there is no exudate noted. Monofilament examination is within normal limits.

31.   Why is it important that the patient had a study to measure the blood flow in her arteries?[11]

32.   Why was an Unna boot used in treatment?[11,18]

33. What is the plan for your Mrs. Williams now?

ONLINE ANSWER SUBMISSION

When you are ready to submit your answers for grading and reflective expert feedback for evaluation, go to http://www.evolve.elsevier.com/DickAndButtaro/ to complete this case.

References

1. Bergan, J. J., Schmid-Schönbein, G. W., Smith, P. D., Nicolaides, A. N., Boisseau, M. R., & Eklof, B. (2006). Chronic venous disease. *The New England Journal of Medicine, 355*(5), 488–498.
2. O'Donnell, T. F., Passman, M. A., Marston, W. A., Ennis, W. J., Dalsing, M., Kistner, R. I., et al. (2014). Management of venous leg ulcers: Clinical practice guidelines of the society for Vascular Surgery® and the American Venous Forum. *Journal of Vascular Surgery, 60*(2 Suppl.), 3S–59S. ISSN 0741-5214.
3. Gosnell, A. L., & Nedorost, S. T. (2009). Stasis dermatitis as a complication of amlodipine therapy. *Journal of Drugs in Dermatology, 8*, 135.
4. Whelton, P. K., Carey, R. M., Aronow, W. S., Casey, D. E., Jr., Collins, K. J., Dennison Himmelfarb, C., et al. (2018). 2017 ACC/AHA/AAPA/ABC/ACPM/AGS/APha/ASH/ASPC/NMA/PCNA guideline for the prevention, detection, evaluation, and management of high blood pressure in adults: A report of the American College of Cardiology/American Heart Association Task Force on Clinical Practice Guidelines. *Journal of the American College of Cardiology.*
5. American Diabetes Association Standards of Medical Care in Diabetes. (2017). Cardiovascular disease and risk management. *Diabetes Care, 40*(Suppl. 1), Online ISSN 1935-5548.
6. Goff, D. C., Jr., Lloyd-Jones, D. M., Bennett, G., Coady, S., D'Agostino, R. B., Sr., Gibbons, R., et al. (2014). 2013 ACC/AHA guideline on the assessment of cardiovascular risk: A report of the American College of Cardiology/American Heart Association Task Force on Practice Guidelines. *Circulation, 129*(Suppl. 2), S49–S73.
7. The Australian Wound Management Association Inc., & the New Zealand Wound Care Society Inc. Australian and New Zealand clinical practice guideline for prevention and management of venous leg ulcers. ISBN Online: 978-0-9807842-2-0; ISBN Print: 978-0-9807842-4-4.
8. Gillespie, D. L. (2010). Venous ulcer diagnosis, treatment, and prevention of recurrences. *Journal of Vascular Surgery, 52*(5 Suppl.), 8S–14S.
9. Ferrence, J. D., et al. (2009). Choosing topical corticosteroids. *American Family Physician, 79*(2), 135–140.
10. Patterson, J. W. (Ed.), (2016). Stasis dermatitis. In *Weedon's skin pathology* (5th ed.). Churchill Livingstone Elsevier.

11. White-Chu, E. F., & Conner-Kerr, T. A. (2014). Overview of guidelines for the prevention and treatment of venoUS leg ulcers: A US perspective. *Journal of Multidisciplinary Healthcare*, *7*, 111–117. (Unna Boot compression bandage).
12. O'Meara, S., Al-Kurdi, D., Ologun, Y., Ovington, L. G., Martyn-St James, M., & Richardson, R. (2014). Antibiotics and antiseptics for venous leg ulcers. *Cochrane Database of Systematic Reviews*, (1), Art. No.: CD003557, doi:10.1002/14651858.CD003557.pub5.
13. del Rio Sola, M. L., Antonio, J., Fajardo, G., & Vaquero Puenta, C. (2012). Influence of aspirin therapy in ulcer associated with venous insufficiency. *Annals of Vascular Surgery*, *26*(5), 620–629.
14. Evangelista, M. T. P., Casintahan, M. F. A., & Villafuerte, L. L. (2014). Simvastatin as a novel therapeutic agent for venous ulcers: A randomized, double-blind, placebo-controlled trial. *The British Journal of Dermatology*, *170*(5), 1151–1157.
15. Jull, A. B., Arroll, B., Parag, V., & Waters, J. (2012). Pentoxifylline for treating venous leg ulcers. *Cochrane Database of Systematic Review*, (12), CD001733, doi:10.1002/14651858.CD001733.pub3.
16. Todd, M. (2011). Venous leg ulcers and the impact of compression bandaging. *British Journal of Nursing (Mark Allen Publishing)*, *20*(21), 1360–1364.
17. Stevens, D. L., Bisno, A. L., Chambers, H. F., Dellinger, P. E., Goldstein, E. J. C., Gorbach, S. L., et al. (2014). 2014 update by the Infectious Diseases Society of America. *Clinical Infectious Diseases*, *59*(2), e10–e52.
18. O'Meara, S., Cullum, N., Nelson, E. A., & Dumville, J. C. (2012). Compression for venous leg ulcers. *Cochrane Database of Systematic Review*, (11), CD000265, doi:10.1002/14651858.CD000265.pub3.

Abdominal Pain

Mary E. Sullivan

Instructions

After reviewing the case study, please jot down your notes or preliminary answers in the spaces provided. When you are ready to submit your answers for grading and reflective expert feedback for evaluation, go to http://www.evolve.elsevier.com/DickAndButtaro/ to complete this case.

Cast Study Scenario/History of Present Illness

Mary Rose (M.R.), a 72-year-old woman, comes to the clinic today for a routine 3-month follow-up blood pressure check. She says she is taking her medications "mostly." She also states she "still doesn't know why she needs a blood pressure pill." She mentions to the nurse who does the intake that she had a "stomach bug" 2 weeks ago with mild abdominal pain and some "diarrhea and cramping," which seems to have resolved. The episode occurred after going to the movies with her daughter where she had the "movie theater" popcorn and a soft drink. She was fine when she went home, but felt crampy and ill the next day. She used Maalox and noted an increase in gas production and had multiple bowel movements that got increasingly looser. She noted terrible cramping when she needed to "go" but felt some relief after emptying her bowels. She has not noted anything like this before. She "pretty much didn't eat for 3 days," then started on that "BRAT diet," and things got better.

Medications:
Coumadin 2.5 milligrams po daily
HCTZ (hydrochlorothiazide) 12.5 milligrams po daily (initiated 6 months ago)
Simvastatin 20 milligrams po daily
Vitamin D 2000 IU po daily,
Calcium 500 milligrams po daily
Fluticasone propionate 50 micrograms/spray 1 spray both nostrils daily prn
Oxybutynin 10 milligrams po daily
Triamcinolone (Kenalog) cream 0.1% applied to affected areas daily
Betamethasone (Diprolene) 0.05% topical ointment two to three times daily as needed

Allergies: Hay fever, Lisinopril causes a cough, and morphine caused her intractable vomiting when she had it after her bladder surgery.

Past medical history: Hypertension (HTN), hyperlipidemia, overactive bladder, psoriasis, and seasonal allergies. Deep vein thrombosis (DVT) diagnosed 2 months ago after taking a trip to Europe 8 weeks ago. Returned with left lower leg edema. A venous duplex revealed a clot in the left leg posterior tibial (distal) vein and she was started on warfarin (Coumadin) for 3 months. She has completed 2 months of therapy so far.

Social history: A widow, M.R. lives on the second floor of a senior community complex with elevator access, which she generally uses. Previous smoker: 1 pack per day (PPD) from age 21 to 35. She drinks one glass of wine nightly with dinner in the community dining room with other residents. Retired from her prior job as an administrative assistant to the president of a large contracting firm 5 years ago. She has three children, one daughter and two sons. Two of her children live nearby, and one son lives in Washington, DC and works for the

Secret Service. Her other son is an architect and travels for business frequently; thus she only sees him about "once a month." Her daughter lives in the next town, about a 10-minute ride, and she sees her multiple times a week. She describes her relationship with her daughter and her three grandchildren as very close.

Past surgical history: Tonsillectomy as a child, age 6; bladder suspension at age 63 for combined stress and urge incontinence.

Family history: Her parents are deceased: her father died at age 79 of prostate cancer, and her mother died at age 85 with past medical history of HTN, osteoporosis. M.R. was the youngest of five children, and three preceded her in death. Her oldest brother was killed in action during the Vietnam War. Her oldest sister died 3 years ago of heart failure. She also had chronic obstructive pulmonary disease (COPD) and was oxygen dependent when she died. "She smoked like a chimney." Her next oldest brother died of a heart attack. He had a lot of bowel trouble, and had a "bag," but that is not what killed him. Sister, age 68 with stage 4 breast cancer, currently on hormone therapy. She has a brother, age 65, with HTN and benign prostatic hypertrophy (BPH).

Review of Systems

General: Feels well today, denies fever/chills.

Skin: Has the usual expected psoriatic skin issues (psoriatic lesions) on knees and elbows.

Head, eyes, ears, nose, and throat (HEENT): Wears bifocals, eye examination up to date per patient. Sees dentist regularly and has native teeth.

Respiratory: Denies cough, wheezing, shortness of breath, or hemoptysis.

Cardiac: Denies chest pain, palpitations, weakness, or syncopal episodes.

Gastrointestinal (GI): Bowel pattern has returned to normal. Usual pattern is one formed stool in the morning after coffee. No return of abdominal pain, no previous episodes, denies nausea/vomiting.

Urinary: No incontinence since surgery and with oxybutynin, and does not require sanitary pad. Up to bathroom once a night.

Musculoskeletal: Some arthritis right hand, especially the thumb, knits to keep the joint loose.

Neurologic: Denies headache, dizziness.

Physical Examination

General: Well-appearing female, looks her stated age, pleasant and cooperative. No acute distress.

Vitals signs: Height 67 inches (170.8 cm), weight 180 pounds (81.8 kg). Blood pressure 168/72 right arm, 170/70 left arm. Heart rate 72, O_2 saturation 98%.

Skin: Warm and dry, raised plaque-like lesions that are erythematous, covered by silvery white scales noted on elbows, knees, and scalp. Skin turgor is fair.

Neck: Supple, no lymphadenopathy, no bruit, thyroid not palpable.

Respiratory: Clear to auscultation, no rales, wheezes, or rhonchi noted.

Cardiac: Regular rate, S1, S2, no S3 or S4, click noted, no murmurs, rubs, or gallops.

Abdomen: Soft, bowel sounds positive. Nondistended, nontender to palpation.

Extremities: Palpable pulses bilateral lower extremities (dorsalis pedis and posterior tibial 2+). No edema, erythema (with the exception of the erythematous skin patches on the knees bilaterally).

ASSESSMENT AND PLAN

1. Based on the history and physical examination results, what are M.R.'s problems that need to be addressed at today's visit?

2. Based on the history and physical examination results, what are the possible causes (differential diagnosis) for the patient's diarrhea complaint?

3. What components of the history and physical are missing?

4. What diagnostics should the health care provider consider necessary at this point in the patient's visit?

Case Study, Continued

With further questioning, M.R. provides more information. She has her blood drawn every Monday at the local Quest Diagnostics office, and the primary care office nurse calls her with her Coumadin instructions. She has been on the same dose of Coumadin 2.5 milligrams po daily for over a month now. She denies bleeding or bruising.

5. What is the length of anticoagulation for a distal deep vein thrombosis?[1,2]

6. How are patients monitored for deep vein thrombosis resolution?[1,2]

Case Study, Continued

M.R. further defines the "mostly" in taking her medications to mean that she missed some doses, and her daughter has been after her to find a way to remember to check that she has taken all her medications each day. She has been writing them down for the last 2 weeks and thinks that system may be the solution for her. She has not had any antibiotics for many years; the last time was when she had "bronchitis" before she retired.

She has no exercise routine except to walk through the entire grocery store when she does her own food shopping twice a week. She is on no specific diet and asks you to further explain why it matters. She uses a salt shaker on the table and only has wine at family events and holidays.

When questioned, she says that her brother had some kind of colon or rectal cancer and ended up with a "bag."

Her last colonoscopy was at age 68, and she was told that she had diverticulosis. She had a bone density when she was 70. Her last mammogram was 6 months ago and it was normal. She has already scheduled her annual mammogram in 7 months.

7. What additional diagnostics would the health care provider consider ordering based on the additional history that M.R. has provided?

8. What is the assessment and plan for each of M.R.'s problems?[3-7]

Basic Metabolic Panel Results

BMP	Patients Results	Reference Range
Sodium	136	136–145 mEq/L
Potassium	4.0	3.5–5.1 mEq/L
Carbon dioxide	25	23–29 mEq/L
Chloride	101	98–107 mEq/L
Glucose	98	74–100 milligrams/dL
Calcium	10.1	8.6–10.2 milligrams/dL
BUN	17	8–23 milligrams/dL
Creatinine	0.9	0.8–1.3 milligrams/dL

BMP, Basic metabolic panel; *BUN,* blood urea nitrogen.

Case Study, Continued

The patient returns in 3 weeks and reports that she feels well and has been taking the new dose of her medication. She is using the medication box and thinks that works very well. She has researched the DASH diet and has increased the frequency of fish in her diet, has limited herself to red meat once a week, and removed the salt shaker from her table at home. She also went shopping with her daughter and bought Mrs. Dash, the salt-free substitute. They are both reading labels, and M.R. decided to switch from canned vegetables to fresh or frozen ones. She has joined the "exercise group" at the community center and is walking for 20 minutes daily, using the "therapy" bands in the exercise group 3 times a week. She asks about seeing a dietician to be sure she is eating the right foods.

Review of System
    General: Feels well today.
    Skin: Psoriasis stable, daily use of topical medications.
    Respiratory: No cough, shortness of breath.
    Cardiac: No chest pain or other cardiac issue.
    Urinary: No episodes of stress or urge incontinence, no difficulties with exercise regimen, voiding every 2 to 3 hours to keep the bladder empty.
    GI: No bowel issues, soft formed stool daily, no further abdominal pain or diarrhea.

Physical Examination
    Vital signs: Blood pressure taken by you is 140/72 right arm and 142/72 left arm, heart rate is 72 and regular, respiratory rate is 18. Temperature 97.8°F. Oxygen saturation 98%. Weight 180 pounds (81.8 kg).
    Skin: Warm and dry, raised plaque-like lesions that are erythematous, covered by silvery white scales noted on elbows, knees, and scalp. Skin turgor is fair.
    Respiratory: Clear to auscultation, no rales, wheezes, or rhonchi noted.
    Cardiac: Regular rate, S1, S2, no S3 or S4, click noted, no murmurs, rubs, or gallops. Point of maximal impulse (PMI) noted to be at fifth intercostal space at the midclavicular line.
    Extremities: Palpable pulses bilateral lower extremities (dorsalis pedis and posterior tibial 2+) no edema, redness, or welling (with the exception of the erythematous skin patches noted on the knees bilaterally).

9. What is the current problem list and management plan?[2,4,5,8]

10. What consults, if any, are indicated for M.R. today?

11. When should M.R. have the next follow-up with the primary care provider?

Case Study, Continued

Three weeks later M.R. calls the office stating, "I have had terrible abdominal pain since yesterday. I have no appetite and have 'terrible pain' in the left side. It even hurts when I pee! She comes into the office for emergent evaluation and notes no recent sick contacts.

12.   What are the priorities for M.R. at this visit?

Case Study, Continued

M.R. states she woke up yesterday morning with abdominal cramping on her left side. She moved her bowels and felt some relief. Then she only had some tea and toast for breakfast and felt nauseous after eating so she limited herself to liquids. She has had three cups of tea since yesterday morning and was up most of the night with terrible pain on the left lower side of her abdomen. She now feels constipated and has trouble voiding. She notes her urine is very dark yellow. She describes no fever that she is aware of, but she did not check it. She describes no chills and states that she has not been near anyone who is ill.

Physical Examination

General: Ill-appearing, pale female.

Skin: Hot and dry, psoriatic patches unchanged, skin tenting consistent with poor skin turgor.

Vital signs: Height 67 inches (170.8 cm). Weight 179 pounds (81.3 kg). Blood pressure 155/72 right arm, 150/70 left arm. Heart rate 104, temperature 98.7°F. O_2 saturation 98%.

Respiratory: Clear to auscultation without adventitious sounds.

Cardiac: Regular rhythm, tachycardic, S1, S2, no S3 or S4, no murmurs, rubs, or gallops.

Abdominal examination: Nondistended, exquisitely tender left lower quadrant (LLQ), no rebound tenderness, no palpable masses or defect.

Rectal examination: Noted positive for tenderness, no masses palpable.

13.   What other history or physical information is needed to manage this patient?

14.   Based on M.R.'s history and physical examination findings, what are the possible causes (differential diagnosis) for the patient's current condition?[9]

15.   What diagnostics are necessary for this patient at this time?[4,5,10]

Case Study, Continued

The laboratory results return and the CBC reveals the following.

Basic Metabolic Panel

Laboratory Test	Laboratory Values
Sodium	144 mEq/L
Potassium	3.9 mEq/L
Chloride	110 mEq/L
Carbon dioxide	28 mEq/L
BUN	30 milligrams/dL
Cre (creatinine)	1.0 milligrams/dL
Glucose	109 milligrams/dL
Calcium	8.9 milligrams/dL
White blood count	11.2
RBC	5.9
Hgb	15.9
Hct	48
Neutrophils	74
Bands	3
Eosinophils	4
Basophils	1
Monocytes	3
Lymphocytes	18

BUN, Blood urea nitrogen; *Cre,* creatinine; *Hct,* hematocrit; *Hgb,* hemoglobin; *RBC,* red blood cell.

Urinalysis

Test	Value
Color	Yellow
Clarity	Clear
Specific gravity	1.020
pH	4.8
Glucose	Negative
Ketones	Trace
Protein	Negative
Urobilinogen	0.2
Blood	Negative
Nitrate	Negative
Leukocyte esterase	Negative

16.   Based on M.R.'s history and physical examination findings, plus the results of her laboratory tests, what differential diagnoses can be eliminated and why?

17.   The health care provider determines that this is a case of diverticulitis. What are the next steps?[4,5]

Case Study, Continued

M.R. presents to sick call 2 days later and now has fever (100.2°F), nausea, increased abdominal pain, and rebound tenderness. The health care provider sends M.R. to the local hospital for emergent evaluation and hydration. She is found to have a significant leukocytosis (14,000) with a neutrophilia, which is common with acute diverticulitis. Leukocytosis can occur with ischemic colitis, diverticulitis, gastroenteritis, or C. difficile colitis and does not discriminate between these diagnoses. She is admitted for intravenous (IV) hydration, given nothing by mouth (NPO), started on IV fluids, and a surgical consult was obtained for her abdominal pain. The surgeon ordered a computed tomography (CT) scan to further assess her abdomen and pelvis for differentiation of the etiology of her abdominal discomfort. Ischemic colitis, diverticulitis, and C. difficile colitis will have different findings on a CT scan. A CT scan is obtained, and the results print off the fax machine in the health care provider's office.

18.   What treatment plan is indicated based on the interpretation of this computed tomography report?

19. This computed tomography scan report shows no fat stranding, perforation, free air, or phlegmon, which indicate that the treatment plan for this episode of diverticulitis does not require surgery. What is the current treatment strategy for diverticulitis at this degree: fever, nausea, pain, dehydration, and constipation?[4,5,11]

Case Study, Continued

M.R. responds to IV fluid and antibiotics (she is treated with metronidazole 1 gram IV every 12 hours and ciprofloxacin 400 milligrams IV every 12 hours) and is pain free in 3 days. She is advanced to a clear liquid diet and oral antibiotics (metronidazole 500 milligrams po three times daily and ciprofloxacin 750 milligrams po every 12 hours for a total of 10 days of antibiotic treatment) and discharged home with follow-up in 1 week with your office.

20. What is the standard length of treatment for diverticulitis and why?[5,10]

Case Study, Continued

During her hospital stay M.R.'s Coumadin was held and she was managed on low-molecular-weight heparin. She has been restarted on her Coumadin with a Lovenox bridge and home care for INR laboratory draws by the visiting nurses.

21. How is an enoxaparin (Lovenox) bridge managed?[1,12]

ONE WEEK LATER

M.R. presents to the clinic for her posthospitalization visit accompanied by her daughter. She states that she is much better. She is eating three low-residue meals daily and has started to "walk outside for 10 minutes at a time." She has been staying with her daughter and has another 5 days of antibiotics left and is taking them as directed. She is eager to "begin to eat more normal food" and return to her home and says she has many questions since being in the hospital. She first asks if she will need to be on Coumadin for the rest of her life. She brings with her a printout from the visiting nurse with her daily INR. Noted on the paper is that her INR was 2.5 yesterday and her Lovenox was discontinued yesterday morning.

M.R. also asks if you think that her increase in blood pressure was caused by her recent bowel illness and finally how will she manage this "diverticular thing" long term.

Review of Systems

General: Feels well, diet history for last 24 hours was a scrambled egg with white toast and coffee for breakfast; a turkey sandwich with peaches for lunch; and chicken, white rice, and green beans for dinner.

Skin: Continues with topical agents. Noticed a flare starting since returning home from hospital, with red and angry patches on her elbows extending to her forearms. Patient notes increase in the itching.

Respiratory: No cough, wheeze.

Cardiac: No chest pain, palpitations, weakness.

Physical Examination

Vital signs: Temperature 98.4°F. Heart rate 72, pulse oximetry 99%. Blood pressure right arm 148/70, left arm 146/68, no orthostatic changes. Weight 177 pounds (76.9 kg).

Respiratory: Lungs clear to auscultation.

Cardiac: Regular rate and rhythms, S1 and S2, no S3, S4. No murmurs or gallops.

Abdominal: Soft, bowel sounds normoactive in all four quadrants. Nontender, no rebound.

Extremities: No edema or calf tenderness. Palpable pulses. Dorsalis pedis and posterior tibial pulses 2+. Increase in erythema and patches on her bilateral arms extending from elbow to forearm, scabbing caused by scratching is noted.

22. What are the priorities for this visit?[1]

23. What is the rationale for a low-residue diet for 3 weeks and then transitioning to a high-fiber diet after a diverticulitis episode?

24. The health care provider also discusses consulting the gastroenterologist for a colonoscopy. Why would the provider counsel M.R. that she will need a colonoscopy in 6 weeks?[4,5]

25. What other recommendations are important for the health care provider to discuss with M.R. and her daughter today?[4,5,10]

26. What is the role of probiotics and active yeast culture in preventing *C. difficile* associated diarrhea in adults?[13]

27. If M.R.'s lower extremity ultrasound is negative, can Coumadin be suddenly stopped or should it be tapered?[1,10]

28. How do health care providers manage a colonoscopy with a patient who is on Coumadin?[1,10,14]

29. When should a follow-up appointment be scheduled for M.R.? Why is further follow-up indicated?

Case Study, Continued

M.R. returns in 4 weeks and reports that she has been busy. She had her venous duplex scan and they "wouldn't give her the results." She had her colonoscopy and was told "things were okay." She describes improvement in her skin and is eager to "stop that blood medicine." She has returned to her walking and exercise program at the community center, is continuing to see the nutritionist, and has "lost 5 pounds." She reports no incontinence and describes a formed stool daily. She has been taking her medications daily using a medication box and feels "great."

You consult her record and see that her lower extremity venous duplex was normal with resolution of the thrombus. Her colonoscopy report is also available and revealed the presence of diverticulosis in the sigmoid colon with no evidence of diverticulitis and no polyps.

Review of Systems

As previously shown. She offers no further information on questioning.

Physical Examination

General appearance: Patient looks well.

Vital signs: Heart rate 74. Temperature 98.2°F. Pulse oximetry 99%. Blood pressure right arm 140/68, left arm 142/64. Weight 176 pounds.

Respiratory: Lungs clear to auscultation. No wheezes, rales, or rhonchi.

Cardiac: Regular rate and rhythm. S1, S2. No S3, S4. No murmurs or rubs.

Abdominal: Soft, bowel sounds positive, normoactive all four quadrants. No organomegaly or tenderness. No rebound.

Extremities: No edema. Palpable pulses. Dorsalis pedis and posterior tibial pulses 2+. Improvement in the affected areas of her skin, minimal erythema, and scant patches on her bilateral arms extending from elbow to forearm.

30. What is the plan for management at today's visit?

31. **What is the plan for follow-up?**

Case Study, Continued

She returns in 3 months and reports that "she is fine NOW." You ask for clarification and she tells you that she had another episode! When questioned further, she tells you that she again went to the movies with her daughter and had popcorn. She thought she would be fine, because she read in the paperwork from the hospital when she had her diverticulitis that seeds and nuts were not an issue. She tells you that she had a repeat episode of the abdominal pain, with no fever or chills. She had some diarrhea and then constipation and immediately switched to a liquid diet. She says it resolved in 48 hours so she did not call and just put herself back on the low-fiber foods. She says she is "back to normal" now and back on her high-fiber foods.

    Review of systems: She is taking her medicine using her medication box and has not missed any doses. She continues in her exercise group at the community center and is active. She offers no other complaints. She has had no swelling in her legs.

    Physical examination: Well-groomed older female in no acute distress. Heart rate 82. Temperature 98.6°F. Pulse oximetry 99%. Blood pressure right arm 138/68, left arm 140/64. No orthostatic blood pressure changes. Weight 175 pounds.

32. **What is the plan for management today?**

33. What ongoing issues will be the focus of future visits?

ONLINE ANSWER SUBMISSION

When you are ready to submit your answers for grading and reflective expert feedback for evaluation, go to http://www.evolve.elsevier.com/DickAndButtaro/ to complete this case.

References

1. Lip, G., & Hull, R. Overview of the treatment of lower extremity deep vein thrombosis. In T. W. Post (Ed.), UpToDate. Waltham, MA: UpToDate.
2. Wigle, P., Hein, B., Bloomfield, H., Tubb, M., & Doherty, M. (2013). Updated guidelines on outpatient anticoagulation. *American Family Physician, 87*(8), 556–566.
3. James, P. A., Oparil, S., Carter, B. L., Cushman, W. C., Dennison-Himmelfarb, C., Handler, J., et al. (2014). 2014 evidence-based guideline for the management of high blood pressure in adults: report from the panel members appointed to the eighth joint national committee (JNC 8). *JAMA: The Journal of the American Medical Association, 311*(5), 507–520.
4. Glass, C. (2016). Gastrointestinal disorders. In J. Cash & C. Glass (Eds.), *Adult-gerontology practice guidelines* (pp. 311–313). New York: Springer Publishing Company.
5. Wilkins, T., Embry, K., & George, R. (2013). Diagnosis and management of acute diverticulitis. *American Family Physician, 87*(9), 612–620.
6. Pardasani, A., Feldman, S., & Clark, A. (2000). Treatment of psoriasis: an algorithm-based approach for primary care physicians. *American Family Physician, 61*(3), 725–733.
7. Uphold, C., & Graham, M. (2013). Dyslipidemia. In C. Uphold & M. Graham (Eds.), *Clinical guidelines in family practice* (5th ed., pp. 539–551). Gainesville, FL: Barmarrae Books.
8. U.S. Department of Health and Human Services and U.S. Department of Agriculture. (2015). 2015–2020 Dietary Guidelines for Americans. Retrieved from https://health.gov/dietaryguidelines/2015/guidelines/.
9. Bickley, L., & Szilagyi, P. G. (2016). *Bates' guide to physical assessment and history taking* (12th ed.). Philadelphia, PA: Lippincott Williams, & Wilkins.
10. Hall, M. (2017). Diverticular disease. In T. Buttaro, J. Trybulski, P. Polgar, P. Bailey, & J. Sandberg-Cook (Eds.), *Primary care: A collaborative practice* (5th ed., pp. 657–663). St. Louis, MO: Elsevier.
11. Shabanzadeh, D. M., & Wille-Jorgensen, P. (2012). *Antibiotics for uncomplicated diverticulitis (review). Cochrane library, Cochrane database of systematic reviews.* John Wiley & Sons Ltd.
12. Lip, G., & Douketis, J. Perioperative management of patients receiving anticoagulants. In T. W. Post (Ed.), UpToDate. Waltham, MA: UpToDate.
13. Boyanova, L., & Mitov, I. (2012). Co-administration of probiotics with antibiotics: Why, when and for how long? *Expert Review of Anti-infective Therapy, 10*(4), 407–409.
14. Daley, B., Taylor, D., & Goicolea, J. (2016). Perioperative anticoagulation management. Medscape, March 28, 2016. Retrieved from https://emedicine.medscape.com/article/285265-overview.

Burning When Urinating

Cathleen Crowley-Koschnitzki

Instructions

After reviewing the case study, please jot down your notes or preliminary answers in the spaces provided. When you are ready to submit your answers for grading and reflective expert feedback for evaluation, go to http://www.evolve.elsevier.com/DickAndButtaro/ to complete this case.

Case Study Scenario/History of Present Illness

- *64-year-old Hispanic female, divorced, lives alone.*
- *Primary problem: Burning with urination for past 3 days with perineal discomfort, frequency.*
- *Comorbidities: Hypertension, type 2 diabetes mellitus (DM).*
- *Care settings: Primary care, urgent care.*

Aria Hernandez is a 64-year-old divorced female who presents to the urgent care setting with complaints of urinary symptoms over the past 3 days. She states she has burning with urination and some perineal discomfort. She also describes mild frequency. She denies pelvic or back pain, and states there is "no itching." She denies seeing blood in her urine, but she adds that she has noted a slight odor since the onset of symptoms. She reports she used to get urinary tract infections(UTIs) quite frequently when she was younger, but states it has been a while since her last urinary infection. She has not taken any over-the-counter medications, but she has been drinking cranberry juice and increased her water intake to eight glasses of water a day, but her symptoms have not decreased.

Medications: Lisinopril 40 milligrams po daily, metformin (Glucophage) ER 500 milligrams po twice a day, multivitamin, CoQ10, and glucosamine.

Allergies: Penicillin (history of rash).

Past medical history: Hypertension, type 2 DM.

Past surgical history: Appendectomy, cholecystectomy, cesarean section × 2, partial hysterectomy at age 42 for heavy uterine bleeding.

Social history: Divorced, one daughter and one son. Currently lives alone. High school graduate. Works full time as a bank teller. Social: She likes to go out with her friends each week. Sexually active, not currently in a monogamous relationship. Habits: Does not smoke, drinks alcohol socially on the weekends. Walks two to three times per week for 30 minutes.

Family history: Grandparent history: All died of old age. Father died from blood sugar problems age 60. Mother died age 72, stroke. Five brothers and sisters, all living. All have hypertension and blood sugar problems.

Review of Systems

General: Reports overall good health. Denies fever, chills, weight loss, confusion, or dizziness.

Skin: Denies rashes or lesions.

Head, eyes, ears, nose, and throat (HEENT): Denies headache, sinus pain, nasal congestion, or sore throat.

Neck: Denies neck pain.

Respiratory: No shortness of breath, no cough.

475

Cardiac: Denies chest pressure, pain, or palpitations.

Gastrointestinal: No difficulty swallowing, no nausea, indigestion, constipation, or diarrhea.

Urinary: As listed previously.

Gynecologic: Hysterectomy 12 years ago, no complaints. Last Pap 3 years ago, no history of abnormal Pap smear. No vaginal bleeding or discharge reported

Musculoskeletal: Denies muscle aches or joint pain, no joint swelling.

Peripheral vascular: Denies swollen legs, calf pain.

Neurovascular: No tingling, pain in hands or feet.

Hematologic: Denies bruising, bleeding gums.

Endocrine: Denies low blood sugar symptoms, denies increased thirst.

Psychiatric: Denies anxiety, depression.

Physical Examination

General: Hispanic female. Appears to be her stated age and in no acute distress. Alert and oriented to person, place, time, and situation.

Vital signs: Height 62.5 inches. Weight 145 pounds. Body mass index (BMI) 26.1. Temperature 98.8°F. Blood pressure 124/82. Heart rate 84 regular. Respiratory rate 16 at rest. O_2 saturation on room air 97% at rest.

Neurologic: Thoughts coherent. Gait smooth, coordinated. No fasciculations or tremors.

Skin: Warm/dry. No jaundice, rash, or acute lesions.

Eyes: Sclera clear; conjunctiva, no injection.

Ears: Pinna and tragus nontender. Auditory canals clear. Tympanic membranes (TMs) pearly gray and intact, no erythema, bulging/retraction.

Nares: Patent bilaterally without exudate. No sinus tenderness.

Oropharynx: Membranes moist, no lesions, or exudate. Tonsils bilateral, no enlargement or exudate. Teeth in fair repair, no cavities noted.

Neck: Supple. No masses, lymphadenopathy noted. Thyroid midline, small and firm without tenderness or palpable masses.

Cardiac: Heart S1 and S2, regular. No S3, S4. No murmurs or rubs noted.

Respiratory: Lungs clear to auscultation. No rales, wheezes, or rhonchi.

Abdomen: Round, soft, bowel sounds positive all four quadrants. +suprapubic tenderness noted on palpation. No costovertebral angle tenderness. No organomegaly.

Gynecologic: Deferred at this time.

Extremities: Pedal pulses present bilaterally, no edema or calf tenderness.

Urine dip: Positive leukocyte esterase: Small. Positive nitrites. Small blood. Trace protein, pH 7.0, specific gravity 1.020, negative ketones, and negative glucose.

1. Based on the history and physical examination results, what are the possible causes (differential diagnosis) of this patient's discomfort?[1,3-7]

2. What criteria are needed for a diagnosis of a urinary tract infection?[8,9]

3. What is the presumptive diagnosis for Mrs. H.?[2,10]

4. Why are postmenopausal women more susceptible to urinary tract infections?[4,11]

5.   What are the American Geriatrics Society criteria related to treatment of bacteriuria?[11-13]

6.   What are the three most common pathogens responsible for urinary tract infections?[10]

7.   What are the preferred treatment options and necessary patient education for uncomplicated urinary tract infection in an older female?[2,7,10,12]

8.   Under what circumstances would TMP-SMX be contraindicated, especially in older adults?[14]

9.   The patient returns to the office in 3 weeks and reports that the urinary symptoms have returned. What approach should the health care provider now take in determining the cause of Mrs. H.'s symptoms?

Physical Examination

   General: Hispanic woman, appears stated age in no acute distress. Alert and oriented to person, place, time, and situation.

   Vital signs: Height 62.5 inches. Weight 144 pounds. BMI 26.1. Temperature 98.6°F. Blood pressure 128/80. Heart rate 84 regular, respiratory rate 16 at rest, O_2 saturation on room air 98% at rest.

   Neurologic: Thoughts coherent. Gait smooth, coordinated.

   Skin: Warm/dry. No jaundice, rash, or acute lesions.

   Cardiac: Heart S1 and S2 regular, no murmurs or noted rubs.

   Respiratory: Lungs clear to auscultation. No rales, wheezes, or rhonchi.

Abdomen: Round, soft, bowel sounds positive all four quadrants. Mild suprapubic tenderness noted on palpation. No other abdominal tenderness, organomegaly, or costovertebral angle tenderness (CVAT) noted.

Gynecologic. Sparse pubic hair noted. Vulva without erythema or excoriation. No external genital lesions noted. Atrophied labia majora and labia minora. Urethra without swelling or discharge noted. Bartholin glands nontender, no enlargement bilaterally. Vaginal tissue or slightly dry, thin, and no rugae noted. No evidence of uterine prolapse. The cervix is pink, midline, and smooth without excoriation. Parous os. Secretions cloudy, thick, and stringy without odor. Bimanual examination: No pain with cervical palpation. Uterus and ovaries not palpated. No abdominal or pelvic tenderness noted.

10.   Based on the patient's physical examination results, what diagnostic testing should be considered?

Case Study, Continued

Laboratory test results: Urine straw colored. Urine dip shows small leukocyte esterase. Positive nitrites. Small blood. Trace protein, pH 7.0, specific gravity 1.020, negative ketones, and negative glucose.

11.   Based on today's examination, what are the differential diagnoses that the health care provider should consider? What, if any, diagnostic testing and/or treatment is necessary at this time for Mrs. H.?

12.   Is this second diagnosis of urinary tract infection considered a chronic or recurrent infection?[2,15,16]

13.   What should the management plan now include for Mrs. H.?[7,10,16,17]

14.   What is the appropriate treatment for atrophic vaginitis?[3,4,12]

15. Now that Mrs. H. is treated for her chief complaint, what health maintenance issues should be addressed as part of routine health care?[2,10,18-26]

ONLINE ANSWER SUBMISSION

When you are ready to submit your answers for grading and reflective expert feedback for evaluation, go to http://www.evolve.elsevier.com/DickAndButtaro/ to complete this case.

References

1. Yu, S., Fu, A. Z., Qiu, Y., Engel, S. S., Shankar, R., Brodovicz, K. G., et al. (2014). Disease burden of urinary tract infections among type 2 diabetes mellitus patients in the U.S. *Journal of Diabetes and Its Complications, 28*, 621–626.
2. Sharma, S., Govind, B., Naidu, S. K., Kinjarapu, S., & Rasool, M. (2017). Clinical and laboratory profile of urinary tract infections in type 2 diabetics aged over 60 years. *Journal of Clinical and Diagnostic Research, 11*(4), OC25–OC28.
3. Kennedy-Malone, L., Fletcher, K., & Martin-Plank, L. (2014). *Advanced practice nursing in the care of older adults.* Philadelphia PA: F.A. Davis Company.
4. Pearson, T. (2011). Atrophic vaginitis. *The Journal for Nurse Practitioners: 7*(6), 502–512.
5. Beaulaurier, R., Fortuna, K., Lind, D., & Emlet, C. (2014). Attitudes and stereotypes regarding older women and HIV risk. *The Journal for Nurse Practitioners: 26*, 351–368.
6. Quinn, M. (2015). Let's talk about sex… and senior citizens. Retrieved from http://www.governing.com/topics/health-human-services/gov-std-senior-citizens-nursing-homes-sex.html.
7. Lee, K. C., Chowdhury, J., Lefevre, M. L., & Myers, D. S. (2016). Sexually transmitted infections: Recommendations from the U.S. Preventive Services Task Force. *American Family Physician, 94*(11), 907–915.
8. Fünfstück, R., Nicolle, L. E., Hanefeld, M., & Naber, K. G. (2012). Urinary tract infection in patients with diabetes mellitus. *Clinical Nephrology, 77*(1), 40–48.
9. Simati, B., Kreigsman, W., & Safranek, S. (2013). Dipstick urinalysis for the diagnosis of acute UTI. *American Family Physician, 87*(10). Retrieved from http://www.aafp.org/afp/2013/0515/od2.html.
10. Capriotti, T. M., & Frizzell, J. P. (2016). *Pathophysiology: Introductory concepts and clinical perspectives.* Philadelphia, PA: F.A. Davis Company.
11. AGS Choose Wisely Workgroup. (2013). American Geriatrics Society identifies five things that healthcare providers and patients should question. *Journal of the American Geriatrics Society, 61*(4), 622–631.
12. Reuben, D. B., Herr, K. A., Pacala, J. T., Pollock, B. G., Potter, J. F., & Semla, T. P. (2016). *Geriatrics at your fingertips* (18th ed.). New York: The American Geriatrics Society.
13. Matsumoto, E., & Carlson, J. R. (2017). Diagnosis and treatment of urinary tract infection: A case-based mini review. *Consultant, 464–467.*
14. Paauw, D. (2017). Six common but underrecognized drug interactions and adverse effects. *Consultant, 454–457.*

15. Nosseir, S. B., Lind, L. R., & Winkler, H. (2012). Recurrent uncomplicated urinary tract infections in women: A review. *Journal of Women's Health*, *21*(3), 347–354.

16. Arnold, J. J., Hehn, L. E., & Klein, D. A. (2016). Common questions about recurrent urinary tract infections in women. *American Family Physician*, *93*(7), 560–569.

17. Corbett, J. V., & Banks, A. (2013). *Laboratory tests and diagnostic procedures with nursing diagnoses* (8th ed.). Boston: Pearson.

18. Kane, R. L., Ouslander, J. G., Abrass, I. B., & Resnick, B. (2013). *Essentials of clinical geriatrics*. New York: McGraw Hill.

19. Center for Disease Control and Prevention. (2017). Adult immunization schedule. Retrieved from https://www.cdc.gov/vaccines/schedules/hcp/imz/adult.html.

20. Croswell, J., & Owings, J. (2016). Screening for breast cancer. *American Family Physician*, *94*(2), 143–144.

21. American Cancer Society. (2017). American Cancer Society recommendations for colorectal cancer early detection. Retrieved from https://www.cancer.org/cancer/colon-rectal-cancer/detection-diagnosis-staging/acs-recommendations.html.

22. American Family Physician. (2012). U.S. Preventive services task force: Screening for osteoporosis: Recommendation statement. *American Family Physician*, *83*(10), 1197–2000.

23. Kato, E., & Beswick-Escanlar, V. (2016). Screening for depression in adults. *American Family Physician*, *94*(4), 305–306.

24. Bajracharya, P., Summers, L., Amatya, A. K., & DeBliek, C. (2016). Implementation of a depression screening protocol and tools to improve screening for depression in patients with diabetes in the primary care setting. *The Journal for Nurse Practitioners: 12*(10), 690–696.

25. McCrudden, J. G. Z., & Hull, B. J. (2015). A practitioner's simple mnemonic for managing diabetes: "GLUCOSE BAD". *The Journal for Nurse Practitioners: 11*(4), 451–455.

26. Bhatt, H. B., & Smith, R. J. (2015). Fatty liver disease in diabetes mellitus. *Hepatobiliary Surgery and Nutrition*, *4*(2), 101–108.

PRACTICE CASE STUDY **11**

Painful Swallowing

Rebecca R. Hill

Instructions

After reviewing the case study, please jot down your notes or preliminary answers in the spaces provided. When you are ready to submit your answers for grading and reflective expert feedback for evaluation, go to http://www.evolve.elsevier.com/DickAndButtaro/ to complete this case.

Case Study Scenario/History of Present Illness

S.M. is a 66-year-old Hispanic male who presents to the primary care office with complaints of altered taste and pain with swallowing for the past 4 days. He states he woke up feeling these symptoms on Monday morning, 4 days ago, after an uneventful prior evening and weekend. This is his first episode, and his symptoms have been relatively constant since onset and are slightly relieved with cool beverages. He does not report any aggravating factors. He has not taken any medications to relieve the symptoms. He denies recent illness or sick contacts, neck pain, swollen or tender lymph nodes, or any other associated symptoms. He rates the painful swallowing as a 4 on a 0 to 10 pain scale. It is pain while swallowing rather than difficulty swallowing that brings him to the office today. This is his first visit to this office; he relocated from out of state 4 months ago and has been receiving episodic care at medical walk-in clinics as needed for medication refills. His last visit to his out-of-state primary care physician (PCP) was more than 5 years ago for a physical examination.

- **Medications:** Zyrtec 10 milligrams daily as needed (prn), albuterol inhaler prn, and omeprazole 20 milligrams po daily.
- **Allergies:** No known drug allergies (NKDA).
- **Past medical history (PMH):** Seasonal allergies, asthma, and gastroesophageal reflux disease (GERD).
- **Past surgical history (PSH):** Tonsillectomy as child. Cholecystectomy 10 years ago.
- **Family history:** Mother died age 88 following cerebrovascular accident (CVA), history of hypertension (HTN), type 2 diabetes mellitus (DM II). Father died age 74 of end-stage renal disease on hemodialysis, coronary artery disease, DM II. One sister, age 62 alive and well. Three children: Son age 36, daughter age 30, and son age 28, all alive and well. Oldest son recently diagnosed with HTN.
- **Social history:** Married, 3 children, works as a car salesman in suburban neighborhood near his home. Lives with his wife and youngest son, age 28. Former 1 pack per day smoker, quit 7 years ago. Social alcohol (ETOH) use approximately 3 to 5 drinks a month. Denies illicit drug use.

Review of Systems

- **General:** Feels well aside from the previous chief complaint. Denies fevers, chills, weakness, and recent weight loss or gain. Reports feeling more fatigued in the past several weeks.
- **Skin:** Denies rashes, lesions, or hair loss.
- **Head, eyes, ears, nose, and throat (HEENT):** Denies headache, visual changes, ear drainage

484

or pain, nasal drainage, or sinus pain. Reports taste change with foods and dysphagia × 4 days. Denies neck pain, swollen lymph nodes, recent sore throat, or infection.

Respiratory: Denies shortness of breath, cough, wheezing, or hemoptysis.

Cardiac: Denies chest pain or palpitations.

Gastrointestinal (GI): Denies nausea/vomiting, abdominal pain.

Genitourinary (GU): Reports nocturia one to three episodes per night. Denies hematuria, dysuria, or urgency.

Musculoskeletal: Denies muscle weakness, pain, or injury.

Neurologic: Denies headaches, confusion, dizziness, or unsteady gait.

Physical Examination

General: Well-appearing, overweight male in no acute distress (NAD). Appears stated age, appropriately dressed for weather.

Vital signs: Height 70 inches. Weight 199 pounds. Blood pressure 158/78. Heart rate (HR) 78 regular, respiratory rate (RR) 18, O_2 saturation 97%. Body mass index (BMI) 30.3.

Skin: Warm, dry, without lesions or ecchymosis.

HEENT: Normocephalic, atraumatic. Pupils equal, round, reactive to light (PERRL), nasal turbinates pink without edema, erythema, or drainage. Tympanic membranes pearly gray with visible landmarks. Good dentition. Oral mucosa moist, erythematous, tonsils absent, white plaque noted on tongue and buccal mucosa. No jugular vein distention noted.

Respiratory: Lung sounds clear throughout. No rales, wheezes, or rhonchi.

Cardiac: S1 S2 regular rate and rhythm (RRR). No S3, S4, murmurs, rubs, or clicks.

Abdomen: Soft, round, nondistended, bowel sounds (BS) present × 4 quadrants, nontender. No organomegaly.

Extremities: Peripheral pulses 2+ bilaterally, no deformity, no edema.

Neurologic: Alert ad oriented × 3, sensation intact.

1. What additional history and/or physical examination information should be obtained?

Case Study, Continued

The patient states he smoked 1 pack per day for 22 years. His last chest x-ray was "about 5 years ago" and "normal" per the patient. The patient denies use of inhaled or oral glucocorticoids in the treatment of his asthma. He reports using his albuterol inhaler one to two times per week as needed for wheezing during his peak asthma symptoms with seasonal allergies. The patient denies headaches, erectile dysfunction, or visual changes and denies elevated blood pressures at past office visits.

Additional physical examination components should include:

- Inspection and palpation for lesions, edema, and erythema of skin.
- Eye examination.
- Assessment of lymph nodes.
- Thyroid palpation and auscultation for bruits.
- Determine presence of carotid bruits.
- Range of motion of the jaw should be tested.

Additional examination revealed no lesions, edema, or erythema noted of skin throughout. Lymph nodes were nonpalpable. The thyroid gland was nonpalpable without bruits. Ophthalmologic examination revealed + red reflex bilaterally, retina visible, vessels without arteriovenous (AV) nicking or copper wiring, optic disc with sharp and well-defined borders bilaterally. Full range of motion of temporomandibular joints bilaterally

2. Based on the history of present illness, review of systems, and physical examination, what are the differential diagnoses for this patient's chief complaint?

3. What diagnostics should be completed for this patient?

Case Study, Continued

The patient declined HIV testing, stating he does not believe he has been exposed because he has been in a monogamous relationship × 35 years. The patient is not currently fasting and will return to the laboratory for a fasting lipid panel within the next few days. Patient reports last laboratory testing "about 5 years ago" was within normal limits.

Complete Blood Count

Tests	Result	Flag	Units	Reference Interval	Lab
CBC With Differential/Platelet					
WBC	5.7		x10E3/uL	4.0–10.5	01
RBC	5.27		x10E6/uL	4.10–5.60	01
Hemoglobin	15.4		grams/dL	12.5–17.0	01
Hematocrit	44.1		%	36.0–50.0	01
MCV	84		fL	80–98	01
MCH	29.2		pg	27.0–34.0	01
MCHC	34.9		grams/dL	32.0–36.0	01
RDW	13.7		%	11.7–15.0	01
Platelets	268		x10E3/uL	140–415	01
Neutrophils	47		%	40–74	01
Lymphs	46		%	14–46	01
Monocytes	6		%	4–13	01
Eos	1		%	0–7	01
Basos	0		%	0–3	01
Neutrophils (Absolute)	2.6		x10E3/uL	1.8–7.8	01
Lymphs (Absolute)	2.6		x10E3/uL	0.7–4.5	01
Monocytes (Absolute)	0.4		x10E3/uL	0.1–1.0	01
Eos (Absolute)	0.1		x10E3/uL	0.0–0.4	01
Baso (Absolute)	0.0		x10E3/uL	0.0–0.2	01
Immature Granulocytes	0		%	0–1	01
Immature Grans (Abs)	0.0		x10E3/uL	0.0–0.1	01

Comprehensive Metabolic Panel

	Result	Flag	Units	Reference Interval	Lab
Glucose, random	247	**High**	milligrams/dL	70–99	01
BUN	16		milligrams/dL	5–26	01
Creatinine, Serum	1.06		milligrams/dL	0.76–1.27	01
eGFR	>59		mL/min/1.73	>59	01
BUN/Creatinine Ratio	15			8–27	01
Sodium, Serum	141		mmol/L	135–145	01
Potassium, Serum	4.4		mmol/L	3.5–5.2	01
Chloride, Serum	101		mmol/L	97–108	01
Carbon Dioxide, Total	23		mmol/L	20–32	01
Calcium, Serum	9.9		milligrams/dL	8.7–10.2	01
Protein, Total, Serum	7.6		grams/dL	6.0–8.5	01
Albumin, Serum	4.9		grams/dL	3.5–5.5	01
Globulin, Total	2.7		grams/dL	1.5–4.5	01
A/G Ratio	1.8			1.1–2.5	01
Bilirubin, Total	**1.8**	**High**	milligrams/dL	0.0–1.2	01
Alkaline Phosphatase, S	65		IU/L	25–150	01
AST (SGOT)	30		IU/L	0–40	01
ALT (SGPT)	32		IU/L	0–55	01
Hemoglobin A1C	10.5%	**High**		<7%	01

Gram stain with 10% KOH wet mount prep: Budding yeast with hyphae and pseudohyphae.

4. Based on the laboratory diagnostics, what is/are the likely diagnosis/diagnoses for this patient?

5. Based on history and physical examination findings, along with diagnostic testing, what differential diagnoses can be eliminated and why?

6. What is the most likely diagnosis and why?

7. What are the recommended treatments for this patient?[1,2]

Case Study, Continued

The patient does not want to begin insulin now. A second agent is added on with metformin. Based on current recommendations by the American Association of Clinical Endocrinologists (AACE)/American College of Endocrinology (ACE),[2] liraglutide (Victoza) 0.6 milligrams subcutaneously daily is prescribed. The patient is instructed to begin this medication at 0.6 milligrams and take it at the same time each day, increasing to 1.2 milligrams daily in 1 week. His Hgb A1C and renal function will be reevaluated in 3 months.

8. What are other second agent medications other than liraglutide that could be added to the metformin?[2]

9.   What additional patient teaching should be conducted based on the diagnoses?[2]

10.   What should the follow-up care include?

11.   Are any referrals necessary at this time?[2]

Case Study, Continued

One month after the initial visit, the patient presents to the primary care provider's office with complaints of urinary frequency, urgency, and dysuria for the past 3 days. He states complete resolution of taste alterations and pain with swallowing after a 10-day course of Nystatin swish and swallow. He reports taking all medications as prescribed without side/adverse effects. He has been checking his blood sugars every 2 to 3 days in the morning before breakfast and sometimes before dinner with the following results:

	Fasting	Before Dinner
Monday	180	150
Wednesday	205	—
Friday	175	—
Monday	201	172
Tuesday	206	—
Thursday	177	145
Sunday	164	—
Tuesday	178	—
Thursday	149	158
Friday	166	—

Random blood sugar in office is 192 milligrams/dL.
The patient completed his fasting lipid panel last week with the following results:

Tests	Result	Flag	Units	Reference Interval
VAP Cholesterol Profile				
Lipids				
LDL Cholesterol	185	High	milligrams/dL	<130
HDL Cholesterol	40		milligrams/dL	>=40
VLDL Cholesterol	34	High	milligrams/dL	<30
Cholesterol, Total	258	High	milligrams/dL	<200
Triglycerides	153	High	milligrams/dL	<150
Non HDL Chol. (LDL+VLDL)	219	High	milligrams/dL	<160
apoB100-calc	150	High	milligrams/dL	<109
LDL-R (Real)-C	142	High	milligrams/dL	<100
Lp (a) Cholesterol	8.0		milligrams/dL	<10
IDL Cholesterol	34	High	milligrams/dL	<20
Remnant Lipo.	55	High	milligrams/dL	<30
(IDL+VLDL3)				
Clinical Consideration				
Probable Metabolic Syndrome	NO			No
Sub-Class Information				
HDL-2 (Most Protective)	11		milligrams/dL	>10
HDL-3 (Less Protective)	29	low	milligrams/dL	>30
VLDL-3 (Small Remnant)	21	High	milligrams/dL	<10
LDL1 Pattern A	28.0		milligrams/dL	
LDL2 Pattern A	20.5		milligrams/dL	
LDL3 Pattern B	77.3		milligrams/dL	
LDL4 Pattern B	16.7		milligrams/dL	
LDL Density Pattern	B	Abnormal		A
	[——————*———] [———] [——————————]			
	Pattern B	Pattern		Pattern A
	Small, Dense LDL	A/B		Large Buoyant LDL

Review of Systems
    General: Feels well aside from the previous chief complaint. Denies weakness, recent weight loss or gain, and fatigue seems to be improving.
    Skin: Denies rashes or lesions.
    HEENT: Reports taste alterations and dysphagia have resolved.
    GI: Denies abdominal pain. Bowel movements (BMs) regular and unchanged.
    GU: Reports nocturia one to three episodes per night, new-onset dysuria, urgency, and frequency × 3 days. Denies hematuria or flank pain.
    Musculoskeletal: Denies muscle weakness or back pain.
    Neurologic: Denies headaches, confusion, dizziness, or unsteady gait.

Physical Examination
    General: Well-appearing, overweight male in NAD.
    Vital signs: Height 70 inches. Weight 197 pounds. Blood pressure 152/92, HR 74 regular, RR 18, O_2 saturation 98%. BMI 30.
    Skin: Warm, dry, without lesions or ecchymosis.
    HEENT: Normocephalic, atraumatic, PERRL. Oral mucosa moist without erythema or lesions.
    Respiratory: Lung sounds clear throughout. No rales, wheezes, or rhonchi.
    Cardiac: S1 S2 RRR. No S3, S4, murmurs, rubs, or clicks.
    Abdomen: Soft, round, nondistended, BS present × 4 quadrants.
    Male GU: Circumcised penis without discharge. Prostate round, symmetric, firm, nontender without masses.
    Extremities: Peripheral pulses 2+ bilaterally. No deformity, edema, or calf tenderness.

12. What additional history and/or physical examination information should be obtained at this visit?

Case Study, Continued

The patient denies fevers, chills, nausea, vomiting, or new sexual partners. The physical examination reveals a nontender abdomen, negative costovertebral angle tenderness bilaterally, and a nonpalpable, nontender bladder. The patient states he has been checking his blood sugar every few days, "when I remember," but he has not checked his blood pressure. He also reports that he has not yet begun an exercise regimen because of a stressful and hectic work schedule, but he has been sleeping well averaging about 7 to 9 hours per night. He has been attempting to decrease his intake of white bread, sugar, and salt, but has not been consistent with these dietary improvements. He has his first appointment with a nutritionist scheduled for next week. He has not completed a food diary, but plans to begin one tomorrow and present it to his visit with the nutritionist.

13. Based on the history of present illness, review of systems, and physical examination, what are the top differential diagnoses?

14. What diagnostics should be completed for this patient based on these data?

Urinalysis Results

Urinalysis—Complete	Result
Color	Yellow
Appearance	Hazy
Specific gravity	1.027
pH	6.5
Glucose	2+
Nitrite	2+
Protein	Negative
Ketones	Negative
Bilirubin	Negative
Occult blood	Negative
Leukocytes	4+
RBC	None
Bacteria	3+

RBC, Red blood cell.

15. What does a finding of glucosuria mean?[3]

16. What is the likely diagnosis?

17. Which differential diagnoses can be ruled out and why?

18. What are the recommended treatment regimens based on the previous data?[4]

19. What doses of atorvastatin and aspirin should be prescribed?[5,6]

20.   What other considerations regarding the plan of care would the provider consider?[9]

21.   What is the plan for follow-up?

Case Study, Continued

Two weeks later, the patient presents for a follow-up of his complicated UTI. Patient reports complete resolution of urinary symptoms. He feels well today and denies concerns. His blood glucose has been trending down per the blood glucose log provided by the patient. S.M. reports he has been taking all medications as prescribed and has not missed any doses. He reports slight muscle pain in his calves since beginning the atorvastatin, which seems to be improving in the past 2 days. The patient has not checked his blood pressure at home.

The results of the urine microalbumin and urine culture and sensitivity are as follows (*S*, sensitivity; *R*, resistance):

- Microalbumin: 45 milligrams (normal range is 30 milligrams or below)
- Urine Culture: *E. coli* greater than 100,000 organisms per milliliter
- Ampicillin $R \geq 32$
- Augmentin $S \leq 4$

- Cefotaxime   S ≤ 4
- Ceftriaxone   S ≤ 8
- Ciprofloxacin   S ≤ 32
- Doxycycline   R ≥ 16
- **Levofloxacin**   **S ≤ 32**
- Tetracycline   R ≥ 16
- Trimethoprim   S ≤ 32

Repeat urinalysis today in the office:

Urinalysis—Complete	
Color	Yellow
Appearance	Clear
Specific gravity	1.013
pH	7.0
Protein (Acid ppt)	Negative
Glucose-Strip	Negative
Ketones	Negative
Bilirubin	Negative
Occult blood	Negative
WBC/HPF	None
RBC/HPF	None
Casts/LPF	None observed

Home blood glucose log:

	Fasting	Before Lunch	Before Dinner
Monday	172	146	—
Tuesday	160	—	188
Friday	164	—	—
Sunday	154	—	172
Tuesday	150	133	—
Thursday	150	—	145
Saturday	148	156	—

Random blood sugar in office: 173 milligrams/dL

Review of Systems

General: Feels well, reports increased energy since completing antibiotic.
Skin: Denies rashes or lesions.
HEENT: Denies pain, dysphagia, or hoarseness.
GI: Denies nausea, vomiting, abdominal pain. BMs regular and unchanged.
GU: Reports nocturia 0 to 1 episodes per night. Denies dysuria, urgency, frequency, or hematuria.
Musculoskeletal: Denies muscle weakness, pain, or injury.
Neurologic: Denies headaches, confusion, dizziness, or unsteady gait.

Physical Examination

General: Well-appearing, overweight male in NAD.
Vital signs: Height 70 inches. Weight 195 pounds. Blood pressure 148/90, HR 68 regular, RR 16, O_2 saturation 98%. BMI 29.6.
Skin: Warm, dry, without lesions or ecchymosis.

HEENT: Normocephalic, atraumatic. Oral mucosa moist without erythema or lesions.
Respiratory: Lung sounds clear throughout.
Cardiac: S1 S2 RRR, no murmurs, rubs, or clicks.
Abdomen Soft, round, nondistended, nontender. BS present × 4 quadrants.
Extremities: No edema, peripheral pulses 2+ bilaterally, no deformities.

22. What other information should be ascertained at this time?

Case Study, Continued

S.M. reports that he has started walking to work when the weather permits, approximately 1 mile to and from work on 3 to 4 days of the week. After his visit with a nutritionist, his wife has made changes to meal preparations and grocery shopping, which has helped him make consistent dietary changes over the past week. He will see the nutritionist in 1 month to discuss additional strategies for improving his diet and learn how to read food labels.

23. Based on the previous data, what are the treatment recommendations?[7]

24. What other diagnostics should be completed for this patient now?[8]

25. What is the plan for follow-up?

References

1. Goroll, A. H., & Mulley, A. G. (2016). *Primary care medicine: Evaluation and management of the adult patient.* Philadelphia, PA: Wolters Kluwer.
2. American Association of Clinical Endocrinologists and American College of Endocrinology. (2015). Comprehensive diabetes management algorithm. *Endocrine Practice, 21*(1 Suppl.), S1–S87.
3. Bhimma, R. (2016). Renal glucosuria. Medscape. Retrieved from http://emedicine.medscape.com/article/983678-overview#a5.
4. Badalato, G., & Kauffman, M. (2016). Adult UTI. American Urological Association. https://www.auanet.org/education/adult-uti.cfm.

5. American Diabetes Association. (2016). Cardiovascular disease and risk management. *Diabetes Care*, *39*(Suppl. 1), S60–S71.
6. Armstrong, C. (2010). Updated recommendations on daily aspirin use in patients with diabetes. *American Family Physician*, *82*(12), 1559–1563.
7. Stone, N. J., Robinson, J. G., Lichtenstein, A. H. et al. (2014). 2013 ACC/AHA guideline on the treatment of blood cholesterol to reduce atherosclerotic cardiovascular risk in adults: A report of the American College of Cardiology/American Heart Association Task Force on Practice Guidelines. *Journal of the American College of Cardiology*, *63*(25 Pt B), 2889–2934.
8. Kibirige, D., & Mwebaze, R. (2013). Vitamin b12 deficiency among patients with diabetes mellitus: Is routine screening and supplementation justified. *Journal of Diabetes and Metabolic Disorders*, *12*(17).
9. James, P. A., Oparil, S., Carter, B. L., et al. (2014). 2014 evidence-based guideline for the management of high blood pressure in adults: report from the panel members appointed to the Eighth Joint National Committee (JNC 8). *JAMA*, Feb 5;311(5):507–520.

Advanced Case Studies

Painful Toe

Nancy S. Morris

Instructions

After reviewing the case study, please jot down your notes or preliminary answers in the spaces provided. When you are ready to submit your answers for grading and reflective expert feedback for evaluation, go to http://www.evolve.elsevier.com/DickAndButtaro/ to complete this case.

Case Study Scenario/History of Present Illness

A 76-year-old African American man called the clinic this morning requesting an urgent appointment for the severe pain he was experiencing in his foot. He walks cautiously into the examination room wearing an open-toe bedroom slipper on his right foot. As he settles into the chair in the examination room, he places his right foot gingerly on the floor in front of him and asks you right away, "Do you think I broke my toe?" He explains that he stubbed his toe on a hallway side-table 2 days ago when he got up during the night to use the bathroom but he did not think much of it at the time. Last night, his toe began to throb and he awoke frequently trying to get into a comfortable position. When he got up this morning, his big toe was reddened, swollen, and so painful he could not even put on a sock. He has never experienced anything like this before. He rates the pain as a 10/10 if anyone or anything touches his toe, but a 5/10 if he just sits still. The pain radiates along the medial side of his foot but does not involve the ankle or heel. He is most comfortable sitting with his bare foot resting on an ottoman. The pain is worse when he walks or if his foot is touched or bumped. He took 1000 milligrams of acetaminophen this morning, but it has not helped at all.

Medications: Acetaminophen 1000 milligrams po every 8 hours if needed for pain, atorvastatin 20 milligrams po daily, chlorthalidone 25milligrams po daily, lisinopril 30 milligrams po daily, and ranitidine 150 milligrams po daily.

Allergies: Erythromycin causes rash.

Habits: Former smoker with 15 pack-year history of tobacco use, quit at age 50; drinks 1 to 2 beers daily.

Past medical history: Gastroesophageal reflux disease (GERD), hyperlipidemia, hypertension (HTN), obesity, and knee osteoarthritis.

Past surgical history: Cholecystectomy, open reduction internal fixation (ORIF) right wrist fracture.

Family history: Father died age 82 after a stroke; mother died age 54 after a car accident.

Personal and social history: Married to his wife of 50 years with whom he lives; resides in his own home. Retired car salesman. Education: Associate's Degree. Independent with driving, plays golf weekly when able, and enjoys playing cards at the senior center weekly. Three adult children live within 30 minutes and visit regularly with their families.

Review of Systems

General: Feels well other than pain. Denies fever or chills.

Skin: Redness and swelling near right great toe noted this morning.

Head, eyes, ears, nose, and throat (HEENT): Denies headaches, change in vision, sinus or nasal symptoms, dysphagia, and sore throat. Hearing has been decreasing over the last several years.

Respiratory: Denies cough, wheeze, hemoptysis, and shortness of breath.

Cardiac: Denies chest pain, palpitations, and syncopal episodes.

Gastrointestinal: Denies nausea/vomiting. Has GERD managed with daily ranitidine and avoidance of aggravating foods. Moves bowels daily.

Urinary: Denies dysuria, hematuria. Has nocturia once nightly.

Musculoskeletal: Bilateral intermittent knee pain that responds to acetaminophen when pain worsens; has gone to physical therapy, which also helped.

Neurologic: Denies headache, dizziness.

Physical Examination

General: Older male, oriented and responding to questions appropriately. Distressed about degree of pain in right big toe.

Vital signs: Height 5 feet 9 inches (175.2 cm). Weight 210 pounds (95.5 kg). Body mass index (BMI) 31. Blood pressure (BP) 152/86 right arm. Heart rate 84 and regular. Respiratory rate 16 and regular, oxygen saturation 98%.

Skin: Dry, few scattered seborrheic keratosis on sides of his face.

Cardiac: Regular rate and rhythm; normal S1, S2 with no murmurs, gallops, or rubs.

Respiratory: Clear to auscultation. No rales, wheezes, or rhonchi.

Right foot: Small abrasion medial side of right foot. Erythema, increased warmth, and swelling proximal end of big toe and around metatarsophalangeal joint and across his forefoot. Tenderness with light palpation over metatarsophalangeal joint and with any movement of big toe. Trace ankle edema. No hair growth below midcalf. Pedal pulse 2+ (Fig. 12.1).

ASSESSMENT AND PLAN

1. Based on the history and physical examination results, what are the possible causes (differential diagnosis) for the patient's current condition?

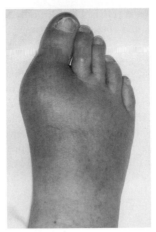

Fig. 12.1   Podagra or acute gout of the first metatarsophalangeal joint is shown. The hyperintense erythema with a dusky hue is characteristic. The area of inflammation usually extends beyond the region of the involved joint. (From Hochberg, M. C., Silman, A. J., Smolen, J. S., & Weisman, M. H. [2015]. *Rheumatology [6th ed.].* Philadelphia: Mosby.)

2.   What components of the history or physical examination are missing?

3. **What diagnostics are necessary for this patient at this time?**

Case Study, Continued

The patient provides more information on further questioning.
- *His father did get "pain in his feet," but he does not remember that a diagnosis of gout was ever made.*
- *Patient denies calf or lower leg pain in either leg. His knees ache often from the osteoarthritis but no change noted recently. Denies recent infections. No history of pedicures; he cuts his own toenails. No recall of recent splinter in foot, although he does walk out on his wooden deck in bare feet at times and has gotten splinters in the past.*
- *He has gained 8 pounds in the last year. Typical daily food intake includes oatmeal; two cups of coffee; two to three cola drinks; soup; fish (preference for shrimp or lobster) or beef; snacking on hard candy; green beans, broccoli, or corn; pasta, rice, or potatoes; and ice cream, cake, or cookies.*
- *Alcohol intake 1 to 2 beers daily and on occasion may have a third.*

Additional findings on examination include body temperature of 99.8°F. No swelling, redness, or warmth in right foot. Right foot with no lateral deviation or rotation of the big toe.

X-ray of right foot: + asymmetric swelling around first metatarsophalangeal joint, preserved joint spaces, no erosions, no lytic lesions, no tophi, and no fracture.

Four weeks ago creatinine was 1.3 and glomerular filtration rate (GFR) was 53.

4. **What additional diagnostics should the provider order based on this additional history?**

5. **What is your working diagnosis?**[1]

6. **What treatment would you recommend for this patient?**[1]

Case Study, Continued

The next day, the practitioner receives the results of the white blood cell (WBC) count, which showed mild leukocytosis. The next day the patient calls the office in the afternoon and says the pain is not letting up despite taking the acetaminophen and the antibiotic. His foot is still swollen and red in about the same spot it was when he saw you in the office. No fever and no chills. No increased swelling or redness.

As the practitioner rethinks the patient's presentation and reviews the possible differential diagnoses, gout comes back to the top of the list, especially because the patient has not responded to the antibiotic prescribed for presumptive cellulitis. A uric acid level is added to the patient's laboratory work and he is asked to return to the office in the morning for follow-up.

The patient returns the next day as requested, and his physical examination is essentially unchanged. His uric acid level is 8.2 milligrams/dL.

7.   What should the practitioner now consider to be the probable cause of this patient's toe pain?[2]

8.   What treatment recommendations are now appropriate for this patient?[3-10]

9. **What are your next steps?**[11]

Case Study, Continued

The patient returns in 10 days and reports that the pain decreased after 2 days once he started the prednisone. The swelling and redness are also gone. His BP today is 142/84 left arm and 140/82 right arm. Additional physical examination findings listed next.

Physical Examination

    Cardiac: Regular rate and rhythm, normal S1, S2 with no murmurs, gallops, or rubs.

    Respiratory: Clear to auscultation.

    Right foot: Skin intact, no erythema, no swelling, and no tenderness with palpation.

10. **What additional history would be helpful here?**

Case Study, Continued

The patient went back to having one to two beers daily once he finished the prednisone and was no longer having any pain. He only used acetaminophen for 1 day because the prednisone really helped the pain settle down quickly. He never used a cane. He is tolerating the new BP medication (losartan) with no side effects.

Further talk of purine-rich foods and alternative food options were discussed. He does not typically add salt to his food, but he eats some prepared foods that have high salt content. He cut back on his soda drinking, and he is willing to work on other dietary changes.

No specific symptoms of thyroid disease noted. Although his uric acid level was high, he is reluctant to consider taking any other medications daily and wants to see if it comes down after the change in BP medications (stopped the diuretic and started losartan). Agrees to have laboratory work to check thyroid-stimulating hormone (TSH). He is currently symptom free from a single gout attack. Scheduled to return in 3 months.

11. What are the priorities for the patient's next visit?

Case Study, Continued

Ten weeks later, the patient called the office and requested an urgent visit because he was experiencing another episode of pain, again in his right big toe. He had not been having any pain until it awoke him last night. He was unable to tolerate the blanket on his foot and came in the office wearing a sandal because it hurt too much to even put a sock on. He denied precipitating trauma, fever, or chills.

Although he made some dietary changes (decreased his intake of shrimp, lobster, and beef), he is back to drinking two colas daily and two beers daily. He has not made any significant progress with efforts to lose weight. He stopped the chlorthalidone and lisinopril and began losartan as suggested.

His laboratory work at last visit confirmed hypothyroidism (TSH was 11.4 mIU/L and free T_4 was 4 micrograms/dL), and he has been taking the levothyroxine daily as prescribed for 8 weeks now.

Physical Examination

General: Somewhat distressed about the recurrent pain in his right foot.

Vital signs: Height 5 feet 9 inches (175.2 cm). Weight 208 pounds (94.3 kg). BMI 31. BP 148/84 right arm. Temperature 98.8°F. Heart rate 86 and regular. Respiratory rate 16 and regular, oxygen saturation 99%.

Cardiac: Regular rate and rhythm; normal S1, S2 with no murmurs, gallops, or rubs.

Respiratory: Clear to auscultation.

Right foot: Redness, increased warmth, and swelling over metatarsophalangeal joint with swelling across the forefoot. Tenderness with palpation of the metatarsophalangeal joint. Worsening pain with motion of great toe. Skin intact. Trace ankle edema. Pedal pulse 2+.

12. Is there an indication for any diagnostic testing at this time?

13. What should the assessment and treatment plan include at this time?[3-8]

Case Study, Continued

This patient wants to avoid another daily medication if possible. He expresses interest in working on weight loss and decreasing his alcohol intake. He is referred to a dietician for guidance with weight loss and asked to reschedule a follow-up appointment in 3 months, or sooner if his symptoms recur or do not subside.

14. What are the priorities for the patient's next visit?

Case Study, Continued

Three months later the patient returns and reports no further gout attacks or pain in his foot. He has made some dietary changes and started walking 3 times a week. He is pleased to tell you he has lost 11 pounds, which he is happy about. He stopped drinking cola and is drinking flavored water instead. He has decreased his alcohol to one beer daily.

His TSH/T$_4$ at his last visit was TSH 4.2 mIU/L and free T$_4$ 5.2 micrograms/dL. He was continued at previous levothyroxine dose.

Last uric acid level remained high at 7.3 milligrams/dL.

Today his weight is 197 pounds, BMI 29. BP 140/78 in the left arm and 138/74 in the right arm.

Additional Physical Examination

Cardiac: Regular rate and rhythm, normal S1, S2 with no murmurs, gallops, or rubs.

Respiratory: Clear to auscultation.

Both feet: Skin intact, no erythema, no swelling, no tenderness with palpation, pedal pulses 2+ bilaterally.

15. What should the health care provider's assessment and treatment plan include at this visit?[3,5-8]

Case Study, Continued

The patient has not had any recurrent gout attacks and is reluctant to take another medication. He plans to continue decreasing his risk factors through weight loss and decreased alcohol use. You ask him to return again in 4 months to reassess BP and gout. He is to call sooner with any acute gout attacks.

Two months later the patient shows up at your office again with an acute gout attack, and this time it is his left great toe that is red and painful. He is requesting another prescription for prednisone. He denies precipitating trauma or infection.

He has lost 5 more pounds, has decreased his beef consumption to one time weekly, and has switched his fish intake to salmon or catfish. He continues to drink one beer almost every day. He is walking for 30 minutes three times a week.

Weight is 192 pounds, BMI is 28. BP is 138/82 right arm. Heart rate is 84 and regular. Respiratory rate 18 and unlabored. Temperature is 98.6°F.

16. What are the priorities for this visit?

17. What is the assessment and treatment plan for this patient now?[3-8]

Case Study, Continued

The patient responded well to prednisone again with complete alleviation of his symptoms in 3 days. He returns to your office 12 weeks later to review uric acid results and discuss options for decreasing frequency of gout attacks. His serum uric acid level is 7.2 milligrams/dL.

Patients with recurrent gout attacks are at risk for developing chronic arthritis and tophaceous disease given the high uric acid levels. Pharmacologic antiinflammatory prophylaxis is recommended with initiation of urate-lowering therapy to prevent acute attacks, which are a common occurrence with the start of urate-lowering drugs. Concurrent with uric acid-lowering therapy, the most recent American College of Rheumatology guidelines[4] recommended colchicine, low-dose NSAIDs, or, if the patient has intolerance, contraindication, or refractoriness to colchicine and NSAIDs, low-dose prednisone (≤10 milligrams/day) for a minimum of 8 weeks to 3 months if no tophi and achievement of target serum urate level <6 milligrams/dL or 6 months if previous tophi and target serum urate level reached. Allopurinol (300 milligrams/day) and febuxostat (40 milligrams/day) are equally effective at decreasing serum urate levels and reducing the risk for acute gout attacks after 12 months.[3] Potential side effects (e.g., rash, lowered WBC and platelet counts, diarrhea, fever with allopurinol and abdominal pain, diarrhea, and musculoskeletal pain with febuxostat) should be discussed.[3]

18.   What additional patient history would be helpful at this time?

Case Study, Continued

This patient has continued his efforts to avoid soda and decrease his meat and candy intake. He has switched from one to two beers daily to one glass of wine with dinner. Still walking for 30 minutes three times a week. He has pain in his knees from arthritis, but it responds to acetaminophen and does not bother him on a daily basis. He lives with his wife who reminds him about his medications if he forgets and he uses a "pill box," which he fills weekly. He is knowledgeable about taking an antiinflammatory medication at the first onset of a gout attack and asks about having some prednisone at home "just in case." Denies known history of being HLA-B*5801 positive and no family history of cutaneous reaction to allopurinol, which his brother and one uncle have taken.

Physical Examination
   Vital signs: Weight 194 pounds, BMI 28. BP 138/76 left arm. Heart rate 86 and regular. Respiratory rate 18 and unlabored.
   Cardiac: Regular rate and rhythm, normal S1, S2 with no murmurs, gallops, or rubs.

Respiratory: Clear to auscultation.

Musculoskeletal: No appreciable tophi at knees, ankles, or feet. Both knees with bony enlargement and slight valgus deformities. No quadriceps atrophy. No erythema or warmth over knee joints. Knees with crepitus and decreased flexion. 125 degrees bilaterally.

Feet: Skin intact, no bony deformities, no erythema, no swelling, no tenderness with palpation, and no pes planus. Full range of motion (dorsi/plantar flexion, inversion, and eversion). Pedal pulses 2+ bilaterally.

19. Are there any indications for any additional diagnostic testing at this time?

20. What are the priorities for this visit?[3]

21.   Describe the assessment and management plan or the patient's visit today.[3,6,12]

Case Study, Continued

Two years later, the patient has not had another gout attack. He is taking allopurinol 300 milligrams po daily. He has modified his diet to decrease meat and shellfish, has eliminated soda altogether, switched from beer to one glass of wine five times a week, and his weight has stabilized.

He asks today if he can stop the allopurinol.

His weight is 186 pounds, BMI 27. BP is 138/76 left arm. Heart rate is 84 and regular, and respiratory rate is 18 and unlabored. Results of laboratory work from last week are nonfasting glucose 95 milligrams/ dL, TSH 3.8 mIU/L, free T4 5 micrograms/dL, alanine transaminase (ALT) 46 U/L, aspartate trans-aminase (AST) 34 U/L, creatinine 1.6, GFR = 41, and uric acid level is 5.2 milligrams/dL.

Additional Focused Physical Examination

Cardiac: Regular rate and rhythm, normal S1, S2 with no murmurs, gallops, or rubs.

Respiratory: Clear to auscultation.

Musculoskeletal: No appreciable tophi at knees, ankles, or feet. Both knees with bony enlarge-ment and slight valgus deformities. No quadriceps atrophy. No erythema or warmth over knee joints. Knees with crepitus and decreased flexion ~120 degrees bilaterally.

Feet: Skin intact, no bony deformities, no erythema, no swelling, no tenderness with palpation, no pes planus. Full range of motion (dorsi/plantar flexion, inversion, and eversion). Pedal pulses 2+ bilaterally.

ASSESSMENT AND MANAGEMENT PLAN AT THIS VISIT

- Gout well controlled. Allopurinol therapy is typically lifelong. Uric acid level acceptable but with worsening renal function may want to consider lowering allopurinol dose to 200 milligrams po daily and recheck uric acid level in 3 to 4 weeks.
- Hypothyroidism is well controlled. Continue current levothyroxine dose.
- BP well controlled. Continue current losartan dose. Avoid adding salt to food.
- Review management of acute gout flare.
- Stage 3B chronic kidney disease. Monitor renal function every 6 months.
- Recognize and support weight loss efforts with goal of getting BMI to less than 25.

22.   What ongoing health care issues will be the focus of future visits?[3]

ONLINE ANSWER SUBMISSION

When you are ready to submit your answers for grading and reflective expert feedback for evaluation, go to http://www.evolve.elsevier.com/DickAndButtaro/ to complete this case.

References

1. Stevens, D. L., Bisno, A. L., Chambers, H. F., Dellinger, E. P., Goldstein, E. J. C., … Wate, J. C. (2014). Practice guidelines for the diagnosis and management of skin and soft tissue infections: 2014 update by the infectious diseases society of American. *Clinical Infectious Disease, 59*(2), e10–e52.
2. Janssens, H. J., Fransen, J., van de Lisdonk, E. H., van Riel, P. L., van Weel, C., & Janssen, M. (2010). A diagnostic rule for acute gouty arthritis in primary care without joint fluid analysis. *Archives of Internal Medicine, 170*(13), 1120–1126.
3. Qaseem, A., Harris, R. P., & Forciea, M. A. (2017). Management of acute and recurrent gout: A clinical practice guideline from the American College of Physicians. *Annals of Internal Medicine, 166*(1), 58–68.
4. Khanna, D., Khanna, P. P., FitzGerald, J. D., Singh, M., Bae, S., … Terkeltaub, R. (2012). 2012 American college of rheumatology guidelines for management of gout part II: Therapy and anti-inflammatory prophylaxis of acute gouty arthritis. *Arthritis Care and Research, 64*(10), 1447–1461.
5. Jamnik, J., Rehman, S., Mejia, S. B., de Souza, R. J., Khan, T. A., … Sievenpiper, J. L. (2016). Fructose intake and risk of gout and hyperuricemia: A systematic review and meta-analysis of prospective cohort studies. *BMJ Open, 6*, e013191. doi:10.1136/bmjopen-2016-013191.
6. Kiltz, U., Smolen, J., Bardin, T., Solal, A. C., Dalbeth, N., … Westhoff, T. H. (2017). Treat-to-target (T2T) recommendations for gout. *Annals of the Rheumatic Diseases, 76*, 632–638.
7. Kolasinski, S. L. (2014). Food, drink, and herbs: Alternative therapies and gout. *Current Rheumatology Reports, 16*, 409–416.
8. Khanna, D., FitzGerald, J. D., Khanna, P. P., Bae, S., Singh, M., … Terkeltaub, R. (2012). 2012 American college of rheumatology guidelines for management of gout part I: Systematic non-pharmacologic and pharmacologic therapeutic approaches to hyperuricemia. *Arthritis Care and Research, 64*(10), 1431–1446.
9. Bruderer, S., Bodmer, M., Jick, S. S., & Meier, C. R. (2014). Use of diuretics and risk of incident gout: A population-based case-control study. *Arthritis and Rheumatology (Hoboken, NJ), 66*(1), 185–196.
10. Wolff, M. L., Cruz, J. L., Vanderman, A. J., & Brown, J. N. (2015). The effect of angiotensin II receptor blockers on hyperuricemia. *Therapeutic Advances in Chronic Disease, 6*(6), 339–346.
11. See, L. C., Kuo, C. F., Yu, K. H., Luo, S. F., Chou, I. J., … Liu, J. R. (2014). Hyperthyroid and hypothyroid status was strongly associated with gout and weakly associated with hyperuricaemia. *PLoS ONE, 9*(12), e114579. https://doi.org/10.1371/journal.pone.0114579.
12. Richette, P., Doherty, M., Pascual, E., Barskova, V., Becce, F., … Bardin, T. (2016). 2016 updated EULAR evidence-based recommendations for the management of gout. *Annals of the Rheumatic Diseases, 76*(1), 29–42.

Cough

Leslie-Faith Morritt Taub

Instructions

After reviewing the case study, please jot down your notes or preliminary answers in the spaces provided. When you are ready to submit your answers for grading and reflective expert feedback for evaluation, go to http://www.evolve.elsevier.com/DickAndButtaro/ to complete this case.

Case Study Scenario/History of Present Illness

Mrs. Manett is a 69-year-old new patient who scheduled an urgent visit in your primary care office for a complaint of a productive cough. She reports that she has been sick for the last 3 weeks with cold symptoms and last night had a temperature of 100°F and shaking chills. She also describes the cough as frequent with green sputum and complains that she has a poor appetite. She reports that she cares for her grandchildren, Sally age 12 and Josh age 9, when her daughter is at work. They both had colds 2 weeks ago, but they are now both well. She had been taking DayQuil and NyQuil, but states she seems to be getting worse rather than better. Her chest hurts from coughing, and she has been feeling like it is harder to breathe. She is worried that she may not be able to care for Sally and Josh while her daughter is working because she feels so tired. She reports she feels less steady on her feet and her daughter, who brought her to the office, reports her Mom seemed a little confused and "off her game" this morning.

Medications: Janumet XR (sitagliptin and metformin extended release) 50 milligrams/1000 milligrams tablets, 2 tablets po daily with the evening meal; Accupril (quinapril) 5 milligrams po daily; Ditropan ER (oxybutynin chloride) 10 milligrams po daily; and Celebrex 100 milligrams po twice daily, prn.

Allergies: Parafon Forte DSC (chlorzoxazone) caused angioedema.

Habits: Smoker with a smoking history of 30 pack-years, denies alcohol use.

Prior medical history: Type 2 diabetes (DM II), urge incontinence (UI), and osteoarthritis (OA).

Prior surgical history: Tonsillectomy age 12, appendectomy age 30.

Family history: Mother died at age 83, myocardial infarction (MI), DM II, OA; father died at age 90 with hypertension (HTN).

Personal and social history: Retired elementary school teacher, widowed 2 years ago (husband had MI). Lives with divorced daughter and two grandchildren.

Review of Systems

General: In usual state of health until 3 weeks ago. Today complains of fatigue and shaking chills.

Skin: Denies noting an exanthem of any kind since this illness started.

Head, eyes, ears, nose, and throat (HEENT): + sensation scratchy throat. Notices dry mouth since starting Ditropan. Denies sinus pain or pressure.

Respiratory: Reports worsening cough, green sputum, dyspnea, and chest discomfort.

Cardiac: Denies palpitations, squeezing sensation in chest or chest heaviness, or prior chest discomfort.

Gastrointestinal: + decrease in appetite. Denies nausea, vomiting, diarrhea, or abdominal pain.

Urinary: Reports fewer episodes of UI with Ditropan. Denies urinary burning or frequency.

Musculoskeletal: Reports bilateral knee pain on occasion, especially in the early morning on awakening. Pain has improved since taking Celebrex prn.

Neurologic: Reports weakness with this illness. Does have some tingling and numbness in both her feet.

Physical Examination

General: Ill-appearing older female, seems anxious and having some problems breathing.

Vital signs: Height: 5'4". Weight 188 pounds. Body mass index (BMI) 32.27. Apical pulse 104, blood pressure (BP) 130/80 left arm and 132/84 right arm. Temperature 100.9°F. Respiratory rate (RR) 24, O_2 saturation 97% on room air.

HEENT: Normocephalic, facies symmetric. Eyes: Sclera clear, no icterus. Ears: External auditory canals clear. Tympanic membranes (TMs): Landmarks visible, no erythema. Nose: No rhinitis or sinus tenderness. Throat mildly erythemic without exudate. Tonsils absent.

Neck: Supple. Thyroid nonpalpable, negative for cervical lymphadenopathy.

Lungs: Coughing frequently. + inspiratory crackles and bronchial breath sounds noted throughout the lung fields bilaterally with dullness to percussion in the right lower lung field.

Cardiac: S1, S2 tachycardic. No S3, S4. No murmur, click, or rub appreciated.

Abdomen: Soft, bowel sounds positive, nondistended. No organomegaly or tenderness.

Extremities: Negative for edema bilaterally. No calf tenderness bilaterally. + crepitus noted on examination of left knee. Monofilament testing of feet demonstrates inability to feel monofilament on right and left dorsal surface of the hallux and second toes and inability to feel the vibrations of a 128-Hz tuning fork over the distal and proximal joints of both halluces. Achilles tendon reflex +1 (hyporeflexic) bilaterally. STAT fingerstick blood sugar 150 milligrams/dL.

ASSESSMENT AND PLAN

1.   Based on the history and physical examination results, what differential diagnoses are you considering for the chief complaint?

2.   What components of the history or physical examination are missing?[1-3]

3.   Based on the information given, what further laboratory or diagnostics will you order and why?[1,4,5]

4.   When considering the etiology of Mrs. Manett's illness, what aspects favor a diagnosis of pneumonia versus an upper respiratory infection or acute bronchitis? Make a chart to help you make a comparative assessment

5.   If Mrs. Manett has no infiltrate on chest x-ray, does a negative chest x-ray exclude the diagnosis of pneumonia? Why or why not? Are there clues in the patient's history that help the provider understand why the chest x-ray might be negative? Are there other diagnostic tests that would indicate pneumonia in a patient with symptoms similar to those of Mrs. Manett?[6]

6. What are the possible causes of pneumonia? If Mrs. Manett has pneumonia, can you explain why her grandchildren had upper respiratory infections that resolved and yet Mrs. Manett appears to be much sicker?[1,7]

7. What is the difference between community-acquired pneumonia and hospital-acquired pneumonia?[4]

8.   Mrs. Manett's laboratory results are as follows. How should the health care provider interpret these results?

CBC: White blood cells (WBCs) 17,000 cells/mm3 (85% neutrophils, 20% lymphocytes).
   Chemistry panel:
   - Sodium: 144 (136–145 mmol/L)
   - Potassium: 4.8 (3.4–5.1 (mmol/L)
   - Chloride: 97 (98–107 mmol/L)
   - Carbon dioxide: 26 (22–32 mmol/L)
   - Blood urea nitrogen (BUN): 19 (5–23 milligrams/dL)
   - Creatinine 0.9: (0.4–1.0 md/dL)
   - Estimated glomerular filtration rate (GFR): >60 mL/min/1.73 m2
   - Random glucose: 147 H (74–118 milligrams/dL)

9.   Based on the patient's history and presentation, which antibiotic is appropriate to use empirically to treat a community-acquired pneumonia caused by *Mycoplasma pneumoniae*?[8]

Case Study, Continued

Mrs. Manett returns to the office in 3 days and does not seem to be responding to the macrolide. She continues to cough, reports extreme malaise, and continues to have a low-grade temperature. The health care provider is concerned and thinking about hospitalizing Mrs. Manett. The Pneumonia Severity Index (PSI) and the CURB-65 are risk assessment tools designed to aid providers in determining whether hospitalization should be a consideration for patients.

10. What important history and physical examination should the health care provider determine in this follow-up visit? What is the benefit of using the Pneumonia Severity Index for pneumonia severity or CURB-65 score for adults and elders with suspected pneumonia?[9-12]

Case Study, Continued

Using the CURB-65 the health care provider calculated Mrs. Manett's score as 2 (age > 65, plus continued confusion reported by her daughter). Based on this score and the fact that Mrs. Manett states that she does not want to be hospitalized, it is decided to continue her outpatient treatment but add another antibiotic to her present regimen.

11.   What antibiotic should be added to Mrs. Manett's regimen, and what would be the appropriate dose based on her creatinine clearance?[1,8]

12.   When should Mrs. Manett be reevaluated if she is treated at home? What social supports are necessary to safely treat her at home?

Case Study, Continued

Mrs. Manett's daughter can take some sick time to be at home with her mother and has also arranged for her brother's wife to stay with Mrs. Manett while she brings her children to school and does outside errands. Mrs. Manett and her daughter have been in close touch with the health care provider, and she has rallied. Her appetite has improved, her cough has resolved in the past few days, her temperature is normal, she has no further episodes of confusion, and she has not smoked since she began treatment for pneumonia.

13. What are the priorities for Mrs. Manett's next visit?[4,13-16]

Case Study, Continued

One week before Mrs. Manett's 3-month visit the health care provider receives her laboratory diagnostic results and notes that her Hgb A1C is 8.9%.

14. What is the recommended hemoglobin A1C for an older adult, and what changes to Mrs. Manett's diabetic regimen should be recommended?[13,17]

Case Study, Continued

Mrs. Manett's total cholesterol was 300, her HDL was 50, and her LDL was 180. Mrs. Manett says she thinks she was "borderline high" at her last provider's laboratory testing, but she decided to try diet and exercise to bring it down. She could not afford a statin medication at that time, and even the copays were too expensive with her Medicare prescription drug coverage plan. She recalls that her HDL was "protective," but her LDL was about 160.

15.   What recommendation will you make for Mrs. Manett today and how will you explain how this recommendation was made?[18]

Case Study, Continued

When you enter Mrs. Manett's information, her 10-year ASCVD risk is 30.7%.

16.   What recommendations will you make for Mrs. Manett to better control her cholesterol?[18]

17. What lifestyle recommendation will you include to promote cholesterol lowering?

18. What referrals should the health care provider recommend for Mrs. Manett today?

Case Study, Continued

Margaret, Mrs. Manett's daughter, accompanies her to her 3-month visit and feels her Mom has been a little depressed since her bout of pneumonia.

19.   Why is this of concern to you? How will you assess Mrs. Manett?

20.   What ongoing issues will need to be addressed in future visits?

ONLINE ANSWER SUBMISSION

When you are ready to submit your answers for grading and reflective expert feedback for evaluation, go to http://www.evolve.elsevier.com/DickAndButtaro/ to complete this case.

References

1. Mandell, L. A., & Wunderink, R. G. (2014). Pneumonia. In D. Kasper, A. Fauci, S. Hauser, D. Longo, J. Jameson, & J. Loscalzo (Eds.), *Harrison's principles of internal medicine* (19th ed.). New York: McGraw-Hill. Retrieved from http://accessmedicine.mhmedical.com/content.aspx?bookid=1130&sectionid=79733578.
2. Fishman, J. A. (2015). Approach to the patient with pulmonary infection. In M. A. Grippi, J. A. Elias, J. A. Fishman, R. M. Kotloff, A. I. Pack, R. M. Senior, et al. (Eds.), *Fishman's pulmonary diseases and disorders* (5th ed.). New York: McGraw-Hill.

3. Mount, D. B. Fluid and electrolyte disturbances. In D. Kasper, A. Fauci, S. Hauser, D. Longo, J. Jameson, & J. Loscalzo (Eds.), *Harrison's principles of internal medicine* (19th ed.). New York: McGraw-Hill.

4. Mandell, L. A., Wunderrink, R. G., Anzueto, A., Barlett, J. G., Campbell, D., Dean, N. C., et al. (2007). Infectious Diseases Society of America/American Thoracic Society consensus guidelines on the management of community-acquired pneumonia in adults. *Clinical Infectious Diseases, 44*, S27–S72.

5. Ebell, M. (2007). Predicting pneumonia in adults with respiratory illness. *American Family Physician, 76*(4), 560–562.

6. Kaysin, A., & Viera, A. J. (2016). Community acquired pneumonia in adults: Diagnosis and management. *American Family Physician, 94*(9), 698–706.

7. Centers for Disease Control and Prevention. (2017a). Mycoplasma pneumoniae infection. Retrieved from https://www.cdc.gov/pneumonia/atypical/mycoplasma/.

8. Centers for Disease Control and Prevention. (2017b). Antibiotic treatment and resistance. Retrieved from https://www.cdc.gov/pneumonia/atypical/mycoplasma/hcp/antibiotic-treatment-resistance.html.

9. Kwok, C. S., Loke, Y. K., Woo, K., & Myint, P. K. (2013). Risk prediction models for mortality in community-acquired pneumonia: A systematic review. *BioMed Research International, 2013*, 504136. http://doi.org/10.1155/2013/504136.

10. Chen, J., Chang, S., Liu, J. J., et al. (2010). Comparison of clinical characteristics and performance of pneumonia severity score and CURB-65 among younger adults, elderly and very old subjects. *Thorax, 65*, 971–977.

11. Fine, M. J., Aubile, T. E., Yealy, D. M., Hanusa, B. H., Weissfeld, L. A., Singer, D. E., et al. (1997). A prediction rule to identify low-risk patients with community acquired pneumonia. *The New England Journal of Medicine, 336*(4), 243–250.

12. Lim, W. S., van der Eerden, M. M., Laing, R., Boersma, W. G., Karalus, N., Town, G. I., et al. (2003). Defining community acquired pneumonia severity on presentation to hospital: An international derivation and validation study. *Thorax, 58*, 377–382.

13. American Diabetes Association. (2017). Standards of medical care in diabetes – 2017. *Diabetes Care, 40*(Suppl. 1).

14. RxList The Internet Drug Index. (2017). Accupril drug interactions. Retrieved from http://www.rxlist.com/accupril-drug/side-effects-interactions.htm.

15. CDC Pneumococcal Disease. (2015). Retrieved from https://www.cdc.gov/pneumococcal/vaccination.html.

16. US Preventive Services Task Force. (2013). Lung Cancer Screening. Retrieved from https://www.uspreventiveservicestaskforce.org/Page/Document/UpdateSummaryFinal/lung-cancer-screening.

17. American Geriatrics Society Expert Panel on the Care of Older Adults with Diabetes Mellitus. (2013). Guidelines abstracted from the American Geriatrics Society guidelines for improving the care of older adults with diabetes mellitus: 2013 update. *Journal of the American Geriatrics Society, 61*(11), 2020–2026.

18. Goff, D. C., Jr., Lloyd-Jones, D. M., Bennett, G., Coady, S., D'Agostino, R. B., Sr., Gibbons, R., et al. (2013). ACC/AHA guideline on the assessment of cardiovascular risk: A report of the American College of Cardiology/American Heart Association Task Force on Practice Guidelines. *Circulation, 135*(11), 3–47.

Nosebleed

Susan G. Henderson ■ Lee Henderson

Instructions

After reviewing the case study, please jot down your notes or preliminary answers in the spaces provided. When you are ready to submit your answers for grading and reflective expert feedback for evaluation, go to http://www.evolve.elsevier.com/DickAndButtaro/ to complete this case.

Case Study Scenario/History of Present Illness

84-year-old Theresa Belanger is a retired homemaker, a part-time office worker, and a widow of 20 years. She is living on her late husband's modest pension along with Social Security retiree benefits. Theresa lives alone in a two-story twin home in a middle-class neighborhood of a major Midwestern American city. The home was bought as a "fixer-upper," but Theresa's husband passed away before he could undertake the planned renovations. Nevertheless, Theresa is adamant that she wants to remain living in her home, often saying, "They'll have to carry me out in a box."

Theresa's younger son (age 55) and daughter-in-law live 10 minutes away by car, but the son travels frequently. Theresa's daughter-in-law, Kate, is a nurse practitioner who works in an OB/GYN clinic and specializes in prenatal care. Theresa's older son (age 56) and his family live about an hour away by car in another state; he and his wife travel frequently, and they have a middle-school-aged son and a college-aged son.

Theresa's home has a powder room on the first floor and a full bathroom on the second floor. Safety features such as bathroom grab bars and double railings on the stairway were added by Theresa's family after she suffered a transient ischemic attack (TIA) 2 years ago, resulting in decreased steadiness when walking. Theresa has been reluctant to have a stair lift installed because of concerns that using the lift will cause her to lose additional mobility. She continues to use the stairs on a limited basis.

Since Theresa's TIA and an episode of confusion approximately 1 year later, the daughter-in-law, Kate, has become increasingly involved in providing supportive care with the activities of daily living, including grocery shopping, laundry, and pouring medications. Theresa's younger sister (age 73) used to drive her for errands and limited social activities but can no longer drive because of worsening rheumatoid arthritis. However, the sister's husband can still drive Theresa on a limited basis. Theresa's next-door neighbors (both in their late 50s) assist her with snow shoveling, lawn mowing, and other outdoor home maintenance.

Theresa's current diagnoses include hypertension and hypercholesterolemia (both controlled medically), osteoarthritis (affecting the shoulders, hips, knees, and hands), and anxiety.

Theresa's past medical history includes:

- Ovarian cancer successfully treated with surgery alone 26 years ago without recurrence.
- Acute anemia treated 12 months ago with 2 units of blood.
- Chronic moderate anxiety.
- Intermittent mild depressive episodes.

Case Study, Continued

After the TIA episode, Theresa was advised by the visiting nurses, the physical therapists, and Kate to use a walker for safety inside and outside the home, but Theresa relies primarily on holding onto furniture in her home and on a quad cane when she is out because of fears that use of the walker will further reduce her mobility. Because of personal preferences and difficulty climbing stairs, Theresa routinely sleeps on her living room sofa with her small dog. She also takes daily naps on the sofa.

Theresa's vital signs at her last visit with her primary care provider approximately 3 months ago were:
- Height 5' 2"
- Weight 210 pounds
- Blood pressure (BP) 122/82
- Temperature 98.3°F
- O_2 saturation 95%

Theresa's medications include:
- Baby aspirin ½ tablet 3 times per week (Monday, Wednesday, and Saturday)
- Citalopram 10 milligrams, po 1 tablet daily
- Lisinopril 10 milligrams po, 1 tablet daily
- Atenolol 25 milligrams po, 1 tablet daily
- Atorvastatin 20 milligrams po, 1 tablet daily
- Vitamin D_3 1000 IU po, 1 tablet daily
- Ferrous sulfate 325 milligrams po, 1 tablet daily
- Meloxicam 15 milligrams po, 1 tablet daily prn for arthritis pain
- Xanax 0.5 milligrams every 4 hours po prn for anxiety

Case Study, Continued

One afternoon, after waking from a nap, Theresa reaches to pick up the newspapers that she routinely leaves on the floor. Then, realizing she needs to go to the powder room quickly to urinate, she quickly stands up, loses her balance, and falls headfirst into her television stand. As Theresa stands back up, she realizes that she is bleeding profusely from her nose. Within a few minutes, her shirtfront is covered in blood, and the bleeding continues, leaving large blood-spattered areas on her throw-rugs, floor, and other clothing.

Recognizing that the bleeding is not slowing, Theresa texts her daughter-in-law, Kate, as follows:

"Just fell + have bloody nose."

Kate, who is working 11 miles away without access to a vehicle, tries to call Theresa, but Theresa does not answer her cell phone because she has gone to the powder room. Kate texts and asks Theresa to call, which Theresa does in the next few minutes. After obtaining Theresa's account of her fall and determining that Theresa seems oriented and that was able to get up without assistance, Kate encourages Theresa to apply ice and pressure and promises to call Theresa back in 10 minutes to see if the bleeding is stopped or slowing down.

When she calls Theresa back, Kate learns that the bleeding has slowed very slightly, but it is still continuing. Kate then contacts her husband, Theresa's younger son, to confer. The younger son is working out of town that day and cannot get to his mother for at least 3 hours. The older son is also out of town that day and cannot reach Theresa until much later. The younger son encourages Kate to have Theresa use her emergency service pendant to call an ambulance.

Kate then calls Theresa again and encourages her to use her emergency service pendant to call emergency services. However, Theresa refuses to do so, saying, "I don't want to press the button because they'll take me to the hospital."

1. How should Kate respond to Theresa?

2. What legal and/or ethical responsibility does Kate have as a health care provider in this situation?[1,2]

3. What aspects of Theresa's health history are of most concern in this episode?[3]

Case Study, Continued

The known history thus far is that Theresa woke from a nap, reached to pick up newspapers, experienced an immediate need to urinate, stood up, lost her balance, and fell head first into the TV stand. The fall resulted in a nosebleed. The need to urinate may or may not be associated with Theresa's subsequent fall, but it seems like her behavior (? rushing/rising quickly), her medications, possible weakness, orthostatic hypotension, imbalance, infection, anemia, dehydration, or even another TIA are possible factors in her injury. The bleeding is likely related to the antiplatelet effects of aspirin, although the bleeding could be associated with an unknown factor. For example, thrombocytopenia can be drug-related and Theresa is on at least one medication (i.e., simvastatin) associated with thrombocytopenia. Additionally, Theresa has a past medical history of anemia

4. What are the immediate priorities and concerns for Theresa's well-being? Given Theresa's desire to avoid hospitalization, what interventions are appropriate now?[3-6]

5. What further assessments are needed?

Case Study, Continued

EMERGENCY ROOM VISIT

Theresa is brought to the emergency room, and the health care provider who first evaluates Theresa is a physician's assistant (PA). The PA conducts the initial primary survey to be certain Theresa's airway, breathing, and circulation are intact, notes the contusion and edema over the nasal bridge and continued nasal bleeding, and then proceeds to the secondary survey to determine whether there are other injuries as well. No other injuries are apparent, and the PA attends to Theresa's history and physical examination.

History of Present Illness. Patient states she was napping, woke up, bent over to pick up some newspapers on the floor, and then noted that she needed to go the bathroom to urinate right away. She quickly stood up, lost her balance, and fell, falling face first into her TV stand. She denies that she was dizzy or the room seemed to be spinning. Denies previous facial injury or facial surgery. Denies loss of consciousness when she fell.

Past Medical History
Distant history of ovarian cancer
Anemia
Hypertension
Hypercholesterolemia
Anxiety/depression
Degenerative arthritis
TIA
Medications: Per patient all taken this morning except atorvastatin, which she takes at night.
Baby aspirin ½ tablet 3 times per week
Citalopram   10 milligrams, po 1 tablet daily
Lisinopril 10 milligrams po, 1 tablet daily
Atenolol 25 milligrams po, 1 tablet daily
Atorvastatin 20 milligrams po, 1 tablet daily
Vitamin D₃ 1000 International units po, 1 tablet daily
Ferrous sulfate 325 milligrams po, 1 tablet daily
Meloxicam 15 milligrams po, 1 tablet daily prn for arthritis pain,
Xanax 0.5 milligrams every 4 hours po prn for anxiety

Review of Systems
General: Feels weak at times. Denies fever or chills.
Skin: Denies rashes or lesions.
Head, eyes, ears, nose and throat (HEENT): + headache and nose pain now, but not usually. Sometimes she does not hear well. Denies dizziness, vision changes.
Neck: Denies neck pain.
Respiratory: Denies cough, wheezing, or shortness of breath.
Cardiac: Denies chest pain, palpitations, dyspnea, or orthopnea.
Gastrointestinal: Occasional problems with constipation. Denies difficulty swallowing, weight loss, nausea, vomiting, or diarrhea.
Urinary: Recent urinary frequency. + urgency today. Denies urinary burning or flank pain.
Musculoskeletal: Some left lower back pain lately. + history of arthritis with pain multiple joints.
Peripheral vascular: Denies swollen legs, calf pain.
Neurovascular: + history TIA. Denies fainting, seizures, or memory loss.

Hematologic: + history of anemia. Denies easy bruising, bleeding gums, or hematuria.

Endocrine: Denies sweating, thirst.

Psychiatric: Reports history of anxiety and depression. "Some days are better than others."

Physical Examination

Vital signs: 142/70, heart rate 88 regular, respiratory rate 22, oxygen saturation 94%.

General: overweight, older female with no acute distress (NAD).

Skin: + nasal contusion. + tenderness nose. No zygomatic tenderness bilaterally. No lacerations, hematomas (Fig. 14.1), or other contusions noted on the body, face, or extremities.

Facies: symmetric.

Eyes: Pupils equal and reactive to light and accommodation (PERLA). Sclera clear, conjunctiva within normal limits.

Ears: Somewhat hard of hearing. External auditory canals clear. Tympanic membranes (TMs): cone of light visualized.

Nose: + contusion nasal bone with some edema. Minimal epistaxis right nostril only.

Mouth: + dentures. No blood noted posterior pharynx. Membranes moist, no obvious lesions tongue or mucosa.

Neck: Supple. Full range of motion (ROM) without pain. No cervical spine tenderness. No masses or lymphadenopathy. No bruits.

Cardiac: S1, S2 regular. No S3 or S4. Electrocardiogram (ECG): Normal sinus rhythm, no ectopy, no QT prolongation or ST changes.

Lungs: Diminished at bases but clear to auscultation without rales, wheezes, or rhonchi.

Abdomen: Soft, bowel sounds +. Nontender, no organomegaly. No costovertebral angle (CVA) tenderness.

Extremities: ROM intact. Pulses present.

Neurologic: Alert, appropriate. Thoughts fluid, congruent. Cranial nerves II to XII intact. Muscle strength symmetric 4/5 upper/lower extremities. Reflexes symmetric bilaterally. Sensation intact. Gait not assessed.

6. What aspects of Theresa's physical examination were concerned with determining possible causes or other potential injuries associated with her fall?

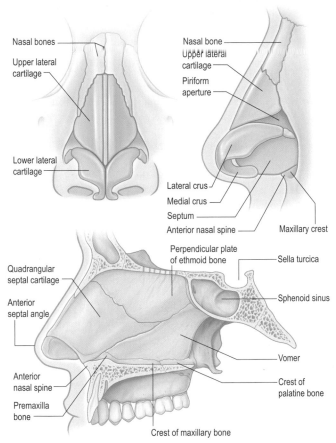

Fig. 14.1 Diagrams of the cartilaginous and bony nose and septum. (From Neligan, P. C. [2013]. *Plastic Surgery* [3rd ed.]. Philadelphia: Saunders.)

7.   Theresa's epistaxis seems to have stabilized. Based on Theresa's history and the physician assistant's evaluation of Theresa, what diagnostics are necessary and why?

8. What are potential reasons that Theresa's diagnostic testing could not be obtained?

Case Study, Continued

Theresa is not orthostatic and her laboratory values are as noted subsequently.

White blood cell count	7.3	4.0–11.0 (K/mm³)
Red blood count	3.95	3.80–5.40 (M/mm³)
Hemoglobin	10.0 L	11.0–16.0 (g/dL)
Hematocrit	33.7 L	35.0–48.0 (%)
Mean cell volume	85.3	80.0–100.0 (fL)
Mean corpuscular hemoglobin	25.3 L	27.0–34.0 (pg)
Mean corpuscular hemoglobin concentrate	29.7 L	31.0–36.0 (g/dL)
Red cell distribution width	16.1 H	11.5–15.0 (%)
Platelet count	469 H	130–400 (K/mm³)
Mean platelet volume	10.0	9.0–11.0 (fL)
Neutrophils %	59.9	37.0–80.0 (%)
Lymphocytes %	30.3	23.0–45.0 (%)
Monocytes %	7.6	2.5–14.0 (%)
Eosinophils %	1.5	0.5–4.0 (%)
Basophils %	0.4	0.0–2.0 (%)
Immature granulocytes %	0.3	0–1 (%)
Nucleated red blood cells%	0.0	0–0 (%)
Neutrophils #	4.4	1.9–7.5 (K/mm³)
Lymphocytes #	2.2	1.2–3.4 (K/mm³)
Monocytes #	0.6	0.0–0.7 (K/mm³)
Eosinophils #	0.11	0.0–0.7 (K/mm³)
Basophils #	0.0	0.0–0.1 (K/mm³)
Immature granulocytes #	0.0	0.0–0.1 (K/mm³)

H, High; *L*, low.

Sodium	143	136–145 (mmol/L)
Potassium	4.1	3.4–5.1 (mmol/L)
Chloride	100	98–107 (mmol/L)
Carbon dioxide	25	22–32 (mmol/L)
Anion gap	16	8–16 (mmol/L)
Glucose	128 H	74–118 (milligrams/dL)
BUN	19	5–23 (milligrams/dL)
Creatinine	1.2 H	0.4–1.0 (milligrams/dL)
Estimated glomerular filtration rate	45.3	(mL/min)
Calcium	9.7	8.6–10.2 (milligrams/dL)

BUN, Blood urea nitrogen.

Urinalysis With Reflex Culture

Name	Value	Reference Range
Urine color	Yellow	Yellow
Urine appearance	Cloudy AA	Clear
Urine glucose (UA)	Negative	Negative (milligrams/dL)
Urine bilirubin	Negative	Negative
Urine ketones	Negative	Negative (milligrams/dL)
Specific gravity, urine	≤1.005	1.005–1.030
Urine blood	Small AA	Negative
pH, urine	6.0	5.0–8.0
Urine protein (UA)	Trace	Negative (milligrams/dL)
Urine urobilinogen	0.2	0.2–1.0 (milligrams/dL)
Urine nitrite	Negative	Negative
Urine leukocyte esterase	Negative	Negative

UA, urinalysis.

9. Based on Theresa's laboratory diagnostics, are there any abnormal findings that the physician assistant should be concerned about?

10.   Theresa's epistaxis now seems to be controlled without further intervention. The physician's assistant discusses Theresa's presentation with the emergency room physician. The discussion should include (1) potential treatments if the epistaxis restarts, (2) computed tomography scan versus facial x-rays, and (3) possible causes of Theresa's fall. Discuss each of these components of Theresa's ongoing care.

Case Study, Continued

The emergency room physician examines Theresa with the PA and decides that a CT scan is appropriate now that the nosebleed has stopped. If the CT scan is negative, Theresa can be discharged home. Based on the urinalysis results, a urine culture and sensitivity will be ordered, and if there is a urinary tract infection, Theresa will be called and started on an antibiotic.

Examination: CT scan of the brain without contrast.

Reason for examination: Fall. + head injury

Comparison examination: None.

Technique: Multiple axial images were obtained of the brain, and 5-mm sections were acquired. The 2.5-mm sections were acquired without injection of intravenous contrast. Reformatted sagittal and coronal images were obtained.

Discussion: No acute intracranial abnormalities appreciated. No evidence for hydrocephalus, midline shift, space-occupying lesions, or abnormal fluid collections. No cortical-based abnormalities appreciated. The sinuses are clear. No acute bony abnormalities identified. Preliminary report given to emergency room at conclusion of examination.

Impression: No acute intracranial abnormalities appreciated.

11. Theresa will be discharged home. (1) Discuss the possible causes of falls in older adults. (2) What physical examination is necessary before Theresa leaves the emergency room? (3) What patient teaching might help prevent additional falls for Theresa?[5,6]

Case Study, Continued

Theresa is discharged home by the physician assistant with instructions to follow up with her primary care provider within the next week. Theresa is told that she can take acetaminophen 500-milligram tablets, 2 tablets three times a day as needed for pain for the next few days, but there are no other medication changes. The PA does explain to Theresa that the Xanax and some of her other medications could have contributed to her fall. Theresa is also encouraged to use a walker at home; sit on the side of her bed, couch, or chair; and move her feet and legs to improve her circulation before standing. She is also advised to return to the emergency room is there is further nasal bleeding.

PRIMARY CARE FOLLOW-UP

Her daughter-in-law, Kate, accompanies Theresa to the office for follow-up. Theresa is using a rolling walker today, and the nurse practitioner notes that Theresa is able to manage the walker in the office hall without difficulty. Theresa states there have been no further episodes, she is feeling well, although still has some facial discomfort. Theresa's vital signs are stable and, aside from the resolving contusion over Theresa's nose, there are no significant physical findings.

1. Discuss the essential components of today's follow-up visit to the primary care provider.
    a. Medication reconciliation: It is important today that the nurse practitioner seeing Theresa asks her what medications and herbals Theresa is taking at home. This list also should include any over-the-counter medications and any alcohol consumption or drugs Theresa might have borrowed from a friend or neighbor.
    b. Theresa needs to be asked about the fall, what medications she took that morning, if she ate, or had been feeling ill in any way before the fall. Learning how many times a day Theresa takes Xanax and how long she has been on the Xanax is also important information. In general, benzodiazepines are medications associated with falls, drowsiness, and confusion in elders and, when possible, should be avoided.[7] However, some patients can have severe anxiety, and the benefit to the patient may outweigh the risk. For patients who have been on benzodiazepines for a long period of time, this category of medications

cannot be abruptly stopped.[8] This is because people who have been taking benzodiazepines for a long period of time are physiologically dependent on the medication and can have severe withdrawal symptoms.

c. The nurse practitioner reviews Theresa's medications and learns Theresa does not take Xanax all the time, but may take it three to four times a week for sleep or if she gets nervous.

   i. Meloxicam, a nonsteroidal antiinflammatory drug (NSAID), is associated with gastrointestinal bleeding, anemia, and hypotension in addition to other concerning side effects when taken at higher doses and for more than short periods of time. It is on the Beers list of medications to avoid for many or most older adults.[8]

   ii. Citalopram, a selective serotonin reuptake inhibitor, is safe in lower doses (20 milligrams a day) but can cause prolonged QT in higher daily doses.[9]

d. Theresa's medications are discussed with Theresa and Kate.

   i. The nurse practitioner tells them that the cause of Theresa's fall is unclear, but it is possible her medications are involved. She explains to Theresa that Xanax can cause confusion and asks Theresa to try not to take Xanax more than three times a week and write down on a piece of paper every time she takes a Xanax and the reason why. They can then discuss it more at the next visit.

   ii. The nurse practitioner also explains that the meloxicam could be causing Theresa's anemia and suggests that Theresa do a fecal immunochemical test (FIT) at home to see if she is still having a problem with gastrointestinal bleeding. She also asks Theresa if she skips taking her iron pill some days because of constipation and checks to see if she takes the iron pill with orange juice. A repeat CBC also will be important before the next visit.

   iii. Finally, she tells both Kate and Theresa that at the next visit they can talk more about the medications to see if these are all necessary.

12. What home accommodations might help prevent additional falls?

Case Study, Continued

Theresa reluctantly states she will keep using the walker for now. "I want to stay in my home and not go to a nursing home, so I'll do it." After asking Theresa and Kate if they have any questions or concerns, an appointment is made for follow-up in another month.

ONLINE ANSWER SUBMISSION

When you are ready to submit your answers for grading and reflective expert feedback for evaluation, go to http://www.evolve.elsevier.com/DickAndButtaro/ to complete this case.

References

1. American Academy of Family Physicians (2013 revision). Recommended curriculum guidelines for family medicine residents risk management and medical liability. Retrieved from http://www.aafp.org/dam/AAFP/documents/medical_education_residency/program_directors/Reprint281_Risk.pdf.
2. Moffett, P., & Moore, G. (2011). The standard of care: Legal history and definitions: The bad and good news. *Western Journal of Emergency Medicine, 12*(1), 109–112.
3. Linxin, L., Geraghty, O. C., Mehta, Z., & Rothwell, P. M. (2017). Age-specific risks, severity, time course, and outcome of bleeding on long-term antiplatelet treatment after vascular events: A population-based cohort study. *The Lancet*, doi:10.1016/S0140-6736(17)30770-5.
4. Pappachan, B., & Alexander, M. (2012). Biomechanics of cranio-maxillofacial trauma. *Journal of Maxillofacial & Oral Surgery, 11*(2), 224–230.
5. Meldon, S. W., & Delaney-Rowland, S. (2010). Subdural hematomas in the elderly: The great neurological imitator. Retrieved from https://www.ahcmedia.com/articles/44955-subdural-hematomas-in-the-elderly-the-great-neurological-imitator.
6. Rubenstein, L. Z., & Dillar, D. (2014). Falls. In R. J. Ham, P. D. Sloane, G. A. Warshaw, J. F. Potter, & E. Flaherty (Eds.), *Ham's primary care geriatrics* (6th ed.). Philadelphia: Elsevier.
7. Marra, E. M., Mazer-Amirshahi, M., Brooks, G., Anker, J., May, L., & Pines, J. M. (2015). Benzodiazepine prescribing in older adults in US ambulatory clinics and emergency departments (2001–10). *Journal of the American Geriatrics Society*.
8. American Geriatrics Society 2015 Beers Criteria Update Expert Panel (2015). American Geriatrics Society 2015 Updated Beers Criteria for Potentially Inappropriate Medication Use in Older Adults. Retrieved from http://onlinelibrary.wiley.com/doi/10.1111/jgs.13702/pdf.
9. Dietle, A. (2015). QTc prolongation with antidepressants and antipsychotics. *U. S. Pharmacist*. Retrieved from https://www.uspharmacist.com/article/qtc-prolongation-with-antidepressants-and-antipsychotics.

Loss of Height

Patricia Bailey

Instructions

After reviewing the case study, please jot down your notes or preliminary answers in the spaces provided. When you are ready to submit your answers for grading and reflective expert feedback for evaluation, go to http://www.evolve.elsevier.com/DickAndButtaro/ to complete this case.

Case Study Scenario

HOME VISIT: ANNUAL HEALTH RISK ASSESSMENT

Debra Taylor is a Caucasian 79-year-old female with a past medical history of chronic obstructive pulmonary disease (COPD), type 2 diabetes, gastroesophageal reflux disease (GERD), hyperlipidemia, and hypertension (HTN). She is being seen today by the health care provider for an annual in-home health and wellness assessment at the request of her health insurance plan. During the visit, Ms. Taylor reports she is concerned that she has been having some back pain.

1. What other information would you like to elicit?

Physical Examination. *On examination, blood pressure is 142/78 mm Hg, heart rate 66 beats per minute, respirations 20 breaths/min, temperature 98.6°F, weight 120 pounds (54.5 kg), and height 61 inches (155 cm). Debra states, "I used to be much taller." Her body mass index (BMI) is 22.7. Her O_2 saturation is 96% on room air.*

    General: Thin. No distress noted. Oriented × 3, with normal mood and affect.

    HEENT: Normocephalic, conjunctiva clear, sclera nonicteric, external ocular movements (EOMs) intact. Pupils equal, round, and reactive to light (PERRL). Tympanic

543

membranes (TMs) translucent and mobile. Hearing intact. No external ear lesions. Septum and turbinates normal. Dentures intact. Mucous membranes moist, no mucosal lesions.

Neck: Supple, without lesions, bruits, or lymphadenopathy. Thyroid nonenlarged and nontender.

Respiratory: Clear, unlabored. No rales, wheezes, or rhonchi.

Cardiac: Regular rate, S1, S2, no S3, S4. No murmurs, rubs, or gallops.

Abdomen: Soft, bowel sounds present. Nondistended, nontender to palpation.

Musculoskeletal: Kyphosis noted. 1+ pitting ankle edema. Generalized weakness in all extremities.

Neurologic: Cranial nerves (CN) II to XII grossly intact. Sensation to pain, touch, and proprioception normal. Deep tendon reflexes (DTRs) normal in upper and lower extremities. Normal reflexes.

Functional: Ms. Taylor is independent in her activities of daily living of bathing and dressing. Her daughters take turns assisting her with shopping, housekeeping, and laundry. Her oldest daughter, who is a nurse, arranges her medications. She currently does not drive and relies on assistance from her children to get to appointments.

Case Study, Continued

Ms. Taylor also reports that she is much shorter now. She reports that she thinks her maximal height was about 5 feet 5 inches, but she is not certain. Each year she has noticed a significant decline in height and this, along with the back pain, is concerning to her.

2. Based on the history and physical examination, what are some potential causes of Ms. Taylor's back pain?[1,2]

Case Study, Continued

Ms. Taylor reports she started smoking at age 14, but quit 10 years ago after her husband passed away from lung cancer. She admits to a sedentary lifestyle since retirement at age 62. She was diagnosed with COPD at age 40 and has been on steroids periodically since that time. She currently eats at least two meals a day and depends on a local community meal service for one of those meals. Ms. Taylor states she does not eat much fruit or vegetables and does not drink any milk.

3. What additional information would it be helpful to learn from Ms. Taylor?

4. What educational and health promotion recommendations would be appropriate for Ms. Taylor at this time?

Case Study, Continued

Ms. Taylor is scheduled to see her health care provider next week and will discuss her back pain concern at her next primary care visit.

PRIMARY CARE OFFICE: ANNUAL VISIT

Seven days has passed since the patient was seen in her home. Today, she presents to primary care clinic for her routine annual visit and increasing back pain. She states that she first noticed the pain 6 months ago, but the discomfort is becoming increasingly worse. The pain is in her lower back. She describes the pain as dull and intermittent. The pain is localized without radiation. Walking and standing for extended periods of time makes the pain worse, but her back pain is relieved with rest. She denies numbness or tingling in her extremities. She rates her pain a 4/10 but states at times it feels like 7/10. She has been taking over-the-counter Advil twice a day with some relief.

Medications: Lisinopril 20 milligrams po daily, hydrochlorothiazide 25 milligrams po daily, aspirin 81 milligrams po daily, multivitamin 1 po daily, simvastatin 40 milligrams po daily, and metformin 500 milligrams po twice a day. Recently tapered off prednisone.

Allergies: No known allergies.

Habits: Former smoker, quit 10 years ago.

Past medical history: COPD, type 2 diabetes, GERD, hyperlipidemia, and HTN.

Past surgical history: C-section ×2.

Family history: Father died age 72 of CAD and MI. Mother died age 80. Medical history included osteoporosis and HTN. Brother died age 48 of CAD and MI.

Personal and social history: Seven children, widowed, lives alone. Retired nurse.

Review of Systems

General: Fatigue.

HEENT: Dizziness, syncope; denies difficulty or changes in his hearing, denies tinnitus. Denies problems or changes in vision. Denies blurred vision.

Respiratory: Denies shortness of breath. Denies cough.

Cardiac: Denies chest pain. Denies palpitations.

Genitourinary: Denies change in bowel or bladder habits.

Musculoskeletal: Reports localized lower back pain.

Neurologic: Denies numbness/tingling in extremities. Reports feeling of generalized weakness.

Physical Examination. *On examination, blood pressure is 126/84 mm Hg, heart rate 70 beats/min, respirations 18 breaths/min, temperature 99.1°F, weight 120 pounds (54.5 kg), and height 61 inches (155 cm). Her BMI is 22.7. O_2 saturation 97% on room air.*

General: Thin; no distress noted. Oriented × 3, normal mood and affect.

HEENT: Pupils round, reactive to light. Moist mucous membranes. No lymphadenopathy. No thyromegaly. No bruits.

Neck: Supple.

Respiratory: Lungs clear on auscultation.

Cardiac: Regular rate, S1, S2, no S3, S4. No murmurs, rubs, or gallops.

Abdomen: Soft, nondistended, nontender to palpation, bowel sounds × 4.

Musculoskeletal: Kyphosis. 1+ pitting ankle edema. Generalized weakness in all extremities. Full range of motion in shoulders, elbows, hands, hips, and knees. Tenderness on palpation of lower spine.

Neurologic: CN II to XII grossly intact. DTRs 2+ throughout. Romberg and pronator drift normal. Normal gait, strength 4/5 bilateral upper and lower extremities.

5.   Based on the history and physical examination, what are your differential diagnoses for Ms. Taylor's presenting complaint?[3-11]

6.   What is the likely cause of this patient's loss in height? What are the differential diagnoses that should be considered and what further diagnostic testing is indicated?[11-13]

7.   What is the diagnostic criteria for osteoporosis? (See Fig. 15.1.)[14-16]

World Health Organization Diagnostic Criteria for Osteoporosis

BMD T-Score	Level of Bone Loss
> 1.0	Normal
−1.0 to >2.5	Osteopenia
<−2.5	Osteoporosis
<−2.5 plus fragility fractures	Severe osteoporosis

BMD, Bone mineral density.

Case Study, Continued

A DEXA was obtained along with the following laboratory testing: CBC/differential to assess for anemia or leukemia (a possible differential in osteoporosis), lipid panel because she is taking a statin, liver function tests (LFTs) to assess liver function, calcium, TSH, and PTH. The results of these were normal. Her calcium and vitamin D levels are lower than normal.

Ms. Taylor's lumbosacral spine films were negative and did not reveal a compression fracture. Her T-score from DEXA of the femoral neck is −3.2 and −2.8 for lumbar. Based on the World Health Organization (WHO) Criteria for Osteoporosis, she meets the criteria for osteoporosis. After hearing the results from this scan, she is willing to start medications now because she "doesn't want to break a bone."

Ca (8.5–10.2)	PTH (0.5–1.4)	TSH (2.0–5.1)	25-Hydroxy Vitamin D (20 and 40 ng/mL)	DEXA (Lumbar) T-Score	DEXA (Femoral) T-Score
7.0	1.3	3.5	16 ng/mL	−2.8	−3.2

Ca, Calcium; *DEXA,* dual-energy x-ray absorptiometry; *PTH,* parathyroid hormone; *TSH,* thyroid-stimulating hormone.

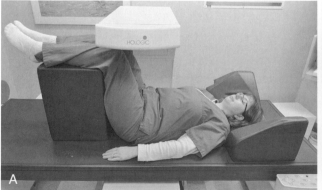
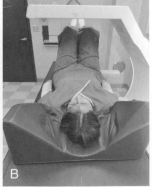

Fig. 15.1 Correct patient positioning for dual-energy x-ray absorptiometry (DEXA) scan of posteroanterior (PA) spine. (A) Lateral photograph shows the positioning block under the subject's feet. (B) Frontal photograph shows that the subject is centered on the scanner table and aligned with the scanner's long axis. (*From Dasher, L. G., Newton, C. D., & Lenchik, L. [2010]. Dual x-ray absorptiometry in today's clinical practice.* Radiologic Clinics of North America, 48[3], 541–560.)

8. **What further diagnostic(s) are indicated for Ms. Taylor?**

9. **In this case what precipitating factors (risk factors) may have contributed to osteoporosis?[17-20]**

10. **Using the FRAX tool, calculate Ms. Taylor's fracture risk (Fig. 15.2)[21,22]**

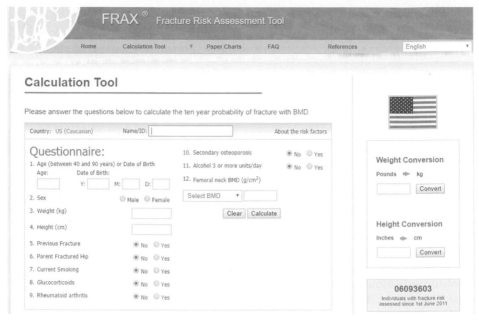

Fig. 15.2 Fracture risk algorithm (FRAX) fracture risk assessment tool. *(Copyright Centre for Metabolic Bone Diseases, University of Sheffield, United Kingdom.)*

11. What lifestyle changes should be recommended?[23,24]

12.   What pharmacologic treatment options should be discussed with the patient?[24-26]

13.   What other issues does Ms. Taylor have that may raise any possible concerns with pharmacologic therapy for osteoporosis?[26]

14. Review the recommended FRAX intervention threshold. What should the treatment plan be for Ms. Taylor's osteoporosis?

15. What are contraindications for the use of bisphosphonates?[27]

Case Study, Continued

TWO-YEAR FOLLOW-UP

Ms. Taylor has been seen on an annual basis for the last 2 years after her diagnosis of osteoporosis. Today, it has been 2 years since her last DEXA. She presents for repeat DEXA. She reports that she has not fallen and has been walking daily. She states that her overall diet has been healthy. A BMD was conducted at this visit. After 2 years of oral treatment with oral bisphosphonates, results revealed a T-score (lumbar spine) of −2.9 and a T-score of total hip of −3.4. You compare the results to her previous DEXA only to find that there was no improvement in Ms. Taylor's bone density.

16. What are possible causes of the decrease in Ms. Taylor's density?[28]

Case Study, Continued

EMERGENCY ROOM VISIT: 2 WEEKS LATER

Ms. Taylor reports today to her local emergency room with her daughter. She reports tripping over a throw rug and falling while entering her bathroom, landing on her right hip. She denies loss of consciousness after the fall. However, she reports severe pain in the right hip and upper thigh, and was unable to get up after her fall. She now has constant pain in her right hip. She rates the pain is 10/10. She is 15 years postmenopausal. Her DEXA results from her last office visit showed a T-score (lumbar spine) of −2.9 and a T-score of total hip of −3.4. On physical examination, Ms. Taylor is alert and oriented to time, place, and date, and she was responding appropriately to questions despite being in considerable pain. An injection of morphine was given to help with pain.

Focused Review of Systems

General: + fatigue, generalized weaknesses. Mild distress caused by pain.

HEENT: Denies headache, dizziness, syncope. Denies difficulty or changes in hearing, denies tinnitus. Denies problems or changes in vision. Denies blurred vision.

Respiratory: Denies shortness of breath.

Cardiac: Denies chest pain. Denies palpitations.

Genitourinary: Denies change in bowel or bladder habits.

Musculoskeletal: Reports localized right hip pain.

Neurologic: Denies numbness/tingling in extremities.

Focused Physical Examination. On examination, Ms. Taylor's blood pressure is 148/80 mm Hg, heart rate 86 beats/min, respirations 20 breaths/min, temperature 98.8°F, weight 122 pounds (55.34 kg), and height 60 inches (153 cm). Her BMI is 23.2. O_2 saturation is 97% on room air.

General: Thin. Oriented × 3, uncomfortable, but normal mood and affect.

Respiratory: Clear, unlabored without rales, wheezes, or rhonchi.

Cardiac: Regular rate, S1, S2, no S3, S4. No murmurs, rubs, or gallops.

Abdomen: Soft, bowel sounds present, nondistended, nontender to palpation.

Musculoskeletal: Moderate kyphosis. 1+ pitting ankle edema. Generalized weakness in all extremities. There are no signs of trauma to the head, neck, torso, arms, or left leg. The right leg and hip are extremely tender.

Neurological: CN II to XII grossly intact. Sensation to pain, touch, and proprioception normal. DTRs normal in upper and lower extremities. Normal reflexes.

Case Study, Continued

Ms. Taylor was transported to the radiology department for an x-ray of her right leg and hip.

Radiology report showed that the x-ray of the right hip revealed a subcapital fracture at the femoral head/neck junction. No other fractures were noted in the right leg. There were also long-term osteoporotic changes in the femur, tibia, and fibula.

After a careful review of Ms. Taylor's radiographs of the fracture with her and her daughter, an orthopedic consultation was requested and surgery was recommended.

17. What concerns should the health care provider caring for Ms. Taylor have when a prolonged period of inactivity is possible after a hip fracture?

Case Study, Continued

The next day, Ms. Taylor underwent surgical fixation. Physical therapy was initiated the day after surgery. On postoperative day seven, Ms. Taylor was discharged to an in-patient rehabilitation facility.

18. What are appropriate treatment recommendations to reduce Ms. Taylor's risk of future falls and fractures?[29,30]

Case Study, Continued

After 4 weeks, Ms. Taylor is ready to be discharged from the in-patient rehabilitation facility. However, rather than returning home, her children convince her to move into an assisted living facility. Ms. Taylor understands her children's concerns and consents to move to a facility near her daughter.

19. What are some of the national recommendations regarding screening for osteoporosis?[30,31]

20. What are recommendations for health care providers?

ONLINE ANSWER SUBMISSION

When you are ready to submit your answers for grading and reflective expert feedback for evaluation, go to http://www.evolve.elsevier.com/DickAndButtaro/ to complete this case.

References

1. National Osteoporosis Foundation (2014). *Clinician's guide to prevention and treatment of osteoporosis.* Washington, DC: National Osteoporosis Foundation.
2. U.S. Preventive Services Task Force. (2011). Screening for osteoporosis: U.S. Preventive services task force recommendation statement. *Annals of Internal Medicine, 154*(5), 356–364.
3. Kalichman, L., Cole, R., Kim, D., Li, L., Suri, P., Guermazi, A., et al. (2009). Spinal stenosis prevalence and association with symptoms: The Framingham Study. *The Spine Journal, 9*(7), 545–550.
4. Siebert, E., Prüss, H., Klingebiel, R., Failli, V., Einhäupl, K., & Schwab, J. (2009). Lumbar spinal stenosis: Syndrome, diagnostics and treatment. *Nature Reviews. Neurology, 5*(7), 392–403.
5. Munagala, R., Vishnu, V., & Tomar, V. (2014). Osteomalacia. *The New England Journal of Medicine, 370*(6), e10.

6. Gifre, L., Peris, P., Monegal, A., de Osaba, M., Alvarez, L., & Guanabens, N. (2011). Osteomalacia revisited: A report on 28 cases. *Clinical Rheumatology, 30*(5), 639–645.

7. Silverberg, S. J., Clarke, B. L., Peacock, M., Bandeira, F., Boutroy, S., Cusano, N., et al. (2014). Current issues in the presentation of asymptomatic primary hyperparathyroidism: Proceedings of the Fourth International Workshop. *Journal of Clinical Endocrinology & Metabolism, 99*(10), 3580–3594.

8. Bilezikian, J. P., & Silverberg, S. J. (2004). Clinical practice: Asymptomatic primary hyperparathyroidism. *The New England Journal of Medicine, 30*(17), 1746–1751.

9. Watts, N., Bilezikian, J., Camacho, P. M., Greenspan, S., Harris, S., Hodgson, S., et al. (2010). American Association of Clinical Endocrinologists and American College of Endocrinology clinical practice guidelines for the diagnosis and treatment of postmenopausal osteoporosis—2016. *Endocrine Practice, 16*(3), 1–37.

10. Fitzpatrick, L. A. (2002). Secondary causes of osteoporosis. *Mayo Clinic Proceedings, 77*(5), 453–468.

11. Cerdá Gabaroi, D., Peris, P., Monegal, A., et al. (2010). Search for hidden secondary causes in postmenopausal women with osteoporosis. *Menopause (New York, N.Y.), 17*(1), 135–139.

12. World Health Organization (2007). *WHO scientific group on the assessment of osteoporosis at the primary health care level: summary meeting report. Brussels, Belgium.* Geneva, Switzerland: World Health Organization. May 5–7, 2004.

13. U.S. Preventative Services Task Force. (2011). U.S. preventative services task force recommendation statement. *Annals of Internal Medicine, 154*, 356.

14. Cosman, F., de Beur, S., LeBoff, M., Lewiecki, E., Tanner, B., & Randall, R. (2014). Clinician's guide to prevention and treatment of osteoporosis. *Osteoporosis International, 25*(10), 2359–2381.

15. International Society for Clinical Densitometry. 2013 Official Positions—Adult. Retrieved from http://www.iscd.org/official-positions/2013-iscd-official-positions-adult/.

16. Schousboe, J. T., Shepherd, J. A., Bilezikian, J. P., & Baim, S. (2013). Executive summary of the 2013 International Society for Clinical Densitometry position development conference on bone densitometry. *Journal of Clinical Densitometry, 16*(4), 455–466.

17. Management of osteoporosis in postmenopausal women. (2010). 2010 position statement of the North American Menopause Society. *Menopause (New York, N.Y.), 17*(1), 25–54.

18. Sweet, M. G., Sweet, J. M., Jeremiah, M. P., & Galazka, S. S. (2009). Diagnosis and treatment of osteoporosis. *American Family Physician, 79*(3), 193–200.

19. Yoon, V., Maalouf, N. M., & Sakhaee, K. (2012). The effects of smoking on bone metabolism. *Osteoporosis International, 23*(8), 2081–2092.

20. Bone Source. Frax Tool. Arlington: National Osteoporosis Foundation; 2016. Retrieved from: https://my.nof.org/frax-tool.

21. Serrano-Montalbán, B., Arias, Á., Friginal-Ruiz, A. B., & Lucendo, A. J. (2017). The use of the WHO facture risk assessment (FRAX®) tool in predicting risk of fractures in patients with inflammatory bowel disease: A systematic review. *Journal of Clinical Densitometry, 20*(2), 180–187.

22. Kanis, J. A. (2011). Task force of the FRAX initiative. Interpretation and use of FRAX^R in clinical practice. *Osteoporosis International, 22*(9), 2395–2411.

23. Body, J. J., Bergmann, P., Boonen, S., Boutsen, Y., Bruyere, O., Devogelaer, J., et al. (2011). Non-pharmacological management of osteoporosis: A consensus of the Belgian Bone Club. *Osteoporosis International, 22*(11), 2769–2788.

24. Cohen, A., Fleischer, J., Freeby, M. J., McMahon, D. J., Irani, D., & Shane, E. (2009). Clinical characteristics and medication use among premenopausal women with osteoporosis and low BMD: The experience of an osteoporosis referral center. *Journal of Women's Health, 18*(1), 79–84.

25. Crandall, C. J., Newberry, S. J., Diamant, A., Lim, Y., Gellad, W., Booth, M., et al. (2014). Comparative effectiveness of pharmacologic treatments to prevent fractures: An updated systematic review. *Annals of Internal Medicine, 161*(10), 711–723.

26. Drugs for postmenopausal osteoporosis. (2014). *The Medical Letter on Drugs and Therapeutics, 56*(1452), 91–96.

27. Pham, A. N., Datta, S. K., Weber, T. J., Walter, L. C., & Colon-Emeric, C. S. (2011). Cost-effectiveness of oral bisphosphonates for osteoporosis at different ages and levels of life expectancy. *Journal of the American Geriatrics Society, 59*, 1642–1649.

28. Siris, E. S., Harris, S. T., Rosen, C. J., Barr, C., Arvesen, J., Abbott, T., et al. (2006). Adherence to bisphosphonate therapy and fracture rates in osteoporotic women: Relationship to vertebral and nonvertebral fractures from 2 US claims databases. *Mayo Clinic Proceedings, 81*(8), 1013–1022.

29. Karinkanta, S., Piirtola, M., Sievänen, H., Uusi-Rasi, K., & Kannus, P. (2010). Physical therapy approaches to reduce fall and fracture risk among older adults. *Nature Reviews. Endocrinology, 6*(7), 396–407.
30. Moyer, V. A. (2012). U. S. Preventive services task force. Prevention of falls in community-dwelling older adults: U.S. Preventive services task force recommendation statement. *Annals of Internal Medicine, 157*(3), 197–204.
31. Giangregorio, L. M., Papaioannou, A., Macintyre, N. J., Ashe, A., Heinonen, K., Shipp, J., et al. (2014). Too fit to fracture: Exercise recommendations for individuals with osteoporosis or osteoporotic vertebral fracture. *Osteoporosis International, 25*(3), 821–835.

Headache

M. Elizabeth Teixeira

Instructions

After reviewing the case study, please jot down your notes or preliminary answers in the spaces provided. When you are ready to submit your answers for grading and reflective expert feedback for evaluation, go to http://www.evolve.elsevier.com/DickAndButtaro/ to complete this case.

Case Study Scenario/History of Present Illness

Chief Complaint: *New patient with headache.*

A 70-year-old white female (Mrs. Collins) comes to the office today as an add-on urgent visit. She reports "not feeling well" over the past couple of days with feelings of fatigue, fever, and having a bad headache. The onset of headache was 2 days ago, is not letting up, and last night it was difficult to fall asleep. Describes headache pain as a sharp, deep ache that throbs at times. Describes the headache as constant with periods of increased intensity. Chewing and sudden movements and activities such as simply washing her hair also aggravate pain. Associated symptoms of headache include nausea with decreased appetite but no vomiting. On a scale of 1 to 10, she rates her pain as a 4 at its best and 8 at its worse. She tried acetaminophen, two 500-milligram tablets, last night with minimal relief. Nothing really makes it better. She admits to a long history of migraine headaches since adolescence but has not had a bad one in years, and she added, "This feels very different." She admits to continued occasional headaches that she attributes to stress, lack of sleep, or eating trigger foods such as dark chocolate. However, these headaches are not the "bad ones" that she refers to as migraines when she needs to lay down in a dark room. Usually a couple of Tylenol or aspirin relieve these types of headaches.

Mrs. Collins is new to the practice, and there are no available records. She states her last physical examination was 2 years ago and reports taking medications daily as prescribed for high blood pressure (BP), high cholesterol, and for her bones and nerves. She denies any recent hospitalizations or surgeries. Her husband drove her here today and is out in the waiting room. She admits to keeping up with preventative screenings such as mammograms and colonoscopy.

Medications: Acetaminophen 1 g po every 6 hours prn for arthritis pain, Fosamax 70 milligrams po weekly, atenolol 50 milligrams daily, atorvastatin 40 milligrams po at bedtime, alprazolam 0.25 milligrams po daily prn for anxiety, calcium citrate with vitamin D 500/400 milligrams twice a day, vitamin D 1000 IU daily, and baby aspirin 81 milligrams daily.

Allergies: Amoxicillin: generalized rash but states no problem with cephalosporin.

Past medical history: Hypertension, osteoporosis, migraine headaches, social anxiety disorder, dyslipidemia, vitamin D deficiency, and generalized osteoarthritis.

Past surgical history: Total abdominal hysterectomy at age 52 because of fibroids and stereotactic biopsy right breast age 40 because of calcifications (findings benign). Tonsillectomy and adenoidectomy as child. Colonoscopy 5 years ago that showed a few diverticula in the sigmoid colon, but otherwise unremarkable.

Family history: Her father died age 75 from complications of amyotrophic lateral sclerosis (ALS) and had a history of hypertension, type 2 diabetes, depression, and coronary artery disease. Denies myocardial infarction (MI) or stents. Her mother died from a subarachnoid hemorrhage and also had history of hypertension and Alzheimer's disease (AD). Grandparent history unknown.

Personal and social history: She is married with 3 grown children and a retired registered nurse and clinical nursing instructor. No prior history of smoking or illicit drugs. She admits to one glass of red wine with dinner. States she has a happy marriage and relationship with her children and is normally active socially with friends and church groups. She volunteers at a local soup kitchen once a week. Denies any history of physical, verbal, or sexual abuse. She does admit to increased stress at times that makes sleep difficult. This has been the same for many years.

Reproductive health: Gravida 3, para 3, all vaginal deliveries without complications, with birth weights between 7 and 8 pounds. Menarche age 13, surgical menopause age 52.

Health maintenance/prevention: Last mammogram 1 year ago, no abnormal findings. Immunizations up to date (Pneumovax age 65, Prevnar-13 age 68, Tdap age 68, receives annual high-dose influenza). Last purified protein derivative (PPD) was around 5 years ago when she was working and was negative.

Review of Systems

General: Positive fatigue, feverish, headache pain. Denies night sweats or chills.
Skin: Denies rashes or lesions.
Head, eyes, ears, nose, and throat (HEENT): + right-sided temporal headache pain. Denies sinus pain, otalgia, and sore throat.
Respiratory: Denies cough, wheeze, hemoptysis, or shortness of breath.
Cardiac: Denies chest discomfort, palpitations, syncope, or near syncope.
Gastrointestinal: Reports nausea with headache but denies vomiting.
Urinary: Denies dysuria, hematuria, and incontinence.
Neurologic: Positive for headache for the past 48 hours. Denies dizziness/vertigo, paresthesias, muscle weakness, or feelings of faintness.
Hematologic: Denies any prior history of anemia or blood dysplasia.

Physical Examination

Vital signs: BP left arm sitting 160/90. Temperature 99°F, heart rate (HR) 82, respiratory rate (RR) 16, SpO$_2$ 99%. Weight 170 pounds. Height 66 inches. Body mass index (BMI) 27.4.
General: Moderate distress caused by pain.
Skin: No lesions, rashes, and no atypical moles/nevi.
Head: + thickened and tender right temporal artery.
Neck: Supple, no lymphadenopathy, and no thyroid nodule or goiter.
Respiratory: Clear to auscultation. No rales, wheezes, or rhonchi.
Cardiac: Regular rate and rhythm, S1, S2 audible, no S3, S4. No murmurs, rubs, or gallops.
Abdomen: Soft, nondistended, bowel sounds positive in all four quadrants, tympanic to percussion, nontender to palpation.
Extremities: No edema, pedal pulses +2 bilaterally.
Neurologic: Oriented to day, time, and place. Cranial nerves (CNs) II to XII intact. Pupils equal, round, react to light and accommodation (PERRLA). Funduscopic examination: No edema of optic disc, no arteriovenous (AV) nicking. Deep tendon reflexes (DTRs) +2 bilaterally.

ASSESSMENT AND PLAN

1. Based on the history and physical examination results, what are the possible causes (differential diagnosis) for the patient's current condition?

2. What components of the history or physical examination are missing?

3. What diagnostics are necessary for this patient at this time?[1]

4.   What is the cause and pathophysiology of giant cell arteritis and who is most at risk?[1]

5.   What is your diagnostic reasoning in determining the most likely cause of Mrs. Collins' symptoms?

Case Study, Continued

The patient provides more information on further questioning. She denies recent symptoms of an upper respiratory infection, gastrointestinal (GI) or genitourologic symptoms (e.g., diarrhea, abdominal pain, dysuria, hematuria, weight loss). She also denies visual changes such as blurred vision, loss of vision, red eye, or diplopia. She reports no associated migraine aura and/or photophobia. Mrs. Collins further denies any recent dental work and states she sees the dentist regularly twice a year. She also denies grinding her teeth or any history of TMJ issues. She denies any recent tick bite, although admits to working in her yard daily mostly gardening and walking dogs. She occasionally does see a tick on her pets, even though she treats them monthly. However, in addition to pain in her right eye, which she associates with the headache, she states she has had increasing achiness in her shoulders and hip areas recently. She especially notices increased pain in her shoulders even with light housecleaning and when reaching for dishes in the upper kitchen cabinets. Mrs. Collins attributes these aches and pains to her arthritis and "old age." She also denies any recent trauma including falls. Additional findings on examination include her extremity strength graded 5, and her active range of motion (ROM) is somewhat limited in her extremities because of discomfort, especially with external shoulder rotation and raising her arms overhead.

6. What additional differentials, if any, should be considered in this case?[2]

7. What is polymyalgia rheumatica?[2]

8. **What diagnostics are indicated based on the complete history provided?**[3,4]

9. **What treatments should the health care provider recommend for this patient?**[4]

10. **What are other appropriate decisions to aid in this patient's care?**

11. What referrals should the health care provider consider for Mrs. Collins?

Case Study, Continued

Mrs. Collins returns in 10 days for follow-up. She did have a temporal artery biopsy, which confirmed the diagnosis of GCA. She is taking prednisone daily as directed and her headache and muscle aches have lessened significantly. Today she rates her pain as 1 to 3 on a daily basis. Her appetite improved, but she still has trouble sleeping because she "worries too much." If she takes an alprazolam, she can sleep, but she does not like to take it regularly. She denies nausea, vomiting, fever, and chills. Her BP today is still elevated at 154/88 in her left arm and 152/84 in her right arm. Additional physical examination findings today include:

General: Afebrile, in no acute distress.

Skin: Wound from temporal biopsy clean and dry, sutures removed.

Eyes: Sclera clear. Pupils equal and reactive to light. Funduscopic exam shows red reflex present. No papilledema or nicking.

Respiratory: Clear to auscultation throughout lung fields. No rales, wheezes, or rhonchi.

Cardiac: Regular rate, S1, S2, no S3, S4. No murmurs, rubs, or gallops.

Initial laboratory results: ESR 90 mm/h. Lyme titer negative. BMP normal. No electrolyte disturbances or renal dysfunction. CRP 5.0 milligrams/L. CBC reveals mild normocytic anemia and slightly elevated platelets, which are common findings with GCA.

12. What additional patient history should be assessed at this time?

13.   What diagnostics are necessary for this patient at this time?

Case Study, Continued

Mrs. Collins' ECG today reveals normal sinus rhythm, rate 70, PR interval 0.12 second, QT interval 0.32 second, no ST elevation or depression, and normal R wave progression. The ECG also was compared with a previous tracing from 2 years ago (old records obtained) with no significant changes.

14.   What options should be considered for improving Mrs. Collins' blood pressure control because her blood pressure remains elevated despite medication adherence?[5]

15.   What is the target blood pressure goal for Mrs. Collins and preferred pharmacologic treatment according to JNC 8?

16.   What is the management plan for today to address Mrs. Collins' uncontrolled hypertension?

17.   What are the priorities for the next visit in 2 weeks?

18. **What referrals or recommendations could be appropriate for Mrs. Collins at this time?**[6]

Case Study, Continued

Mrs. Collins presents today in a cheerful mood. She states her headache is only occasional now and she is able to complete her daily activities as she did before this all started. She states the biopsy site is still tender to touch so she is careful when showering. Denies falls or near falls, confusion, dizziness, chest pain, or dyspnea on exertion. Her muscle aches have lessened and some days are better than others but she does not really think about it so much now. Has an appointment with the rheumatologist in 3 weeks.

Her physical examination reveals the following:

General: Well-appearing older female, in no acute distress, pleasant.

Vital signs: Weight 152 pounds. Temperature 98.4°F. BP 136/80 left arm. HR 68, O_2 saturation 99%.

Respiratory: Clear to auscultation without wheezes or crackles.

Cardiac: Regular rate, S1, S2, no S3, S4. No murmurs, rubs, or gallops.

Extremities: No edema, pedal pulses 2+ bilaterally.

Musculoskeletal: Full active ROM of all extremities with mild discomfort in both shoulders with external rotation.

Neurologic: No focal deficits.

Other: Home BP log of four readings ranging from 128 to 138 systolic and 70 to 84 diastolic.

19. **What ongoing issues will be the focus of future visits?**[7,8]

20.   What are your concerns about long-term management with prednisone?[9]

21.   What are the long-term effects of glucocorticoid hormones such as prednisone?[10]

Case Study, Continued

The rheumatologist followed Mrs. Collins for 9 months and she is in to see you today and wants to know if the health care provider can take over all her care. She is feeling so much better and is comfortable with your care and knowledge. She states it is much easier to get an appointment here and you spend more time with her at each visit.

22. What are the guidelines for tapering prednisone for patients with giant cell arteritis and/or polymyalgia rheumatica and recommendations for follow-up including laboratory inflammatory markers?[3,7,11]

23. Is it within the scope of practice as an adult/gerontology primary care nurse practitioner or physician's assistant to follow Mrs. Collins as she requested?

ONLINE ANSWER SUBMISSION

When you are ready to submit your answers for grading and reflective expert feedback for evaluation, go to http://www.evolve.elsevier.com/DickAndButtaro/ to complete this case.

References

1. Vorvick, L., & Reinhardt, R. (2013). A differential guide to 5 common eye complaints. *The Journal of Family Practice, 62*(7), 345–355.
2. Kennedy, S. (2012). Polymyalgia rheumatica and giant cell arteritis: An in-depth look at diagnosis and treatment. *Journal of the American Academy of Nurse Practitioners, 277–285*
3. Smith, J., & Swanson, J. (2014). Giant cell arteritis. *Headache, 54*, 1273–1289.
4. Center for Disease Control and Prevention (CDC). (2017). Tickborne diseases of the United States: A reference manual for healthcare providers. Retrieved from https://www.cdc.gov/lyme/resources/tickbornediseases.pdf.
5. James, P., Oparil, S., Carter, B., et al. (2014). 2014 evidence-based guideline for the management of high blood pressure in adults: Reports from the panel members appointed to the eighth joint national committee (JNC 8). *JAMA: The Journal of the American Medical Association, 311*(5), 507–520.
6. Cosman, F., de Beur, S. J., LeBoff, M. S., Lewiecki, E. M., Tanner, B., Randall, S., et al. (2014). Clinician's guide to prevention and treatment of osteoporosis. *Osteoporosis International, 25*(10), 2359–2381.
7. American Geriatrics Society. (2015). American Geriatrics Society 2015 updated Beers criteria for potentially inappropriate medication use in older adults. *Journal of the American Geriatrics Society, 63*(11), 2227–2246.
8. Sheikh, J., & Yesavage, J. (1986). Geriatric depression scale (GDS): Recent evidence and development of a shorter version. *Clinical Gerontologist, 5*, 165–173.
9. Leuppi, J. D., Schuetz, P., Bingisser, R., Bodmer, M., Briel, M., Drescher, T., et al. (2013). Short-term vs conventional glucocorticoid therapy in acute exacerbations of chronic obstructive pulmonary disease the REDUCE randomized clinical trial. *JAMA: The Journal of the American Medical Association, 309*(21), 2223–2231.
10. Nakasato, Y. R., & Carnes, B. A. (2009). Myopathy, polymyalgia rheumatic, and temporal arteritis. In J. Halter, J. Ouslander, M. Tinetti, S. Studenski, K. High, & S. Asthana (Eds.), *Hazzard's geriatric medicine and gerontology* (6th ed., pp. 1445–1452). New York: McGraw Hill Medical.
11. Freeman, A., & Rappoport, R. (2013). Polymayalgia rheumatica and giant cell arteritis: How best to approach these related diseases. *Family Practice, 62*(6), S5–S9.

Blood in the Urine

Jean Boucher

Instructions

After reviewing the case study, please jot down your notes or preliminary answers in the spaces provided. When you are ready to submit your answers for grading and reflective expert feedback for evaluation, go to http://www.evolve.elsevier.com/DickAndButtaro/ to complete this case.

Case Study Scenario/History of Present Illness

R.K. is a 63-year-old African American male who presents to a primary care clinic with increasing urinary urgency with incomplete bladder emptying, nocturia three to four times nightly, a weak stream, and lower back pain. He describes the lower back pain as an intermittent, dull ache with no radiation to the legs. R.K. is currently taking nonsteroidal antiinflammatory drugs (NSAIDs) around the clock for this pain, with limited relief. The patient also admits to seeing blood in his urine over the last few months. He states these symptoms have been getting worse over the past 6 months. He denies any fever or chills and does note some increasing fatigue over the last few months.

Allergies: Sulfa (shellfish).

Medications: Metformin 1000 milligrams po daily, Flomax 0.4 milligrams po daily, and ibuprofen 400 milligrams po every 4 to 6 hours.

Past medical history: Type 2 diabetes mellitus (DM), osteoarthritis.

Past surgical history: Right knee meniscus repair, age 38.

Family history: Mother died of breast cancer at age 70. Father died age 60, type 2 DM and renal failure. Paternal uncle, prostate cancer diagnosed age 50, died age 54. Two brothers, age 40 and 45, alive and well.

Social history: Married, lives at home with wife and son, age 16. Works as a maintenance person at a public high school. Smoker: 1 pack per day (PPD) smoker × 10 years, quit at age 35. Alcohol: 1 to 2 drinks (beer) on the weekend.

Review of Systems

General: Reports fatigue that has been increasing in recent months. Denies fever, chills, or recent illness.

Skin: Denies rashes or bruising.

Head, eyes, ears, nose, and throat (HEENT): Wears glasses, no vision changes, no dysphagia.

Pulmonary: Notes some dyspnea on exertion with work. Denies recent respiratory illnesses (i.e., no pneumonia, no asthma, no chronic obstructive pulmonary disease [COPD]).

Cardiac: Denies chest pain, no palpitations, no history of cardiac murmurs.

Gastrointestinal: Occasional reflux with spicy foods, denies nausea or vomiting.

Genitourinary: Complains about incomplete bladder emptying with nocturia three to four times a night, a weak stream, and occasional hematuria over the past few months.

Musculoskeletal: Chronic right knee and right hip pain from osteoarthritis. Lower back pain described as a dull, intermittent ache.

Neurologic: Denies dizziness or headaches.

Physical Examination

    General: Well-groomed, overweight male presents in no acute distress, afebrile.

    Vital signs: Height 68 inches. Weight 210 pounds. Blood pressure 140/78. Heart rate (HR) 78 regular, respiratory rate (RR) 12, O_2 saturation 98% on room air. Body mass index (BMI) 31.

    Skin: Intact, warm, dry, without lesions or ecchymosis or bleeding

    HEENT: Normocephalic, atraumatic, pupils equal, round, reactive to light (PERRL), no scleral icterus bilaterally. Good dentition. Oropharynx clear with moist mucous membranes, no lesions. Tonsils intact, no erythema or enlargement.

    Neck: Supple. No thyromegaly, no nodularity.

    Respiratory: Lung sounds clear bilaterally, no adventitious sounds.

    Cardiac: S1, S2, regular rate and rhythm (RRR). No S3, S4, murmurs, or gallops.

    Abdomen: Soft, bowel sounds (BS) present × 4 quadrants. Nontender, no hepatosplenomegaly.

    Genitourinary: Digital rectal examination (DRE) reveals a nontender, smooth prostate gland with bilateral asymmetric enlargement (right greater than left), no masses in rectum.

    Extremities: Moves upper and lower extremities, noted stiffness and crepitus in the right knee and right hip with flexion. No edema.

    Neurologic: Alert, oriented, appropriate.

ASSESSMENT AND PLAN

1. Based on the history and physical examination results, what are the possible causes (differential diagnosis) for the patient's current condition?

2. What components of the history are missing?

3. **What components of the physical examination are missing?**

4. **What diagnostics are necessary for this patient at this time?**

Case Study, Continued

R.K.'s presenting urinary symptoms cause the health care provider to suspect a UTI. The associated complaints of back pain suggest the possibility of prostate cancer and indicate the importance of obtaining the alkaline phosphatase to assess for bone turnover (indicated by an elevated finding), which is associated with prostate cancer.[1]

R.K.'s urine is tested by dipstick and is positive for 1+ leukocytes, 50 red blood cells (RBCs), and negative for nitrates and blood. The decision is made to treat R.K. for a UTI. R.K. does not complain of a fever and chills, and the rectal examination did not reveal prostate tenderness, which might otherwise support a diagnosis of acute prostatitis. The health care provider considers fosfomycin 3 grams po, which is a one-time dose given the presentation of an uncomplicated cystitis characterized by urinary symptoms and microscopic hematuria without upper UTI symptoms (i.e., no fever or costovertebral angle (CVA) tenderness) in an older man with type 2 DM. The patient cannot have trimethoprim-sulfamethoxazole (Bactrim) because he is allergic to sulfa, and fluoroquinolones are presumed to have higher risk for bacterial resistance in UTIs.[2,3] However, the health care provider is concerned about the cost of fosfomycin knowing that not all health insurances will cover it and asks R.K. if he has had any antibiotic therapy in the past 3 months. Learning that the patient has not had antibiotics for even longer than that, the provider decides to prescribe ciprofloxacin 500 milligrams po twice a day for 7 days.[4]

In a review of his chart, a previous PSA was normal with mild enlargement bilaterally of the prostate noted without nodularity or discomfort. The patient had been placed on Flomax at that time

Patient teaching should include.

- The importance of laboratory testing being done today.
- Instructions to explain how to take the prescribed medication appropriately.
- Information explaining the importance of calling the health care provider if R.K. develops any fever, nausea, vomiting, worsening urinary symptoms, or flank pain.
- Return to clinic for follow-up in 2 weeks, but sooner if he feels worse.

R.K. returns to clinic in 2 weeks with the same genitourinary symptoms unresolved. His laboratory results from his previous visit include:

Visit	Previous Visit 6 Months Ago	Normal Ranges
CBC:	*CBC:*	*CBC:*
WBC 5.4	WBC 6.0	4.5–11.0
RBC 3.0	RBC 3.9	3.5–5.5
HGB 11.8	HGB 14	12–15
HCT 32	HCT 38	36–48
MCV 78	MCV 85	80–100
MCH 24	MCHC 34	25–35
MCHC 30	MCHC 36	31–37
PLT 155	PLT 200	150–420
RDW 18.4	RDW 13	11–14.5
Neutrophils 50	Neutrophils 60	40–80
Lymphocytes 26	Lymphocytes 28	20–50
Monocytes 5	Monocytes 7	2–12
Eosinophils 0	Eosinophils 0	0–0.5
Basophils 0	Basophils 0	0–0.2
CMP:	*CMP:*	
Na 140	Na 140	
K 3.9	K 3.9	
Cl	Cl	65–100 (fasting)
CO_2	CO_2	8–25
Glucose 180 (nonfasting)	Glucose 160 (nonfasting)	0.8–1.3
BUN 12	BUN 12	8.5–10.5
Creatinine 1.2	Creatinine 1.2	3.0–5.0
Ca 9.0	Ca 9.0	5–35
Albumin 3.5	Albumin 3.5	17–45
AST 18	AST 18	0.1–1.3
ALT 30	ALT 30	30–132
Total bilirubin 0.6	Total bilirubin 0.6	
Alkaline phosphatase 157	Alkaline phosphatase 140	
PSA 4.0	PSA 2.0	0–4
Urine culture less than 20,000 colonies	—	—

ALT, Alanine transaminase; *AST*, aspartate transaminase; *BUN*, blood urea nitrogen; *CBC*, complete blood count; *CMP*, comprehensive metabolic panel; *HGB*, hemoglobin; *HCT*, hematocrit; *MCH*, mean corpuscular hemoglobin; *MCHC*, mean corpuscular hemoglobin concentration; *MCV*, mean corpuscular volume; *PLT*, platelet; *PSA*, prostate-specific antigen; *RBC*, red blood count; *RDW*, red cell distribution width; *WBC*, white blood count.

The health care provider explains to R.K. that based on his urinary culture findings, R.K. did not have a UTI. The provider also discusses with R.K. that his laboratory tests reveal that he is somewhat anemic, which may be related to a chronic disease condition. Additionally, R.K.'s laboratory results indicate a concerning rise in his PSA level and alkaline phosphatase blood tests, which could indicate that his symptoms are caused by a different problem. The provider explains that further workup to evaluate R.K. for the possibility of prostate cancer as the cause of his health problem is necessary, even though he has hematuria, which is not commonly associated with prostate cancer.

5. What additional factors and findings in the clinical presentation would justify the health care provider's consideration of prostate cancer as a potential diagnosis for this patient?[5-9]

6. What are the current screening guidelines for prostate cancer?[10-12]

7.   What should health care providers know about prostatic-specific antigen levels in African American males?[8]

8.   What factors are important to discuss with R.K. about his suspected prostate cancer?[13-15]

9.   What diagnostic tests and consultations should be considered for this patient (R.K.) to evaluate him for prostate cancer?[9]

10. What should informed consent and patient education for R.K. include? (See Box 17.1)[16]

BOX 17.1 ■ Patient Education: Prostate Cancer Screening

The American College of Physicians and the American Cancer Society have suggested useful discussion points to consider when counseling patients about prostate cancer, including a summary of key points:

- Prostate cancer is a leading cause of death in men, thus prostate cancer screening is an important consideration. However, screening for prostate cancer is controversial, so it is important that men be involved in deciding whether to screen or not screen for this disorder.
- Prostate cancer screening may reduce the chance of prostate cancer mortality, but the evidence is mixed with a small absolute benefit.
- Most men who choose not to have PSA testing will not be diagnosed with prostate cancer and will die of another cause. However, some men who choose not to be screened with PSA testing will die of prostate cancer.
- Both false-positive and false-negative results can occur from PSA testing and DRE. A prostate biopsy may be required to evaluate an abnormal finding for cancer, and this procedure can miss finding a cancer and can rarely cause serious infections.
- Patients who choose PSA testing are much more likely than those who decline testing to be diagnosed with prostate cancer. This is associated with a risk for being "overdiagnosed."
- Aggressive therapy is necessary to realize any benefit from finding an early-stage prostate cancer; however, studies show men with a high PSA or Gleason Score are most likely to benefit.
- Surgery and radiation treatments most commonly offered with the intent to cure prostate cancer can lead to problems with urinary, bowel, and sexual function.
- Active surveillance may be appropriate for men who are at low risk for progression from prostate cancer (PSA < 10 ng/mL and Gleason < 7). PSA tests, DRE, and repeating biopsies can be planned to determine whether aggressive treatment is warranted because of cancer progression.

DRE, *Digital rectal examination;* PSA, *prostate-specific antigen.*

11.   What does clinical evaluation and management for prostate cancer include?[11,17]

Recommended therapies for prostate cancer are based on several factors such as the patient's health status, age, local versus advanced-stage disease, risk stratification (Box 17.2), castration-sensitive versus castration-resistant disease, and quality of life. Treatments include surgery to remove the prostate (i.e., a radical prostatectomy [RP]), radiation therapy (e.g., external beam or seed implants), hormone ablation (using medications or surgical orchiectomy) or with medications known as androgen deprivation therapy (ADT) (e.g., antiandrogens, luteinizing hormone-releasing hormone [LHRH] antagonists), chemotherapy for advanced-stage disease, newer oral agents for metastatic castrationresistant cancer, and bone-directed therapies (biphosphonates).

Other nontreatment options discussed with patients with prostate cancer can involve watchful waiting and active surveillance to be considered based on individual risk and health factor considerations.

The Cancer of the Prostate Risk Assessment (CAPRA) score of 0 to 10 is calculated based on the PSA level, biopsy Gleason Score, clinical T stage, positive biopsy score, and age, which can also be used by urologists and oncologists for disease risk and prognosis.[18]

BOX 17.2 ■ Risk Stratification Groups[18]

Very low:
T1c (tumor identified by needle biopsy), PSA < 10, GS 6, <3 cores and no cores >50%, PSAD < 0.15

Low:
T1 (T1 clinically inapparent tumor, T1a and b tumor histologic finding, to T1c tumor identified)
T2a (tumor involves one half of one lobe or less), PSA < 10, GS 6

Intermediate:
T2b (tumor involves more than one-half of one lobe but not both lobes)
T2c (tumor involves both lobes) or GS 7 or PSA 10–20

High
T3a (extracapsular extension [unilateral or bilateral]) or GS 8–10, or PSA > 20

Very high:
T3b (tumor invades seminal vesicle(s)
T4 (tumor is fixed or invades adjacent structures other than seminal vesicles)

Note: Information is based on tumor stage, PSA level, Gleason Score, and core biopsy findings for cancer.
GS, Gleason Score; PSA, prostate-specific antigen; PSAD, prostate-specific antigen density.

Follow-Up Urology. *R.K. was seen by the urologist and had the prostate TRUS biopsy.*

- **Pathology report:** 10 of 12 cores positive, 50% of cancer in cores noted in both lobes indicating T2c clinical stage.
- **Histology:** Adenocarcinoma.
- **Gleason Score:** 4/3 indicating a more aggressive tumor.
- **Abdominal pelvic CT scan:** No lymphadenopathy, normal abdominal and pelvic structures, and no evidence of metastatic disease.
- **Bone scan:** Negative for bone lesions indicating cancer.

Case Study, Continued

R.K. is referred to a medical genitourinary oncologist who specializes in prostate cancer for a second opinion and further evaluation. The medical oncologist consults with the radiation oncologist and provides recommendations to R.K. and his wife about potential treatment options.

After talking with the oncologist, R.K. opts to start on androgen hormonal therapy with Lupron (LHRH agonist) and bicalutamide po (antiandrogen therapy) to treat his prostate cancer before starting radiation therapy with the ADT therapy he will need to undergo for 6 months. Antiandrogen therapy is indicated to block testosterone production, which is known to contribute to the development of prostate cancer cells.

12. What important medication side effects and other patient education does the health care provider need to discuss with R.K before he starts his therapy?[5,19]

13. What advice should the health care provider discuss with R.K. about working while the prostate cancer is being treated?

Case Study, Continued

While R.K. is on prostate cancer therapy, he comes to see his primary care provider 2 months into his prostate cancer therapy for his diabetes checkup. R.K. describes increasing urinary incontinence associated with lower back pain radiating down his left leg to his foot. He also complains of weakness in his left leg with ambulation. He has been taking Tylenol 500 milligram tablets, 2 tablets po every 6 hours without any relief of pain and describes the pain as an "8" on a scale of 1 to 10.

Review of Systems

General: Denies fever, chills. Describes some appetite loss but denies known weight change.

HEENT: Denies vision changes, dysphagia.

Pulmonary: No recent cough, sputum production, or shortness of breath.

Cardiac: No chest pain or palpitations.

Gastrointestinal: He describes two episodes when he was unable to make it to bathroom and lost control of his bowels. Denies nausea, vomiting, reflux, abdominal pain, diarrhea, or blood in stools.

Genitourinary: Notices increased urinary incontinence, wears incontinence pads and changes them every few hours. Denies hematuria.

Musculoskeletal: Describes increasing lower back pain radiating down his left buttock to left leg and foot.

Neurologic: Describes pain and difficulty lifting left foot and leg to tie shoes, and when going up stairs.

Physical Examination

General: R.K. presents walking into the examination room with a cane borrowed from a friend and with notable discomfort.

Vital signs: Blood pressure 148/88. HR 80, RR 14, pulse ox 97% on room air resting.

HEENT: Moist mucous membranes, oropharynx is clear without erythema or lesions.

Neck: Supple. No cervical or supraclavicular lymphadenopathy.

Lungs: Clear to auscultation, no adventitious sounds bilaterally.

Abdomen: Soft, BS present. Nontender, no organomegaly.

Rectal examination: Anal reflex decreased. Negative blood or masses on examination.

Musculoskeletal: Unable to stand upright on both lower extremities because of left leg weakness, noted discomfort from lower back pain. Spine: Tender to palpation at lumbar region lower back. Unable to walk toe to heel because of unsteady gait related to leg weakness and pain.

Neurologic: Motor strength 5/5 upper extremities bilaterally, 4/5 right leg, 3/5 left leg. Deep tendon reflexes 2+ bilaterally upper arms, negative lower extremities. Sensation intact upper extremities, and right leg; decreased to left leg and foot.

Extremities: No peripheral edema and no calf pain tenderness bilaterally. Lower extremities warm to touch.

14. Based on R.K.'s prostate cancer diagnosis and diagnostic results, what oncological emergent condition should the health care provider suspect and what diagnostics are now indicated?

Case Study, Continued

R.K. is admitted to the hospital diagnosed with a spinal cord compression caused by positive metastatic disease in his L4 and L5 spine regions. A multidisciplinary team (surgery, radiation, and medical oncology) decide that the cord compression is not operable and not the best option for R.K. The preferred emergent treatment in this case is radiation plus dexamethasone (Decadron), 16 milligrams po daily in divided doses (i.e., 4 milligrams po every 6 hours). After stabilization R.K. is discharged on Decadron 4 milligrams po every 6 hours with a rapid taper to decrease the Decadron by 2 milligrams (½ tablet) po every 3 to 4 days until finished. It is also noted that R.K.'s Vitamin D level is noted to be 20 and he rarely eats dairy.[20-23]

15. What follow-up is warranted for R.K. after hospital discharge?[24,25]

Case Study, Continued

R.K. returns to clinic for his diabetes checkup 1 month later. He reports he is stable, after therapy for prostate cancer, but asks if his son or brother would be at risk for prostate cancer and need to be tested.

16. What would an appropriate response be to R.K.'s question?

17. R.K. also asks if he should be tested for the BRCA mutation because his mother died of breast cancer and he read on the Internet that breast cancer with the BRCA mutation can lead to prostate cancer in men.[26-30]

Case Study, Continued

R.K. calls the primary care office a month later reporting that he has been experiencing hematuria with blood clots over the past 3 days. He denies fever, nausea, vomiting, burning, or new frequency on urination.

18. Based on what the health care provider knows about R.K.'s recent history, which of the following should the provider consider the likely cause of R.K's current symptoms?

A. Bladder cancer
B. Kidney cancer
C. Radiation cystitis
D. Urinary tract infection

Case Study, Continued

The urology consultation reveals that R.K's has radiation cystitis from radiation therapy. He will be treated by Urology with observation and potential sclerotherapy if medical management fails.[31]

19. What will R.K. require for further follow-up monitoring?[32]

References

1. Jung, K., Lein, M., Stephan, C., Von Hosslin, K., Semjonow, A., Sinha, P., et al. (2004). Comparison of 10 serum bone turnover markers in prostate carcinoma patients with bone metastatic spread: Diagnostic and prognostic implications. *International Journal of Cancer*, *11*(5), 783–791.
2. Gupta, K., Hooton, T., Naber, K. G., Wullt, B., Colgan, R., Miller, L. G., et al. (2011). International clinical practice guidelines for the treatment of acute uncomplicated cystitis and pyelonephritis in women: A 2010 update by the Infectious Diseases Society of America and the European Society for Microbiology and Infectious Diseases. *Clinical Infectious Diseases*, *52*(5), e103–e120.
3. Grigoryan, L., Trautner, B. W., & Gupta, K. (2014). Diagnosis and management of urinary tract infections in the outpatient setting a review. *Journal of the American Medical Association*, *312*, 1677–1684.
4. Drekonja, D. M., Rector, T. S., Cutting, A., & Johnson, J. R. (2013). Urinary tract infection in male veterans: Treatment patterns and outcomes. *JAMA Internal Medicine*, *173*(1), 62–68.
5. CDC. (2017). Centers for Disease Control and Prevention. Cancer in men. Retrieved from https://www.cdc.gov/cancer/dcpc/data/men.htm.
6. Siegel, R. L., Miller, K. D., & Jemal, A. (2017). Cancer statistics. *CA: A Cancer Journal for Clinicians*, *67*(1), 7.
7. Wilson, K. M., & Mucci, L. A. (2015). Epidemiology of prostate cancer. In E. J. Trabulsi (Ed.), *Prostate cancer, A multidisciplinary approach to diagnosis and management* (pp. 11–24). New York: Demos Medical Publishing.
8. Shenoy, D., Packianathan, S., Chen, A. M., & Vijayakumar, S. (2016). Do African-American men need separate prostate cancer screening guidelines? *BioMed Central Urology*, *16*, 19. Retrieved from https://www.ncbi.nlm.nih.gov/pmc/articles/PMC4862049/#CR8.

9. Odedina, F. T., Akinremi, T. O., Chinewundoh, F., Roberts, R., Yu, D., Reams, R. R., et al. (2009). Prostate cancer disparities in black men of African descent: A comparative literature review of prostate cancer burden among black men in the United States, Caribbean, United Kingdom, and west Africa. *Infectious Agents and Cancer, BioMed Central.*, *4*(1), S2, 1–8.

10. American Urological Association (2015). Early detection of prostate cancer. Retrieved from http://www.auanet.org/guidelines/early-detection-of-prostate-cancer-(2013-reviewed-and-validity-confirmed 2015).

11. National Comprehensive Cancer Network (NCCN) (2017). National Comprehensive Cancer Network Guidelines. Retrieved from https://www.trikobe.org/nccn/guideline/urological/english/prostate_detection.pdf.

12. US Preventive Services Task Force (USPSTF). (2017). USPSTF Screening for prostate cancer. Retrieved from http://www.screeningprostatecancer.org.

13. Hoffman, R. M. (2017). Screening for prostate cancer. *Uptodate*. Retrieved from https://www.uptodate.com/contents/screening-for-prostatecancer?source=see_link&sectionName=Referrals%20to%20urology%20to%20evaluate%20abnormal%20results&anchor=H37#H37.

14. Qaseem, A., Barry, M. J., Denberg, T. D., Owens, D. K., & Shekelle, P. (2013). Screening for prostate cancer: A guidance statement from the clinical guidelines committee of the American College of Physicians. *Annals of Internal Medicine*, *158*(10), 761–769.

15. Wolf, A. M., Wender, R. C., Etzioni, R. B., Thompson, I. M., D'Amico, A. V., Volk, R. J., et al. (2010). American Cancer Society guideline for the early detection of prostate cancer. American cancer society Prostate Cancer Advisory Committee. *CA: A Cancer Journal for Clinicians*, *60*(2), 70–98.

16. Rasuli, P., & Hammond, D. (1998). Metformin and contrast media: Where is the conflict? *Canadian Association of Radiologists Journal*, *49*(3), 161–166.

17. Pearson, R., Williams, P. M., & O'Callaghan, M. (2014). Common questions about the diagnosis and management of benign prostatic hyperplasia. *American Family Physician*, *90*(11), 769–774. Retrieved from http://www.aafp.org/afp/2014/1201/p769.pdf.

18. Reichard, C. A., & Klein, E. A. (2015). Current approaches to prostate cancer staging and risk stratification: In the midst of a paradigm shift. In E. J. Trabulsi (Ed.), *Prostate cancer, a multidisciplinary approach to diagnosis and management* (pp 67–76). New York: Demos Medical Publishing.

19. National Cancer Institute. (NCI). (2017). Prostate cancer, nutrition, and dietary supplements (PDQ®)–Patient Version. Questions and Answers about Soy. Retrieved from https://www.cancer.gov/about-cancer/treatment/cam/patient/prostate-supplements-pdq#section/_95.

20. Byrne, T. N. (1992). Spinal cord compression from epidural metastases. *New England Journal of Medicine*, *327*(9), 614–619.

21. Osowski, M. (2002). Spinal cord compression: An obstructive oncologic emergency. *Topics in Advanced Practice Nursing eJournal*, *2*(4). Retrieved from http://www.medscape.com/viewarticle/442735_6.

22. Huff, S. J. (2001). Neoplasms, spinal cord. *eMedicine Journal [serial online]*, *2*, 1–11. Retrieved from http://www.emedicine.com/emerg/topic337.htm.

23. L'Espérance, S., Vincent, F., Gaudreault, M., Ouellet, J. A., Li, M., Tosikyan, A., et al. (2012). Treatment of metastatic spinal cord compression: CEPO review and clinical recommendations. *Current Oncology*, *19*(6), e478–e490.

24. Datta, M., & Schwartz, G. G. (2012). Calcium and vitamin D supplementation during androgen deprivation therapy for prostate cancer: A critical review. *The Oncologist*, *17*(9), 1171–1179.

25. Mennen-Winchell, L. J., Grigoriev, V., Alpert, P., Dos Santos, H., & Tonstad, S. (2015). Determinants of vitamin D levels in men receiving androgen deprivation therapy for prostate cancer. *Journal of the American Association of Nurse Practitioners*, *27*(1), 39–47.

26. Agalliu, I., Karlins, E., Kwon, E. M., Iwasaki, L. M., Diamond, A., Ostrander, E. A., et al. (2007). Rare germline mutations in the *BRCA2* gene are associated with early-onset prostate cancer. *British Journal of Cancer*, *97*, 826–831.

27. Edwards, S. M., Kote-Jarai, Z., Meitz, J., Hamoudi, R., Hope, Q., Osin, P., et al. (2003). Two percent of men with early-onset prostate cancer harbor germline mutations in the BRCA2 gene. *American Journal of Human Genetics*, *72*, 1–12.

28. Giri, V. N., Gross, L., Gomella, L. G., & Hyatt, C. (2016). How I do it: Genetic counseling and genetic testing for inherited prostate cancer. *The Canadian Journal of Urology*, *23*(2), 8247–8253.

29. NCCN Clinical Practice Guidelines in Oncology (NCCN Guidelines®): Genetic/familial high-risk assessment: Breast and Ovarian (Version 2.2017). Retrieved from http://www.nccn.org/professionals/physician_gls/pdf/genetics_screening.pdf.

30. Klein, E. A., Cooperberg, M. R., Magi-Galluzzi, C., Simko, J. P., Falzarano, S. M., Maddala, T., et al. (2016). A 17-gene assay to predict prostate cancer aggressiveness in the context of gleason grade heterogeneity, tumor multifocality, and biopsy undersampling. *European Urology*, *66*(3), 550–560.
31. Muruve, N. A. (2017). Radiation cystitis treatment & management. Retrieved from http://emedicine.medscape.com/article/2055124-treatment.
32. Gralow, J. R., Sybil Biermann, J., Farooki, A., Fornier, M. N., Gagel, R. F., Kumar, R., et al. (2013). NCCN task force report: Bone health in cancer care. *Journal of National Comprehensive Care Network*, *11*(3), S1–S50.

Falling

Dawn Carpenter

Instructions

After reviewing the case study, please jot down your notes or preliminary answers in the spaces provided. When you are ready to submit your answers for grading and reflective expert feedback for evaluation, go to http://www.evolve.elsevier.com/DickAndButtaro/ to complete this case.

Case Study Scenario/History of Present Illness

Mr. Smith is an 80-year-old man admitted after a fall at home. He has had a prolonged hospital stay, including 10 days in the medical intensive care unit (ICU). The following is his discharge summary from the hospital. You will be the health care provider receiving this patient into your care post hospital discharge.

Discharge Summary. This is an 80-year-old gentleman admitted April 1 who is being discharged today April 14. This dictation covers his hospital stay, including ICU days from April 1 through April 9, and his time on the general care floor from April 9 through today's discharge.

History of Present Illness. Mr. Smith presented to the emergency department (ED) reporting he tripped over his O_2 tubing and fell, hitting his head on the table, but he is unclear of the exact events surrounding his fall. He does admit to increased weakness and complaints of increasing shortness of breath (SOB) over the previous 2 to 3 days, despite escalating doses of his albuterol inhaler. He denied fevers and chills but admits to cough and increased sputum production. He admitted to being thirsty with poor po intake × 48 hours before admission. He denied sick contacts or recent hospitalizations.

> **Past medical history:** Chronic obstructive pulmonary disease (COPD) and is O_2 and steroid dependent, Stage 3 chronic kidney disease (CKD) (baseline creatinine 1.5), hypertension (HTN), hyperlipidemia, coronary artery disease (CAD), diet-controlled diabetes mellitus (DM), anxiety, osteoarthritis, and obesity. One to two hospitalizations per year for pneumonia and flu over the last 5 years.
>
> **Past surgical history**: Appendectomy 1940. Right total knee replacement age 66.
>
> **Allergies**: Ibuprofen (Motrin).
>
> **Medications on Admission:**
> Albuterol 90 micrograms, 2 puffs four times a day
> Fluticasone/salmeterol (Advair) 500/50 1 puff twice daily
> Tiotropium (Spiriva) 18 micrograms inhaled daily
> Prednisone 10 milligrams po daily
> Lisinopril (Zestril) 10 milligrams po daily
> Aspirin 325 milligrams po daily
> Atorvastatin (Lipitor) 40 milligrams po daily
> Metoprolol 50 milligrams po twice a day

Ativan 0.5 milligrams po every 8 hours as needed.

Pneumovax and influenza immunization at his primary care provider's office.

Social history: Retired farmer, married with three children. Remote history of smoking (60 pack-year history). Alcohol (ETOH): Two beers per day, denies illicit substances.

Family history: Mother died of myocardial infarction (MI) age 78. Father died of kidney disease age 82. Sister alive and well age 62, but past history of breast cancer (CA). Brother alive age 64 with COPD. Three children alive and well, with no known health issues.

Review of symptoms: On arrival to the ED positive for right hip pain, mild headache, but denies vision changes, photophobia, or nausea/vomiting. Denies weight gain/loss, vision changes, hearing problems, sore throat, chest pain, palpitations, diarrhea, constipation, or leg swelling.

Physical Examination on Presentation to Emergency Department

General: Cachectic, anxious, older male sitting semirecumbent on stretcher with pursed lip breathing on 4 L oxygen via nasal cannula (NC).

Neurologic: Awake, alert, male. Oriented on arrival but became somnolent during examination.

Head, eyes, ears, nose, and throat (HEENT): Ecchymosis right temporal area. Sclera clear. Mucous membranes dry, no jugular vein distention (JVD).

Pulmonary: Barrel chested, tachypneic, scattered wheezing noted throughout.

Cardiovascular: Clear S1 S2, no murmurs, rubs, or gallops. Palpable dorsalis pedis (DP) and posterior tibial (PT) pulses.

Abdomen: Abdomen soft, bowel sounds +, nontender, nondistended.

Extremities: Thin skin, fragile with small ecchymotic area near IV attempts, + clubbing of fingers bilaterally. Right hip area mildly ecchymotic and tender to palpation. Right lower extremity: No external rotation or shortening.

Laboratory results on ED admission:

Sodium: 145 (136–145 mmol/L)

Potassium: 4.0 (3.4–5.1 (mmol/L)

Chloride: 102 (98–107 mmol/L)

Carbon dioxide: 30 (22–32 mmol/L)

Blood urea nitrogen (BUN): 40 (5–23 milligrams/dL)

Creatinine: 1.8 (0.4–1.0 md/dL)

Estimated glomerular filtration rate (eGFR) (mL/min): 35 mL/min/1.73 m^2

Random glucose: 152 H (74–118 milligrams/dL)

Magnesium: 1.5

Phosphorous: 1.5

White blood cell (WBC): 10.5

Hemoglobin: 16.0

Hematocrit: 50

Platelets: 160,000

Radiology:

Head computed tomography (CT) scan: 5-mm subdural hemorrhage (SDH) in right temporoparietal area.

Chest x-ray: No infiltrates, flattened diaphragm consistent with COPD. Right rib fractures. Right hip and femur and pelvis x-rays are negative for fracture.

Hospital Course by System

Pulmonary: Mr. Smith was admitted directly to the ICU from the ED for observation related to rib fractures and COPD history. He required a high-flow NC briefly and then BiPAP for respiratory support for presumed COPD exacerbation. After 36 hours of BiPAP, the decision was made that he needed to be intubated because he was beginning to fatigue and was becoming more hypercarbic. He was subsequently intubated and ventilated for the majority of his ICU stay. During his ICU stay he was treated for pneumonia. Initial treatment was with piperacillin-tazobactam (Zosyn) and vancomycin, but was then changed to ceftriaxone (Rocephin) and completed a total of 7 days of treatment.

Cardiac: Mr. Smith had an elevated troponin the day he was intubated. Troponin peaked at 0.8 ng/dL. Electrocardiogram (ECG) showed left ventricular hypertrophy (LVH), but no infarction. An echocardiogram was performed and his ejection fraction (EF) was 55%. Cardiology was consulted. He remained hemodynamically stable throughout his hospital course. His HTN was managed with his metoprolol because his lisinopril was held because of his deteriorating renal status (acute chronic renal failure). Lisinopril was subsequently added back after his renal function improved.

Neurology:
- Right SDH: Seen by neurosurgery and observed. No operative intervention indicated.
- Delirium: Hospital course was complicated by delirium while he was intubated, but the delirium resolved 24 hours after extubation. This resolved with intermittent doses of haloperidol (Haldol) and quetiapine (Seroquel), which have since been discontinued.
- Moderate headache since injury. Treated with scheduled acetaminophen (Tylenol) 6 milligrams po every 8 hours and fentanyl intravenously (IV) prn for severe pain.
- His anxiety has been a challenge to manage, but it is better with lorazepam (Ativan) scheduled around the clock.

Genitourology/electrolytes:
- **Renal:** Mr. Smith's hospital course was complicated by acute kidney injury (AKI) related to dehydration in the setting of a high vancomycin level of 25.5. This resolved with hydration and withholding the vancomycin and he is now back to his baseline creatinine level of 1.5. In addition, Mr. Smith has had hypophosphatemia and hypomagnesemia requiring aggressive replacement.

Gastrointestinal: Malnutrition has been an issue and was managed with tube feeding of Pivot 1.5 at 50 mL/h while intubated and is now tolerating po diet after extubation. We have continued bowel regimen of docusate sodium (Colace) and sennosides (Senokot).

Hematology: Mr. Smith has been anemic during this hospitalization, and this is thought to be multifactorial related to his critical illness. He has not received a transfusion and current hemoglobin/hematocrit is 10.2/32.

Infectious disease: Mr. Smith became septic because of his pneumonia and required fluid boluses but never needed vasopressors. Antibiotics were given as noted previously in the pulmonary section.

Endocrine: Mr. Smith has DM at baseline and was hyperglycemic during this admission. While in the ICU he was treated with an insulin infusion, which was weaned off on transfer to the floor. He is now being managed with an insulin sliding scale.

Musculoskeletal: Right hip negative for fracture. Hematoma and contusion and pain are resolving. Mr. Smith has ICU-acquired weakness. He has no focal deficits, but is deconditioned.

Integumentary: Skin is intact but fragile with multiple ecchymosis over his bilateral arms. A few small skin tears are noted on the left antecubital area.

Review of Symptoms at Time of Discharge
Neurologic: Mild headache at times.
Pulmonary: + SOB, ambulating in hallways. Denies SOB with rest.

Cardiovascular: Denies chest pain/pressure, palpitations.

Gastrointestinal: Complains of urgency with diarrhea and does not always make it to the bathroom in time.

Extremities: Complains of generalized weakness, "not quite myself yet."

Physical Examination at Time of Discharge

General: Thin, frail elderly man.

Vital signs: Temperature 98.0°F (36.7°C). Heart rate (HR) 68, respiratory rate (RR) 20. Blood pressure (BP) 138/76. O_2 saturation 94% on 4 L via NC.

Neurologic: Awake, alert, interactive.

HEENT: Sclera clear. Mucous membranes moist (MMM). No JVD.

Pulmonary: Scattered rhonchi and wheezing throughout; sputum light yellow, small amount.

Cardiovascular: Clear S1, S2, no murmurs, rubs, or gallops.

Abdomen: Abdomen soft, bowel sounds +, nontender, nondistended.

Extremities: Mild edema bilateral lower extremities (BLEs). Pedal and PT pulses 2+ bilaterally.

Laboratory tests done the day before discharge include:

Sodium: 140 (136–145 mmol/L)

Potassium: 4.0 (3.4–5.1 (mmol/L)

Chloride: 100 (98–107 mmol/L)

Carbon dioxide: 30 (22–32 mmol/L)

BUN: 15 (5–23 milligrams/dL)

Creatinine: 1.5 (0.4–1.0 md/dL)

eGFR (mL/min): >40 mL/min/1.73 m^2

Random glucose: 180 H (74–118 milligrams/dL)

Magnesium 1.8

Phosphorous: 2.2

WBC count: 8.8

Hemoglobin: 10.2

Hematocrit: 32

Platelets: 158,000

Medications on discharge include:

Albuterol nebulizer 2.5 milligrams every 4 hours

Advair 500/50 1 puff twice daily

Prednisone 40 milligrams po daily

Lisinopril (Zestril) 10 milligrams po daily

Atorvastatin (Lipitor) 40 milligrams po daily at bedtime

Ativan 0.5 milligrams IV every 8 hours

Metoprolol 75 milligrams po twice daily; hold for HR < 60 or systolic BP (SBP) < 100

Sennosides 2 tablets po daily

Docusate sodium (Colace) 100 milligrams po daily

Heparin 5000 units subcutaneously (SC) every 8 hours

Chlorhexidine swish and spit every 6 hours

Nystatin powder to groin every 8 hours

Acetaminophen 650 milligrams po per 8 hours prn mild pain

Fentanyl 25 micrograms IV every 2 hours prn moderate to severe pain

Insulin sliding scale

There are no outstanding tests. He is being discharged in stable condition. He has remained full code throughout this admission.

1. What are the discharge options for Mr. Smith and what are the criteria for admission to each?[1-6]

2. What is the level of care Mr. Smith needs? Why?[1,2,5]

3. Define Mr. Smith's skilled needs.[4]

4.   What essential details are missing from the discharge summary? What additional information do you need to assume care for this patient?

5.   How would you obtain the previously identified missing data?

6.   What is the definition of pneumonia and what are the possible types of his pneumonia?[7,8]

7.   Why is it important for primary care providers to understand the different types of pneumonia?[7]

8.   Which of the medications on discharge should be changed early on in the admission to the facility?[9]

Case Study, Continued

During Mr. Smith's initial physical examination at your facility you find that you agree with much of the examination except for the following findings:

- 2+ edema left upper extremity (LUE).
- Moisture-associated skin damage (MASD) to coccyx.
- The patient is incontinent of liquid brown diarrhea.

9. Given these new examination findings, what are the differential diagnoses and plan?

Case Study, Continued

During Mr. Smith's first 4 days of acute rehabilitation admission, everything has gone well and he has been receiving nursing assessments, physical therapy, and occupational therapy every day. The admitting provider made the following changes to his plan of care:

- *Senna was stopped, but docusate sodium (Colace) was continued.*
- *Pain medication was changed to acetaminophen 650 milligrams po prn for mild pain and oxycodone 2.5 milligrams po every 4 hours prn for moderate pain and 5 milligrams po every 4 hours prn for severe pain.*
- *Ativan was changed back to his home dose of 0.5 milligrams po every 8 hours prn anxiety.*
- *Oxygen was weaned to 2 L via NC, which family reported is his home dose.*
- *A Prednisone taper had begun and the patient had been tapered down to 30 milligrams po daily with a plan to taper down to his usual home dose of 10 milligrams po daily.*
- *LUE was elevated and warm compresses were applied.*

The following assessments have been noted:

- *His MASD is improved with nystatin powder and frequent toileting.*
- *Breath sounds are decreased in the right lower lung fields and he has persistent, scattered wheezing, but he denies SOB at rest or complaints of dyspnea on exertion. Denies paroxysmal nocturnal dyspnea.*
- *Diarrhea has improved and he is having regular soft stools daily.*
- *LUE appears slightly better but not fully resolved. There is no redness. No induration or warmth noted, but patient remains slightly weaker on the left side 4/5 for both LUE and left lower extremity (LLE).*

This morning the night nurse reports Mr. Smith has been progressively more short of breath since yesterday afternoon and is now hypoxic despite an additional albuterol nebulizer treatment and increase in oxygen. Vital signs are temperature 37.7°F, HR 100, RR 28, BP 110/48, O_2 saturation 88% to 90% on 6 L via NC. On examination he has scattered wheezes throughout and crackles in the right lower lung fields. He denies increase in sputum production. He is sleepy but is easily aroused to voice commands.

10.   What are the most likely differential diagnoses for Mr. Smith's change in condition?[10]

11.   What should the health care provider's next course of action when considering the previous differential diagnoses?[11-16]

Case Study, Continued

Mr. Smith continued to become progressively more hypoxic (i.e., oxygen saturation 86%–88%), despite additional albuterol nebulizers, and the decision is made to transfer him to the ED.

12. What categories of information do you as Mr. Smith's current health care provider need to communicate to the receiving facility emergency department?[17,18]

13. Write a concise transfer summary for this patient.

14. In retrospect, what were Mr. Smith's risk factors for readmission to the hospital?[19]

Case Study, Continued

Mr. Smith was readmitted to your acute rehabilitation center 2 days later. The medical resident dictated a brief discharge summary as follows:

> Mr. Smith was admitted in hypoxic respiratory failure. CXR revealed right middle lobe and right lower lobe collapse because of mucous plugging. A bronchoscopy was performed and a bronchoalveolar lavage was performed. Cultures are pending. He was subsequently observed for 48 hours and is now back to his baseline O_2 on 2 L via NC. He was also mildly dehydrated on admission, which is most likely related to his tachypnea. He was rehydrated with IV fluids and his BUN and creatinine have returned to his baseline. All home medications have been continued. He remains a full code.

15. In reviewing Mr. Smith's case, what aspects of his care could have prevented these complications and avoided his readmission to the hospital?[11]

16. Why is it important to try to prevent hospital readmissions?[6]

Case Study, Continued

Over the course of the next 4 days, the nurses note that Mr. Smith's pulmonary status has been stable. The therapists are concerned that he has not really progressed with his therapy, and at times he seems to be confused about where he is, but he realizes he has been in multiple facilities in 1 week.

Today the nursing assistant noted that Mr. Smith was lethargic and this morning he was difficult to get dressed. She also shared that he was incontinent of urine overnight, which is not normal for him.

The health care provider was then called and asked to evaluate Mr. Smith and found him to be difficult to arouse, oriented to self, but confused to place, month, year, and answered that Jimmy Carter is the president. He immediately goes back to sleep when not verbally stimulated.

Vital signs are temperature 98.6°F (37.0°C), HR 88, RR 22, BP 160/88, O₂ saturation 94% on 2 L via NC. On examination, he is weaker on the left side 3/5 for both LUE LLE and does not have coordinated movements with his left side. No facial droop or ptosis noted. Speech is clear.

17. What are the most likely causes of Mr. Smith's change in mental status?[20]

18. What important steps should the health care provider take to determine which of the previous potential diagnoses is the most likely cause of Mr. Smith's confusion and weakness?

19. The health care provider calls the family to let them know the ambulance has been called to take Mr. Smith to the ED. The family asks what additional workup should be expected. What should the health care provider include in response?[20]

Case Study, Continued

Mr. Smith is evaluated in the ED. Results of the workup show:

- *CT scan head: Increased size of subdural hematoma now with midline shift.*
- *ABG: pH 7.36, CO_2 45, PaO_2 80, bicarb 28, saturation 94%, base excess +2.*
- *CBC: WBC 9.0, hemoglobin 12, hematocrit 36, platelets 158,000, and differential shows no bandemia.*
- *BMP: Na 140, K 3.8, Cl 100, bicarb 28, BUN 24, and creatinine 1.5.*

Neurosurgery was consulted and he underwent emergent operative intervention with burr hole and hematoma evacuation. He was admitted to the step-down unit with a Jackson–Pratt drain that was removed at 48 hours. Repeat CT scan shows expected resolution of hematoma with midline shift resolved and brain reexpanded. Then the nurse noted the patient was coughing while drinking water. He underwent a formal speech and swallow evaluation and passed for regular diet with nectar-thick liquids. Physical therapy and occupational therapy evaluated him and determined that Mr. Smith needs acute rehabilitation for strength training and ADLs. He was resumed on the following medications at the time of discharge on day 3:

- *Albuterol nebulizers per protocol*
- *Advair 500/50 1 puff twice daily*
- *Prednisone 30 milligrams po daily*
- *Atorvastatin (Lipitor) 40 milligrams po daily at bedtime*
- *Metoprolol 75 milligrams po daily; hold for HR < 60 or SBP < 100*
- *Docusate sodium (Colace) 100 milligrams po daily*
- *Senna 2 tablets po daily at bedtime*
- *Acetaminophen 650 milligrams po every 4 hours prn mild pain*
- *Oxycodone 5 milligrams po every 4 hours prn moderate pain*
- *Oxycodone 10 milligrams po every 4 hours prn severe pain*
- *po at bedtime prn insomnia*
- *Regular Insulin sliding scale*

20.   What are potential problems with the previous discharge medications?[21]

21.   Please reconcile Mr. Smith's medications. What should he be on?[21]

22.   What additional orders are needed on readmission?

23.   What ongoing issues will need to be addressed before Mr. Smith can be discharged home?

24.   What discharge planning needs to be addressed?

ONLINE ANSWER SUBMISSION

When you are ready to submit your answers for grading and reflective expert feedback for evaluation, go to http://www.evolve.elsevier.com/DickAndButtaro/ to complete this case.

References

1. National Council on Aging. (2016). Medicare Rights Center; Getting Medicare right. Hospital Transitions and Discharge Planning; Frequently Asked Questions. Retrieved from https://www.ncoa.org/wp-content/uploads/Hospital-Transitions-FAQ.pdf.
2. Medicare Benefit Policy Manual Chapter 8—Coverage of Extended Care (SNF) Services Under Hospital Insurance Updated 10/13/16. Retrieved from https://www.cms.gov/Regulations-and-Guidance/Guidance/Manuals/downloads/bp102c08.pdf.

3. Harvard Pilgrim Medical Review Criteria Skilled Nursing Facility & Subacute Care Effective Date. (February 23, 2017). Retrieved from https://www.harvardpilgrim.org/pls/portal/docs/PAGE/PROVIDERS/MEDMGMT/MEDICAL_REVIEW_CRITERIA/SNF%20SUBACUTE_PUBLICATION_022317A.PDF.

4. Department of Health and Human Services, Centers for Medicare & Medicaid Services. (July 2012). Medicare learning services, Inpatient Rehabilitation Therapy Services: Complying with Documentation Requirements. ICN 905643. Retrieved from https://www.cms.gov/Outreach-and-Education/Medicare-Learning-Network-MLN/MLNProducts/downloads/Inpatient_Rehab_Fact_Sheet_ICN905643.pdf.

5. Harvard Pilgrim. Medical Review Criteria Inpatient Rehabilitation & Long-Term Acute Care. Effective Date: October 12, 2016. Retrieved from https://www.harvardpilgrim.org/pls/portal/docs/PAGE/PROVIDERS/MEDMGMT/MEDICAL_REVIEW_CRITERIA/IRF_LTAC%20FINAL_101416.PDF.

6. American Hospital Association Special Bulletin. CMS Releases Fy 2016 Final Rules For Three Post-Acute Care Settings: LTCHs, IRFs & SNFs. Retrieved from http://www.aha.org/content/15/ltch-aug19call-150803specialbulletin.pdf.

7. Kalil, A. C., Metersky, M. L., Klompas, M., Muscedere, J., Sweeney, D. A., Palmer, L. B., et al. (2016). Management of adults with hospital-acquired and ventilator-associated pneumonia: 2016 clinical practice guidelines by the Infectious Diseases Society of America and the American Thoracic Society. *Clinical Infectious Diseases*, *63*, 1–51.

8. Mandell, L. A., Wunderink, R. G., Anzueto, A., Bartlett, J. G., Campbell, G. D., Dean, N. C., et al. (2007). Infectious Diseases Society of America/American Thoracic Society consensus guidelines on the management of community-acquired pneumonia in adults. *Clinical Infectious Diseases*, *44*(Suppl. 2), S27–S72.

9. Andrus, B., & Lacaille, D. (2014). 2013 ACC/AHA guideline on the assessment of cardiovascular risk. *Journal of the American College of Cardiology*, *63*, 2886.

10. Campbell, M. L. (2017). Dyspnea. *Critical Care Nursing Clinics of North America*, *29*, 461–470.

11. Carver, T. W., Milia, D. J., Somberg, C., Brasel, K., & Paul, J. (2015). Vital capacity helps predict pulmonary complications after rib fractures. *Journal of Trauma and Acute Care Surgery*, *7*, 413–416.

12. Kritek, P. A., & Choi, A. M. (2015). Approach to the patient with diseases of the respiratory system. In D. Kasper, S. Hauser, J. Jameson, A. Fauci, D. Longo, & J. Loscalzo (Eds.), *Harrison's principles of internal medicine* (19th ed., pp. 1661–1663). New York: McGraw-Hill Companies.

13. Maier, R. V. (2015). Approach to the patient in shock. In D. Kasper, S. Hauser, J. Jameson, A. Fauci, D. Longo, & J. Loscalzo (Eds.), *Harrison's principles of internal medicine* (19th ed., pp. 1744–1751). New York: McGraw-Hill Companies.

14. Munford, R. S. (2015). Severe sepsis and septic shock. In D. Kasper, S. Hauser, J. Jameson, A. Fauci, D. Longo, & J. Loscalzo (Eds.), *Harrison's principles of internal medicine* (19th ed., pp. 1751–1759). New York: McGraw-Hill Companies.

15. O'Gara, P. T., & Loscalo, J. (2015). Physical examination of the cardiovascular system. In D. Kasper, S. Hauser, J. Jameson, A. Fauci, D. Longo, & J. Loscalzo (Eds.), *Harrison's principles of internal medicine* (19th ed., pp. 1442–1450). United States of America: McGraw-Hill Companies.

16. Goldhaber, S. Z. (2015). Deep venous thrombosis and pulmonary thromboembolism. In D. Kasper, S. Hauser, J. Jameson, A. Fauci, D. Longo, & J. Loscalzo (Eds.), *Harrison's principles of internal medicine* (19th ed., pp. 1631–1637). New York: McGraw-Hill Companies.

17. Health Information and Quality Authority. (2013). National Standard for Patient Discharge Summary Information. Retrieved from https://www.hiqa.ie/sites/default/files/2017-01/National-Standard-Patient-Discharge-Summary.pdf.

18. Jack, B., Paasche-Orlow, M., Mitchell, S., Forsythe, S., & Martin, J. (2013). Re-Engineered Discharge (RED) Toolkit. Agency for Healthcare Research and Quality. Publication No. 12(13)-0084. Retrieved from https://www.ahrq.gov/sites/default/files/publications/files/redtoolkit.pdf.

19. Peters, J. S. (2017). Role of transitional care measures in the prevention of readmission after critical illness. *American Association of Critical Care Nurses*, *37*, e10–e17.

20. Josephson, S. A., & Miller, B. (2015). Confusion & delirium. In D. Kasper, S. Hauser, J. Jameson, A. Fauci, D. Longo, & J. Loscalzo (Eds.), *Harrison's principles of internal medicine* (19th ed., pp. 166–170). New York: McGraw-Hill Companies, Inc.

21. American Geriatrics Society. (2015). Updated Beers criteria for potentially inappropriate medication use in older adults. *Journal of the American Geriatrics Society*, *63*, 227–2246.

Weight Loss

Brianna Morgan

Instructions

After reviewing the case study, please jot down your notes or preliminary answers in the spaces provided. When you are ready to submit your answers for grading and reflective expert feedback for evaluation, go to http://www.evolve.elsevier.com/DickAndButtaro/ to complete this case.

Case Study Scenario/History of Present Illness

Chief Complaint: Weight loss, fatigue, and asthenia in established patient.

Mrs. Murphy is a 78-year-old Irish American woman presenting for a scheduled annual health maintenance appointment with her daughter, Cathy. Mrs. M has been a patient in the nurse practitioner-run Patient-Centered Medical Home for the last 7 years since her gynecologist discharged her from her practice saying she "no longer needed primary care for women's issues."

Today Cathy reports concern that over the past several weeks she has noticed her mom has lost her "get up and go." She volunteers at the local art museum, but has since reduced her hours. Mrs. M states that since she retired from her job as a paralegal last year she spends most of her time in her apartment reading, doing crossword puzzles, or watching TV. She has lost "some weight" over the past 2 months, noting that her clothes are fitting her more loosely. She reports that her appetite has been "just fine." She eats most meals alone.

She continues to manage her apartment including cooking and cleaning independently, but this takes her more time than usual because she needs frequent rest periods. She uses a pill manager for medications, which she takes regularly without difficulty or error. She walks one block to a corner grocery story weekly for groceries. However, over the past 2 months she has been going less frequently. She uses a straight walking cane for long distances at baseline because of osteoarthritis, but Cathy notes that recently she has been using the furniture in her apartment to get around.

When prompted, Mrs. M reports that she feels weaker and fatigued. She reports having fallen "a few times" in the apartment without injury. She sleeps 7 hours a night and wakes well rested. She has had two urinary tract infections (UTIs) in the past year and more frequent upper respiratory infections that have taken a longer time than normal to resolve.

Medications: Levothyroxine 75 micrograms po daily in the morning, lisinopril 10 milligrams po daily, atorvastatin 40 milligrams po daily, omeprazole 40 milligrams po daily in the morning, mirabegron ER 25 milligrams po daily, Fosamax 70 milligrams po once a week, aspirin 81 milligrams po daily, acetaminophen 650 milligrams every 6 hours as needed for arthritis pain, one multivitamin po daily.

Allergies: Penicillin caused urticaria as a child.

Past medical history: Hypertension, hyperlipidemia, hypothyroidism, melanoma, osteoarthritis bilateral knees, osteoporosis, and urge incontinence.

Past surgical history: Thyroidectomy for goiter at age 25 and MOHS procedure for melanoma at age 75 with clear margins. Cataract repair in right eye at age 73.

Family history: Mother died at 81 of "senility" and had "memory loss" for many years. She also had a history of depression and breast cancer. Father died at 73 after an acute myocardial infarction (MI) and had a history of hypertension, type 2 diabetes, and coronary artery disease with stents. Brother is living with bipolar disorder and history of suicide attempt.

Personal and social history: Mrs. M immigrated to the United States when she was 5 years old. She is widowed with one grown daughter, Cathy, who lives 20 minutes away. Her husband died 6 years ago from lung cancer and he had a 100-pack-year history of tobacco use. She retired last year from her job as a paralegal where she had worked for nearly 60 years. She lives alone in a small one-bedroom apartment on the 11th floor of a high-rise. The building has an elevator and a doorman. She has a new boyfriend, Earl, who lives in her building. He has been coming over on occasion to cook dinner with her when he takes a break from caring for his wife who is in a nursing home with advanced dementia. She denies a history of smoking or illicit drug use. She denies any history of physical, verbal, or sexual abuse.

Reproductive health: Gravida 1, para 2, with one miscarriage. Vaginal delivery without complications, breastfed until her daughter was age 1. Menarche age 12, menopause at age 54.

Health maintenance/prevention: Last gynecologic examination was at age 71. All previous Pap smears had been normal. Last colonoscopy at age 75 was normal. Last mammogram 7 years ago with no abnormal findings. Last dual-energy x-ray absorptiometry (DEXA) scan was 4 years ago with a T-score of −2.6. Last ophthalmology examination was this past year. She wears reading glasses only. Regular visits to the dentist for the past 7 years. She wears dentures.

Immunizations: Up to date (PCV-13; Zostavax and Tdap at age 71; PPSV-23 at age 72; and influenza vaccine yearly for the past 7 years, last was this year). Last purified protein derivative (PPD) was last year through her workplace and was negative.

Review of Systems

General: Progressive weight loss over the past 2 months, associated with fatigue and increasingly worsening activity intolerance. Denies fevers, night sweats, or chills. No pain.

Skin: No rashes or lesions.

Eyes: No changes in vision.

Head, ears, nose, and throat (HENT): No headache. No tinnitus, ear pain, or discharge. No sinus pressure or nasal discharge. No sore throat.

Respiratory: No shortness of breath, cough, or wheezing. No dyspnea on exertion.

Cardiac: No chest pain. No edema.

Gastrointestinal: Soft brown bowel movements once daily. No diarrhea or constipation. No nausea or vomiting. No early satiety.

Urinary: No change in baseline urge incontinence. Improved since starting mirabegron. Wears incontinence pads for occasional "accidents." No urgency, frequency, or dysuria. Last UTI was 4 months prior.

Musculoskeletal: No muscle pain. Baseline joint stiffness and pain in the morning in bilateral knees. Relieved with acetaminophen and activity. No diarrhea or constipation.

Neurologic: Reports mild progressive muscle weakness. Denies dizziness/vertigo, paresthesia, or syncope.

Hematologic: No easy bleeding or bruising.

Lymphatic: No noticeable lymph nodes.

Psychological: Reports depressed mood, irritability, and difficulty concentrating since retirement more than a year ago. States, "I just feel slower than normal." Denies suicidal ideation.

Physical Examination

Vital signs: Blood pressure (BP) right arm seated is 124/73. Temperature 97.2°F. Heart rate (HR) 77, respiratory rate (RR) 16, SpO_2 99%. Weight 102 pounds. Weight 2 months prior was 115 pounds. Height: 5 feet 1 inch. Body mass index (BMI) today is 19.3.

General: Appears older than stated age. Thin with clavicular wasting. No acute distress.

Skin: Good turgor. No lesions or rashes. No changes in nevi since last examination.

Eyes: Geriatric ectropion. No exudate. Conjunctiva without redness or icterus.

HENT: Head is atraumatic and normocephalic. Ear canals are clear with minimal yellow cerumen. Tympanic membranes pearly and intact. Unable to hear whisper bilaterally. Nares are patent without exudate. Mucous membranes are pink and moist. No oral lesions. Thyroid nonpalpable.

Respiratory: Clear to auscultation bilaterally. No wheezes, rhonchi, or rales.

Cardiac: Regular rate and rhythm, S1, S2 audible, no S3 or S4. No murmurs, rubs, or gallops.

Gastrointestinal: Soft, bowel sounds present in all four quadrants. Tympanic to percussion, nondistended, nontender. Liver and spleen nonpalpable.

Musculoskeletal: Sarcopenia throughout. Strength 4/5 throughout. Range of motion intact.

Neurologic: Oriented to person, place, and time. Cranial nerves (CNs) II to XII intact. Pupils equal, round reactive to light and accommodation (PERRLA). Deep tendon reflexes (DTRs) +2 throughout. Gait with cane is wide and slowed with varus thrust right greater than left on weight bearing. Fluent, coherent speech. Speaking loudly.

Hematologic: No widespread bruising.

Lymphatic: No palpable lymph nodes.

Psychological: Slightly withdrawn. Flat affect.

ASSESSMENT AND PLAN

1. Based on the history and physical examination, what are the possible causes of Mrs. M's symptoms?

2.   What components of the history and physical examination are missing?

3.   What additional diagnostics are appropriate at this time?

Case Study, Continued

On further investigation Mrs. M reveals that she has been feeling so fatigued that she has started eating mostly prepared meals, like TV dinners. She often only finishes around half of the meal. Yesterday she had black coffee and one piece of dry toast for breakfast, 1 cup of split pea soup for lunch, and 75% of a TV dinner. She wants to put on weight. She is not binge eating or regurgitating her food.

She does not drink alcohol. Denies dark or bloody stool and reports no difficulty swallowing, no dyspepsia, and no epigastric discomfort.

Additional physical examination reveals:

- *Timed up and go (TUG) test is 23 seconds (normal <15).*
- *Romberg is negative.*

- *Her grip strength is 30 pounds (average = 47.6 pounds) in her right hand and 28 pounds (average 42.5 pounds) in her left hand using the Jamar dynamometer.*
- *Montreal Assessment of Cognition is 28/30 (>26 is normal cognition), losing one point for delayed recall and one for calculations.*
- *Geriatric Depression Screen is 9/15 (>5 is suggestive of depression).*
- *BP is 123/76 seated and 120/73 standing*
- *Gag and swallow are intact.*
- *No suspicious nevi or lesions.*
- *Clinical breast examination is negative for masses. She declines vaginal examination.*
- *Chest x-ray: No evidence of disease*
- *Stool jemoccult: Negative*

Diagnostics are as follows:

Glucose	80	70-99 milligrams/dL
Urea Nitrogen	15	8-20 milligrams/dL
Creatinine	0.97	0.44-1.03 milligrams/dL
Sodium	139	136-144 mmol/L
Potassium	3.9	3.6-5.1 mmol/L
Chloride	105	101-111 mmol/L
Carbon Dioxide	27	22-32 mmol/L
Anion Gap	7	3-12
Calcium	9.6	8.9-10.3 milligrams/dL
Albumin	4.1	3.5-5.1 g/dL
Protein Total	7.3	6.1-7.9 g/dL
Bilirubin, Total	0.3	0.3-1.2 milligrams/dL
Alkaline Phosphatase	52	38-126 U/L
AST	26	15-41 U/L
ALT	23	14-54 U/L

White Blood Cells	5.1	4.0-11.0 THO/uL
Red Blood Cells	4.08	3.80-5.3 MIL/uL
Hemoglobin	13.8	12.0-160 g/dL
Hematocrit	40	36-46%
RDW	15.5 (H)	11.5-14.5%
MCH	34 (H)	27-33 pg
MCHC	34	31-36 g/dL
MCV	98	80-100 fL
Platelets	312	150-400 THO/ul

TSH	2.49	0.27-4.20 uIU/mL
Hemaglobin A1C	5.3	4.0%-5.6%
Sedimentation rate	5	0-30 mm/h
CRP	0.8	<7.4 milligrams/L
Vitamin B_{12}	154 (L)	211-946 pg/mL
25OH vitamin D_2 and D_3 total	18 (L)	25-80 ng/mL
Creatine kinase	113	96-145 U/L (females)

Prealbumin	11 (L)	16-35 milligrams/L
HIV	Negative	—
HCV	Negative	—

4. What cancer-related risk factors are present and for which malignancy?

5. What is the likely cause for Mrs. M's vitamin B deficiency and recommended treatment?[1,2]

6. What is the evidence for and against screening and treating Mrs. M for vitamin D deficiency?[3-5]

7. What role does vitamin D deficiency and subsequent supplementation play in the various multimorbid aspects of Mrs. M's case?

8. What are some of the factors that may contribute to Mrs. M's weight loss and possible targeted interventions?[3,6]

9. **What are pharmacologic interventions for weight loss and muscle wasting? Is there a role for them in this case?[7,8]**

10. **What role does aging play in protein metabolism?[8]**

11. **What are some of the evidence-based interventions for fatigue?[7]**

12.   What are the pertinent positives and negatives that support a differential diagnosis of depression?

13.   What are treatment options for Mrs. M's mood, including the risks and benefits?[9,10]

14.   What is the definition of frailty in clinical practice?[11-13]

15.   Explain the pathophysiology behind the frailty spiral.[11-13] (See Fig. 19.1)

16.   What are some of the reversible causes of frailty in Mrs. M's case?

Case Study, Continued

Mrs. M returns 8 weeks later for a problem-focused visit. She has completed her vitamin D course. She is stable on 15 milligrams of mirtazapine each day and has completed 4 weeks of interpersonal therapy. She has had 2 months of vitamin B_{12} injections. She also has new dentures and completed audiology testing; hearing aids were recommended. Today she is wearing bilateral hearing aids.

She reports that she has gained 3 pounds and her energy level and depression are improving. She has been getting Meals on Wheels for 4 weeks and now eats lunch with the volunteer who drops off her meals. She has been supplementing the meals with one Boost daily. She is happy to report that she is volunteering with the art museum more regularly and is considering taking a volunteer position on their board.

However, she also notes 3 days of painless, pink-tinged urine without nocturia, urgency, dysuria, or worsening incontinence. She denies fever, chills, or pain. No changes in medications or recent consumption of beets. No recent trauma. All other review of systems (ROS) is noncontributory. Her vital signs and physical examination, including a vaginal examination, are normal.

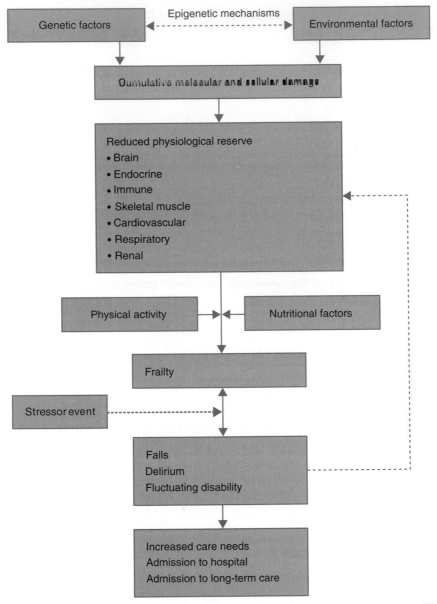

Fig. 19.1 Schematic representation of the pathophysiology of frailty. (From Clegg, A., Young, J., Iliffe, S., Rikkert, M. O., & Rockwood, K. [2013]. Frailty in elderly people. *Lancet,* 381[9868], 752–762.)

17.   What is the differential for painless hematuria?

18.   What additional diagnostic testing would be helpful in determining a cause of Mrs. M's hematuria at this time?

Case Study, Continued

Urine dipstick shows pink-tinged urine with visible clots positive for blood. All else negative. Urine microscopy shows red blood cell (RBC) 20 per high power field (hpf) (normal 0–2 hpf). Urine culture shows no growth.

Repeat CBC and CMP are normal.

19.   What are the appropriate next steps?

Case Study, Continued

Mrs. M returns 2 weeks later after visiting the urologist. She had a cystoscopy with pathology that revealed transitional cell carcinoma. CT showed a 2.3 × 1.5-cm bladder lesion highly suspicious for malignancy, but no signs of metastatic disease or other structural abnormalities. Follow-up transurethral resection of bladder tumor (TURBT) revealed low-grade noninvasive transitional cell carcinoma without residual. Her oncologist is recommending treatment with mitomycin for the bladder cancer. Treatment is with curative intent. Mrs. M states, "My husband had chemotherapy and he was very sick. I'm not sure I would want that for myself."

20.   Is it appropriate for a primary care provider to discuss treatment options and goals of care with a patient?[14]

Case Study, Continued

After significant discussion, Mrs. M agrees that it is consistent with her goals to start treatment.

21. What are some things to consider in maintaining her wellness as she chooses to pursue treatment?

References

1. Langan, R. C., & Zawistoski, K. J. (2011). Update on vitamin B12 deficiency. *American Family Physician, 83*(12), 1425–1430.
2. Stover, P. J. (2010). Vitamin B12 and older adults. *Current Opinion in Clinical Nutrition and Metabolic Care, 13*(1), 24–27.
3. Holick, M. F., Binkley, N. C., Bischoff-Ferrari, H. A., Gordon, C. M., Hanley, D. A., Heaney, R. P., et al. (2011). Evaluation, treatment, and prevention of vitamin D deficiency: An endocrine society clinical practice guidelines. *Journal of Clinical Endocrinology & Metabolism, 96*, 1911–1930.
4. Ross, A. C., Manson, J. E., & Abrams, S. A. (2010). The 2011 report on dietary reference intakes for calcium and vitamin D from the Institute of Medicine: what clinicians need to know. *Journal of Clinical Endocrinology and Metabolism, 96*(1), 53–58.
5. LeFevre, M. L. (2015). Screening for vitamin D deficiency in adults: U.S. Preventative Services Task Force recommendation statement. *Annals of Internal Medicine, 162*(2), 133–140.
6. Zhou, J., Huang, P., Liu, P., Hao, Q., Chen, S., Dong, B., et al. (2016). Association of vitamin D deficiency and frailty: A systematic review and meta-analysis. *Maturitas, 94*, 70–76.
7. Rolland, Y., Dupuy, C., van Abellan Kan, G., Gillete, S., & Vellas, B. (2011). Treatment strategies for sarcopenia and frailty. *The Medical clinics of North America, 95*, 427–438.
8. Gaddey, H. I., & Holder, K. (2014). Unintentional weight loss in older adults. *American Family Physician, 89*(9), 718–722.
9. Taylor, W. D. (2014). Depression in the elderly. *The New England Journal of Medicine, 371*(13), 1228–1236.

10. Marcum, Z. A., Perera, S., Thorpe, J. M., Switzer, G. E., Castle, N. G., Strotmeyer, E. S., et al. (2016). Antidepressant use and recurrent falls in community-dwelling older adults: Findings from the health ABC study. *The Annals of Pharmacotherapy, 50*(7), 525–533.
11. Cesari, M., Calcani, R., & Marzetti, E. (2017). Frailty in older persons. *Clinics in Geriatric Medicine, 33,* 293–303.
12. Ko, D. C. (2011). The clinical care of frail, older adults. *Clinics in Geriatric Medicine, 27,* 89–100.
13. Fried, L., Tangen, C. M., Walston, J., Newman, A. B., Hirsch, C., Gottdiener, J., et al. (2001). Frailty in older adults: Evidence for a phenotype. *Journals of Gerontology, 56*(3), M146–M156.
14. Morgan, B., & Tarbi, E. (2016). The role of the advanced practice nurse in geriatric oncology care. *Seminars in Oncology Nursing, 32*(1), 33–43.

Confusion

Danielle Shih ▮ Terry Mahan Buttaro

Instructions

After reviewing the case study, please jot down your notes or preliminary answers in the spaces provided. When you are ready to submit your answers for grading and reflective expert feedback for evaluation, go to http://www.evolve.elsevier.com/DickAndButtaro/ to complete this case.

Case Study Scenario/History of Present Illness

Mr. B is an 88-year-old man who presents to the clinic with his son with complaints of intermittent confusion and increasing fatigue. He fell approximately 4 days ago and broke two ribs but did not hit his head. He went to the emergency room (ER) after the fall and was discharged home. Since Mr. B came home, his son states that his father has not been acting like himself. He has not been eating or drinking much, and his confusion is getting worse. His son is his historian for a majority of the visit.

Medications:
Levothyroxine 75 micrograms po daily
Pantoprazole 40 milligrams po daily
Sertraline 75 milligrams po daily
Apixaban 2.5 milligrams po twice a day
Nephrocaps 1 milligram po daily at 4 p.m.
Mirtazapine 15 milligrams po daily at bedtime
Finasteride 5 milligrams po daily
Amiodarone 100 milligrams po daily
Donepezil 5 milligrams po daily at bedtime
Vitamin C 500 milligrams po daily
Vitamin D 2000 IU po daily
Vitamin B$_{12}$ 1000 micrograms po daily
Calcium 500 milligrams po daily
Coenzyme Q10 300 milligrams po daily
Acetaminophen 650 milligrams po two to three times a day as needed for pain
Lidocaine patch 5% apply to left rib area twice a day

Allergies: Penicillin.

Past medical history: Depression; ventricular fibrillation; deep vein thrombophlebitis; colon cancer; small cell lung cancer, stage 4, basal cell carcinoma on bilateral ears; frequent urinary tract infections (UTIs); pneumonia; fractured ribs related to falls; and frequent falls.

Past surgical history: Colectomy at age 68. Lobectomy at age 72. Skin biopsies. Lasik eye surgery.

Personal history: Married with four adult stepchildren, no biological children. All four children live in the same town and are able to care for both him and his wife often.

Family history: Has one sister who lives locally but does not know her medical history. Does not remember any other family history, but his parents were both old when they died.

Review of Systems

General: Denies pain, fevers, sweating, or chills. Reports sleeping more often. Has history of some confusion but not to people or places.

Skin: Denies skin abnormalities other than scarring from skin cancer.

Head, eyes, ears, nose, and throat (HEENT): Denies headache, sinus pain, eye pain, mouth pain, or difficulty swallowing. Denies difficulty with hearing, but wears hearing aids occasionally. Does not wear glasses, and denies difficulty with vision.

Cardiac: Denies any chest pain other than his fractured ribs. Denies palpitations. Denies peripheral edema.

Respiratory: Reports some shortness of breath (SOB) with exertion, but has always had this problem. No other respiratory symptoms or recent illness. Uses oxygen at home during periods of SOB.

Gastrointestinal: Reports some difficulty with swallowing. Denies diarrhea, constipation, abdominal pain, or changes in bowel habits. Has had some episodes of incontinence during the past week. Reports some nausea, no vomiting. No recent weight loss, but has been losing weight over time.

Genitourinary: Denies any difficulty with urination. Denies pain or burning. Usually gets up one to two times per night to urinate. Usually uses urinal at home, but for the past 2 days has been incontinent of urine. Denies odorous urine.

Musculoskeletal: Reports pain on left side from fractured ribs. Denies muscle pain. Is slow to change position or get up from chair, but is able. Often unsteady on feet.

Psychosocial: Lives with stepson since his most recent fall. Has a large family to assist in his care. His wife is often sick and unable to care for him since his fall. Is a former smoker, but quit smoking 25 years ago. Drinks an occasional beer. Denies depression, but "my wife says I am."

Physical Examination

Vital signs: Pulse 97. Blood pressure (BP) 122/84. SpO$_2$ 97% on room air (RA). Temperature 100.8°F. Respiratory rate (RR) 22.

Height: 5 feet 8 inches. Weight 115 pounds.

General: Ill-appearing older man. Appears agitated during the examination.

Neurological: Slow unsteady gait. Alert and oriented to self and place. Able to engage in conversation but often answers inappropriately. Unable to test cranial nerves because patient is somewhat agitated and uncooperative.

Skin: Skin warm, dry, and intact. Areas of redness on pinna but no open areas. Stage 1 pressure ulcer on coccyx.

HEENT: Head normocephalic, no palpable lymph nodes. Pupils equal, round reactive to light (PERRL). Conjunctiva pale, sclera white, no discharge. Skin on ears reddened and some scarring. Tympanic membranes (TMs) pearly gray. No rhinitis. Mouth and lips dry.

Cardiac: Pulse 97, regular. Capillary refill <3 seconds. No murmurs, gallops, or rubs. No peripheral edema.

Respiratory: Breathing easily, not labored. No retractions. No wheezing or adventitious sounds. No cough during examination.

Gastrointestinal: Abdomen flat, nondistended. Positive bowel sounds in all four quadrants. No tenderness with palpation. No masses, hernias, or pulsations.

Genitourinary: No masses or lesions noted. No redness or inflammation. No discharge noted. No costovertebral angle tenderness (CVAT).

Musculoskeletal: Unsteady gait, limited active range of motion (ROM) in all extremities. Some muscle atrophy associated with age and lack of activity. No joint swelling.

1.   What further information would the health care provider need to diagnose the cause of Mr. B's confusion, weakness, and possible relationship to his recent fall? What tools are available to assist the health care provider in obtaining a systematic and thorough history of patient illness? Why is this information important?

2.   What questions should the health care provider ask the family member to elicit a better history of present illness?

Case Study, Continued

Mr. B's stepson explains Mr. B has fallen in the past but did not have a recent fall until 4 days ago. He states that no one really saw Mr. B's fall the other day, but heard a loud thump and found him on the floor. He thinks maybe Mr. B was going to look for something, but is not sure. He states, "Mr. B is confused at times, but he has 'not been himself' for the past week. He is eating less, sleeping more. He told me he was at the beach yesterday with my mother and he was really surprised when I told him that he has not been to the beach in years! We never had to take him to the ER before the other day. This was the worst fall, that's for sure!"

Mr. B's stepson also tells the health care provider that Mr. B only takes the prescribed medications and does not drink alcohol very often, but he has had urinary incontinence the past week or so. His also tells the health care provider that "He is usually pretty good about using the bathroom. He just is not himself right now."

3. Can any of Mr. D's medications be implicated in his current symptoms, or his recent fall? Are there any potential drug–drug interactions that could cause his symptoms?[1]

4. Based on the information so far, what concerns should the health care provider consider when caring for Mr. B? Why are these concerns important?

Emergency Department Capetown General Hospital 9/10/2017

History of Present Illness
Chief Complaint: *Fall*

88-year-old gentleman with past medical history of depression, ventricular fibrillation, deep vein thrombophlebitis, colon cancer, small cell lung cancer stage 4, and basal cell carcinoma on both ears found on floor by family. Fall was not witnessed, although family heard the fall. Patient was alert when found, immediately complained of acute left-sided chest pain, and was brought to the ER by family. Patient states he thinks he "tripped over his own two feet," and complains of pain in left chest that increases in severity with breathing. Denies chest pain before fall, jaw or arm pain, or diaphoresis. Admits he has not been feeling well in general but denies fever, chills, headache, dizziness, back or other pain, abdominal pain, nausea, vomiting, diarrhea, melena or hematochezia, urinary symptoms, or decreased sensation or movement in his extremities.

Past Medical History
Nurses' notes reviewed.

Review of Systems
Additional findings: Poor appetite per stepson who brought him to the ER. Head: Denies head injury, loss of consciousness. Eyes and ears: Patient denies change in vision, photophobia, or change in hearing. Neck pain: Denies neck pain, stiffness, or limitation in range of motion. Cardiac: Denies known irregular heartbeat/palpitations, chest pain before fall, or sweating. Respiratory: Denies cough or recent infection. Gastrointestinal: Denies abdominal pain, diarrhea. Musculoskeletal: Denies joint pain or swelling.

Physical Examination
Vital signs: Temperature 98.2°F, blood pressure 91/75, heart rate 95, oxygen saturation 95% on room air.

General: Alert older male, oriented to person and place. No acute distress.

HEENT: Atraumatic. PERLA. EOMI. Nose: No contusion or tenderness. Mouth: Membranes moist, no evidence of bleeding.

Neck: Supple, nontender, full ROM.

Cardiac: S1, S2 regular. No murmur or rub.

Lungs: + chest wall tenderness left anterior chest wall. Breath sounds clear. No rales, wheezes, or rhonchi bilaterally.

Abdomen: Soft, bowel sounds +, no bruits or tenderness.

Extremities: Full ROM upper and lower extremities. Normal hand grip strength. Sensation intact. Pedal pulses present bilaterally. No edema or calf pain.

Neurologic: Cranial nerves II to XII intact. Motor strength/sensation grossly intact. Speech is clear. Mentation appropriate. Gait not observed.

Course/Decision-Making
Patient is alert, holding left chest wall. Immediately placed on cardiac monitor: + NSR without ectopy.

Plan: ECG, CBC/differential, Chem 8, x-rays, and chest film.

ECG Interpretation: NSR. Borderline first degree AV block. No signs of ischemia/infarction.

Chest x-ray: Rib fracture fourth and fifth left ribs. No pneumothorax or pneumonia.

Laboratory:
- WBC: 11 (4.0–11.0 K/mm^3)
- Hemoglobin: 14 (11–16 g/dL)
- Hematocrit: 39 (35–48%)
- Platelets: 210 (130–400 K/mm^3)
- Neutrophils %: 80 (37–80)

Chemistry:
- Sodium: 138 (136–145 mmol/L)
- Potassium: 3.8 (3.4–5.1 (mmol/L)
- Chloride: 101 (98–107 mmol/L)
- Carbon dioxide: 25 (22–32 mmol/L)
- BUN: 19 (5–23 milligrams/dL)
- Creatinine: 1.2 (0.4–1.0 md/dL)
- Glucose: 124 (74–118 milligrams/dL)
- eGFR: 54 mL/min/1.73 m^2

Disposition
Clinical Impression: Status post mechanical fall with fracture of fourth and fifth right ribs.
Discharge home: Lidocaine patch, 5% to left chest wall area every 12 hours as needed for chest pain.
Referrals: Follow-up primary care next week.
Electronically Signed: M. Quinn, PA

AV, Atrioventricular; *BUN,* blood urea nitrogen; *CBC,* complete blood count; *ECG,* electrocardiogram; *eGFR,* estimated glomerular filtration rate; *EOMI,* extraocular movements intact; *ER,* emergency room; *NSR,* normal sinus rhythm; *PERLA,* pupils equal and reactive to light and accommodation; *ROM,* range of motion; *WBC,* white blood cell.

5. The primary care provider reviews Mr. B's hospital report and contemplates the next steps in determining what is going on with Mr. B. Are there missing physical findings that the health care provider should consider while contemplating the cause of Mr. B's symptoms?

6. What is Mr. B's most likely diagnosis? What are three top differential diagnoses that should be considered in this gentleman?[2-4]

7. Which diagnostics are initially indicated for Mr. B? Support each of your diagnostic choices.[5-6]

MR. B'S DIAGNOSTIC RESULTS

- **Chest x-ray posteroanterior (PA)/lateral:** Wet read. Right lower lobe lobectomy. Left rib fractures, ribs 4 and 5. Negative for infiltrates or suspicious lesions.
- **Noncontrast CT head:** There is no intracranial hemorrhage. There are chronic white matter hypodensities consistent with microvascular disease. There has been no interval change since previous scan. The ventricles are normal in size and configuration. The bony calvarium appears intact. There is mucosal thickening in several ethmoid air cells. Impression: No acute intracranial disease. Gliotic changes of microvascular disease.
- **ECG:** Normal sinus rhythm (NSR), rate 80. No ectopy or ST changes. QTc 440 ms.
- **Urine dipstick:**
  - + leukocytes
  - + nitrates
  - Small blood
  - Trace protein
  - pH 7.0
  - Specific gravity 1.027
  - No glucose or ketones
- **CBC:**
  - White blood cell (WBC): 13.8 H (4.0–11.0 K/mm^3)
  - Hemoglobin: 13.4 (11–16 g/dL)
  - Hematocrit: 38.6 (35%–48%)
  - Platelets: 212 (130–400 K/mm^3)
  - Neutrophils %: 83.3 H (37–80)
- **Chemistry:**
  - Sodium: 146 (136–145 mmol/L)
  - Potassium: 3.8 (3.4–5.1 mmol/L)
  - Chloride: 101 (98–107 mmol/L)
  - Carbon dioxide: 25 (22–32 mmol/L)
  - Blood urea nitrogen (BUN): 24 H (5–23 milligrams/dL)
  - Creatinine: 1.4 H (0.4–1.0 md/dL)
  - Estimated glomerular filtration rate (GFR): 35 (mL/min)
  - Glucose: 76 (74–118 milligrams/dL)

8.   Based on Mr. B's diagnostic results, what is/are possible causes of his confusion and weakness? What recommendations would be appropriate for Mr. B? Support your choices with evidence.[1,7-10]

9.   Are there specific renal dosing considerations necessary for the pharmacologic treatments indicated for Mr. B's urinary tract infection? Write a sample prescription for Mr. B's treatment.[11,12]

Case Study, Continued

The medication risks and options are discussed with Mr. B and his stepson. The side effects of the fluoroquinolones are concerning to the stepson, and the decision is made to try TMP/SMZ 160 milligrams/800 milligrams po twice a day for 5 days. The health care provider also explains to Mr. B's stepson that the prescription will only be for 5 days because it is unclear if Mr. B has prostatitis. An appointment is made for the urology consult in 2 days, and the urologist will decide if the prescription should be continued at that time. The health care provider also explains the importance of a repeat chemistry profile in 2 days to assess Mr. B's fluid status.

MARCUS BEAN, PhD, AGPCNP-BC
Seaside Associates
Beach Street
Capetown, SC

Patient Name: Mr. B.
Date of Birth: January 15, 1929
Address: 12 Parker Way, Capetown SC
Date: 03/16/2018
Trimethoprim/sulfamethoxazole
160 milligrams/800 milligrams
Take one tablet by mouth
every 12 hours for 5 days
Dispense: 10 tablets
Diagnosis: Urinary tract infection
Refill: O times

Marcus Bean, NP

10. What potential complications are important for the health care provider to monitor in this patient?

11. What would be appropriate patient education for Mr. B and his family before he is discharged home?

Case Study, Continued

The health care provider faxes the office note to the urologist and asks the urologist to call if there are any concerns after Mr. B is seen later in the week.

The next day, the provider calls Mr. B's home and speaks to another family member who states Mr. B is taking the medications and drinking water "pretty well." Mr. B had a temperature of 100°F last night, but today his temperature was 98.2°F.

Two days later, Mr. B has a repeat chemistry profile and is seen by urology.

The urologist calls the office after Mr. B's visit and explains that Mr. B does have prostatitis, some prostatic hypertrophy, and urinary retention. Mr. B could continue with a lower dose of TMP/SAMZ 80 milligrams/400 milligrams by mouth once or twice a day for 6 weeks depending on cardiogram concerns (i.e., QT prolongation) and renal status. Cephalexin is another option for treatment, but it is contraindicated in patients with a penicillin allergy.[13] The urologist also tells the health care provider that even with treatment, some patients continue to have chronic prostatitis. The urologist also recommends stopping the mirtazapine, if possible, because it causes urinary retention in some patients.

- Sodium: 139 (136–145 mmol/L)
- Potassium: 4.2 (3.4–5.1 (mmol/L)
- Chloride: 102 (98–107 mmol/L)
- Carbon dioxide: 28 (22–32 mmol/L)
- BUN: 20 (5–23 milligrams/dL)
- Creatinine: 1.3 H (0.4–1.0 md/dL)
- Estimated GFR: 42 (mL/min)
- Glucose: 92 (74–118 milligrams/dL)

12. Discuss Mr. B's current chemistry profile results. What changes have occurred and why?

FOLLOW-UP PRIMARY CARE

History of Present Illness

Mr. B returns to the clinic 2 weeks later and is now taking trimethoprim/sulfamethoxazole 80 milligrams/400 milligrams by mouth a day, which the urologist prescribed for him. Mr. B's stepson states Mr. B is less agitated and less confused. The urinary incontinence has improved.

Mr. B himself says he feels better.

Medication reconciliation:

TMP/SMZ 80 milligrams/400 milligrams po daily

Levothyroxine 75 micrograms po daily

Pantoprazole 40 milligrams po daily
Sertraline 75 milligrams po daily
Apixaban 2.5 milligrams po twice daily
Nephrocaps 1 milligram po daily at 4 p.m.
Mirtazapine 15 milligrams po daily at bedtime
Finasteride 5 milligrams po daily
Amiodarone 100 milligrams po daily
Donepezil 5 milligrams po daily at bedtime
Vitamin C 500 milligrams po daily
Vitamin D 2000 IU po daily
Vitamin B_{12} 1000 micrograms po daily
Calcium 500 milligrams po daily
Coenzyme Q10 300 milligrams po daily
Lidoderm patch, 5% twice daily as needed
Acetaminophen 650 milligrams po twice or three times daily as needed for pain
Allergies: Penicillin.

Review of Systems

General: Feels good. Denies pain, fevers.

Skin: Denies rash.

HEENT: Wears hearing aids. Denies headache, eye pain, nasal discharge, mouth pain, difficulty swallowing, or neck or throat pain.

Cardiac: Denies chest pains, palpitations.

Respiratory: Still has some SOB with exertion but the same as always. Denies cough.

Gastrointestinal: Feels like his swallowing is better. Denies nausea, diarrhea, constipation, abdominal pain, or changes in bowel habits.

Genitourinary: Denies urinary pain, burning. Nocturia × 1. No urine incontinence.

Musculoskeletal: Pain better from fractured ribs. Denies falls. Denies other muscle pain.

Psychosocial: Lives with stepson. Wife has health problems. Former smoker, quit smoking 25 years ago. Drinks an occasional beer. Denies depression today.

Physical Examination

Vital signs: Pulse 88. BP 136/84 sitting and 142/80 standing (no heart rate changes when stands). SpO_2 97% on RA. Temperature 97.8°F. RR 18. Height 5 feet 8 inches. Weight 118 pounds.

General: Alert male using rolling walker in no acute distress (NAD).

Neurologic: Alert, appropriate. Thoughts coherent today.

Skin: Skin warm, dry, intact. Stage 1 pressure ulcer on coccyx, clean, no exudate.

HEENT: Head normocephalic. Eyes: Sclera clear, conjunctiva within normal limits. PERRL. Ears: Some scarring pinna. TMs: Landmarks visible. Nose: No rhinitis or sinus tenderness. Mouth: + dentures. Membranes moist, no lesions.

Cardiac: S1, S2 regular. No S3, S4, murmurs, or rubs. Capillary refill <3 seconds. No peripheral edema. ECG shows NSR. First degree block, but no evidence of prolonged QT.

Respiratory: Breathing easily, not labored. Clear to auscultation. No retractions. No wheezing or adventitious sounds. No cough.

Gastrointestinal: Abdomen flat. + bowel sounds positive. Nondistended. No tenderness with palpation. No masses, hernias, or pulsations.

Genitourinary: No masses or lesions noted. No redness or inflammation. No discharge noted. No CVAT.

Musculoskeletal: Using rolling walker smoothly. + muscle atrophy upper and lower extremities. No joint swelling.

Extremities: No edema or calf tenderness.

13. Based on his medication reconciliation, what other health care problems does Mr. B have? How would these problems influence treatment recommendations for Mr. B? Should his medications all be continued and, if so, for how long?

Case Study, Continued

The health care provider talks with Mr. B and his stepson. Physical therapy will be started to help Mr. B regain some strength, and the health care provider explains the urologist's recommendation to stop the mirtazapine. However, the health care provider opts to decrease Mr. B's mirtazapine to 7.5 milligrams po daily for 2 weeks to see how he does and then discontinue the medication. The side effects of mirtazapine are discussed with Mr. B and his stepson so they will understand the reasoning. Mirtazapine is often used for weight gain but it does cause confusion, dizziness, and depression, so it is worthwhile trying to stop it. Mr. B does not think he needs the lidocaine patch anymore so that and the vitamin C and Coenzyme Q 10 will be discontinued.

Mr. B will return for follow-up in 2 weeks and the stepson can discuss any changes at that time. A new medication sheet is given to Mr. B and the stepson along with the follow-up appointment. The new mirtazapine prescription (with the dose change noted) is faxed to the local pharmacy.

Mr. B's Medication List

TMP/SMZ 80 milligrams/400 milligrams po daily
Levothyroxine 75 micrograms po daily
Pantoprazole 40 milligrams po daily
Sertraline 75 milligrams po daily
Apixaban 2.5 milligrams po twice a day
Nephrocaps 1 milligram po daily
Mirtazapine 7.5 milligrams po daily at bedtime
Finasteride 5 milligrams po daily
Amiodarone 100 milligrams po daily
Donepezil 5 milligrams po daily at bedtime
Vitamin D 2000 IU po daily
Vitamin B^{12}, 1000 micrograms po daily
Calcium 500 milligrams po daily
Acetaminophen 650 milligrams po two to three times daily as needed for pain

References

1. Lexicomp. In UpToDate. UpToDate. Waltham, MA. Retrieved from https://www.uptodate.com/contents/donepezil-drug-information?search=aricept&source=panel_search_result&selectedTitle=1~44&usage_type=panel&kp_tab=drug_general&display_rank=1.

2. Papa, L., Mendes, M. E., & Braga, C. F. (2012). Mild traumatic brain injury among the geriatric population. *Current Translational Geriatrics and Experimental Gerontology Reports*, *1*(3), 135–142.

3. Ropper, A. H. (2014). Concussion and other traumatic brain injuries. In D. Kasper, A. Fauci, S. Hauser, D. Longo, J. Jameson, & J. Loscalzo (Eds.), *Harrison's principles of internal medicine* (19th ed.). New York: McGraw-Hill. Retrieved from http://accessmedicine.mhmedical.com.ezproxy.simmons.edu:2048/content.asp x?bookid=1130&sectionid=79756215.

4. Dick, K. (2016). Delirium. In T. M. Buttaro, J. Trybulski, P. Polgar-Bailey, & J. Sandberg-Cook (Eds.), *Primary care: A collaborative practice* (5th ed., pp. 1016–1019). St. Louis, MO: Elsevier.

5. Goldblatt, D., & O'Brien, K. L. (2014). Pneumococcal infections. In D. Kasper, A. Fauci, S. Hauser, D. Longo, J. Jameson, & J. Loscalzo (Eds.), *Harrison's principles of internal medicine* (19th ed.). New York: McGraw-Hill. Retrieved from http://accessmedicine.mhmedical.com.ezproxy.simmons.edu:2048/content.asp x?bookid=1130&sectionid=79756215.

6. Fisher, A. A., & Davis, M. W. (2008). Prolonged QT interval, syncope, and delirium with galantamine. *The Annals of Pharmacotherapy*, *42*(2), 278–283.

7. Han, J. H., & Wilber, S. T. (2013). Altered mental status in older emergency department patients. *Clinics in Geriatric Medicine*, *29*(1), 101–136.

8. Buttaro, T. M. (2016). Hypernatremia and hyponatremia. In T. M. Buttaro, J. Trybulski, P. Polgar-Bailey, & J. Sandberg-Cook (Eds.), *Primary care: A collaborative practice* (5th ed., pp. 1112–1119). St. Louis, MO: Elsevier.

9. Gupta, K., & Trautner, B. W. (2014). Urinary tract infections, Pyelonephritis, and prostatitis. In D. Kasper, A. Fauci, S. Hauser, D. Longo, J. Jameson, & J. Loscalzo (Eds.), *Harrison's principles of internal medicine* (19th ed.). New York: McGraw-Hill. Retrieved from http://accessmedicine.mhmedical.com.ezproxy.simmons.edu:2048/content.aspx?bookid=1130&sectionid=79756215.

10. Hooton, T. M. (2017). Acute complicated cystitis and pyelonephritis. In T. E. Post (Ed.), *Uptodate*. Waltham, MA: UpToDate.

11. FDA Drug Safety Communication: FDA advises restricting fluoroquinolone antibiotic use for certain uncomplicated infections; warns about disabling side effects that can occur together. Retrieved from https://www.fda.gov/Drugs/DrugSafety/ucm500143.htm.

12. Meyrier, A., & Fekete, T. (2017). Acute bacterial prostatitis. In T. E. Post (Ed.), *Uptodate*. Waltham, MA: UpToDate.

13. Meng, M. V., Walsh, T. J., & Chi, T. D. (2018). Urologic disorders. In M. A. Papadakis, S. J. McPhee, & M. W. Rabow (Eds.), *Current medical diagnosis & treatment 2018*. New York. Retrieved from http://accessmedicine.mhmedical.com/content.aspx?bookid=2192&sectionid=168019217#1145404629.

Leg Numbness

M. Elizabeth Teixeira

Instructions

After reviewing the case study, please jot down your notes or preliminary answers in the spaces provided. When you are ready to submit your answers for grading and reflective expert feedback for evaluation, go to http://www.evolve.elsevier.com/DickAndButtaro/ to complete this case.

Case Study Scenario/History of Present Illness

Chief Complaint: Newly established patient "here for follow-up."

An 80-year-old black female (Mrs. Jones) is here today for a routine office visit for ongoing management of chronic medical conditions including type 2 diabetes mellitus (DM II), hypertension, persistent atrial fibrillation, congestive heart failure, stage B chronic kidney disease (CKD), and dyslipidemia. She initially states she has no new complaints, but on further questioning specifically regarding pain, she does admit to "numbness and discomfort in her lower extremities." She denies chest pain, worsening shortness of breath, palpitations, or decreased appetite. Her shortness of breath is usually only after much exertion such as walking long distances or climbing a flight of stairs. She does state she is having more difficulty sleeping because her legs are increasingly bothersome and worse at night. Mrs. Jones tried taking two Tylenol before bed the past couple of nights, with minimal relief. Once she falls asleep, however, she awakes maybe once to go to the bathroom. She denies any recent falls, although she had a near fall a couple days ago when getting up during the night. Mrs. Jones does have a walker that she states she uses for ambulation but does not always have it nearby.

Note: Mrs. Jones is a fairly new patient to your practice, having transferred only 3 months ago. She was living alone in Florida but recently relocated to live with her daughter. She states she is adjusting and likes being closer to her children and grandchildren. Mrs. Jones brought her old medical records; however, there are no recent labs or ECG available from the previous 6 months.

Medications: Carvedilol (Coreg) 25 milligrams po twice daily, furosemide (Lasix) 40 milligrams po in the morning, ramipril (Altace) 10 milligrams po daily, Janumet (sitagliptin/metformin) 50/1000 milligrams po twice daily, glargine/Lantus insulin (Solostar Pen) 10 units subcutaneously at bedtime, amiodarone 200 milligrams po daily, atorvastatin (Lipitor) 40 milligrams po at bedtime, vitamin D 1000 IU twice daily, rivaroxaban (Xarelto) 15 milligrams po with evening meal, sertraline (Zoloft) 50 milligrams po daily, and omeprazole 40 milligrams po in the morning.

Allergies: No know allergies (NKA).

Past medical history: Mrs. Jones has a history of DM II for the past 20 years; gastroesophageal reflux disease (GERD); hypertension; coronary artery disease (CAD) (<50% occlusion of left anterior descending [LAD] artery per heart catheterization 2 years ago); dyslipidemia; vitamin D deficiency; nonvalvular atrial fibrillation; CKD stage 2; depression; and left breast cancer T1N1M0 with surgery, radiation, and chemotherapy 10 years ago.

Surgical history: Left partial mastectomy age 70, appendectomy as child, and last colonoscopy at age 70 with no significant findings.

Family history: Parents are both deceased. Father died from liver cirrhosis caused by alcohol use in the early 1960s. Mother died in her nineties from heart disease.

Personal and social history: Lives now with daughter in her home. Her bedroom is located on the first floor with a full bathroom. Mrs. Jones is able to manage all activities of daily living with minimal assistance. She uses a walker for ambulation. Grab bars were installed in the bathroom, and halls and rooms are lit at night with nightlights per patient. Instrumental activities of daily living do require more assistance mainly for preparing meals, shopping, and finances. Mrs. Jones continues to drive short distances during the day without any reports of accidents or getting lost. Mrs. Jones' daughter is retired but does have a live-in caretaker for her mom when she travels approximately twice a year. Never smoked, but exposure to secondhand smoke as a child (father smoked in the home).

Health maintenance/ prevention: Immunizations up to date (Pneumovax age 65, Prevnar-13 age 68, Tdap age 68, receives annual high-dose influenza). Mrs. Jones refused a mammogram for the past 2 years. Her last full eye examination with an ophthalmologist was 2 years ago. Her last mammogram was 2 about years ago. Mrs. Jones agrees that routine colonoscopy is no longer advised.

The following assessments are from this visit including her new symptoms/problem.

Diabetes follow-up: Denies symptoms of hyperglycemia or hypoglycemia. Self-monitoring of blood glucose (SMBG) daily in the morning, and she reports readings range between 110 and 140. Takes medications as prescribed and has no problems administering insulin at bedtime. She states she is not on any special diet, and eats small meals with a couple of snacks during the day. She states she saw a specialist when first diagnosed years ago and attended a few classes at that time. She denies any visual problems and had a dilated eye examination with the ophthalmologist about 2 years ago.

Hypertension follow-up: Mrs. Jones is taking medications as prescribed and denies any adverse effects such as cough, facial swelling, or weakness in her extremities. She denies headache, dizziness, or a history of stroke. She does not monitor her blood pressure at home. She states she does not add salt to her foods and tries to avoid canned foods unless marked "no salt added."

Congestive heart failure: Mrs. Jones denies weight gain or increase in shortness of breath. She does report shortness of breath with exertion such as climbing one flight of stairs or walking long distances when shopping, but this has not changed in the past year. She sleeps on one or two pillows mainly for comfort. She denies orthopnea, chest pain, and palpitations. She does state ankles swell more so in the evening but no more than usual. She last saw a cardiologist in Florida before the move and reports no change in medications.

CKD: Denies oliguria, hematuria, or dysuria. Denies frothy urine. Does not note any change in urinary frequency and states her urine is light yellow in color without odor; however, it is somewhat darker with the first void in the morning. She has not seen a nephrologist.

Pain and numbness in lower extremities: Mrs. Jones describes her foot and leg discomfort as a burning sensation, sometimes sharp shooting pain that is noticeable some hours of the day and worse at night. Sometimes calves and legs feel itchy. Mrs. Jones rates the discomfort as a 5/10 at its worse but she states, "It is always there."

Review of Systems

General: Denies fatigue, fever, night sweats, and weight loss or gain.

Skin: Denies rashes or lesions, denies calluses on feet.

Head, eyes, ears, nose, and throat (HEENT): Denies visual changes, hearing loss, otalgia, or sore throat. She has her own teeth and sees a dentist twice a year.

Cardiac: Denies chest discomfort, palpitations, syncope, or near syncope. Positive for lower extremity swelling.

Urinary: Denies dysuria, hematuria, and incontinence.

Neurologic: Denies dizziness, headaches, or memory loss. Positive for numbness and pain in lower extremities.

Psychiatric: Denies depression or anxiety, but positive for recent sleep difficulty.

Hematologic: Denies any prior history of anemia or blood dysplasia.

Endocrine: History of diabetes, no symptoms of hyperglycemia or hypoglycemia.

Physical Examination

Vital signs: Blood pressure (BP) left arm sitting 130/82. Temperature 97°F. Heart rate (HR) 82, respiratory rate (RR) 14, SpO$_2$ 99%. Weight 170 pounds. Height 64 inches. Body mass index (BMI) 29.2.

General: Alert and oriented, no acute distress.

Skin: No lesions, rashes, and no atypical moles/nevi.

Neck: Supple. No lymphadenopathy, no thyroid nodule or goiter, carotid pulses brisk, no bruits.

Respiratory: Clear to auscultation throughout. No rales, wheezes, or rhonchi.

Cardiac: Irregularly, irregular rate rhythm, 78 beats/min, S1, S2 audible, no S3, S4. No murmurs, rubs, or gallops.

Abdomen: Soft, bowel sounds + in all four quadrants, tympanic to percussion, no distension, nontender to palpation.

Extremities: +1 nonpitting edema bilaterally. Pedal pulses +2 bilaterally.

Diabetic foot examination: No calluses, fissures, or corns noted. Mild hammertoes third and fourth digits of right foot. Vibratory sense decreased in both feet. Nails of large toes both thickened and yellowed.

Neurologic: Oriented to day, time, and place. Cranial nerves (CNs) II-XII intact. Pupils equal, round reactive to light and accommodation (PERRLA). Funduscopic examination: No edema of optic disc, no arteriovenous (AV) nicking or cotton wool patches noted, deep tendon reflexes (DTRs) +2 bilaterally, decreased sensation to both extremities as noted previously.

ASSESSMENT AND PLAN

1.   Based on the presented history and physical examination results, what are the possible causes (differential diagnosis) for Mrs. Jones' symptoms of pain and numbness in the lower extremities?

2.   What components of the history or physical examination are missing?

3.   What diagnostics are necessary for this patient at this time?[1]

4.   What are the possible causes of peripheral neuropathy in this patient that the health care provider should consider in the differential diagnosis?[2]

5. Describe the underlying pathology of diabetic peripheral neuropathy.[3,4]

6. How can diabetic peripheral neuropathy be prevented?

7. What is the diagnostic reasoning involved in determining the most likely cause of Mrs. Jones' symptoms?[1]

Case Study, Continued

The patient provides more information on further questioning.

Mrs. Jones tells you that she has had numbness in her feet for over a year but only recently has it gotten worse. She never mentioned her symptoms before because no one asked and she did not think it was important because it was not really interfering with her daily routine until now. Recently though, she has been experiencing painful discomfort, especially at night. In terms of her diabetes management, she was started on bedtime insulin a couple of years ago because she was told her numbers were up. She does not recall her most recent laboratory values, but she was told they were better. She denies a history of substance use disorder including alcohol and only has a glass of wine on holidays or special occasions.

Mrs. Jones also tells you about her near falls and that she did have a fall about 6 months ago while living in Florida. She states that both times "she lost her balance." She denies dizziness, vertigo, faintness, or syncope.

The health care provider also asks her to describe further her symptoms at night to elicit any signs of RLS and mainly any urge to move legs during the night in response to dysesthesias. RLS is considered a movement disorder with symptoms often described previously, and they occur mostly at night or during long periods of rest.[5]

Further physical examination findings are given.

On further examination, the health care provider notes that Mrs. Jones has no difficulty or pain with lateral bending or pain with palpation of lumbar and sacral spinal processes. Her straight leg test is negative and she has +4 quad strength bilaterally. Her TUG test using her walker was completed in 20 seconds, indicating a higher risk for falls.

8. What treatments should the health care provider recommend for this patient?[2,6]

Case Study, Continued

After discussing possible causes for her symptoms with long-standing diabetes being the most likely, Mrs. Jones states she would like to "hold off on more pills," check her blood work, and return for a follow-up visit in 2 weeks. Mrs. Jones is willing to try the over-the-counter capsaicin cream in the meantime at bedtime for her leg symptoms.

9.   **What are other appropriate decisions to aid in this patient's care?**

10.   **What referrals should the health care provider consider for Mrs. Jones?**

Case Study, Continued

Mrs. Jones returns in 2 weeks to discuss her laboratory results and as a follow-up for her leg pain. She reports some help from the capsaicin cream but rates pain still at 3 to 4 out of 10. During the day she reapplies the cream once or twice, which gives her some relief.

- Laboratory results are as follows:
  - CBC within normal limits.
  - Vitamin B_{12} and folate within normal range.
  - Chemistry shows fasting glucose 150, creatinine 1.3, blood urea nitrogen (BUN) 22 milligrams/dL, and estimated glomerular filtration rate (eGFR) 36, otherwise unremarkable.

- TSH 6.0.
- Hemoglobin A1C 7.5%.
- Lipid panel shows total cholesterol 180, triglycerides 210, low-density lipoprotein (LDL) 90, and high-density lipoprotein (HDL) 50.
- 25-hydroxy vitamin D level 25 ng/mL.
- Celiac panel negative.
- RPR nonreactive.

Physical Examination
  General: Afebrile, older female in no acute distress.
  Eyes: Sclera clear. Pupils equal and reactive to light, red reflex present. No papilledema or nicking noted.
  Respiratory: Clear to auscultation throughout lung fields. No rales, wheezes, or rhonchi.
  Cardiac: Irregularly irregular rhythm with rate of 80 beats/min. No S3, S4. No murmurs, rubs, or gallops.

11. Based on the current laboratory results, what treatment changes do you recommend?

12. What options should be considered for improving Mrs. Jones' glucose control, and what is your target goal for A1C?[7]

13. Any other laboratory tests or diagnostics that should have been ordered?

Case Study, Continued

The provider orders these additional tests and the results are as follows:
- Spot urine reveals a ratio greater than 300 milligrams/g.
- Free T_4 within normal range.
- ECG interpretation: Normal QRS complex but with absent P waves throughout all leads. Partial right bundle branch block (RBBB) also noted in chest leads.

14. What referrals should be considered at this time?[8]

15. What are the priorities for the next visit in 6 weeks?

Case Study, Continued

Mrs. Jones returns for a follow up visit in 6 weeks after an appointment with the nephrologist and cardiologist and twice-a-week physical therapy. She is alert and oriented and in no acute distress. She states that the cardiologist sent her for an echocardiogram and did not change any medications but will see her back in 3 months. The nephrologist also made no changes to her medications and wants her to collect a 24-hour urine if possible. Regarding her diet, she is trying to have an egg for breakfast or a high-fiber/high-protein cereal with low-fat milk that the provider had recommended.

Her physical examination reveals the following:

General: Well groomed and dressed, pleasant.

Vital signs: Weight 167. Temperature 98.4°F. BP 136/84 left arm. HR 78. O_2 saturation 99%.

Respiratory: Clear to auscultation.

Cardiac: Regular rate, S1, S2, no S3, S4. No murmurs, rubs, or gallops.

Extremities: Minimal edema bilaterally. Pedal pulses 2+ bilaterally.

Neurologic: Decreased sensation, unchanged from last visit. PSQI score is 6 (a total score of 5 or greater suggests poor sleep quality during the prior month).

The provider discusses results with Mrs. Jones and reassesses her neuropathy symptoms. She is agreeable to try medication because it will replace another drug. The plan is to wean Mrs. Jones off the sertraline over a week's time (reducing dose to half) and start duloxetine 30 milligrams daily (duloxetine is indicated for both depression and neuropathic pain). The dose of duloxetine can be increased to 60 milligrams after 1 week; however, given Mrs. Jones' age, it is best to start low and go slow, reassessing in 4 to 6 weeks.

16. **What ongoing issues will be the focus of future visits?**[9]

ONLINE ANSWER SUBMISSION

When you are ready to submit your answers for grading and reflective expert feedback for evaluation, go to http://www.evolve.elsevier.com/DickAndButtaro/ to complete this case.

References

1. Kane, R., Ouslander, J., Abrass, I., & Resnick, B. (2015). *Essentials of clinical geriatrics* (7th ed.). McGraw-Hill Education.
2. American Geriatrics Society Beers Criteria Update Expert Panel. (2015). American Geriatrics Society 2015 Updated Beers Criteria for Potentially Inappropriate Medication Use in Older Adults. Retrieved from http://onlinelibrary.wiley.com/doi/10.1111/jgs.13702/pdf.

3. Centers for Disease Control and Prevention (2014). *National diabetes statistics report: Estimates of diabetes and its burden in the United States, 2014*. Atlanta, GA: US Department of Health and Human Services. Retrieved from cdc.gov/diabetes/data/statistics/2014statisticsreport.html.

4. Staff, N., Grisold, A., Grisold, W., & Windebank, A. (2017). Chemotherapy-induced peripheral neuropathy: A current review. *Annals of Neurology, 81*, 772–781.

5. Winkelman, J., et al. (2016). Practice guideline summary. Treatment of restless legs syndrome in adults. Report of the guideline development, dissemination, and implementation subcommittee of the American Academy of Neurology. *Neurology, 87*, 2585–2593.

6. Walfogel, J. M., et al. (2017). Pharmacotherapy for diabetic peripheral neuropathy pain and quality of life: A systematic review. *Neurology, 88*, 1958–1967.

7. American Geriatrics Society Expert Panel on the Care of Older Adults with Diabetes Mellitus. (2013). Guidelines abstracted from the American geriatrics society guidelines for improving the care of older adults with diabetes mellitus: 2013 update. *Journal of the American Geriatrics Society, 61*, 2020–2026.

8. Vassalotti, J., Centor, R., Turner, B., Greer, R., Choi, M., Sequist, T., et al. (2016). Practical approach to detection and management of chronic kidney disease for the primary care clinician. *The American Journal of Medicine, 129*, 153–162.

9. James, P., Oparil, S., & Carter, B. (2014). 2014 evidence-based guideline for the management of high blood pressure in adults: Reports from the panel members appointed to the eighth joint national committee (JNC 8). *JAMA: The Journal of the American Medical Association, 311*(5), 507–520.

Wooziness

Karen L. Dick ▪ Nancy S. Morris

Instructions

After reviewing the case study, please jot down your notes or preliminary answers in the spaces provided. When you are ready to submit your answers for grading and reflective expert feedback for evaluation, go to http://www.evolve.elsevier.com/DickAndButtaro/ to complete this case.

Case Study Scenario/History of Present Illness

The daughter of an 86-year-old woman called the office requesting an appointment for her mother because she declined an invitation to come to her house for dinner yesterday saying she had been recently feeling "woozy." Her daughter was concerned because this was not her mother's typical response. The office is able to schedule an appointment for her mother in 2 days.

At the visit, the patient tells the provider right away that she has not had any "woozy spells" for a week so maybe it is nothing to worry about because she feels fine now. Two weeks ago it was particularly bad. She had been cleaning the bathroom and had just started to wipe the bathroom mirror when she got woozy and was even afraid she might fall because she felt so off-balance. She held onto the sink until the feeling passed; it only took a minute. All that afternoon it seemed to come and go as she was busy straightening up things in her apartment. At times she even felt weak and nauseated so she thought she must be coming down with something. The woozy feeling happened frequently for a few days. She never vomited and never had a headache or fever. She tried drinking more water because she thought that seemed to help. However, she started a trial of furosemide about a month ago for worsening lower extremity edema and feels like she is in the bathroom all day anyway, so that did not really work very well. She states she has not had any symptoms now for a week.

Medications: Acetaminophen 1000 milligrams po two to three times a day for knee and back pain, amlodipine 5 milligrams po daily, atorvastatin 20 milligrams po daily, calcium carbonate 500 milligrams po twice daily, furosemide 20 milligrams po daily, levothyroxine 75 micrograms po daily, timolol 0.25% drops once daily both eyes, and vitamin D 1000 units po daily.

Allergies: Penicillin causes hives.

Habits: Nonsmoker; drinks one glass of wine every Sunday.

Past medical history: Glaucoma, hyperlipidemia, hypothyroidism, hypertension (HTN), osteoarthritis (bilateral knees), osteopenia, spinal stenosis, and mild sensorineural hearing loss bilaterally.

Past surgical history: Hysterectomy for fibroids, appendectomy.

Family history: Father died age 77 from pneumonia. Mother died age 80 from colon cancer.

Personal and social history: Widow for 7 years. Lives in an apartment building for seniors. High school graduate, worked part time in a bank opening new accounts for many years, retired age 65. Has three adult children, one son and one daughter live nearby and one daughter lives out of state. Only drives during the day. Her daughter helps with grocery shopping. The patient is independent with activities of daily living (ADLs), housework, laundry, and meal preparation.

Review of Systems

General: Feels well today, no fever, no chills.

Skin: Denies rash, pruritus.

Head, eyes, ears, nose, and throat (HEENT): Denies blurred vision, ear pain or fullness, tinnitus, nasal stuffiness, and sore throat.

Respiratory: Mild shortness of breath on stairs if she goes up fast. Denies cough.

Cardiac: Denies chest pain or pressure, palpitations.

Gastrointestinal: Denies abdominal pain, has daily bowel movement.

Urinary: Denies dysuria. She feels like she is in the bathroom "all the time" when she takes the furosemide in the morning. She skips it on days she has errands to do. Has nocturia once nightly.

Musculoskeletal: Bilateral knee pain, managed well with acetaminophen two to three times daily.

Neurologic: Denies difficulty speaking or swallowing, headaches, paresthesia, or arm/leg weakness.

Physical Examination

General: Older female, oriented and responding to questions appropriately, speech clear.

Vital signs: Height 5 feet, 1 inch (154.9 cm). Weight 121 pounds (54.9 kg). Body mass index (BMI) 23. Blood pressure (BP) 116/68 right arm. Heart rate 88 and regular, respiratory rate 18 and regular, oxygen saturation 96%.

Skin: Scattered seborrheic keratosis on upper back, two skin tags on right side of neck.

HEENT: no facial asymmetry. Tongue midline. Eyes: Funduscopic examination normal, extraocular movements (EOMs) intact, visual fields normal. No cervical adenopathy.

Cardiac: Regular rate and rhythm. Normal S1, S2 with no murmurs, gallops, or rubs.

Respiratory: Clear to auscultation. No rales, wheezes, or rhonchi.

Abdomen: Soft, bowel sounds +, nondistended.

Lower extremities: Trace edema in both ankles, pedal pulses 2+ bilaterally.

Neurologic: Cranial nerves (CNs) II to XII intact with no focal deficits, gait steady with no assistive device, Romberg negative.

ASSESSMENT AND PLAN

1. Based on the history and physical examination results, what are the possible causes (differential diagnosis) for the patient's current condition?

2. What components of the history or physical examination are missing?[1-6]

Case Study, Continued

On further questioning, the patient clarifies that the woozy feeling was sometimes one of feeling off-balance and sometimes feeling as if the room was spinning around her. It was better when she sat still. She does have decreased hearing, but that has come on gradually over the years and is not new. She denies ringing in the ears. She wears bifocal glasses and has not noticed any change in her vision. Denies diaphoresis and dysarthria. One of her grandsons had bronchitis and she saw him about a week before the woozy feeling began, but no other sick contacts. When asked what time of the day she takes the furosemide, she comments that she takes it in the morning but is only able to take it some days because if she has to go somewhere, she does not want to have to look for a bathroom. She did, however, take it today. She also reports she knows she does not drink enough even though she knows she should drink more.

Additional findings on examination include normal otoscopic examination both ears. Both tympanic membranes (TMs) are visualized. There is trace cerumen in both canals. On the Rinne test, air conduction is heard longer than bone conduction, and on the Weber test she reports hearing the same in both ears. Finger-to-nose test is normal. Alternating hand movements normal. Lying BP is 128/74 and pulse 80. Standing BP is 110/62 and pulse 88.

3. What additional diagnostics should the health care provider order based on the patient's additional history?

4.   What is the working diagnosis?

5.   What treatment recommendation is appropriate for this patient?

6.   What are further recommendations that the health care provider should consider?[7-9]

Case Study, Continued

The patient returns in 2 weeks and reports she is very happy not to have to urinate so often during the day since she stopped the furosemide. However, she had the "dizzy" sensation again 2 days this past week. Each episode lasted for less than 1 minute, but it happened several times throughout the day, and sometimes the episodes were associated with nausea. It was frequent enough that she was afraid to drive anywhere. Even at night she would feel dizzy if she rolled on her side, so she tried to lie quietly. The feeling would go away if she would stop what she was doing and be still.

The patient provides more information with further questioning. She reflects back over the years and comments that she used to get these "spells" every once in a while even 8 or 10 years ago. She used to think it was because the weather was very hot and she had not been drinking enough water. They never lasted long, seconds or maybe a full minute. She would just stand still until the feeling passed, have a drink of water, and then carry on with whatever she was doing. The first time it happened she had been looking for gloves that were on the shelf in her entry closet. She remembers it clearly because she was almost late getting to her granddaughter's dance recital because she waited about 15 minutes wanting to be sure the dizzy feeling had passed before she started driving.

Because the patient is able to describe her symptoms as a "sensation of movement," with sudden onset, short duration, episodic, and with visceral symptoms (nausea), the provider is able to categorize the cause as most likely peripheral and not central. This allows the provider to rule out many of the differentials initially considered.

The blood test results from 2 weeks ago are sodium 134, potassium 4.1, creatinine 1 milligram/dL, and estimated glomerular filtration rate (eGFR) 52.

Physical Examination Findings Today

> **Vital signs:** Weight 122.5 pounds. Lying BP is 136/84 and pulse 84. Standing BP is 132/82 and pulse 88. Respiratory rate 18 unlabored. Oxygen saturation 96%.
>
> **General:** Elderly female, pleasant, in no distress.
>
> **Cardiac:** Regular rate and rhythm. Normal S1, S2 with no murmurs, gallops, or rubs.
>
> **Respiratory:** Clear to auscultation. No rales, wheezes, or rhonchi.
>
> **Ears:** Bilateral ear canals clear with no erythema and good visualization of TMs. On Rinne test air conduction is heard longer than bone conduction. On Weber test she reports hearing the same in both ears.
>
> **Neurologic:** CNs II to XII intact, gait steady, Romberg negative, finger-to-nose test normal, rapid alternating hand movement normal.
>
> **Lower extremities:** 1+ pedal edema.

7. What additional diagnostics or testing should the provider consider based on the additional history provided?[10,11]

For this patient, the Dix–Hallpike maneuver (Fig. 22.1) reveals positive nystagmus in the right eye only (slow phases clockwise and down, fast phases counterclockwise and up). The nystagmus begins after a few seconds, increases in velocity, and fades away within 60 seconds.

To perform the Dix Hallpike maneuver[3] the provider has the patient sit up on an examination table with his or her head rotated 45 degrees. The patient then quickly lies back in a supine position with the head still rotated and slightly extended (about 20 degrees) so that it "hangs" supported off the edge of the examination table. The provider observes the eyes for torsional upbeating nystagmus that may take 20 seconds to appear, intensify, and then resolve within 60 seconds. The provider should check the patient with his or her head rotated to the right and to the left. A positive Dix–Hallpike test indicates posterior canal BPPV in the dependent ear.[3]

- To perform the supine roll test, the patient begins by lying supine with his or her head in a neutral position facing the ceiling. The provider quickly moves the patient's head 90 degrees to one side and monitors the eyes for nystagmus. If present, the nystagmus will typically be a geotropic type with horizontal and beating toward the lower ear, or an ageotropic nystagmus, with horizontal and beating toward the upper ear. For geotropic nystagmus, the side associated with the stronger nystagmus is the affected ear causing BPPV. For ageotropic nystagmus, the side associated with the weaker nystagmus is the affected ear causing BPPV.[10]

---

8. What should the health care provider now consider to be the probable cause of this patient's symptoms?

9. What treatment recommendations are now appropriate for this patient?[3,10-14] (See Fig. 22.2)

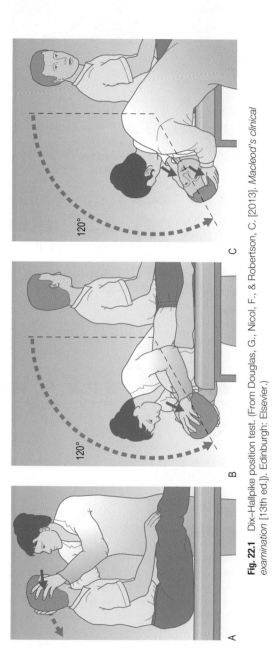

Fig. 22.1 Dix–Hallpike position test. (From Douglas, G., Nicol, F., & Robertson, C. [2013]. *Macleod's clinical examination* [13th ed.]). Edinburgh: Elsevier.)

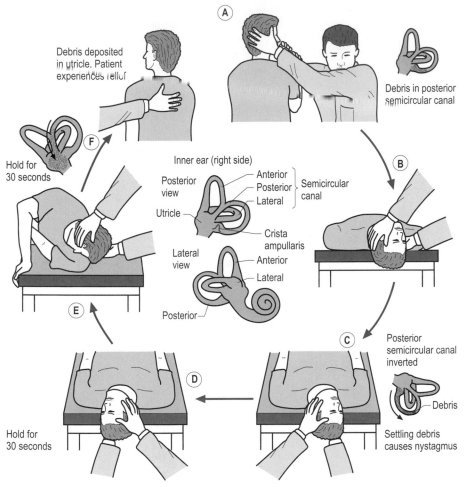

Fig. 22.2 Epley maneuver. (From Beck, R. [2012]. *Functional neurology for practitioners of manual medicine* [2nd ed.]. Edinburgh: Churchill Livingstone.)

Case Study, Continued

The health care provider performs the Epley maneuver during that visit and follows up with the patient 4 days after the visit. The patient reports that she has not had any more woozy episodes. She agrees to keep checking her BP at home and to wearing compression stockings and elevating her legs while sitting.

The patient returns in 2 weeks and reports that she has been checking her BP at home and the top number is always between 132 to 146 and the bottom number is always in the 80s. She has stopped adding salt when cooking. She is taking her BP medication as prescribed. She also has been able to take a walk a couple of times a week, but she feels like her balance is not as good as it was. She denies vertigo. She has had a few "almost" falls but was always able to grab onto something nearby and never actually fell. She denies numbness in her legs or feet. Her knees are not bothering her "too much" because she continues taking acetaminophen 1000 milligrams two to three times a day.

Physical Examination

    Vital signs: Weight: 122 pounds. Lying BP is 134/80 and pulse 84. Standing BP is 130/82 and pulse 88. Respiratory rate 18 and unlabored, oxygen saturation 98%.

    HEENT: Bilateral canals clear, trace cerumen. EOMs intact, tongue midline.

    Cardiac: Regular rate and rhythm. Normal S1, S2 with no murmurs, gallops, or rubs.

    Respiratory: Clear to auscultation. No rales, wheezes, or rhonchi.

    Neurologic: Difficulty maintaining balance with toe-to-heel walking. Veers a bit to the left when trying to walk a straight line. Finger-to-nose is normal and rapid alternating hand movement normal. Romberg negative.

    Lower extremities: Trace pedal edema.

10.   What additional history would be helpful to determine?

Case Study, Continued

The patient has had no further issues with orthostatic hypotension. She is able to prepare foods from the DASH diet, following salt restrictions. Denies change in vision and new glasses. Home safety features addressed.

    In some patients, the Epley maneuver eliminates the vertigo, but the patient may still feel off-balance or unsteady for a few weeks.[11] The health care provider explains this to the patient and recommends vestibular rehabilitation to improve her balance and safety with ADLs, all with a goal of increasing her safety at home.[15]

11.   Is there an indication for any diagnostic testing at this time?[11,16]

12. What should the patient's assessment and treatment plan include at this time?[11,17]

13. What are the priorities for the patient's next visit?

Case Study, Continued

Three months later the patient returns and reports no further vertigo and states that her balance has improved. She denies falls and has completed the vestibular therapy. Her BP is well controlled.

Six months later the primary care office is notified of the patient's recent admission to the local hospital for dizziness. She had been out shopping with her daughter when she began to feel lightheaded and nauseous. She complained that any change in the position of her head made her woozy and nauseous. She was admitted, treated with intravenous (IV) fluids, monitored on telemetry, and evaluated by Physical Therapy. She had no neurologic deficits. All laboratory work including a complete blood count (CBC) and complete metabolic profile was normal. A urinalysis was negative. She was discharged home with visiting nurse and physical therapy services. She was given a prescription for meclizine 25 milligrams to be taken orally up to three times a day for dizziness.

A computed tomography (CT) of the head without contrast was done and read as follows:

Clinical history: Nausea, vertigo.

Exam: Axial 5-mm noncontrast sections were obtained from above the vertex through the foramen magnum.

Findings: There are no prior examinations available for comparison. There is mild age-appropriate generalized volume loss. Cerebral hemispheres, deep gray nuclei, brainstem, and cerebellum appear normal. There is no evidence of hemorrhage. There is no evidence of edema, mass-effect, or mass. No abnormality of the cerebrospinal fluid (CSF) spaces or ventricles is shown. No localized sulcus effacement and gyral swelling or attenuation change is evident. Paranasal sinuses, petromastoids, globes, orbits, and skull are unremarkable.

Conclusion:

1. Mild generalized age-appropriate involution or volume loss; otherwise unremarkable noncontrast CT scan of the head.

2. No CT evidence of hemorrhage, edema, mass, or acute ischemic insult.

Case Study, Continued

During her posthospital visit to the primary care provider, the patient asks about taking meclizine, saying she does not like the way it makes her feel.

14. How does meclizine work and is it appropriate to use for patients with vertigo?[11]

Case Study, Continued

One year later, the patient calls for an urgent visit because her vertigo is back and she is very nauseated. She comes in the following day. The patient reports that she was out of town visiting her daughter for a week and the arthritis in her knees acted up. Although she took the acetaminophen she had with her, it was not adequate, and her daughter gave her some ibuprofen 600 milligrams three times a day to take. This really worked well and she was doing much better until the day before she left to come home when the vertigo started up again. Every time she moves her head, up or down, she gets queasy and dizzy. It does not last long, only about a minute at the most, but it happens so often throughout the day that she is really bothered and worries about falling. Denies vomiting, headache, tinnitus, and vision or hearing changes. Reports no falls and no recent viral illness.

Physical Examination

Vital signs: Weight 123 pounds. BP 138/84. Pulse 88, respiratory rate 18 and unlabored, oxygen saturation 96%.

General: Speech clear, she is oriented and alert.

Skin: Dry overall. Scattered seborrheic keratosis on upper back, two skin tags right sign of neck.

HEENT: Facies symmetric bilaterally, no facial asymmetry. Eyes: EOMs intact. Visual field normal. Ears: Canals clear and normal visualization of TM.

Neck: Supple, no cervical adenopathy.

Cardiac: Regular rate and rhythm. Normal S1, S2 with no murmurs, gallops, or rubs.

Respiratory: Clear to auscultation. No rales, wheezes, or rhonchi.

Abdomen: Flat, positive bowel sounds in all four quadrants. No hepatosplenomegaly, no tenderness with palpation, no guarding, no rebound tenderness.

Neurologic: CNs II to XII intact. EOMs intact. Finger-to-nose normal. Rapid alternating hand movement normal. Romberg negative, gait steady. Dix–Hallpike positive on right side.

Lower Extremities: Pedal pulses 2+ bilaterally. No ankle edema.

15. What additional testing should the health care provider consider at this visit?[18,19]

Case Study, Continued

The provider conducts the TUG test and the Tinetti Balance Assessment and finds the patient to be at a moderate increased risk for falls.

16. What should the health care provider's assessment and treatment plan include at this visit?[1,11,20]

Case Study, Continued

The patient called back in 1 week and reported that she was still feeling the vertigo. The provider arranged for an office visit the following day. Her description of her symptoms is the same. There is the possibility that she had some movement of the otoconia with the first Epley maneuver and the otoconia may have shifted and could now be located in the lateral canal instead of the posterior canal. BBPV can sometimes be in more than one canal and can be in both the right and left ear at the same time. The provider should perform a Dix–Hallpike to assess for posterior canal BPPV and the supine roll test to assess for lateral canal BPPV.[10,11]

17.   What additional patient history would be helpful at this time?

Case Study, Continued

The patient did stop using ibuprofen, and her knee pain is manageable at this time with acetaminophen. Her activity level this week has been limited because she pretty much stayed home. The vertigo was too frequent and she did not feel safe leaving the house.

> **Physical examination:** No changes in physical examination findings. The Dix–Hallpike is again positive on the right side confirming a diagnosis of BPPV.

18.   Are there any indications for any additional diagnostic testing at this time?[11]

19.   What are the priorities for this visit?

20.   What ongoing health care issues will be the focus of future visits?

References

1. Kutz, J. W. (2010). The dizzy patient. *The Medical Clinics of North America*, *94*(5), 989–1002.
2. Nguyen-Huynh, A. (2012). Management of vertigo. *Otolaryngologic Clinics of North America*, *45*, 925–940.
3. Wipperman, J. (2014). Dizziness and vertigo. *Primary Care*, *41*, 115–131.
4. Hogue, J. (2015). Office evaluation of dizziness. *Primary Care*, *42*(2), 249–258.
5. Lüscher, M., Theilgaard, S., & Edholm, B. (2014). Prevalence and characteristics of diagnostic groups amongst 1034 patients seen in ENT practices for dizziness. *The Journal of Laryngology and Otology*, *128*(2), 128–133.

6. Karlberg, M., Hall, K., Quikert, N., Hinson, J., & Halmagyi, G. (2000). What inner ear diseases cause benign paroxysmal positional vertigo? *Acta Oto-Laryngologica, 120*(3), 380–385.

7. Appel, L. J., & American Society of Hypertension Writing Group. (2009). ASH position paper: Dietary approaches to lower blood pressure. *Journal of the American Society of Hypertension, 3*(5), 321–331.

8. Castro, I., Waclawovsky, G., & Marcadenti, A. (2015). Nutrition and physical activity on hypertension: Implication of current evidence and guidelines. *Current Hypertension Reviews, 11*(2), 91–99.

9. Rosendorff, C., Lackland, D. T., Allison, M., Aronow, W. S., Black, H. R., ... White, W. B. (2015). Treatment of hypertension in patients with coronary artery disease. AHA/ASH Scientific Statement. *Journal of the American Society of Hypertension, 9*(6), 453–498.

10. Fife, T. D., Iverson, D. J., Lempert, T., Furman, J. M., Baloh, R. W., ... Gronseth, G. S. (2008). Practice parameter: Therapies for benign paroxysmal positional vertigo (an evidence-based review): Report of the Quality Standards Subcommittee of the American Academy of Neurology. *Neurology, 70*(22), 2067–2074.

11. Bhattacharyya, N., Gubbels, S. P., Schwartz, S. R., Edlow, J. A., El-Kashlan, H., ... Corrigan, M. D. (2017). Clinical practice guidelines: Benign paroxysmal positional vertigo (Update). *JAMA Otolaryngology–Head & Neck Surgery, 156*(3S), S1–S47.

12. Epley, J. M. (1992). The canalith repositioning procedure: For treatment of benign paroxysmal positional vertigo. *JAMA Otolaryngology– Head & Neck Surgery, 107*, 399–404.

13. Semont, A., Freyss, G., & Vitte, E. (1988). Curing the BPPV with a liberatory maneuver. *Advances in Oto-Rhino-Laryngology, 42*, 290–293.

14. Hilton, M. P., & Pinder, D. K. (2014). The Epley (canalith repositioning) manoeuvre for benign paroxysmal positional vertigo. *Cochrane Database Systematic Reviews*, (12), CD003162, doi:10.1002/14651858.CD003162. pub3.

15. Han, B. I., Song, H. S., & Kim, J. S. (2011). Vestibular rehabilitation therapy: Review of indications, mechanisms, and key exercises. *Journal of Clinical Neurology, 7*(4), 184–196.

16. Bakhit, M., Heidarian, A., Ehsani, S., Delphi, M., & Laatifi, S. M. (2014). Clinical assessment of dizzy patient: the necessity and role of diagnostic tests. *Global Journal of Health Science, 6*(3), 194–199.

17. McDonnell, M. N., & Hiller, S. L. (2015). Vestibular rehabilitation for unilateral peripheral vestibular dysfunction. *Cochrane Database of Systematic Reviews*, (1), Art. No.: CD005397, doi:10.1002/14651858. CD005397.pub4.

18. Mathias, S., Nayak, U. S., & Isaacs, B. (1986). Balance in elderly patients: The "get up and go" test. *Archives of Physical Medicine and Rehabilitation, 67*(6), 387–389.

19. Tinetti, M. E., Williams, T. F., & Mayewski, R. (1986). Fall risk index for elderly patients based on number of chronic disabilities. *The American Journal of Medicine, 80*, 429–434.

20. Chimirri, S., Aiello, R., Mazzitello, C., Mumoli, L., Palleria, C., Altomonte, M., et al. (2013). Vertigo/ dizziness as a drugs' adverse reaction. *Journal of Pharmacology & Pharmacotherapeutics, 4*(Suppl. 1), S104–S109.

Page numbers followed by "*f*" indicate figures, "*t*" indicate tables, and "*b*" indicate boxes.

Quick Reference to Diagnostic Reasoning for Older Adults

Diagnostic Reasoning Is a Learned Skill That Involves:

1. Pleasant professionalism
2. Reflection and ability to critically assess one's decisions
3. Ability to readily establish the patient–provider relationship:
   a. Introduce yourself if this is a new patient.
   b. Sit across from the patient and face the patient directly so the patient can hear you and you can see and hear the patient's responses clearly.
4. Attentively listening to the patient history:
   a. Ask the patient, "How can I help you today?" or "What brings you here today?"
   b. Ask the patient to explain the problem in his or her own words, starting from when the problem was first noticed.
   c. Ask how the patient's complaint is affecting his or her quality of life or affecting activities during the day or night.
5. Questioning skills that are systematic and persistent:
   a. Have all components of OLDCARTS (*O*nset, *L*ocation/radiation, *D*uration, *C*haracter, *A*ggravating factors, *R*elieving factors, *T*iming, and *S*everity) been answered?
   b. Have all medications (including over-the-counter [OTC] medications) been reviewed with the patient?
6. Understanding the importance of repeating back your understanding of the patient's problem for clarification:
   a. For older adults especially, it may be useful to perform a brief cognitive screen to determine whether there is any evidence of cognitive impairment.
   b. In some instances, speaking with family members or other caregivers might be helpful to get more information regarding the patient's baseline cognitive status.
7. A relevant but complete "Review of Systems" to further elucidate the problem
8. A tailored diagnostic examination that searches for clues and elicits pertinent patient findings:
   a. Clinical measurements
   b. General appearance
9. Developing more than one diagnostic hypothesis (usually a minimum of three):
   a. Reviewing the patient history and focused physical examination to determine and justify the priority diagnoses
   b. Rationally choosing the diagnosis
   c. Reconsidering other possibilities (i.e., STAR: Stop, Think, Act, Review)
10. Comparing hypotheses by reviewing the information, asking further questions: Which of the primary hypotheses/potential diagnoses can be eliminated based on the patient history and the physical examination findings?
11. Establishing a hypothesis:
    a. What is your perception of the patient's degree of illness?
       i. Remember that older adults often have an atypical presentation of illness compared with younger adults.
       ii. Older adults (and their caregivers) may also minimize symptoms, attributing them to older age.
    b. What is the most likely cause of the patient's complaint? Is there a cluster of clues from the history and physical examination that best explains the chief complaint?
    c. Could the patient's problem be related to one or more comorbidities?
    d. Could a medication or medication interaction (prescribed, herbal, or OTC) be the source of the patient's problem?
       i. Has the patient stopped, started, or missed doses of existing or new medications?
       ii. What are the risks/benefits of deprescribing a medication that is a potential cause of the patient's symptoms?